STATISTICAL DESIGN AND ANALYSIS IN PHARMACEUTICAL SCIENCE

STATISTICS: Textbooks and Monographs

A Series Edited by

D. B. Owen, Founding Editor, 1972–1991

W. R. Schucany, Coordinating Editor
Department of Statistics
Southern Methodist University
Dallas, Texas

R. G. Cornell, Associate Editor
for Biostatistics
University of Michigan

W. J. Kennedy, Associate Editor
for Statistical Computing
Iowa State University

A. M. Kshirsagar, Associate Editor
for Multivariate Analysis and
Experimental Design
University of Michigan

E. G. Schilling, Associate Editor
for Statistical Quality Control
Rochester Institute of Technology

Additional Volumes in Preparation

STATISTICAL DESIGN AND ANALYSIS IN PHARMACEUTICAL SCIENCE

Validation, Process Controls, and Stability

edited by

SHEIN-CHUNG CHOW
Bristol-Myers Squibb Company
Plainsboro, New Jersey

JEN-PEI LIU
Berlex Laboratories, Inc.
Wayne, New Jersey

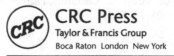

CRC Press
Taylor & Francis Group
Boca Raton London New York

CRC Press is an imprint of the
Taylor & Francis Group, an **informa** business

CRC Press
Taylor & Francis Group
6000 Broken Sound Parkway NW, Suite 300
Boca Raton, FL 33487-2742

First issued in paperback 2019

© 1995 by Taylor & Francis Group, LLC
CRC Press is an imprint of Taylor & Francis Group, an Informa business

No claim to original U.S. Government works

ISBN-13: 978-0-8247-9336-4 (hbk)
ISBN-13: 978-0-367-40187-0 (pbk)

Library of Congress Cataloging-in-Publication Data

Chow, Shein-Chung
    Statistical design and analysis in pharmaceutical science :
validation, process controls, and stability / Shein-Chung Chow, Jen
-pei Liu.
        p.   cm. — (Statistics, textbooks and monographs ;   143)
    Includes bibliographical references and index.
    ISBN 0-8247-9336-6 (hardcover : alk. paper)
    1. Pharmacy—Statistical methods.   I. Liu, Jen-pei
II. Title   III. Series: Statistics, textbooks and monographs ; v.
143.
        [DNLM: 1. Drugs—standards.   2. Chemistry, Pharmaceutical—
methods.   3. Statistics.   QV 771 C552 1995]
    RS122.2.C48   1995
    615'.1'072—dc20
    DNLM/DLC
    for Library of Congress   94-43570
                                                                                      CIP

Visit the Taylor & Francis Web site at
http://www.taylorandfrancis.com

and the CRC Press Web site at
http://www.crcpress.com

Preface

Current Good Manufacturing Practice (CGMP) requires that valid sampling plans, acceptance criteria, and statistical methods be employed to ensure the identity, strength, quality, and purity of pharmaceutical compounds developed according to *United States Pharmcopeia* and *National Formulary* (USP/NF) standards. This book provides a comprehensive and unified presentation of designs and analyses employed at various stages of pharmaceutical development. In addition, it is intended to give a well-balanced summary of current and recently developed statistical methods in stability analysis.

It is our goal to provide a useful reference book for the chemical scientist, pharmaceutical scientist, development pharmacist, and statisticians in the pharmaceutical industry, regulatory agencies, and academia. This book can also serve as a textbook for graduate courses in the areas of pharmacy, pharmaceutical development, stability studies, and biostatistics. The primary emphasis in this book is on biopharmaceutical applications. All statistical methods and their interpretations are illustrated through real examples that have occurred during various stages of pharmaceutical development.

This book covers statistical designs and analyses in pharmaceutical development and stability studies. It covers three areas in detail: pharmaceutical validation, quality assurance, and stability study. Chapter 1 deals with definitions, background, and regulatory requirements. Chapters 2 and 3 cover statistical designs and methods for assay development and validation. In Chapter 4 we summarize screening and optimization designs in scaleup programs, and in Chapter 5 we introduce specification limits and USP tests for various dosage forms. Also included in this chapter are their statistical interpretations. Chapter 6 is devoted to validations of a manufacturing process, which include prospective, concurrent, and retrospective validations and revalidation. Statistical issues regarding multiple-stage sampling and validation designs are also addressed in Chapter 6. In Chapter 7 we discuss useful statistical methods for quality assurance and release targets, while in Chapter 8 we provide fundamental concepts of stability, overage, and expiration dating. Accelerated stability testing and long-term stability study are also described in Chapter 8. Chapter 9 covers chemical kinetic models used in accelerated stability testing, statistical analysis, and prediction through the Arrhenius equation. In Chapter 10 we compare several stability designs, including the complete factorial design and fractional factorial designs such as matrixing and bracketing designs. In Chapter 11 we introduce various types of statistical analysis of stability data based on fixed effects models, and in Chapter 12 we review various statistical methods for determination of drug shelf life using random effects models.

In each chapter, real-world examples are given to illustrate the concepts, appropriate applications, and limitations of statistical methods. Comparisons of the relative merits and disadvantages of these statistical methods are also discussed. Where applicable, topics for possible future research development are noted at the ends of chapters.

From Marcel Dekker, Inc., we would like to thank M. Allegra for providing us with the opportunity to work on this book and A. Berin and T. Finnegan for their outstanding efforts in preparing this book for publication. We are deeply indebted to the Bristol-Myers Squibb Company and Berlex Laboratories, Inc., for their support, in particular S. A. Henry, M. Loberg, S. Barker, S. Weiss, and W. Holyoak. We are grateful to H. L. Ju, K. W. Chen, and H. T. Chang for many helpful discussions and for reviewing the manuscript. We also wish to thank E. Norbrock for his support and encouragement, and Dr. James Bergum for providing us with his unpublished work (in-house seminar, workshop, and short course), research papers, and SAS programs which were used for Chapters 4 and 5 of the book.

Finally, we are fully responsible for any errors remaining in the book. The views expressed are those of the authors and are not necessarily those of Bristol-Myers Squibb Company or Berlex Laboratories, Inc.

Shein-Chung Chow
Jen-pei Liu

Contents

STATISTICAL DESIGN
AND ANALYSIS
IN PHARMACEUTICAL
SCIENCE

1

Introduction

1.1. BACKGROUND

In the pharmaceutical industry, the development of a new drug is a lengthy process involving drug discovery, laboratory development, animal studies, clinical trials, and regulatory registration. As indicated in *USA Today* (Feb. 3, 1993), 26 drugs were introduced in 1992. The average time that a pharmaceutical company spent getting each drug to market was 12 years, 8 months. Three years and 6 months were devoted to laboratory development. Six years and 8 months were spent in human testing. The U.S. Food and Drug Administration (FDA) review took 2 years and 6 months. This lengthy process is necessary to assure the efficacy and safety of the drug product. After the drug is approved, the FDA also requires that the drug product be tested for identity, strength, quality, and purity before it can be released for use.

Statistical methods are usually employed as a useful tool in design and analysis in various stages of drug development. Applications of statistics to drug development can be classified as nonclinical, preclinical, or clinical. *Clinical* applications involve human testing, such as bioavailability or bioequivalence studies, and clinical trials. *Preclinical* studies include short- and long-term toxicology studies, carcinogenecity studies, and reproductive (or teratological) studies. *Nonclinical* applications are mainly for pharmaceutical validation (e.g., the calibration of an instrument, assay validation, and process validation), quality assurance (e.g., scaleup design, specifications, in-process quality control, and release targets), and stability analysis for determination of the drug expiration dating period. In this book our primary emphasis is placed on a discussion of statistical issues that may occur during the process of drug development in nonclinical applications. To provide a better understanding, Fig. 1.1.1 summarizes some key components of nonclinical biostatistical applications in the process of drug development. We describe these key components below.

When a new drug is discovered, it is important to design an appropriate pharmaceutical dosage form (or formulation) for the drug so that it can be delivered efficiently to the site of action of the body for the optimal therapeutic effect for the intended patient population. The pharmaceutical dosage forms include tablet, capsule, powder, liquid suspension, aerosol, cream, gel, solution, inhalation, lotion, paste, suspension, and suppository. The FDA requires that an appropriate assay methodology for the active ingredients of the designed formulation be developed and validated before it can be applied to animal or human subjects. To assess pharmacological characteristics, efficacy, and drug safety, a number of animal studies are usually conducted first. Having demonstrated efficacy and safety in animals, the drug is then applied to human subjects, generally in the form of bioavailability studies and phase I to III clinical trials. The results are usually submitted to the FDA as either a *new drug application* (NDA) or a *product license application* (PLA) for regulatory review and approval. For completion of the submission, the FDA also requires that a stability study be conducted to establish an expiration dating period for the drug product.

Before a drug is approved, the drug samples used in laboratory development, animal studies, and clinical trials are often obtained from laboratory batches. A laboratory batch is usually relatively small compared to the usual production batch. To ensure that the production batch can maintain the identity, strength, quality, and purity of the drug product, a scaleup experiment must be performed. For this purpose, various tests are usually conducted to establish standards (or specifications) for certain characteristics of the drug, such as potency and dissolution. The specifications of drug products currently on the market are given in the *United States Pharmacopeia* and the *National Formulary* (USP/NF). Before a drug can be released for sale, the FDA requires that it be tested to ensure that the product conforms to USP/NF specifications. This is essential to assure the identity, strength, quality, and purity of the product. For this purpose, the manufacturing process is usually validated according to established in-house acceptance criteria which assure that the batches produced meet USP/NF or other predetermined specifications by the end of the established drug expiration dating period. At each stage of the pharmaceutical development of a drug product there is a set of regulatory requirements to ensure its identity, strength, quality, and purity. These requirements are discussed in detail in the following section.

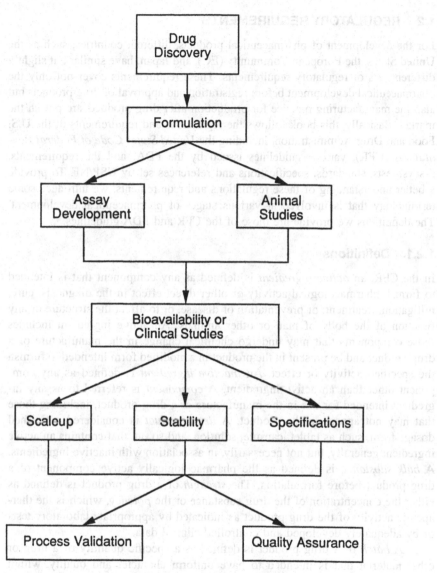

FIGURE 1.1.1 Flowchart for drug development.

1.2. REGULATORY REQUIREMENTS

For the development of pharmaceutical products, different countries, such as the United States, the European Community (EC), and Japan, have similar but slightly different sets of regulatory requirements. These requirements cover not only the pharmaceutical development before registration and approval of drug products but also the manufacturing practice for production after drug products are put on the market. Basically, this book follows the regulations and requirements of the U.S. Food and Drug Administration, including the *United States Code of Federal Regulations* (CFR), various guidelines issued by the FDA, and the requirements, assays, tests, standards, specifications and references set by USP/NF. To provide a better understanding of these regulations and requirements, we introduce some terminology that is involved at various stages of pharmaceutical development. The definitions we provide are those of the CFR and FDA guidelines.

1.2.1. Definitions

In the CFR, an *active ingredient* is defined as any component that is intended to furnish pharmacological activity or other direct effect in the diagnosis, cure, mitigation, treatment, or prevention of disease, or to affect the structure or any function of the body of man or other animals. An active ingredient includes those components that may undergo chemical change in the manufacture of a drug product and be present in the product in a modified form intended to furnish the specified activity or effect. An *inactive ingredient* is defined as any component other than an active ingredient. A *component* is referred to as any ingredient intended for use in the manufacture of a drug product, including those that may not appear in the product. A *drug product* is considered a finished dosage form, such as tablet, capsule, solution, and so on, that contains an active ingredient generally, but not necessarily, in association with inactive ingredients. A *bulk substance* is defined as the pharmacologically active component of a drug product before formulation. The *strength* of a drug product is defined as either the concentration of the drug substance or the *potency*, which is the therapeutic activity of the drug product as indicated by appropriate laboratory tests or by adequately developed and controlled clinical data.

A *batch* of a drug product is defined as a specific quantity of a drug or other material that is intended to have uniform character and quality, within specific limits, and is produced according to a single manufacturing order during the same cycle of manufacture. A *lot* can be interpreted as a batch, or a specific identified portion of a batch, having uniform character and quality within specified limits; or, in the case of a drug product produced by continuous process, a lot is a specific identified amount produced in a unit of time or quantity in a manner that assures its having uniform character and quality within specified limits.

A *quality control unit* can be restated as any person or organizational element designated by the firm to be responsible for the duties relating to quality control. A set of *acceptance criteria* is defined as the product specifications and acceptance/rejection criteria, such as acceptable quality level and unacceptable quality level, with an associated sampling plan, that are necessary for making a decision to accept or reject a lot or a batch. A *representative sample* is a sample that consists of a number of units that are drawn based on rational criteria such as random sampling and intended to assure that the sample accurately portrays the material being sampled.

1.2.2. Code of Federal Regulations

The U.S. federal requirements for manufacture, processing, packing or holding of a drug product during various stages of pharmaceutical development can be summarized as follows:

CFR number	Stage of pharmaceutical development
21 CFR 312	Investigational new drug application (IND)
21 CFR 314	New drug application (NDA)
21 CFR 314	Abbreviated new drug application (ANDA)
21 CFR 314	Supplements
21 CFR 601	Product license application (PLA)
21 CFR 210 and 211	Current good manufacturing practice (CGMP)

Before the registration and approval of a drug product, at the minimum, the FDA requires that the following information about the drug substance and drug products be provided:

1. Physical and chemical characteristics and stability
2. Such specifications and analytic methods as are necessary to assure the identity, strength, quality, and purity of the drug substance and all components used in the manufacture of the product
3. Stability data with a proposed expiration date
4. A description of manufacturing, packaging procedures, and in-process control of the drug product.

The information above is usually included in the technical section on chemistry, manufacturing, and controls (CMC) in an IND and/or NDA submission. Note that as production changes from pilot-scale to large-scale production, sponsors must also submit information on all modifications in chemistry, manufacturing, or controls. The CMC section may be checked by both chemical and statistical reviewers at the FDA.

1.2.3. Current Good Manufacturing Practice

CGMP is codified in 21 CFR 211 provides minimum requirements for the manufacture, processing, packing, and holding of a drug product. Its purpose is to assure that the drug product meets the requirements of the federal Food, Drug, and Cosmetic Act as to the safety, identity, strength, quality, and purity characteristics that it purports to possess. CGMP covers the regulations with respect to requirements for organization and personnel, buildings and facilities, equipment, control of components and drug product containers and closures, production and process control, packaging and process control, holding and distribution, laboratory controls, records and reports, and returned and salvaged drug products.

The major responsibilities of a quality control unit as specified by CGMP is to approve or reject drug products manufactured, processed, packaged, or held under contract by another company and to approve or reject all procedures or specifications affecting the identity, strength, quality, and purity of a drug product. CGMP also requires that all equipment used in the manufacture, processing, packing, and holding of a drug product be routinely calibrated, inspected, or checked. In addition, all computerization systems used in master production, process controls, and laboratory analysis should be checked routinely for accuracy and be validated by written documentation.

CGMP requests that representative samples and quantities of material from each component for testing or examination be based on appropriate criteria, such as statistical criteria for component variability, confidence levels, and degree of precision desired. Sometimes, a particular component is sampled from the top, middle, and bottom of the container. However, subsamples should not be composited together for testing. In addition, each component of the drug product should be verified for identity and be tested for conformity with written specifications for purity, strength, and quality by validated tests and analyses. On the other hand, CGMP requires that the in-process controls be conducted on appropriate samples of in-process material of each batch to assure batch uniformity and integrity of drug products. These control procedures include tablet or capsule weight; disintegration time; adequacy of mixing to assure uniformity and homogeneity; dissolution time; dissolution rate; and clarity, completeness, of pH of solutions. Based on the previous acceptable process average and variability, appropriate statistical methods can be applied to set up valid in-process specifications so that the finished drug product will meet its final specifications.

Before the release for distribution of any drug product, appropriate laboratory testing should be conducted for satisfactory conformance to final specifications of identity and strength for each active ingredient of the drug product. The method of sampling and the number of units per batch should be described fully in the sampling and testing plan of the written procedures. Adequate acceptance criteria for the sampling and testing before approval and release of batches should be based on appropriate statistical quality control criteria to meet appropriate specifications. The statistical quality control criteria should include appropriate acceptance level (i.e., type II error) and/or appropriate rejection level (i.e., type I error). The sponsors should establish, validate, and document the accuracy, sensitivity, specificity, and reproducibility of test methods. In addition, CGMP requires that all drug products bear an expiration date determined by an appropriate stability testing method, which will be described in more detail later in this chapter.

Finally, it should be noted that record keeping is also a very important part of CGMP. In general, all records should be retained for at least one year after the expiration date of the batch. These records include equipment and use logs; component, drug product container, closure, and labeling records; laboratory records; distribution records; and complaint files. Failure to comply with CGMP may trigger stiff legal action by the FDA. For example, as reported in the *Star Ledger* of New Jersey on July 9, 1993, a New Jersey drug company agreed to a consent decree with the FDA for a dispute over record keeping at its two manufacturing plants. This settlement is expected to cost the company at least $50 million in lost sales in the first and second quarters of 1993. However, a consent decree is less severe than such alternative actions as injunctive relief and product seizure or recalls by the FDA. For example, according to NatWest Securities, if the FDA requires the company to remove all multisource drugs made by the two plants of the company, it may cost as much as $350 million in annual sales.

1.2.4. The *United States Pharmacopeia* and *National Formulary*

The *United States Pharmacopeia* and *National Formulary* (USP/NF) are compendia of legally public standards for drug identity, strength, quality, purity, packaging, and labeling of drug products in the United States recognized as official compendia in the federal Food, Drug and Cosmetic Act. Since the standards described in the USP/NF are frequently cited by both CGMP (see, e.g., 21 CFR 211.194) and NDA [see, e.g., 21 CFR 314.50 (d) (1)], in this book all the standards for drug development considered will be based on the USP/NF (i.e., USP XXII and NF XVII, 1990).

The USP/NF describes not only the legally recognized standard testing methods and assay procedures for drug identity, strength, quality, and purity but also the number of samples to be tested and the acceptance criteria of various tests for release standards. In addition, USP/NF specifies the requirements for assay validation. Assay validation should examine the performance characteristics expressed in terms of analytical parameters. Typically, there are eight analytical parameters that should be examined in assay validation. These parameters include precision, accuracy, limit of detection, limit of quantitation, selectivity, range, linearity, and ruggedness. The definitions of these analytical parameters, which are given in the USP/NF, are summarized below. We discuss these analytical parameters in more detail in Chapter 3.

Precision is defined as the degree of agreement among individual test results when the procedure is applied repeatedly to multiple samplings of a homogeneous sample. Precision is a measure of the degree of reproducibility of the analytical method under normal operating circumstances. *Accuracy* is considered as the closeness of test results obtained by that method to the true value. Accuracy is a measure of the exactness of the analytical method.

Limit of detection is referred to as the lowest concentration of analyte in a sample that can be detected, but not necessarily quantitated, under the experimental conditions stated. The *limitation of quantitation* is interpreted as the lowest concentration of analyte in a sample that can be determined with acceptable precision and accuracy under the experimental conditions stated.

Selectivity (or *specificity*) is defined as the ability of an analytical method to measure the analyte accurately and specifically in the presence of components expected to be present in the sample matrix. Selectivity is sometimes considered a measure of the degree of interference as expressed by bias in the presence of a complex sample mixture.

Linearity is the ability of an analytical method to elicit test results that are directly, or by a well-defined mathematical transformation, proportional to the concentration of analyte in samples within a given range. *Range* is the interval between the upper and lower levels of analyte that have been demonstrated to be determined with precision, accuracy, and linearity using the method as written.

The *ruggedness* of an analytical method is the degree of *reproducibility* of test results obtained by an analysis of the same samples under a variety of normal test conditions, such as different laboratories, different analysts, different instruments, different lots of reagents, different elapsed assay times, different assay temperatures, and different days. Ruggedness can be interpreted as a measure of reproducibility of test results under normal, expected operational conditions from laboratory to laboratory and from analyst to analyst.

1.3. PHARMACEUTICAL VALIDATION

Pharmaceutical validation includes the validation of laboratory instruments such as gas chromatography (GC) or high-performance liquid chromatography (HPLC), and test procedures such as a specific assay method based on GC or HPLC, bioassay, or manufacturing processes for specific compounds. CGMP requires that pharmaceutical manufacturers establish the reliability of test results through appropriate validation of the test results at appropriate intervals. More specifically, the CGMP requires that the accuracy, precision, limit of detection, limit of quantitation, specificity, linearity, range, and reproducibility of test methods employed be established and validated. The validation of an instrument, a test procedure, or a manufacturing process is very important since statistical analyses depend heavily on test results of samples obtained from the instrument, the test procedure, or the manufacturing process. If the instrument, the test procedure, or the manufacturing process is not validated, the conclusions drawn from these tests results may lack reliability and may even be misleading. In the following we discuss some statistical issues that may occur in the validation of an instrument, a test procedure (e.g., an assay method), or a manufacturing process.

1.3.1. Calibration of an Instrument

For product testing the test procedure involves the accuracy and precision of an instrument. Therefore, the calibration of an instrument is essential for obtaining reliable measurement of a sample. For the calibration of an instrument, several standard concentration preparations are usually put through the instrument to obtain the corresponding responses (e.g., absorbances). A calibration curve can then be obtained based on these responses by fitting an appropriate statistical model. A linear regression model is usually employed under the normality assumption with equal variances. The fitted calibration curve is usually referred to as the standard curve or matrix curve. For a given sample, the concentration (or assay result) can then be determined using the standard curve.

For many compounds, however, it is expected that high concentration preparations have larger variability in their responses. In this case the usual ordinary least-squares method may not be appropriate for determining the standard curve. In this case, a weighted least-squares method is suggested with appropriate weights for determining the standard curve. This raises an interesting question: What weights should be used in the weighted least-squares approach? Furthermore, in many cases, although a linear regression model is preferred, the model may not be appropriate even with appropriate weights. Another question of interest: What statistical model should be used for calibration? Currently, there are five different statistical models with three commonly used weights. Therefore, how to select an appropriate model with appropriate weights is an important issue in the instrument calibration. Selection of weight and model for the standard curve in the calibration of an instrument is discussed in detail in Chapter 2.

Once an appropriate statistical model with appropriate weights is selected, an interesting question is: Should the same statistical model be used for all future samples? It should be noted that the standard curve based on the same statistical model may vary from time to time due to the variability of the reference material and instrument aging. Therefore, it may be desirable to recalibrate the instrument over a fixed time period, say every 3 months, or according to the calibration standard operating procedure (SOP).

Note that the problem of linear calibration of an instrument has been studied extensively in the past several decades [see, e.g., Krutchkoff (1967, 1969), Draper and Smith (1981), Lwin and Maritz (1982), Oman (1985), Sundberg (1985), and Fisch and Strehlau (1993)]. Under a linear regression model, the scientist may, for convenience, reverse the dependent variable (response) and the independent variable (standard concentration preparation). This approach is usually referred to as the *inverse method*. In practice, it is of great concern that switching the dependent and independent variables (i.e., switching from the classical method to the inverse method) may have an impact on determination of the unknown sample and thus may alter the conclusion drawn. Chow and Shao (1990b) studied the difference between the two methods of calibration in terms of the probability that the ratio of the assay results from the two methods differs from unity by more than a specified small constant. The results show that this probability increases as the absolute value of the ratio of the regression slope and error standard deviation decreases.

1.3.2. Assay Validation

As indicated earlier, assay validation involves eight analytical parameters. Among these parameters, accuracy and precision are usually considered to be the primary parameters for validation. Therefore, an assay method may be considered validated if the *accuracy* (unbiasedness) and *precision* (variability) of an assay meet acceptable limits. For the validation of an assay method, pharmaceutical manufacturers usually perform three or five assays on each of three separate runs (days) to evaluate the accuracy and precision of an assay. The estimates of mean and variability of an assay are then obtained to assess its accuracy and precision. For example, for accuracy, with 95% assurance, the bias of an assay must not be significant and has to be less than a certain percentage of a given standard under worst-case conditions (say, 5%). For precision, the total variability of an assay, which is the sum of the between-run and within-run variabilities, should not be greater than a specified allowable limit (say, 6%). The estimated total variability is usually expressed in terms of the *relative standard deviation* (RSD) or the *coefficient of variation* (CV). The most commonly used method for estimation of the total variability is estimation of individual variance components (i.e., the between-run and within-run variabilities) using the method of *analysis of variance* (ANOVA). However, the ANOVA method may lead to a negative estimate for the between-run variability when the true between-run variability is relatively small compared to the within-run variability. To avoid negative estimates, we may use such estimators as the maximum likelihood (ML) estimator (Herbach, 1959), the restricted maximum likelihood (REML) estimator (Thompson, 1962; Corbeil and Searle, 1976; Hocking, 1985), Searle et al. (1992), or the estimator proposed by Chow and Shao (1988). However, it is unclear whether the sum of two good individual variance component estimates constitutes a good estimate of the total variability. As an alternative, Chow and Tse (1991) proposed an estimate of the total variability rather than taking the sum of individual estimates of the between-run and within-run variabilities. The proposed estimator is preferred in the sense of lower mean-squared error.

Note that if the assay method involves complicated equipment that needs daily adjustment and may be performed by different analysts, the usual assay validation design (i.e., one-way random effects model) may not be appropriate. In this case, an appropriate validation design that can account for the analyst-to-analyst variation should be used. The design should be chosen such that analyst-to-analyst variation is not confounded with run-to-run variation. More details regarding a complicated assay validation design are given in Chapter 3.

1.3.3. Process Validation

The purpose of process validation is to demonstrate the reliability and reproducibility of manufacturing processes. To assure batch uniformity and integrity of drug products, CGMP requires validation of the manufacturing processes for finished pharmaceuticals. It should be noted that due to recent emphasis on preapproval inspection by the FDA, the pharmaceutical industry is also taking formal steps to validate the manufacturing processes for *bulk pharmaceutical chemicals* (BPCs). Without process validation, the FDA district office will withhold approval of an application.

A validation program is to establish documented successful evaluation of several full-scale production batches (usually three batches): that is, that the process will consistently meet predetermined specifications based on a validation protocol. The validation protocol is a written document that defines and gives details of the critical parts of the manufacturing process, states how the validation program will be conducted, and lists criteria for successful validation. The procedure will be followed to monitor the performance of those manufacturing steps that may be responsible for causing variability in the characteristics of in-process materials and finished drug products. For solid dosage forms, the tests usually include potency, content uniformity, dissolution, weight variation, and disintegration time. Testing of samples assures that drug products conform to USP/NF specifications.

Manufacturing process *validation* provides assurance that a process does what it purports to do. A manufacturing process is considered validated if the attributes of a sample meet USP/NF specifications. A common approach to process validation is to obtain a single sample and test the attributes of interest to see whether USP/NF specifications are met. It should be noted that there is no guarantee that if the test is performed again, it will have a high probability of meeting the specification even through the process is validated. Bergum (1990) proposed a way to construct acceptance limits which guarantee that future samples from a batch meet a given product specification a given percentage of the time. The idea is to consider a multiple-stage test. If the criteria for the first stage are met, the test is passed. If the criteria for the first stage are not met, additional testing is done. The test is passed when all the criteria at a particular stage are met. Acceptance limits for a validation sample are then constructed to assure that a future sample will have at least a certain chance of passing a multiple-stage test.

1.4. QUALITY ASSURANCE

CGMP recommends that every pharmaceutical company have a quality control unit to approve or reject all procedures or specifications that affect the identity, strength, quality, and purity of every drug product based on tests for such drug characteristics as potency and dissolution. Any lot or batch of product that meets USP/NF specifications for identity, strength, quality, and purity, and related tests, may be approved and released for use. Any lot or batch of such material that does not meet such specifications will be rejected.

Quality assurance involves quality control of raw material inspection, in-process material testing, and product testing. For each testing procedure, an appropriate sampling scheme is employed to assure that representative samples of each lot or batch are collected for testing. CGMP recommends that the number of samples to be tested be chosen based on appropriate statistical criteria for variability, confidence levels, and degree of precision desired. Acceptance criteria for the sampling and testing should be selected so that the drug product meets established in-house statistical quality control criteria and leads to meeting USP/NF specifications during the expiration dating period. If the test results meet all the in-house acceptance criteria, the quality control unit may approve and release the drug for sale.

During each stage of manufacturing, a commonly used approach for in-process quality control is to construct a cumulative sum (CUSUM) quality control chart over time. The CUSUM chart is useful in identifying a potential problem that may occur during the manufacturing process. If a problem is identified by the CUSUM chart, the quality control unit will issue a warning and an action will be taken to investigate the possible causes of the problem.

Note that a drug product which fails to meet USP/NF specifications during the expiration dating period of the drug is subject to recall even if it meets the in-house release targets. Therefore, an important statistical issue in quality assurance is how to construct a set of in-house acceptance criteria (or release targets) so that future samples will have a high level of assurance of meeting USP/NF specifications during the expiration dating period. This statistical issue is explored in Chapters 5 and 7. We summarize below several key components in quality assurance which have a great impact on the quality of the final product.

1.4.1. Scaleup

Before a drug is approved, most samples used for laboratory tests, animal studies, and clinical trials are from a laboratory batch. The scale of a laboratory batch is usually relatively small compared to that of a regular production batch. It is important for pharmaceutical companies to conduct a scaleup experiment so that the production batch can maintain the same identity, strength, quality, and purity of the drug. Various statistical designs are available in the literature.

A scaleup experiment usually involves many process factors. For example, the process factors for the manufacture of tablets of a drug may include the blender, use of preblend granulating water level, granulating blending procedure, granulating blend time, wet screen size, drying conditions, dry screen size, slug hardness, roll speed, degree of compaction, and lubricant blend time. The response variables of interest include particle size, flow, bulk density, moisture, hardness, ejection force, dissolution, weight variation, disintegration, and friability.

The purposes of a scaleup design are to (1) maximize information with minimal cost, (2) determine the effects of critical factors efficiently, (3) provide an organized approach, (4) determine optimum ranges, and (5) answer future questions. Scaleup designs include screening designs and optimization designs. The objective of a screening design is not only to identify critical factors but also to determine operating ranges provided that the basic formula is satisfactory. A typical 2^{K-P} fractional factorial is usually considered for a screen design. When the basic formula is not satisfactory, an optimization design is often employed to estimate the response surface and to identify levels that optimize the formula or process. Typically, a central composite design is considered for this purpose.

To reduce the cost within a fixed time frame requires the selection of an optimal design for achieving the objectives desired. Note that a design should be chosen to show that there are no interaction and confounding effects among factors. Other basic design considerations, such as ranges, sample size, response variables, and special problems, should also be taken into account when selecting an optimal design. Optimal scaleup designs are considered in detail in Chapter 4.

1.4.2. Raw Material Inspection

To ensure that the final product meets approved specifications, it is important to test the material at each stage of manufacture. The raw materials are often stored in drums. Typically, one selects a number of drums (say, the square root of the total number of drums) at random. For each drum sampled, CGMP suggests that a grain thief be used to draw random samples from the top, middle, and bottom parts of the drum. In practice, the strength contained in each drum may differ from the labeled strength and may vary from drum to drum. How to mix the raw materials from each drum uniformly so that the blended material can meet the desired strength becomes an important issue. To achieve the desired strength, each drum may contribute a different volume of materials for mixing. In practice, a V-blender has a certain capacity. Therefore, it is necessary to develop a statistical methodology for selecting the number of drums and the corresponding volumes for mixing such that the capacity of the V-blender is fully utilized and the mixed raw materials meet the targeted strength.

1.4.3. In-Process Materials Testing

The in-process materials include any material fabricated, compounded, blended, or derived by chemical reaction that is produced for, and used in, preparation of the drug product. At each stage of manufacturing, the in-process materials should be tested to control the expected and unexpected sources of variation. As an example, consider a procedure for manufacturing tablets of a pharmaceutical compound. The procedure may involve various critical stages, such as the active preblending, primary blending, lubricant preblending, milling, final blending, blending in transport, and compression. Suppose that the blender used in the manufacturing process is a 150-ft^3 V-blender with an intensifier bar. The major concerns are to establish that (1) the ingredients are uniformly mixed, (2) segregation does not occur in the blending process, and (3) no significant losses of active ingredients are encountered. When blending is completed, the material is transferred to conical transport devices. At each blending stage and blending-in-transport stage, the quality control unit evaluates potency and content uniformity and establishes acceptance limits that will ensure statistically that the tablets in the batch meet USP/NF specifications for dosage uniformity. For the primary and final blending processes, 12 samples are usually drawn from the top, middle, and bottom and front and back of the right and left sides of the V-blender after blending the material for a certain period with the intensifier bar running (see Fig. 1.4.1) for content uniformity testing. For blending in transport, a composite sample may be taken with a grain thief from each transport device for potency testing (see Fig. 1.4.2) and 12 samples from each quadrant of the filling port from the top, middle, and bottom of each transport device for content uniformity testing (see Fig. 1.4.3).

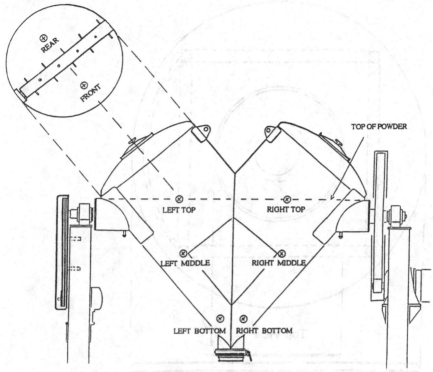

FIGURE 1.4.1 Sampling plan for V-blender.

1.4.4. Product Testing

Before the manufacturer can release a batch for sale, the batch needs to be tested for potency, content uniformity, dissolution, weight variation, and disintegration time to assure that the batch conforms to USP/NF specifications. Such tests are usually referred to as *release testing*. A common approach to release testing is to obtain a single random sample and test the attributes or variables of interest. If the specifications for the tested attribute are met, the batch is released. For each test, the quality control unit may construct acceptance limits based on other experiments, such as assay validation and stability study. The acceptance limits constructed are also known as *release targets*. These quarantee that future samples from a batch meet a given product specification within a given percentage of time. For example, for potency testing, the USP/NF requires that the average drug potency of the batch be within an interval (L, U), where $0 < L < U$ represents the USP/NF specification limits. Since the average potency is unknown, the release test is based on the potency assay result of a sample (or the average

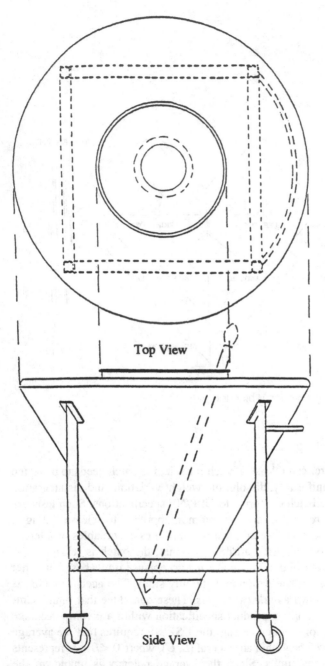

Top View

Side View

FIGURE 1.4.2   Sampling plan for conical transport (potency).

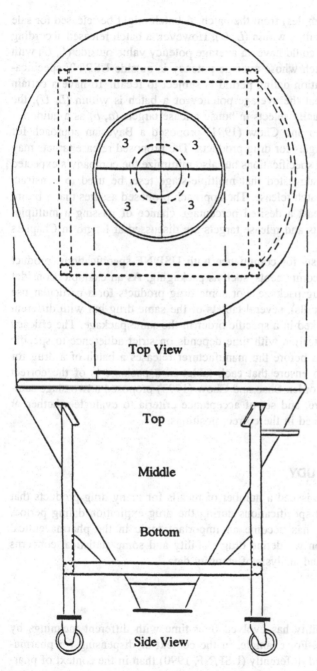

FIGURE 1.4.3 Sampling plan for conical transport (content uniformity).

potency results of n samples) from the batch. A batch might be released for sale if its potency assay result is within (L, U). However, a batch released according to such a test criterion could have an average potency value outside (L, U) with high probability. A batch whose average potency is outside USP/NF specifications during the expiration dating period is subject to recall. To have a certain degree of assurance that the average potency of a batch is within (L, U), the quality control unit usually selects in-house release targets (a, b) as a guide for releasing a batch. Shao and Chow (1991) proposed a Bayesian approach for constructing release targets for drug products. The proposed release targets may not only meet USP/NF specifications but also minimize the company's expected loss. Bergum (1990) suggested that multiple-stage tests be used to construct acceptance limits for batch release. The approach proposed assures that a future sample will have at least a desired percentage chance of passing a multiple-stage test. USP/NF tests and release targets are discussed at length in Chapters 5 and 7.

In addition to tests for compliance with USP/NF specifications, product testing involves other components, such as packaging. As an example, consider the evaluation of a drug package. For some drug products for a particular use (such as birth control pills), several tablets of the same drug but with different strengths are often packed in a specific order in the same package. The efficacy and safety of the medication with time depends on strict adherence to specific dosing schedules. Thus before the manufacturer releases a batch of a drug for sale, it is important to ensure that each tablet in a package is of the correct strength in the correct order. Shao and Chow (1993) proposed a two-stage sampling, testing procedure, and set of acceptance criteria to evaluate whether or not the tablets are packed in the correct positions.

1.5. STABILITY STUDY

Recently, the FDA has issued a number of recalls for many drug products that failed to meet product specifications during the drug expiration dating period. The study of stability has become an important topic in the pharmaceutical industry. In this section we define drug stability and some statistical concerns regarding the design and analysis of stability data.

1.5.1. Definition

The definition of stability has evolved over time with different meanings by different organizations. For example, in the context of dispensing for pharmacists, stability is defined differently (USP/NF, 1990) than in the context of pharmaceutical dosage forms for manufacturers. In this book we adopt the definition given in the 1987 U.S. Food and Drug Administration guideline (FDA, 1987). It should be noted that the European Community (EC) and Japan provide similar but slightly different definitions in their respective guidelines (Helboe, 1992). *Stability* is defined as the capacity of a drug product to remain within specifications established to ensure its identity, strength, quality, and purity. As stated in the FDA guideline, manufacturers should establish stability not only for drug products but also for bulk drug substances.

One major objective of a stability study is to characterize the degradation of a drug product over time and then to establish an expiration dating period for the product. The expiration dating period or *shelf life* is defined as the interval that a product is expected to remain within the approved specifications after manufacture.

1.5.2. Accelerated Testing and Long-Term Stability

In practice, since it may take a long time to observe the degradation of a drug product, for stability studies a pharmaceutical company usually first conducts an accelerated test (or stress test) to speed up the rate of chemical or physical degradation of the product under exaggerated storage conditions. The purpose of accelerated testing is to study the performance of essential kinetic parameters so as to establish a tentative drug shelf life. A long-term stability study is then conducted under ambient conditions to support the shelf life claimed in an NDA or a PLA.

Generally, there are different criteria for acceptable levels of stability with respect to chemical, physical, microbiological, therapeutic, and toxicological characteristics of drug products (USP/NF, 1990). The requirements for stability of these five characteristics differ from dosage form to dosage form. The FDA guideline summarizes specific requirements of the tests for different properties of different dosage forms. For example, a stability study of tablets should include tests for appearance, friability, hardness, color, odor, moisture, strength, and dissolution. The expiration dating period should be established based on degradation of quantitative drug product characteristics such as strength. As indicated earlier, the strength of a drug product is defined as either (1) the concentration of the drug substance or (2) the potency (i.e., the therapeutic activity) of the drug product, which can be determined by an appropriate laboratory test or by adequately developed and controlled clinical data. However, in the FDA guideline, the strength of a drug product is interpreted as a quantitative measure of the active ingredient of a drug product, as well as other ingredients requiring quantitation, such as alcohol and preservatives. For an analysis of stability data, the FDA requires that percent of label claim, not percent of initial average value, be used as the primary variable for strength.

1.5.3. Storage Conditions and Sampling

The stability of the characteristics of a drug product for a particular dosage form may be influenced by storage conditions, such as temperature, humidity, light, or air and by package type, such as high-density polyethylene (HDPE). The FDA guidelines recommend that a long-term stability study be conducted to generate stability data on a drug product stored in the proposed container or closure for marketing under storage conditions that support the shelf life proposed. Stability data obtained from a long-term stability study are usually referred to as the *primary stability data*. The data obtained from accelerated testing are classified as *supportive stability data*.

In a long-term stability study, FDA guidelines require that at least three batches of the product be tested under ambient conditions every 3 months the first year, every 6 months the second year, and annually thereafter. For accelerated testing, the stress conditions include temperature (e.g., 5, 50, and 75°C), relative humidity (e.g., 75%), and exposure to various wave lengths of electromagnetic radiation.

Suppose for a particular dosage form such as a tablet that there are three dose levels, 5 mg, 10 mg, and 20 mg, and three package containers, HDPE with 40 tablets (HDPE40), HDPE with 120 tablets (HDPE120), and blisters. Suppose further that the stability plan for this dosage form calls for a 5-year long-term stability study at two temperatures, 20 and 30°C, as well as accelerated testing at temperature 45°C, relative humidity 75%, and at 2, 4, and 6 months. Table 1.5.1 shows that there are a total of 27 batch–dose–package combinations at each time point. As a result, this stability plan has a total of 621 tests (540 for the long-term study and 81 for accelerated testing). Moreover, different regions (e.g., the United States, the EC, and Japan) have different requirements for stability studies. As a result, if a pharmaceutical company is interested in registering the drug in these countries, it may require a total of $3 \times 621 = 1863$ tests to establish the stability of the drug.

1.5.4. Factorial, Bracketing, and Matrixing Designs

To achieve a sound statistical implication of drug stability, the FDA guideline requires that a random sample of containers be chosen from each of three batches and that dosage units be sampled randomly from each of at least two containers at each time point. Therefore, to characterize the degradation of a drug product requires an enormous number of assays, such as for potency and dissolution. A traditional full-length test of long-term stability or an accelerated test may involve such factors as time, batch, temperature, humidity, container, and dose level, which may be very time consuming and/or costly to complete. Therefore, it is of interest to reduce the number of assays while achieving the same precision. Recently, the question of how to reduce the number of assays

TABLE 1.5.1 Example of a Stability Plan

Factor	Level
	Long-term stability study
Strength	5, 10, 20 mg
Batch	1, 2, 3
Temperature	20°C, 30°C
Package	HDPE40, HDPE120, blister
Sampling time points	0, 3, 6, 9, 12, 18, 24, 36, 48, 60 months
Total number of assays	540
	Accelerated testing
Strength	5, 10, 20 mg
Batch	1, 2, 3
Temperature	45°C
Package	HDPE40, HDPE120, blister
Sampling time points	2, 4, 6 months
Total number of assays	81

with desired precision using a fractional factorial design has received much attention [see, e.g., Chow (1992), Lin (1990), Lin (1994), Nordbrock (1992), Nakagaki (1990), Helboe (1992), and ICH (1993)].

One fractional factorial design that is of particular interest is *bracketing design* (Nakagaki, 1990; Chow, 1992; Helboe, 1992; ICH, 1993, Lin, 1994). The basic assumption of a bracketing design is that the stability of different levels of a factor in stability studies can be determined by the stability of the extremes (Nakagaki, 1990). Therefore, if one of the factors considered in the design is bracketed, only the lowest and highest levels of the factor are included for study. For example, suppose that there are four package containers: HPDE20, HPDE80, HPDE160, and HPDE320. A bracketing design requires only that HPDE20 and HPDE320 be included in the study. Bracketing design may reduce the number of assays and consequently, reduce the cost substantially. For example, only 50% of assays in a full factorial design need to be performed in the example above. It should be noted however, that the fundamental assumption for the bracketing design is very difficult or impossible to verify. Moreover, a solid statistical justification is needed for using a bracketing design.

Another popular design is *matrixing design*, which is actually a fractional factorial design (Nakagaki, 1990; Chow, 1992; Helboe, 1992; ICH, 1993; Lin,

1994). The underlying assumption of a matrixing design is that the stability from a fractional factorial design can be representative of that from a full factorial design. Unlike bracketing design, this assumption can be verified if the levels of the factors employed in the fractional factorial design are balanced in a manner similar to that of a completely balanced block design. Moreover, statistical criteria can be imposed in the stability plan when a matrixing design is used.

When the drug product degrades over time in a linear fashion, the slope of the degradation curve is generally used as an indicator of the stability loss over time. Different batches may have different stability losses (slopes) for different strengths and package types. Nordbrock (1992) compared 10 different fractional factorial designs, including the full factorial design, some bracketing designs, and matrixing designs, in terms of power for detection of a significant difference between slopes. Chow (1992) and Ju and Chow (1994b), however, pointed out that the primary objective of a stability study is to estimate the drug shelf life rather than detecting a difference between stability losses among batches. Therefore, it is recommended that fractional factorial designs be evaluated based on whether they can provide an estimate of drug shelf life with the best precision.

1.5.5. Determination of Drug Shelf Life

As mentioned earlier, the purpose of accelerated testing is to estimate the rate of chemical or physical degradation and to provide a prediction of a tentative expiration dating period. To do this, first, one needs to determine the order of a reaction. For example, a zero-order equation describes a linear relationship between the drug characteristics and time, while the first-order equation indicates that a logarithmic transformation of the drug characteristic is a linear function of time. Once the order of the reaction is determined empirically, the relationship between the rate of degradation and the temperature can be characterized through the *Arrhenius equation*, which describes the linear relationship between log(degradation) and the reciprocal of the absolute temperature. A prediction of a tentative expiration dating period can then be obtained. For an analysis of accelerated testing, both the weighted least-squares procedure (Bohidar and Peace, 1988) and a standard nonlinear regression procedure (Davies and Hudson, 1981) have been suggested. In either case the assumption of the Arrhenius equation should be verified by a lack-of-fit test.

For long-term stability studies, assuming that drug strength decreases with time, the FDA guideline suggests that the expiration dating period be determined as the time at which the 95% one-sided lower confidence limit for the mean degradation curve intersects the acceptable lower specification limit. In addition, the FDA requires a peliminary test for batch similarity before the results of different batches can be pooled for estimation of a single expiration dating period. However, the test suggested in the FDA guideline is the one for detecting the difference of slopes and intercepts among batches to be performed at a level of significance of 25% (Bancroft, 1964). Furthermore, acceptance of the null hypothesis of no difference in slopes among batches does not guarantee that the batches have similar degradation rates, because the problem of similarity is formulated incorrectly by the wrong hypothesis of difference. The interval hypothesis for bioequivalence problems (Chow and Liu, 1992) can be applied to test the batch similarity. However, this approach assumes that the batch effect is fixed. One can argue that by the time the sponsor files an NDA or a PLA, only three batches of the product have been manufactured. Therefore, the batch effect should be considered fixed. The 1987 FDA guideline states clearly and precisely that "the design of a stability is intended to establish, based on testing a limit number of batches of a drug product, an expiration dating period applicable to all future batches of the drug product manufactured under similar circumstances" (p. 24). Within this context, the batch effect must be considered random; otherwise, the proposed expiration dating period is applicable only to the three batches used for filing the NDA, not to any future production batches. If the batch is assumed random, the shelf life can be estimated without any preliminary test for batch similarity. Recently, several methods for combining information from different batches have been proposed. Under the assumption of the fixed batch effect, Ruberg and Hsu (1992) proposed the use of a multiple comparison procedure for pooling with the worst batch. Estimation procedures for shelf life under the assumption of a random batch effect can be found in Murphy and Weisman (1990), Chow and Shao (1990a, 1991), and Shao and Chow (1994). Simulation results for comparing various methods under either fixed or random effects, including the FDA approach, can be found in Ho et al. (1992). Morris (1992) also examined the consequences of using an incorrect linear model rather than the true exponential model in an estimation of drug shelf life.

1.6. AIMS AND STRUCTURE OF THE BOOK

The goal of this book is to provide a comprehensive and unified presentation of statistical methods employed during various stages of pharmaceutical development. In addition, it is intended to give a well-balanced summary of current and recently developed statistical methods in stability analysis.

It is our goal to provide a useful reference book for chemical scientists, pharmaceutical scientists, development pharmacists, and statisticians in the pharmaceutical industry, regulatory agencies, and academia. The book can also serve as a textbook for graduate courses in the areas of pharmacy, pharmaceutical development, stability studies, and biostatistics. Our primary emphasis in this

book is on biopharmaceutical applications. All statistical methods and their interpretations are illustrated through real examples that have occurred during
various stages of pharmaceutical development.

The scope of the book is restricted to statistical designs and analyses in
pharmaceutical development and stability studies. Basically, the book consists
of three parts: pharmaceutical validation, quality assurance, and stability study.
In Chapter 1 we give the background and regulatory requirements for various
stages of pharmaceutical development. Chapters 2 and 3 cover statistical designs
and methods for assay development and validation. In Chapter 4 we summarize
screening and optimization designs for scaleup programs. In Chapter 5 we introduce the USP/NF specification limits and the corresponding tests for different
dosage forms. Also included in Chapter 5 are their statistical interpretations.
Chapter 6 is devoted to the validation of manufacturing processes: prospective,
concurrent, retrospective, and revalidation. Statistical issues regarding multiple-
stage sampling and validation designs are also addressed in Chapter 6. In Chapter 7 we discuss useful statistical methods for quality assurance and release
targets. In Chapter 8 we provide fundamental concepts of stability, overage, and
drug expiration dating periods. Accelerated stability testing and long-term stability study are also discussed in Chapter 8. Chapter 9 covers chemical kinetic
models used in accelerated stability testing, statistical analysis, adequacy of
models, and prediction through the Arrhenius equation. In Chapter 10 we compare several stability designs, including the complete factorial design and matrixing and bracketing designs. In Chapter 11 we introduce statistical analysis
of stability data based on fixed effects models. In Chapter 12 we review statistical methods for determination of drug shelf life using random effects models.

For each chapter, real examples are given to illustrate the concepts, appropriate applications, and limitations of statistical methods. Comparisons of the
relative merits and disadvantages of these statistical methods are also discussed.
When applicable, topics for possible future research development are provided
at the end of the chapter.

2

Assay Development

2.1. INTRODUCTION

When a new pharmaceutical compound is discovered, assay and test procedures are developed for determining the active ingredient of the compound in compliance with USP/NF standards for the identity, strength, quality, and purity of the compound. An assay method is usually developed based on instruments such as gas chromatography (GC) and high-performance liquid chromatography (HPLC). CGMP indicates that an instrument must be suitable for its intended purposes and be capable of producing valid results. The instrument is to be calibrated, inspected, and checked routinely according to written procedures. In the next two chapters we focus on statistical issues commonly encountered in the development of an assay method for a pharmaceutical compound. These issues include instrument calibration, statistical methods for the standard curve, determination of an unknown sample, and design and analysis of assay validation.

In Sec. 2.2, instrument calibration and the establishment of standard curves for assay methods are outlined. In Sec. 2.3 we provide a brief review of simple linear regression analysis, which is often employed in assay development. Statistical methods for determination (estimation) of an unknown sample based on an established standard curve are described in Sec. 2.4. Weight and model selections for establishing standard curves in the calibration of an instrument are discussed in Sec. 2.5. Some statistical considerations in assay development are provided in Sec. 2.6.

2.2. CALIBRATION AND STANDARD CURVE

For the development of an assay method, CGMP [see, e.g., 21 CFR 211.194 (a)] requires that the assay method for assessing compliance of pharmaceutical products with established specifications meet proper standards of accuracy and reliability. An assay method not meeting established specifications cannot be used. To meet the established specifications, instrument calibration is essential.

A common approach to instrument calibration is to have a number of known standard concentration preparations put through the instrument to obtain the corresponding responses (e.g., absorbance and peak response). On the basis of these standards and their corresponding responses, an estimated calibration curve can be obtained by fitting an appropriate statistical model between these standards and their corresponding responses. The estimated calibration curve is usually referred to as the *standard curve*. For a given unknown sample, the concentration can be determined based on the standard curve by replacing the dependent variable with its response. As can be seen, the calibration of an instrument involves the selection of a set of standard preparations (*standards*, hereafter). CGMP indicates that, where practical, the calibration standards used for assay development must be in compliance with USP/NF standards. If USP/NF standards are not practical for the parameter being measured, an independent reproducible standard must be used. If no applicable standards exist, an in-house standard must be developed and used.

CGMP also indicates that instrument calibration must include specific directions and limits for accuracy, precision, and other analytical parameters. If the accuracy, precision, and other parameter limits are not met, the instrument must have provisions for remedial action. The instrument used for assay must be calibrated, inspected, and checked routinely. Note that if the assay method is described in the USP/NF, validation of accuracy and reliability is not required. However, the suitability of the instrument under actual conditions of use must be verified. If computers are used as part of an automated system, the computer software programs must be validated by adequate, documented testing.

Note that a linear regression model is often employed in instrument calibration to determine the standard curve. The standard curve is then used to determine the unknown sample. Standard linear calibration involves two commonly used methods, the classical method and the inverse method (Krutchkoff, 1967, 1969). The method described in the second paragraph of this section is usually referred to as the *classical method*. For the *inverse method*, a similar standard curve can be obtained by switching the dependent variable (response) and the independent variable (standard) in the classical method. The concentration of the unknown sample can then be determined similarly. In Sec. 2.3 we provide a brief review of simple linear regression models that are widely used when calibrating the standard curve.

2.3. SIMPLE LINEAR REGRESSION

For instrument calibration, a simple linear regression model that involves only one independent variable (standard) and one dependent variable (response) is probably the most widely applied statistical model. Statistical methods for such a model are well established and are described in many introductory statistical texts [see, e.g., Draper and Smith (1981) and Ott (1984)]. In this section we provide a brief review of statistical inferences such as estimation, confidence interval, and hypothesis testing for simple linear regression models.

Let $X_i > 0$ be the ith known standard (e.g., concentration) and Y_i be its corresponding response (e.g., absorbance or peak response) obtained from the instrument, where $i = 1, \ldots, n$. The simplest model for empirical description of the relationship between X_i and Y_i is a linear regression model:

$$Y_i = \alpha + \beta X_i + e_i, \qquad i = 1, \ldots, n, \tag{2.3.1}$$

where α is the Y intercept, which is the value of the response when the standard is zero; β is the slope of the straight line that measures the change in response per unit change in standard; and e_i is the random error in observing Y_i. It is assumed that e_i are independent and identically distributed (i.i.d.) as a normal distribution with mean zero and variance σ^2.

Under the normality assumption of random error e_i, the distribution of Y_i is also a normal distribution with mean

$$E(Y_i) = \alpha + \beta X_i \tag{2.3.2}$$

and variance

$$\mathrm{var}(Y_i) - \sigma^2. \tag{2.3.3}$$

From (2.3.2) and (2.3.3) it can be seen that three unknown parameters (i.e., α, β, and σ^2) need to be estimated from the data. Let $\hat{\alpha}$ and $\hat{\beta}$ be estimators of α and β, respectively. Then the predicted response $\hat{Y}_i$ at X_i is given by

$$\hat{Y}_i = \hat{\alpha} + \hat{\beta} X_i \tag{2.3.4}$$

and the deviation of the predicted response $\hat{Y}_i$ from the observed response Y_i is

$$Y_i - \hat{Y}_i. \tag{2.3.5}$$

Therefore, the sum of squares of the deviations of the predicted response $\hat{Y}_i$ from the observed response Y_i is given by

$$\sum_{i=1}^{n} (Y_i - \hat{Y}_i)^2 = \sum_{i=1}^{n} (Y_i - \hat{\alpha} - \hat{\beta} X_i)^2. \tag{2.3.6}$$

The method of ordinary least squares provides the ordinary least-squares estimates (LSEs), which minimize the sum of squares of the deviation given in
(2.3.6).

Define the sample means of the standards and the responses as

$$\bar{X} = \frac{1}{n} \sum_{i=1}^{n} X_i,$$
$$\bar{Y} = \frac{1}{n} \sum_{i=1}^{n} Y_i. \tag{2.3.7}$$

The corrected sum of squares and cross products are given by

$$S_{XX} = \sum_{i=1}^{n} (X_i - \bar{X})^2,$$

$$S_{XY} = \sum_{i=1}^{n} (X_i - \bar{X})(Y_i - \bar{Y}), \tag{2.3.8}$$

$$S_{YY} = \sum_{i=1}^{n} (Y_i - \bar{Y})^2.$$

The LSEs of the intercept α and the slope β in model (2.3.1), which can be
obtained by minimizing (2.3.6), are given by

$$a = \bar{Y} - b\bar{X}, \tag{2.3.9}$$
$$b = \frac{S_{XY}}{S_{XX}},$$

respectively. The predicted value of Y_i is then given by

$$\hat{Y}_i = a + bX_i \tag{2.3.10}$$
$$= \bar{Y} + b(X_i - \bar{X}).$$

The deviation of the response from the sample mean can be expressed in terms
of the sum of the deviation of the predicted value from the observed response
and the deviation of the predicted value from the sample mean:

$$Y_i - \bar{Y} = (Y_i - \hat{Y}_i) + (\hat{Y}_i - \bar{Y}), \qquad i = 2, \ldots, n. \tag{2.3.11}$$

It can then be shown that

$$S_{YY} = \sum_{i=1}^{n} (Y_i - \bar{Y})^2$$

$$= \sum_{i=1}^{n} (Y_i - \hat{Y}_i)^2 + \sum_{i=1}^{n} (\hat{Y}_i - \bar{Y})^2 \qquad (2.3.12)$$

$$= \text{SSE} + \text{SSR},$$

where SSR and SSE are the sum of squares due to the regression and the sum of squares of residuals, respectively. Note that SSR is the total variability explained by the standards, while SSE represents the variability that cannot be explained by the standards. Note that the relationship among the total sum of squares, the sum of squares due to regression, and the sum of squares of residuals can be summarized in the analysis of variance table as given in Table 2.3.1.

It can easily be verified that

$$\text{SSR} = \frac{S_{XY}^2}{S_{XX}}, \qquad (2.3.13)$$

$$S_{YY} = \text{SSR} + \text{SSE}$$

$$= \frac{S_{XY}^2}{S_{XX}} + \left(S_{YY} - \frac{S_{XY}^2}{S_{XX}} \right). \qquad (2.3.14)$$

Define the coefficient of determination as follows:

$$R^2 = \frac{\text{SSR}}{\text{SSR} + \text{SSE}} = \frac{S_{XY}^2}{S_{XX}S_{YY}}. \qquad (2.3.15)$$

Then R^2 represents the proportion of the total variability of the response explained by the standards.

TABLE 2.3.1 ANOVA Table for Simple Linear Regression

Source of variation	df	Sum of squares[a]	Mean sum of squares	F value
Regression	1	SSR	MSR = SSR	F_b = MSR/MSE
Residual	$n - 2$	SSE	MSE = SSE/$(n - 2)$	
Total	$n - 1$	SST		

[a] SSR = S_{XY}^2/S_{XX}; SSE = $S_{YY} - S_{XY}^2/S_{XX}$

Under the normality assumption, an unbiased estimator of σ^2 can be obtained as

$$\hat{\sigma}^2 = \frac{1}{n-2} \, \text{SSE}$$

$$= \frac{1}{n-2} \sum_{i=1}^{n} (Y_i - \hat{Y}_i)^2 \tag{2.3.16}$$

$$= \frac{1}{n-2} \sum_{i=1}^{n} (Y_i - a - bX_i)^2.$$

The variance of a and b are given by

$$\text{var}(a) = \left(\frac{1}{nS_{XX}} \sum_{i=1}^{n} X_i^2 \right) \sigma^2,$$

$$\text{var}(b) = \frac{1}{S_{XX}} \sigma^2. \tag{2.3.17}$$

From (2.3.17), unbiased estimators of $\text{var}(a)$ and $\text{var}(b)$ can be obtained simply by replacing σ^2 with its unbiased estimator, $\hat{\sigma}^2$. This gives

$$\widehat{\text{var}}(a) = \left(\frac{1}{nS_{XX}} \sum_{i=1}^{n} X_i^2 \right) \hat{\sigma}^2,$$

$$\widehat{\text{var}}(b) = \frac{1}{S_{XX}} \hat{\sigma}^2. \tag{2.3.18}$$

Let $\text{SE}(a)$ and $\text{SE}(b)$ be the standard errors of a and b,

$$\text{SE}(a) = \sqrt{\widehat{\text{var}}(a)} \quad \text{and} \quad \text{SE}(b) = \sqrt{\widehat{\text{var}}(b)}.$$

Then, under the hypotheses that $\alpha = 0$ and $\beta = 0$, both

$$T_a = \frac{a}{\text{SE}(a)} \quad \text{and} \quad T_b = \frac{b}{\text{SE}(b)}$$

follow a central t distribution with $n - 2$ degrees of freedom. As a result, the $(1 - \alpha) \times 100\%$ confidence intervals for α and β are given by

$$a \pm t(\tfrac{1}{2}\alpha, n - 2)\text{SE}(a), \tag{2.3.19}$$

$$b \pm t(\tfrac{1}{2}\alpha, n - 2)\text{SE}(b),$$

where $t(\tfrac{1}{2}\alpha, n - 2)$ is the $(\tfrac{1}{2}\alpha)$th upper quantile of a central t distribution with $n - 2$ degrees of freedom.

To test for zero intercept, consider the following hypotheses:

$$H_0: \alpha = 0 \quad \text{vs.} \quad H_a: \alpha \neq 0. \tag{2.3.20}$$

The null hypothesis of (2.3.20) is rejected at the α level of significance if

$$|T_a| = \left| \frac{a}{SE(a)} \right| > t(\tfrac{1}{2}\alpha, n - 2).$$

Similarly, we may test for zero slope based on the following hypotheses:

$$H_0: \beta = 0 \quad \text{vs.} \quad H_a: \beta \neq 0. \tag{2.3.21}$$

The null hypothesis of (2.3.21) is rejected at the α level of significance if

$$|T_b| = \left| \frac{b}{SE(b)} \right| > t(\tfrac{1}{2}\alpha, n - 2). \tag{2.3.22}$$

Note that the null hypothesis of zero slope can also be tested using the technique of analysis of variance (ANOVA). From Table 2.3.1 the null hypothesis of (2.3.21) is rejected at the α level of significance if

$$F_b > F(\alpha, 1, n - 2), \tag{2.3.23}$$

where $F(\alpha, 1, n - 2)$ is the upper αth quantile of a central F distribution with 1 and $n - 2$ degrees of freedom. It should be noted that $T_b^2 = F_b$.

After having obtained the LSEs of α and β, we can predict the response of a given standard through the following least-squares predictor:

$$\hat{Y} = a + bX. \tag{2.3.24}$$

It can be seen that $\hat{Y}$ is an unbiased estimator of $\alpha + \beta X$. Its variance can be estimated by

$$\widehat{\text{var}}(\hat{Y}) = \left[1 + \frac{1}{n} + \frac{(X - \bar{X})^2}{S_{xx}} \right] \hat{\sigma}^2.$$

Therefore, the $(1 - \alpha) \times 100\%$ confidence interval for Y is given by

$$\hat{Y} \pm t(\tfrac{1}{2}\alpha, n - 2) \, \hat{\sigma} \left[1 + \frac{1}{n} + \frac{(X - \bar{X})^2}{S_{xx}} \right]^{\frac{1}{2}}. \tag{2.3.25}$$

Example 2.3.1

To illustrate the statistical methodology for a simple linear regression, consider the following example concerning the calibration of an instrument of a pharmaceutical compound. Twelve concentrations of standard preparations were chosen at 80% [$L = 17.65 \, \mu M$ (micromolar)], 100% ($M = 22.06 \, \mu M$), and 120% ($H = 26.43 \, \mu M$) of that expected from the sample being assayed. The standard preparations and the unknown sample S were put through the instrument in the order LLMMHHSHHMMLL to obtain the corresponding absorbances in the same run. The standard preparations and their corresponding absorbances are listed in Table 2.3.2. Figure 2.3.1 gives the scatter plot of the data.

From Table 2.3.2, the sample means of the standards and responses, and the corrected sum of squares and cross products, can be obtained as

$$\overline{X} = \frac{264.72}{12} = 22.060,$$

$$\overline{Y} = \frac{1408.869}{12} = 117.406,$$

$$S_{XX} = 155.585,$$

$$S_{XY} = 844.705,$$

$$S_{YY} = 4744.613.$$

The LSEs of the intercept and slope are then given by

$$a = \overline{Y} - b\overline{X}$$
$$= 117.406 - (5.429)(22.06) = -2.363,$$
$$b = \frac{S_{XY}}{S_{XX}} = \frac{844.705}{155.585} = 5.429.$$

TABLE 2.3.2 Calibration Data Display

Concentration, X_i	Absorbance, Y_i
17.65 (L)	97.485
17.65 (L)	95.406
22.06 (M)	121.200
22.06 (M)	121.968
26.47 (H)	142.346
26.47 (H)	145.464
S	90.044
26.47 (H)	141.835
26.47 (H)	135.625
22.06 (M)	113.814
22.06 (M)	112.890
17.65 (L)	89.872
17.65 (L)	90.964

Source: Chow and Shao (1990b).

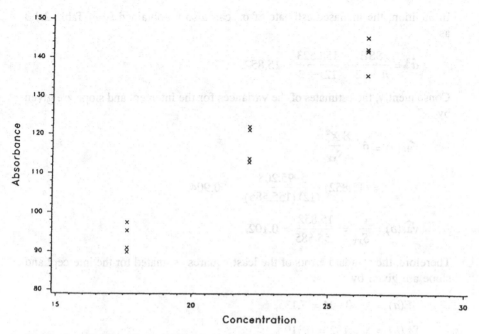

FIGURE 2.3.1 Scatter plot of data set in Table 2.3.2.

Therefore, the least-squares predictor for a given concentration X (i.e., the estimated standard curve) is given as

$$Y = -2.363 + 5.429X.$$

The ANOVA table for the data given in Table 2.3.2 is summarized in Table 2.3.3. It can be verified from Table 2.3.3 that the coefficient of determination is given by

$$R^2 = \frac{SSR}{S_{YY}} = \frac{4586.090}{4744.613} = 0.967.$$

TABLE 2.3.3 ANOVA Table for Data in Table 2.3.2

Source of variation	df	Sum of squares	Mean square	F value	p value
Regression	1	4586.090	4586.090	289.302	<0.0001
Residual	10	158.523	15.852		
Total	11	4744.613			

In addition, the unbiased estimate of σ^2 can also be obtained from Table 2.3.3 as

$$\hat{\sigma}^2 = \frac{SSE}{n-2} = \frac{158.523}{12-2} = 15.852.$$

Consequently, the estimates of the variances for the intercept and slope are given by

$$\widehat{var}(a) = \hat{\sigma}^2 \frac{\sum X_i^2}{nS_{xx}}$$

$$= (15.852)\frac{5995.208}{(12)(155.585)} = 50.904,$$

$$\widehat{var}(b) = \frac{\hat{\sigma}^2}{S_{xx}} = \frac{15.852}{155.585} = 0.102.$$

Therefore, the standard errors of the least-squares estimated for the intercept and slope are given by

$$SE(a) = \sqrt{50.904} = 7.135,$$

$$SE(b) = \sqrt{0.102} = 0.319.$$

It follows that the 95% confidence intervals for the intercept and slope are $(-18.260, 13.533)$ and $(4.718, 6.140)$, respectively. The hypothesis of zero intercept can be tested using the following statistic:

$$|T_a| = \left|\frac{-2.363}{7.135}\right| = 0.331,$$

which is less than $t(0.025, 10) = 2.228$. Thus we fail to reject the null hypothesis of zero intercept at the 5% level of significance. This result is consistent with the fact that the 95% confidence interval for the intercept contains zero. For testing the hypothesis of zero slope, it can be verified that

$$|T_b| = \left|\frac{5.429}{0.319}\right| = 17.009,$$

which is greater than $t(0.025, 10)$. Hence the hypothesis of zero slope is rejected at the 5% level of significance. This result conforms to the fact that the 95% confidence interval for the slope does not contain zero. It should be noted that

$$(T_b)^2 = (17.009)^2 = 289.302,$$

which is the same as the value of F_b in the ANOVA table in Table 2.3.3.

Based on the estimated curve, the predicted value for an observed absorbance at a specified standard concentration can also be obtained. For example, for the low standard concentration 17.65 μM, we have

$$\hat{Y} = -2.363 + (5.429)(17.65) = 93.463.$$

The estimate of the corresponding variance is given by

$$var(\hat{Y}) = (15.852)\left[1 + \frac{1}{12} + \frac{(17.65 - 22.06)^2}{155.585}\right]$$
$$= 19.155.$$

Hence the 95% confidence interval for an observed absorbance at 17.65 μM is obtained as

$$93.463 \pm (2.228)\sqrt{19.155} = 93.463 \pm 9.752$$
$$= (83.712, 103.215).$$

To provide better understanding, the estimated regression line or the estimated standard curve, as well as its 95% confidence band, are presented in Fig. 2.3.2.

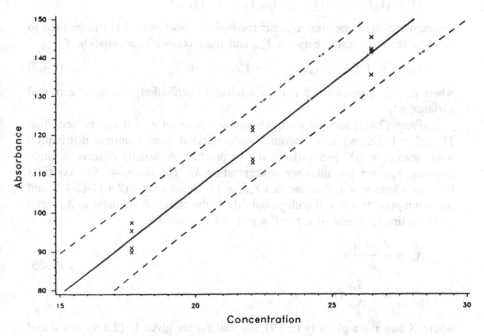

FIGURE 2.3.2 Regression line and 95% CI for data set in Table 2.3.2.

2.4. STATISTICAL METHODS FOR CALIBRATION

As indicated earlier, an instrument is calibrated to establish a standard curve which can describe the empirical relationship between known standards and their corresponding responses obtained from the instrument. In most cases the relationship between the known standards and their responses is linear within the range under study. Therefore, in this section, for simplicity, we assume that the relationship between the standards and their responses is linear. This permits us to introduce two statistical methods, the classical and inverse methods, for calibration. The relative merits and disadvantages of these two methods are also examined.

2.4.1. Classical and Inverse Methods

Let X_i and Y_i be the ith standard and its corresponding response from the instrument, where $i = 1, \ldots, n$. In addition to the assumption that the relationship between Y_i and X_i is linear, we assume that there are m additional responses $Y_{n+j}, j = 1, \ldots, m$ observed from an unknown concentration X_0. As a result, we have the following data structure:

$$\begin{pmatrix} X_1 \\ Y_1 \end{pmatrix}, \begin{pmatrix} X_2 \\ Y_2 \end{pmatrix}, \ldots, \begin{pmatrix} X_n \\ Y_n \end{pmatrix}, \begin{pmatrix} X_0 \\ Y_{n+1} \end{pmatrix}, \ldots, \begin{pmatrix} X_0 \\ Y_{n+m} \end{pmatrix}. \tag{2.4.1}$$

Furthermore, the same simple linear regression model in (2.3.1) can be used to describe the relationship between Y_{n+j} and the unknown concentration X_0:

$$Y_{n+j} = \alpha + \beta X_0 + e_{n+j}, \qquad j = 1, 2, \ldots, m, \tag{2.4.2}$$

where e_{n+j} are also assumed i.i.d. as a normal distribution with mean zero and variance σ^2.

From (2.4.2) and the distribution assumption of e_{n+j}, it can be seen that $\{Y_{n+j}, j = 1, \ldots, m\}$ is a random sample selected from a normal distribution with mean $\alpha + \beta X_0$ and variance σ^2. In practice we usually observe a single response Y_{n+1} for the unknown concentration X_0. Therefore, we first consider the case where $m = 1$. Assume that $Y_{n+1} = Y_0$. Under model (2.4.1)–(2.4.2) and the assumption that $b \neq 0$ with probability 1, the classical estimator of X_0 based on the estimated standard curve $Y = a + bX$ is given by

$$\hat{X}_C = \frac{Y_0 - a}{b} \tag{2.4.3}$$

$$= \bar{X} + \frac{S_{XX}}{S_{XY}} (Y_0 - \bar{Y}),$$

where $\bar{X}$ and $\bar{Y}$ are given in (2.3.7), S_{XX} and S_{XY} are given in (2.3.8), and a and b are the LSEs of α and β, which are also given in (2.3.9).

Under the normality assumption of e_i, the classical estimator is the maximum likelihood estimator of X_0 (Graybill, 1976), which is the ratio of two correlated normal random variables. As a result, the population mean, variance, and any other higher moments of $\hat{X}_C$ generally do not exist. However, it is interesting to note that $\hat{X}_C$ converges to X_0 with probability 1. In other words, $\hat{X}_C$ and X_0 differ by a negligibly small quantity for sufficiently large n. Since the variance of the classical estimator does not exist, we cannot directly estimate the precision (variability) of X_0. However, we can still construct a $(1 - \alpha) \times 100\%$ confidence interval for X_0. The precision and reliability of $\hat{X}_C$ can then be assessed based on the width of the $(1 - \alpha) \times 100\%$ confidence interval. In addition, the width of the constructed confidence interval may provide useful information as to the range where X_0 is most likely to locate.

Note that if X_0 were known, the deviation $Y_0 - a - bX_0$ follows a normal distribution with mean zero and variance

$$\text{var}(Y_0 - a - bX_0) = \left[1 + \frac{1}{n} + \frac{(X_0 - \bar{X})^2}{S_{xx}} \right] \sigma^2. \tag{2.4.4}$$

In this case, an unbiased estimator of $\text{var}(Y_0 - a - bX_0)$ can be obtained by replacing σ^2 in (2.4.4) with its unbiased estimator $\hat{\sigma}^2$ given in (2.3.16):

$$\widehat{\text{var}}(Y_0 - a - bX_0) = \left[1 + \frac{1}{n} + \frac{(X_0 - \bar{X})^2}{S_{xx}} \right] \hat{\sigma}^2. \tag{2.4.5}$$

Since $Y_0 - a - bX_0$ and $\hat{\sigma}^2$ are independent and $(n - 2)\hat{\sigma}^2/\sigma^2$ is distributed as a chi-square with $n - 2$ degrees of freedom, it follows that

$$T = \frac{Y_0 - a - bX_0}{\hat{\sigma} \left[1 + 1/n + (X_0 - \bar{X})^2/S_{xx} \right]^{1/2}} \tag{2.4.6}$$

is distributed as a central t distribution with $n - 2$ degrees of freedom. Thus if the null hypothesis of zero slope given in (2.3.21) is not rejected at the α level of significance, there exists no finite $(1 - \alpha) \times 100\%$ confidence interval for X_0. However, if the null hypothesis of zero slope given in (2.3.21) is rejected at the α level of significance, the lower and upper limits of the $(1 - \alpha) \times 100\%$ confidence interval are the two roots of the following quadratic equation of X_0:

$$(Y_0 - a - bX_0)^2 = t^2 \left(\tfrac{1}{2}\alpha, n - 2 \right) \hat{\sigma}^2 \left[1 + \frac{1}{n} + \frac{(X_0 - \bar{X})^2}{S_{xx}} \right]. \tag{2.4.7}$$

Solving (2.4.7) gives

$$\hat{X}_U(\hat{X}_L) = \bar{X} + \frac{1}{1 - g^2} \left\{ (\hat{X}_C - \bar{X}) \right.$$

$$\left. \pm \frac{t(\tfrac{1}{2}\alpha, n - 2) \, \hat{\sigma}}{b} \left[\frac{n + 1}{n} (1 - g^2) + \frac{(\hat{X}_C - \bar{X})^2}{S_{xx}} \right]^{\frac{1}{2}} \right\}, \tag{2.4.8}$$

where

$$g^2 = \frac{t^2(\frac{1}{2}\alpha, n - 2)\,\hat{\sigma}^2}{b^2 S_{XX}}.$$

Now consider the case where there are m responses from an unknown concentration X_0. Define

$$\bar{Y}_0 = \frac{1}{m} \sum_{j=1}^{m} Y_{n+j},$$

$$S_0^2 = \frac{1}{m-1} \sum_{j=1}^{m} (Y_{n+j} - \bar{Y}_0)^2.$$

Then the classical estimator and a $(1 - \alpha) \times 100\%$ confidence interval of X_0 are given by

$$\hat{X}_c = \frac{\bar{Y}_0 - a}{b}, \tag{2.4.9}$$

$$\hat{X}_U(\hat{X}_L) = \bar{X} + \frac{1}{1 - g^2} \left\{ (\hat{X}_c - \bar{X}) \pm \frac{t(\frac{1}{2}\alpha, n - 2)}{b} \right. \tag{2.4.10}$$

$$\left. \left[\left(S_0^2 + \frac{\hat{\sigma}^2}{n} \right)(1 - g^2) + \frac{\hat{\sigma}^2\,(\hat{X}_c - \bar{X})^2}{S_{XX}} \right]^{\frac{1}{2}} \right\}.$$

Alternatively, for determination of the unknown concentration X_0, we may obtain an estimator of X_0 by switching X_i and Y_i in the classical linear regression model. This leads to

$$X_i = \alpha' + \beta' Y_i + e_i', \qquad i = 1, \ldots, n. \tag{2.4.11}$$

Under model (2.4.11), Krutchkoff (1967) derived the following estimator of X_0:

$$\hat{X}_I = \bar{X} + (Y_0 - \bar{Y}) \frac{S_{XY}}{S_{YY}}. \tag{2.4.12}$$

The estimator above is usually referred to as the *inverse estimator*. Dunsmore (1968) and Halperin (1970) also recognized $\hat{X}_I$ as Bayes's estimators of X_0, corresponding to different distribution assumptions with various priors. The inverse estimator has been used widely because of its simplicity in that the estimate of the unknown concentration X_0 can be obtained directly from replacing Y in the standard curve (2.4.11) with its response Y_0.

The classical method and the inverse method have been widely accepted and applied to instrument calibration. In practice, it is of interest to study which method provides a better estimate in terms of accuracy and precision of the resulting assay of the unknown sample. In the past several decades, several researchers have studied the difference in mean-squared errors of estimators obtained by these two methods [see, e.g., Krutchkoff (1967), Berkson (1969), Lwin and Maritz (1982), Oman (1985), and Sundberg (1985)]. Figure 2.4.1 is a large-sample comparison of classical and inverse estimators in terms of their mean-squared error. It can be seen that the inverse estimate is preferred with a smaller mean-squared error within a certain range of X_0, say (X_L, X_U). The classical estimate, however, has a smaller mean-squared error outside the range of (X_L, X_U).

For a comparison of the two estimators, Halperin (1970) suggested the use of Pitman's nearness as a criterion to assess the closeness of the two estimators to the true unknown. However, Halperin's results apply only for large samples. As an alternative, Chow and Shao (1990b) assessed the closeness between the two estimators in terms of their ratio (i.e., $\hat{X}_I/\hat{X}_C$) and/or relative ratio [i.e., $(\hat{X}_I - \overline{X})/(\hat{X}_C - \overline{X})$].

From (2.3.15) we have

$$R^2 = \frac{S_{XY}^2}{S_{XX}S_{YY}}.$$

Combining this fact with (2.4.3) and (2.4.12), the relative ratio of estimates and the ratio of estimates can be obtained as follows:

$$\frac{\hat{X}_I - \overline{X}}{\hat{X}_C - \overline{X}} = R^2, \tag{2.4.13}$$

$$\frac{\hat{X}_I}{\hat{X}_C} = 1 + (1 - R^2)\left(\frac{\overline{X}}{\hat{X}_C} - 1\right), \tag{2.4.14}$$

respectively. From (2.4.13) and (2.4.14) we have the following observations:

1. The difference between the two estimates is zero if and only if $R^2 = 1$ (i.e., there is a perfect fit between X and Y or $Y_0 = \overline{Y}$).
2. Since $R^2 \leq 1$, the inverse estimate is always closer to $\overline{X}$ than the classical estimate.
3. The distribution of the relative ratio is independent of the unknown concentration X_0.

Chow and Shao (1990b) evaluated the closeness between $\hat{X}_i$ and $\hat{X}_C$ in terms of the probabilities that $(\hat{X}_I - \overline{X})/(\hat{X}_C - \overline{X})$ and $\hat{X}_I/\hat{X}_C$ differ from unity by the small amount δ. Next, we summarize these two probabilities.

2.4.2. Relative Ratio of Estimates

Let $\theta = \beta^2/\sigma^2$. Then the probability that $(\hat{X}_I - \overline{X})/(\hat{X}_C - \overline{X})$ differs from unity

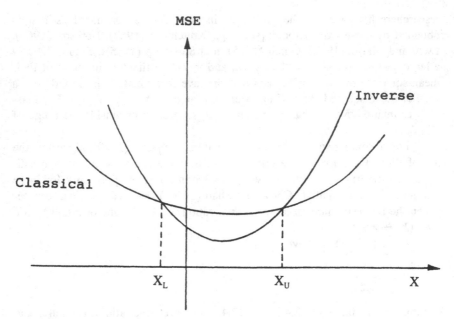

FIGURE 2.4.1   Comparison of classical and inverse estimators.

by δ can be expressed as

$$p(\theta) = P\left\{1 - \frac{\hat{X}_I - \overline{X}}{\hat{X}_C - \overline{X}} > \delta\right\} = P\left\{F < \frac{(n-2)(1-\delta)}{\delta}\right\}, \qquad (2.4.15)$$

where

$$F = \frac{(n-2)R^2}{1-R^2}$$

has a noncentral F distribution with degrees of freedom 1 and $n-2$ and non-central parameter $S_{xx}\theta$. Note that $\hat{X}_C$ is derived from the regression of Y on X, where X is assumed fixed, while $\hat{X}_I$ can be viewed as it can be obtained from the regression of X and Y, where X is assumed random and Y is fixed. It can be verified that

$$\frac{R^2}{1-R^2} = \frac{\text{SSR}}{\text{SSE}},$$

where

$$\text{SSR} = \frac{S_{XY}^2}{S_{XX}},$$

$$\text{SSE} = S_{YY} - \text{SSR}.$$

The probability given in (2.4.15) is a decreasing function of θ. Therefore, the probability is small if the ratio $|\beta|/\sigma$ is large. To examine the closeness between $\hat{X}_I$ and $\hat{X}_C$, Chow and Shao (1990b) provided a table of $p(\theta)$ with respect to $\lambda = S_{XX}\theta/n$ (with $n = 12$) for various values of δ (see Table 2.4.1). From Table 2.4.1 it can be seen that the difference between the classical and inverse methods is not appreciable $[p(\theta) \le 0.05]$ when $\lambda \ge 152$ for $\delta = 1\%$. To provide a better understanding, plots of $p(\theta)$ vs. λ for $\delta = 1\%$ and 3% are presented in Fig. 2.4.2.

TABLE 2.4.1 Various Values of δ, $\lambda = S_{XX}\theta/n$, and $p(\theta)$

$p(\theta)$	0.01	0.02	0.03	0.04	0.05	0.06	0.07	0.08	0.09	0.10
1.00	3	1	1	0	0	0	0	0	0	0
0.95	32	16	10	8	6	5	4	3	3	3
0.90	40	20	13	9	7	6	5	4	4	3
0.85	46	23	15	11	9	7	6	5	4	4
0.80	51	25	16	12	10	8	6	6	5	4
0.75	55	27	18	13	11	9	8	7	6	5
0.70	60	30	19	14	11	9	8	7	6	6
0.65	64	32	21	16	12	10	9	7	6	6
0.60	68	34	23	17	13	11	9	8	7	6
0.55	73	36	24	18	14	12	10	8	7	7
0.50	77	38	25	19	15	12	10	9	8	7
0.45	82	40	27	20	16	13	11	10	8	8
0.40	87	43	28	21	17	14	12	10	9	8
0.35	92	45	30	23	18	15	12	11	10	9
0.30	98	48	32	24	19	16	13	12	10	9
0.25	104	52	34	25	20	17	14	12	11	10
0.20	111	55	37	27	22	18	15	13	12	10
0.15	120	60	40	30	23	19	17	14	13	11
0.10	133	66	44	33	26	21	18	16	14	13
0.05	152	75	50	38	30	25	21	18	16	15
0.01	193	96	64	48	38	31	27	23	21	19

Source: Chow and Shao (1990b).

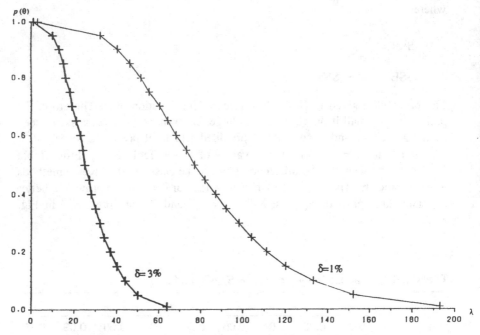

FIGURE 2.4.2   Plot of $p(\theta)$ vs. λ. [From Chow and Shao (1990b).]

Note that since θ is unknown, it is crucial to have a good estimate of θ or to have a lower (or upper) bound for θ. If $\hat{\theta}$ is an estimate of θ, $p(\hat{\theta})$ is also an estimate of $p(\theta)$. Suppose that we estimate θ based on the data

$$Z_i = \alpha + \beta X_i + \epsilon_i, \qquad i = 1, \ldots, m,$$

where $m \geq n$. The Z_i's may or may not be the same as the Y_i's. In practice, we may need to collect new data using the same X_i's under the same experimental conditions if the Y_i's are not available. When n is small, we may need to collect more data to increase the accuracy of the estimate of θ by repeating the same experiment k times at each X_i. In this case $m = kn$. Let b be the least-squares estimate of β based on Z_i's and

$$\hat{\sigma}^2 = \frac{\{\text{sum of residual squares}\}}{m - 2}$$

be an estimator of σ^2. Then the adjusted maximum likelihood estimator (MLE) of θ is given by

$$\hat{\theta}_0 = \frac{b^2}{\hat{\sigma}^2}.$$

Note that $kS_{xx}\hat{\theta}_0$ has a noncentral F distribution with degrees of freedom 1 and $m - 2$ and noncentral parameter $kS_{xx}\theta$. Hence the expected value and standard deviation of $\hat{\theta}_0$ are given by

$$E(\hat{\theta}_0) = \frac{m}{m-2}\left(\theta + \frac{1}{kS_{xx}}\right) \qquad \text{for } m > 2,$$

$$SD(\hat{\theta}_0) = \frac{2^{1/2}\, m}{(m-2)\,(m-4)^{1/2}}\left[\left(\theta + \frac{1}{kS_{xx}}\right)^2 + (m-2)\left(\frac{2\theta}{kS_{xx}} + \frac{1}{k^2S_{xx}^{\,2}}\right)\right]^{\frac{1}{2}},$$

respectively. Thus $\hat{\theta}_0$ is upward biased. An unbiased estimator of θ can be obtained as follows:

$$\hat{\theta} = \frac{m-2}{m}\,\hat{\theta}_0 - \frac{1}{kS_{xx}}.$$

The standard deviation of $\hat{\theta}$ is then given by

$$SD(\hat{\theta}) = \frac{m-2}{m}\,SD(\hat{\theta}_0),$$

which is smaller than that of $\hat{\theta}_0$. In practice, we may consider $p(\hat{\theta})$ as an estimate of $p(\theta)$ and $p_+ = p(\theta_-)$ [or $p_- = p(\theta_+)$] as an upper (or lower) bound for $p(\theta)$, where

$$\theta_\pm = \hat{\theta} \pm t(\tfrac{1}{2}\alpha, m-2)\,SE(\hat{\theta}),$$

where $SE(\hat{\theta})$ is the standard error of $\hat{\theta}$ which is given by

$$SE(\hat{\theta}) = \frac{2^{1/2}}{(m-4)^{1/2}}\left[\left(\hat{\theta} + \frac{1}{kS_{xx}}\right)^2 + (m-2)\left(\frac{2\hat{\theta}}{kS_{xx}} + \frac{1}{k^2S_{xx}^{\,2}}\right)\right]^{\frac{1}{2}}.$$

2.4.3. Ratio of Estimates

Chow and Shao (1990b) also examined the closeness between $\hat{X}_I$ and $\hat{X}_C$ in terms of the following probability:

$$P\left\{\left|\frac{\hat{X}_I}{\hat{X}_C} - 1\right| \geq \delta\right\}.$$

Since there exists no closed form for the distribution of $\hat{X}_I/\hat{X}_C$, it is difficult to evaluate the probability above. As an alternative, Chow and Shao (1990b) suggested using the following approximation:

Theorem 2.4.1 Suppose that as $n \to \infty$, $\bar{X} \to \mu_x$ and $n^{-1}S_{XX} \to \Sigma$, where Σ is some positive number. Let $r = (1 + \theta^{-1}\Sigma^{-1})^{-1}$ and X_0 be the true X value corresponding to Y_0. Then as $n \to \infty$,

$$
P\left\{ \left| \frac{\hat{X}_I}{\bar{X}_C} - 1 \right| \geq \delta \right\}
$$

$$
\approx \begin{cases} t(\theta,X_0) + s(\theta,X_0) & \text{if } \delta < 1 - r \\ t(\theta,X_0) & \text{if } \delta = 1 - r, \quad (2.4.16) \\ t(\theta,X_0) + s(\theta,X_0) - 1 & \text{if } \delta > 1 - r \end{cases}
$$

where

$$
t(\theta,X_0) = \Phi\{[(1 - r + \delta)^{-1}(1 - r)\bar{X} - X_0]\,\theta^{\frac{1}{2}}\},
$$
$$
s(\theta,X_0) = \Phi\{[X_0 - (1 - r - \delta)^{-1}(1 - r)\bar{X}]\,\theta^{\frac{1}{2}}\},
$$

and $\Phi(x)$ is the standard normal distribution function.

Proof From the consistency of the least-squares estimator and the law of large numbers, we have as $n \to \infty$,

$$
b \xrightarrow{\text{a.s.}} \beta,
$$
$$
\frac{S_{YY}}{S_{XX}} \xrightarrow{\text{a.s.}} \beta^2 + \frac{\sigma^2}{\Sigma}
$$

where a.s. denotes almost surely. Therefore,

$$
R^2 = \frac{S_{XY}^2}{S_{XX}S_{YY}} = \frac{\hat{b}^2 S_{XX}}{S_{YY}} \xrightarrow{\text{a.s.}} \frac{\beta^2}{\beta^2 + \sigma^2/\Sigma} = r. \qquad (2.4.17)
$$

Let $e_0 = Y_0 - (\alpha + \beta X_0)$. Then e_0 is distributed as $N(0,\sigma^2)$ and

$$
\hat{X}_C - X_0 = (b^{-1} - \beta^{-1})Y_0 - (ab^{-1} - \alpha\beta^{-1}) + \beta^{-1}e_0. \qquad (2.4.18)
$$

From $b \to \beta$ and $a \to \alpha$, almost surely, it follows that as $n \to \infty$,

$$
\hat{X}_C - X_0 \to N(0,\theta^{-1}) \quad \text{in distribution.}
$$

By (2.4.14),

$$
P\left\{ \left| \frac{\hat{X}_I}{\hat{X}_C} - 1 \right| > \delta \right\} = P\left\{ \left| \frac{\bar{X}}{\hat{X}_C} - 1 \right| > \frac{\delta}{1 - R^2} \right\},
$$

which can be approximated by

$$P\left\{\left|\frac{\bar{X}}{\hat{X}_C} - 1\right| > \frac{\delta}{1-r}\right\}$$

under (2.4.16). From expression (2.4.17)

$$P\left\{\frac{\bar{X}}{\hat{X}_C} - 1 > \frac{\delta}{1-r}\right\}$$

$$= P\left\{0 < \hat{X}_C < \frac{(1-r)\bar{X}}{1-r+\delta}\right\}$$

$$\approx t\,(\theta,\,X_0) - P\{\hat{X}_C < 0\}.$$

If $\delta = 1 - r$,

$$P\left\{\frac{\bar{X}}{\hat{X}_C} - 1 < \frac{-\delta}{1-r}\right\} = P\left\{\frac{\bar{X}}{\hat{X}_C} < 0\right\} = P\{\hat{X}_C < 0\}.$$

Also, if $\delta < 1 - r$,

$$P\left\{\frac{\bar{X}}{\hat{X}_C} - 1 < \frac{-\delta}{1-r}\right\}$$

$$= P\left\{\hat{X}_C > \frac{(1-r)\bar{X}}{1-r-\delta}\right\} + P\{\hat{X}_C < 0\}$$

$$\approx s(\theta,X_0) + P\{\hat{X}_C < 0\},$$

and if $\delta > 1 - r$,

$$P\left\{\frac{\bar{X}}{\hat{X}_C} - 1 < \frac{-\delta}{1-r}\right\}$$

$$= P\left\{\frac{(1-r)\bar{X}}{1-r-\delta} < \hat{X}_C < 0\right\}$$

$$= P\{\hat{X}_C < 0\} - P\left\{\hat{X}_C < \frac{(1-r)\bar{X}}{1-r-\delta}\right\}$$

$$\approx s(\theta,X_0) + P\{\hat{X}_C < 0\} - 1.$$

The results follow.

Let $q(\theta,X_0)$ be the function given on the right-hand side of (2.4.16). Then $q(\theta,X_0)$ is a continuous function of δ since $s(\theta,X_0) \to 0$ as $\delta \uparrow 1 - r$ and $s(\theta,X_0) \to 1$ as $\delta \downarrow 1 - r$. Furthermore, since $r \to 1$ as $\theta \to \infty$ (Σ is fixed), $t(\theta,X_0) \to 0$ and $s(\theta,X_0) \to 1$ for any $\delta > 0$. Hence $q(\theta,X_0)$ is small if θ is large. Figure 2.4.3 gives the plot of $q(\theta,X_0)$ versus θ for $X_0 = 18$, 20, and 25. Note that

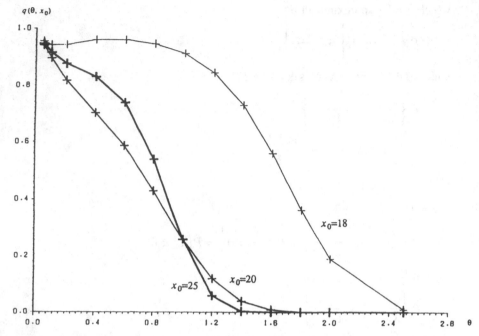

FIGURE 2.4.3 Plot of $q(\theta, X_0)$ vs. θ (δ = 1%). [From Chow and Shao (1990b).]

probabilities (2.4.16) can be approximated by

$$q(X_0) = \begin{cases} t(\hat{\theta}, X_0) + s(\hat{\theta}, X_0) & \text{if } \delta < 1 - R^2 \\ t(\hat{\theta}, X_0) & \text{if } \delta = 1 - R^2, \\ t(\hat{\theta}, X_0) + s(\hat{\theta}, X_0) - 1 & \text{if } \delta > 1 - R^2 \end{cases}$$

where $\hat{\theta}$ is an estimator of θ. It can be seen that $q(X_0)$ also depends on the unknown X_0. In practice, we may examine $q(X_0)$ over a range of reasonable X_0 values to assess the probability of the closeness between $\hat{X}_C$ and $\hat{X}_I$.

Example 2.4.1

From Example 2.3.1 the estimated standard curve based on the classical method is given by

$$Y = -2.363 + 5.429X.$$

Similarly, it can easily be verified from the information given in Example 2.3.1 that the estimated standard curve based on the inverse method is given by

$$X = 1.162 + 0.178Y.$$

Note that the observed absorbance of the unknown sample is 90.044, which is the lowest among all 13 samples. Consequently, we would expect that the estimates of the concentration of the unknown sample might be lower than the low concentration of standard preparation, 17.65 μM.

Based on the estimated standard curves obtained from the classical method and the inverse method, we have

$$\hat{X}_C = \frac{90.044 - (-2.363)}{5.429} = 17.02,$$

$$\hat{X}_I = 22.06 + (90.044 - 117.406) \left(\frac{844.705}{4744.613}\right)$$

$$= 22.06 - 4.871$$

$$= 17.19.$$

It can be seen from above that both methods produce similar estimates. As expected, both estimates are outside the range of the standard preparations used in the experiment. As a result, these estimates might not be reliable. Furthermore, the 95% confidence interval for the concentration of the unknown sample with an observed absorbance 90.044 based on the classical methods is given by (15.090,18.774). This interval is rather wide and a large portion of the interval is outside the range of the standard preparation employed in the experiment. Therefore, it is recommended that the same experiment be repeated with a different set of standard preparations if the unknown sample is still available.

The differences between $\hat{X}_C$ and $\hat{X}_I$ in terms of ratio (2.4.13) and relative ratio (2.4.14) are about 1% and 3%, respectively. For the relative ratio,

$$\hat{\lambda} = \frac{S_{xx}\hat{\theta}}{n} = 24.11.$$

From Table 2.4.1 or Fig. 2.4.3 ($\delta = 1\%$), $p(\hat{\theta}) = 0.97$. A lower bound for $p(\theta)$ is $p_- = 0.92$ (or $\theta_+ = 2.856$). Therefore, from Table 2.4.1, $p(\theta)$ is negligible if $\delta \geq 8\%$. In this case, $p(\theta)$ is about 5% or lower.

On the other hand, Fig. 2.4.4 gives the plot of the probability $q(X_0)$ versus X_0 for $\delta = 1\%$. The probability $q(X_0)$ is unacceptably high when $X_0 \leq 18.5$, a large range of X_0 values containing both $\hat{X}_C$ and $\hat{X}_I$.

From the discussion above it can be seen that the probabilities that the ratio and relative ratio differ from unity by 1% are not negligible. Hence the classical and inverse methods are not interchangeable in this case.

2.5. WEIGHT AND MODEL SELECTIONS

As indicated earlier, the accuracy and precision of an assay depends on the estimate of the unknown concentration. The determination of the unknown con-

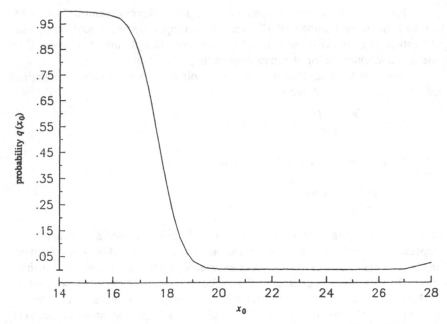

FIGURE 2.4.4 Plot of the probability $q(X_0)$ vs. X_0 for $\delta = 1\%$. [From Chow and Shao (1990b).]

centration is based on the standard curve, which relies on the selection of an appropriate statistical model. Therefore, it is important to select an appropriate statistical model for instrument calibration. In the following we introduce five commonly used statistical models for standard curves in assay development which are acceptable to the FDA.

The most commonly used statistical model for standard curves is the following simple linear regression model:

$$\text{Model 1:} \quad Y_i = \alpha + \beta X_i + e_i. \tag{2.5.1}$$

Based on model 1, the unknown sample can be determined by (2.4.3):

$$\hat{X}_c = \frac{Y_0 - a}{b}.$$

When the standard curve passes through the origin (i.e., there is zero intercept), model 1 reduces to

$$\text{Model 2:} \quad Y_i = \beta X_i + e_i. \tag{2.5.2}$$

In this case the concentration of the unknown sample can be estimated by

$$\hat{X}_C = \frac{Y_0}{b},$$

where b is the LSE of β under model (2.5.2)

In some cases the relationship between X_i and Y_i may be quadratic:

Model 3: $Y_i = \alpha + \beta_1 X_i + \beta_2 X_i^2 + e_i.$ (2.5.3)

In this case the concentration of the unknown sample X_0 can be determined by solving the quadratic equation

$$b_2 X^2 + b_1 X + (a - Y_0) = 0,$$

where a, b_1, and b_2 are LSEs of α, β_1, and β_2 under model (2.5.3), respectively. This leads to

$$\hat{X}_C = (2b_2)^{-1} [-b_1 \pm \sqrt{b_1^2 - 4b_2 (a - Y_0)}].$$

Another model of particular interest is

Model 4: $Y_i = \alpha X_i^\beta e_i.$ (2.5.4)

This model is equivalent to a simple linear regression model after a logarithmic transformation, that is,

$$\log(Y_i) = \log(\alpha) + \beta \log(X_i) + e_i',$$ (2.5.5)

or

$$Y_i' = \alpha' + \beta X_i' + e_i',$$

where $Y_i' = \log(Y_i)$, $X_i' = \log(X_i)$, $\alpha' = \log(\alpha)$, and $e_i' = \log(e_i)$. Let a' and b' be the LSEs of α' and β' under model (2.5.5). Then the concentration of the unknown sample can be obtained as

$$\hat{X}_C = \exp\left[\frac{\log(Y_0) - \log(a')}{b'}\right].$$

A similar model that is also often considered is the following:

Model 5: $Y_i = \alpha e^{\beta X_i} e_i.$ (2.5.6)

Model 5 can be linearized by taking a log transformation:

$$\log(Y_i) = \log(\alpha) + \beta X_i + e_i',$$ (2.5.7)

where $e_i' = \log(e_i)$. Therefore, the concentration of the unknown sample can be determined as

$$\hat{X}_C = \frac{\log(Y_0) - \log(a)}{b},$$

where $\log(a)$ and b are the LSEs of $\log(\alpha)$ and β under model (2.5.7).

It can be seen that under each model, the standard curve can be obtained by fitting an ordinary linear regression. The question of particular interest to researchers deals with how to select an appropriate statistical model for determining the standard curve based on the observed calibration data. To address this problem, Chow (1989) and Ju and Chow (1994a) proposed an ad hoc criterion for selecting an appropriate statistical model among the foregoing five models. We describe their idea below.

Since models 1 to 4 are polynomials and model 5 can be approximated by a polynomial, Chow (1989) and Ju and Chow (1994a) recommend the following selection procedure.

Step 1: If the level of standard concentration is below 4, go to step 2. Otherwise, start with the linear model

$$Y_i = \alpha + \beta_1 X_i + \beta_2 X_i^2 + \beta_3 X_i^3 + \beta_4 X_i^4 + e_i.$$

Let p_{34} be the p value for testing H_{034}: $\beta_3 = \beta_4 = 0$. If p_{34} is greater than a predetermined level of significance, go to step 2; otherwise, go to step 4.

Step 2: Since β_3 and β_4 are not significantly different from zero, the model above reduces to model 3. That is,

$$Y_i = \alpha + \beta_1 X_i + \beta_2 X_i^2 + e_i.$$

We then select a model among models 1 to 3. Let p_2 be the p value for testing H_{02}: $\beta_2 = 0$. If p_2 is less than the predetermined level of significance, model 3 is chosen; otherwise, go to the next step.

Step 3: If β_2 is not significantly different from 0, model 3 reduces to

$$Y_i = \alpha + \beta X_i + e_i.$$

In this case we choose between models 1 and 2 by testing H_{01}: $\alpha = 0$. If the p value for testing H_{01} is smaller than the predetermined level of significance, model 1 is chosen; otherwise, model 2 is selected.

Step 4: We select model 4 or model 5. Since models 4 and 5 have the same number of parameters, we would select the model with a smaller residual sum of squares.

A flowchart for model selection is given in Fig. 2.5.1.

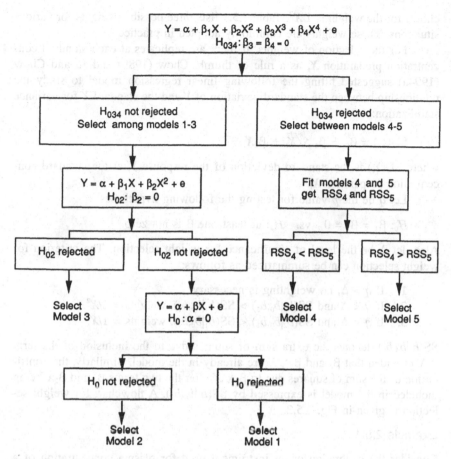

FIGURE 2.5.1   Model selection.

For the calibration of an instrument, since the response of a higher standard concentration preparation usually has a larger variability, the ordinary least-squares approach may not be appropriate. In this case a weighted least-squares method is often considered to remove the heterogeneity of the variability. The weight is selected so that the variance of the response at each standard concentration preparations is stabilized (i.e., the variance of Y_i at each standard concentration preparation remains a constant). Selection of an appropriate weight depends on the pattern of the standard deviation of the response at each standard concentration preparation. For example, if the standard deviation of the response at standard concentration preparation X is proportional to X, an appropriate choice for the weight is $1/X^2$. Table 2.5.1 lists three possible weights for various situations. These weights are commonly adopted in practice.

For the selection of weights, if there are replicates at each standard concentration preparation X, as a rule of thumb, Chow (1989) and Ju and Chow (1994a) suggested fitting the following linear regression model to study the relationship between the standard deviation of Y and the standard X for variance stabilization.

$$SD(Y_i) = \beta_0 + \beta_1 \sqrt{X_i} + \beta_2 X_i + e_i,$$

where $SD(Y_i)$ is the standard deviation of the response Y_i at the standard concentration preparation X_i.

Let q be the p value for testing the following hypotheses:

$$H_0: \beta_1 = \beta_2 = 0 \quad \text{vs.} \quad H_a: \text{at least one } \beta \text{ is not zero.}$$

Also, let Δ be the level of significance for weight selection. The criterion for weight selection can be summarized as follows:

1. If $q > \Delta$, no weighting is necessary.
2. If $q < \Delta$ and $SS(b_2|b_0,b_1) > SS(b_1|b_0,b_2)$, weights $= 1/X^2$.
3. If $q < \Delta$ and $SS(b_2|b_0,b_1) < SS(b_1|b_0,b_2)$, weights $= 1/X$.

$SS(b_2|b_0,b_1)$ denotes the extra sum of squares due to the inclusion of the term $\beta_2 X$ provided that β_0 and $\beta_1\sqrt{X}$ are already in the model. Similarly, the contribution of the sum of squares due to $\beta_1\sqrt{X}$ after the two terms β_0 and $\beta_2 X$ being included in the model is expressed by $SS(b_1|b_0,b_2)$. A flowchart for weight selection is given in Fig. 2.5.2.

Example 2.5.1

Consider the calibration of an instrument used for plasma concentration of a pharmaceutical compound. The calibration was done on three separate days. Nine standard concentration preparations ($X = 0.0, 0.5, 1.0, 2.0, 5.0, 10.0, 15.0,$

TABLE 2.5.1 Appropriate Weights for Various Situation

SD(Y) is proportional to:	Weight
Constant	1[a]
$\sqrt{X}$	$1/X$
X	$1/X^2$

[a]No weights.

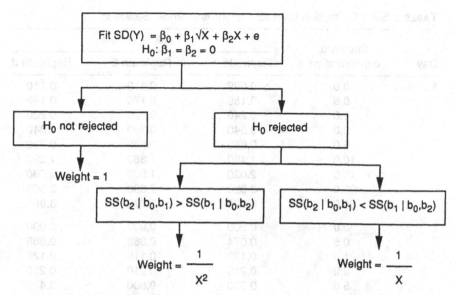

FIGURE 2.5.2 Weight selection. *Note*: b_0, b_1 and b_2 are estimates of β_0, β_1, and β_2, respectively.

20.0, and 30.0) were chosen. The response of interest is peak response. For each level of standard concentration preparation, three responses (replicates) were obtained on each day. Table 2.5.2 lists the responses of these standard concentration preparations. The standard deviations of the responses at each level of standard concentration preparation are given in Table 2.5.3. It can be seen from Table 2.5.3 that the standard deviation of the response at higher levels of standard concentration preparation tends to be higher. Therefore, a weighted least-squares method is necessary for determining the standard curve.

For weight selection we use the data from the three days. The p value for the null hypothesis that $\beta_1 = \beta_2 = 0$ is less than 0.0001. This implies tht the standard deviation of the peak response is highly correlated to the concentration. Therefore, a weight that is a function of X is needed to stabilize the variance of the response. Since

$$SS(b_1|b_0,b_2) < SS(b_2|b_0,b_1),$$

weights $= 1/X^2$ is selected.

Following the procedure for model selection, we first fit the following model:

$$Y_i = \alpha + \beta_1 X_i + \beta_2 X_i^2 + \beta_3 X_i^3 + \beta_4 X_i^4 + e_i.$$

TABLE 2.5.2   Calibration Data for Weight and Model Selection

Day	Standard concentration	Peak response		
		Replicate 1	Replicate 2	Replicate 3
1	0.0	0.086	0.110	0.110
	0.5	0.160	0.170	0.160
	1.0	0.240	0.220	0.200
	2.0	0.340	0.350	0.340
	5.0	0.650	0.630	0.770
	10.0	1.400	1.360	1.290
	15.0	2.030	1.920	2.030
	20.0	3.020	2.830	2.360
	30.0	3.730	3.770	3.960
2	0.0	0.000	0.039	0.000
	0.5	0.074	0.088	0.069
	1.0	0.130	0.110	0.120
	2.0	0.210	0.210	0.250
	5.0	0.530	0.500	0.470
	10.0	1.100	1.060	1.000
	15.0	1.690	1.480	1.310
	20.0	2.290	2.170	2.160
	30.0	3.250	3.410	3.030
3	0.0	0.032	0.030	0.000
	0.5	0.073	0.081	0.083
	1.0	0.110	0.100	0.100
	2.0	0.190	0.210	0.170
	5.0	0.430	0.430	0.400
	10.0	0.920	0.920	0.870
	15.0	1.380	1.280	1.280
	20.0	1.840	1.800	1.950
	30.0	2.820	2.690	2.380

Table 2.5.4 summarizes the results from the model selection procedure. For day 1 and day 2, model 1 is selected since hypotheses H_{034} and H_{02} are both not rejected at the 5% level of significance sequentially. Although the null hypothesis that H_{034}: $\beta_3 = \beta_4 = 0$ is rejected at the 5% level of significance for day 3, which suggests that either model 4 or model 5 may be appropriate, it should be noted that the adjusted R^2 value for the model with higher-order terms included (approximation to model 4 or 5) and the first-order term (model 1) included are 0.9888 and 0.9816, respectively. The small difference in the adjusted R^2 of the two models indicates that variation in the peak response could be explained reasonably

TABLE 2.5.3 Standard Deviations at Each Standard Concentration Preparation

Standard concentration	SD(Y)		
	Day 1	Day 2	Day 3
0.0	0.014	0.023	0.018
0.5	0.006	0.010	0.005
1.0	0.020	0.010	0.006
2.0	0.006	0.023	0.020
5.0	0.076	0.030	0.017
10.0	0.056	0.050	0.029
15.0	0.063	0.190	0.058
20.0	0.340	0.072	0.078
30.0	0.123	0.191	0.226

well by model 1. The model with the higher-order terms of the concentration included does not improve much more in explaining the variation of the peak response than model 1. Therefore, model 1 is considered adequate for day 3. As a result, model 1 appears to be the most appropriate model. The result is also confirmed by applying the model selection procedure to the 3 days of combined data.

2.6. STATISTICAL CONSIDERATIONS

From the discussions given in previous sections, we have the following observations. First, the classical and inverse estimators of the unknown concentration X_0 are derived under the assumption that the relationship between the standards and their corresponding responses is linear and the random errors are i.i.d. normal with mean zero and variance σ^2. In practice it is often of interest to evaluate whether these assumptions are met before a standard curve is estimated. Second,

TABLE 2.5.4 p Values of Test Results at Steps 1 to 3

Day	$Y = \beta_0 + \beta_1 X + \beta_2 X^2 + \beta_3 X^3 + \beta_4 X^4$ H_{034}: $\beta_3 = \beta_4 = 0$	$Y = \beta_0 + \beta_1 X + \beta_2 X^2$ H_{02}: $\beta_2 = 0$	$Y = \beta_0 + \beta_1 X$ H_0: $\beta_0 = 0$
1	0.39	0.29	<0.01
2	0.84	0.08	<0.01
3	0.03	0.02	<0.01
Three-day combined	0.86	0.46	<0.01

the classical and inverse estimates for the unknown concentration given in Example 2.5.1 are 17.02 and 17.19, respectively, which are both outside the range of standards used for the calibration. In addition, the 95% confidence interval based on the classical estimator may be too wide to be of practical interest. These are the consequences of a poorly designed experiment with the wrongly chosen design points for the standards. In practice, calibration experiments may be conducted on separate days. It is then of interest to combine standard curves obtained from different days. In this section we discuss these issues and provide some basic design considerations for conducting a calibration equipment.

2.6.1. Tests of Assumptions

To test whether the assumptions are met, we may apply the technique of lack of fit for adequacy of the postulated straight-line relationship between the standards and their corresponding responses provided that there are repeated runs at each standard (Draper and Smith, 1981).

Let Y_{ij} be the jth repeated response at X_i, where $j = 1, \ldots, n_i$ and $i = 1, \ldots, I$. Also, let $\bar{Y}_{i\cdot}$ be the sample mean at X_i:

$$\bar{Y}_{i\cdot} = \frac{1}{n_i} \sum_{j=1}^{n_i} Y_{ij}, \qquad i = 1, \ldots, I.$$

Then the deviation of the predicted response $\hat{Y}_{ij}$ from the observed response can be expressed as

$$Y_{ij} - \hat{Y}_{ij} = (Y_{ij} - \bar{Y}_{i\cdot}) - (\hat{Y}_{ij} - \bar{Y}_{i\cdot}). \tag{2.6.1}$$

Note that all repeated responses at X_i have the same predicted response $\hat{Y}_{ij}$. Define the sum of squares of pure error (SSPE) and the sum of squares of lack of fit (SSLF), respectively, as

$$\text{SSPE} = \sum_{i=1}^{I} \sum_{j=1}^{n_i} (Y_{ij} - \bar{Y}_{i\cdot})^2, \tag{2.6.2}$$

$$\text{SSLF} = \sum_{i=1}^{I} n_i (\hat{Y}_{ij} - \bar{Y}_{i\cdot})^2. \tag{2.6.3}$$

It can be seen from (2.6.1) that the sum of squares of residuals can be further decomposed in terms of SSPE and SSLF as follows:

$$\sum_{i=1}^{I} \sum_{j=1}^{n_i} (Y_{ij} - \hat{Y}_{ij})^2 = \sum_{i=1}^{I} \sum_{j=1}^{n_i} (Y_{ij} - \bar{Y}_{i\cdot})^2 + \sum_{i=1}^{I} n_i (\hat{Y}_{ij} - \bar{Y}_{i\cdot})^2. \tag{2.6.4}$$

The degrees of freedom for SSPE and SSLF are given by

$$df\ (SSPE) = \sum_{i=1}^{I} (n_i - 1) = n - I,$$

$$df\ (SSLF) = (n - 2) - (n - I) = I - 2,$$ (2.6.5)

where

$$n = \sum_{i=1}^{I} n_i.$$

Therefore, the mean squares of pure error and lack of fit can be obtained by dividing the respective sum of squares by their corresponding degrees of freedom as follows:

$$MSPE = \frac{1}{n - I} \sum_{i=1}^{I} \sum_{j=1}^{n_i} (Y_{ij} - \bar{Y}_{i\cdot})^2,$$ (2.6.6)

$$MSLF = \frac{1}{I - 2} \sum_{i=1}^{I} n_i\ (\hat{Y}_{ij} - \bar{Y}_{i\cdot})^2.$$ (2.6.7)

Table 2.6.1 gives the ANOVA table that incorporates SSPE and SSLF. In practice, whether the linear regression model is adequate or not can be tested based on the lack-of-fit test. The model is considered adequate if we fail to reject the null hypothesis of no lack of fit. We would reject the null hypothesis of no lack of fit at the α level of significance if

$$F_{LF} = \frac{MSLF}{MSPE} > F\ (\alpha, I - 2, n - I),$$ (2.6.8)

where $F(\alpha, I - 2, n - I)$ is the αth upper quantile of a central F distribution with degrees of freedom $I - 2$ and $n - I$.

If we fail to reject the null hypothesis of no lack of fit at the α level of significance, SSPE and SSLF can be pooled (i.e., SSE = SSPE + SSLF) to

TABLE 2.6.1 ANOVA Table for Lack of Fit

Source of variation	df	Sum of squares	Mean square	F value
Regression	1	SSR	MSR = SSR	F_b = MSR/MSE
Residual	$n - 2$	SSE	MSE = SSE/$(n - 2)$	
Lack of fit	$I - 2$	SSLF	MSLF = SSLF/$(I - 2)$	F_{LF} = MSLF/MSPE
Pure error	$n - I$	SSPE	MSPE = SSPE/$(n - I)$	
Total	$n - 1$	SST		

provide an unbiased estimator for σ^2 by dividing SSE by $n - 2$. However, if the null hypothesis of no lack of fit is rejected, the linear regression model is inadequate. In this case it is recommended that the possible causes be investigated or an alternative model be considered. In practice, the lack of fit can also be examined by various plots of studentized residuals. The studentized residuals are defined as the deviations of the predicted values from the observed responses divided by the corresponding standard errors:

$$\hat{e}_i = \frac{Y_i - \hat{Y}_i}{\hat{\sigma}[1 + 1/n + (X_i - \overline{X})^2/S_{xx}]^{\frac{1}{2}}}. \tag{2.6.9}$$

Note that the examination of residuals in regression analysis can be found in many books. For example, see Draper and Smith (1981). In summary, we recommend the following residual plots for calibration experiments:

1. Scatter diagram of the responses versus standards
2. Plots of studentized residuals against predicted values
3. Plots of studentized residuals against standards

The scatter diagram may provide a visual examination of a choice of all possible models for a standard curve, the homogeneity of variances of responses across different levels of standards, and the existence of potential outlying data. For residual plots, the vertical axis is usually centered at zero and two horizontal lines are drawn at -2 and 2. If the model is adequate and there are no outlying data, the studentized residuals should scatter randomly between -2 and 2 across the range of standards considered for the calibration [see, e.g., Fig. 2.6.1(a)]. Any studentized residuals outside the range of -2 and 2 should be closely examined because there might be potential outliers or influential responses. Figure 2.6.1(b) indicates that the variances are not homogeneous. Therefore, the methods for variance stabilization discussed in Sec. 2.5 should be considered to select an appropriate weight. Figure 2.6.1(c) suggests that the intercept may be wrongly omitted in the model. Figure 2.6.1(d) reveals that the model is inadequate and that additional terms should be considered.

Example 2.6.1

For the data given in Table 2.3.2, the ANOVA table with the sum of squares for lack of fit and pure errors is given in Table 2.6.2. The sum of squares due to lack of fit is 0.023. As a result, we fail to reject the null hypothesis of no lack of fit because

$$F = 0.001 < F(0.05,1,9) = 5.117.$$

Based on the empirical evidence of no lack of fit and $R^2 = 0.967$, the simple linear regression is an adequate model for describing the relationship between

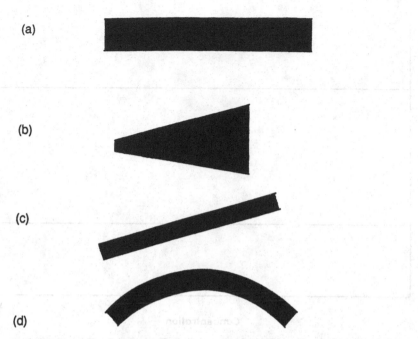

(a)

(b)

(c)

(d)

FIGURE 2.6.1 Patterns of residual plots. [From Draper and Smith (1981).]

absorbances and standard concentrations. Furthermore, the sum of squares of lack of fit and pure errors can be pooled to provide an unbiased estimate of σ^2 which is given by 15.852.

To examine the adequacy of the fitted model, some residual plots, such as studentized residuals vs. concentrations, studentized residuals vs. predicted values, and studentized residuals vs. observed absorbances, are given in Figs. 2.6.2 to 2.6.4. It can be seen from these figures that all studentized residuals are

TABLE 2.6.2 ANOVA Table for Lack of Fit for Data in Table 2.3.2

Source of variation	df	Sum of squares	Mean square	F value	p value
Regression	1	4586.090	4586.090	289.302	<0.0001
Residual	10	158.523	15.852		
Lack of fit	1	0.023	0.023	0.001	0.972
Pure error	9	158.500	15.845		
Total	11	4744.613			

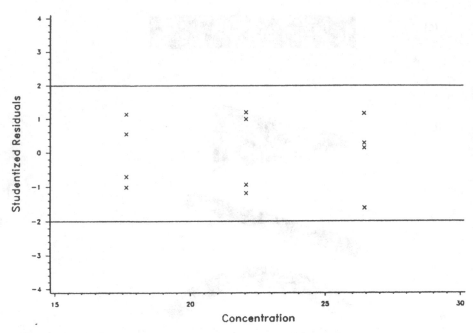

FIGURE 2.6.2   Studentized residuals for data set in Table 2.3.2.

randomly scattered within -2 and 2. Moreover, the patterns of these plots are similar to Fig. 2.6.1(a). This also suggests that the linear regression model is adequate.

2.6.2   Basic Design Considerations

In previous sections, a regression analysis technique is applied to characterize empirically the relationship between the standards and their corresponding responses. However, this empirical relationship is limited to the range of standards used in the experiment. The relationship might not be the same outside the range. The classical estimator $\hat{X}_C$ provides its best precision when $X_0 = \overline{X}$ because the width of the corresponding $(1 - \alpha) \times 100\%$ confidence interval is shortest at $X_0 = \overline{X}$. The confidence interval becomes wider and wider as $\hat{X}_C$ moves away from $\overline{X}$. However, the data from the calibration experiment described in Example 2.4.1 give estimated concentrations of 17.02 and 17.19, which were obtained by the classical and inverse methods, respectively. Both estimates are outside the range (17.65,26.47) which was used in the experiment. As a result these two estimates might not be accurate for determination of the unknown concentration. In practice it may be desirable to conduct the calibration experiment repeatedly

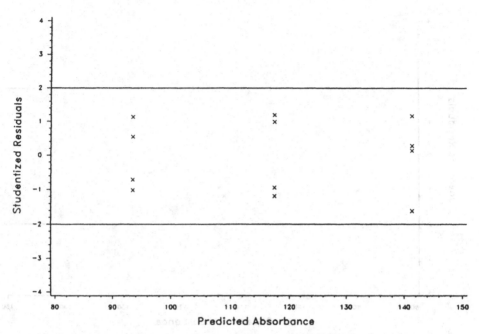

FIGURE 2.6.3 Studentized residuals vs. predicted values for data set in Table 2.3.2.

with different ranges of standards to ensure that the resulting estimate is within a reasonable range of X_0 and consequently, to have the estimate close to the mean of the standards with certain assurance.

In the following we provide some basic statistical considerations for conducting a calibration experiment. Our recommendations are made based on the assumption that the classical method will be used for determination of an unknown concentration. For simplicity, consider the three levels of standards (i.e., L, M, and H) design for linear calibration described in Example 2.3.1. The following is a list of basic statistical considerations when designing the three standards:

1. Sample-size determination (i.e., the determination of total number of standards)
2. Choice of standards and its range
3. Distribution of the number of runs at each standard.

As indicated earlier, the distribution of $\hat{X}_C$ generally does not have any moments greater than or equal to the first. However, under the normality assumption of

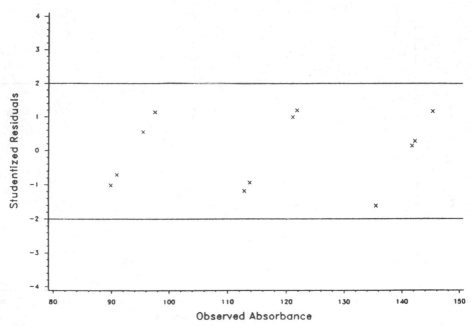

FIGURE 2.6.4 Studentized residuals vs. observed values for data set in Table 2.3.2.

random errors, the mean and variance of the classical estimator do exist provided that the unknown slope is bounded away from zero (Buonaccorsi, 1986). It can easily be verified that

1. $\hat{X}_C$ converges to X_0 with probability 1.
2. One of the asymptotic variance under normality assumption is given by

$$\text{var}(\hat{X}_C) = \sigma^2 \left[1 + 1/n + (\hat{X}_C - \overline{X})^2/S_{XX}\right]/\beta^2, \qquad (2.6.10)$$

as n becomes large.

The purpose of a calibration experiment is to estimate the unknown concentration. Therefore, a good calibration design needs to satisfy criteria concerning the estimation of X_0. All of these criteria involve the variance of the estimate. For the classical method, we have to use the asymptotic variance because the variance of $\hat{X}_C$ either does not exist or is very difficult to find. Buonaccorsi (1986) and Buonaccorsi and Iyer (1986) considered the following three criteria for choosing a calibration design:

1. V optimality, which minimizes $\text{var}(\hat{X}_C)$
2. AV optimality, which minimizes an average asymptotic variance with respect to prior distribution of X_0
3. M optimality, which minimizes the maximum asymptotic variance $\text{var}(\hat{X}_C)$ over a range of X_0.

It is then suggested that the design with the same number of runs at each standard (i.e., equally weighted endpoint design) will achieve the optimalities listed above if the mean standard is equal to the unknown concentration (V optimality) and the average of the high and low standards is the mean of any prior distribution of X_0 (AV and M optimalities). For illustration, the following are the recommended steps for selection of a calibration design with three levels of standards for estimation of the unknown concentration using the classical method based on simple linear regression.

Step 1: Make a guess of X_0, say $\bar{X}_0$. Then $\bar{X}_0$ is used as the middle level of standards (M).

Step 2: Make low and high level of standards (i.e., L and M) be symmetric about $\bar{X}_0$.

Step 3: Select X_i, $i = 1, \ldots, n$ such that S_{xx} is as large as possible. As mentioned before, a good design should place the unknown slope as far away from zero as possible to produce a finite closed $(1 - \alpha) \times 100\%$ confidence interval for X_0. Recall that the variance of b is σ^2/S_{xx}. Therefore, we need to select X_i such that S_{xx} is as large as possible.

Note that the steps above suggest not only the choice of the low and high standards symmetric about X_0 but also the choice of the standards as far away from X_0 as possible.

Step 4: The condition for the existence of a closed interval for the $(1 - \alpha) \times 100\%$ confidence interval for X_0 is that the null hypothesis of the zero slope given in (2.3.21) is rejected at the α level of significance. Consequently, the sample size should provide sufficient power to reject the null hypothesis of (2.3.21). However, for most calibration experiments conducted in the pharmaceutical industry, the range of standards is usually chosen so that there is a positive linear relationship between the responses and the standards. Therefore, the hypothesis of interest in terms of slope for sample-size determination at the planning stage should be based on the following one-sided hypothesis:

$$H_0: \beta = \beta_0 \quad \text{vs.} \quad H_a: \beta > \beta_0, \tag{2.6.11}$$

where β_0 is a positive expected slope. In general, the sample size required for hypothesis (2.6.11) will provide sufficient power for hypothesis (2.3.21) of zero slope. The sample size can be determined by the traditional method based on the following t statistic:

$$n_0 \geq [t\,(\alpha, n - 2) + t(\eta, n - 2)]^2 \frac{\sigma^2}{S_{xx}\,(\beta - \beta_0)^2}, \qquad (2.6.12)$$

where α and η are the probabilities of type I and type II errors, and S_{xx} can be determined from the choice of low, middle, and high standards. However, Buonaccorsi (1986) suggested that

$$\left| \frac{\beta S_{xx}}{\sigma^2} \right| > 3$$

is a necessary condition for the unimodality of the distribution of $\hat{X}_C$. These factors allow us to incorporate information about the variability of responses and the expected slope from previous experiments. However, in (2.6.12), the degrees of freedom $n - 2$ is unknown, so a numerical iterative procedure is required to solve for n_0. In practice, a few iterations are usually required.

Step 5: Round n_0 up to a multiple of 3, say n_C.

Step 6: The equally weighted endpoint design can be achieved by putting $n_C/3$ runs at each of L, M, and H standard concentration preparations.

Example 2.6.2

For the data set in Table 2.3.2, both classical and inverse methods give an estimated concentration of the unknown sample outside the range of standards. It is recommended that another experiment be performed to provide a better estimate of the unknown sample. Based on the results from Table 2.3.2, the unknown concentration is approximately 17. Hence we may choose 17 as the middle design point. As a result, the low and high design points may be chosen as 12 and 22, respectively. Also, from Example 2.3.1, the estimated slope and mean-squared error are 5.43 and 15.85, respectively. Suppose that the expected slope is 5. Based on this information, the sample size required to yield 90% power for hypothesis (2.3.11) at the 2.5% level of significance can be determined as follows.

Suppose we guess that the sample size is 9. Then $S_{xx} = 150$, $t(0.025,7) = 2.365$, and $t(0.1,7) = 1.415$. According to (2.6.12), we have

$$n \geq (2.365 + 1.415)^2 \frac{(15.85)^2}{(150)\,(5.43 - 5)^2}$$

$$= 8.24$$

$$\cong 9.$$

Thus we choose the sample size to be 9. Hence there are three replicates at each of the three standards [i.e., 12(L), 17(M), and 22(H)].

2.6.3. Combining Calibration Lines

The data given in Table 2.5.2 for Example 2.5.1 are the plasma concentrations of a pharmaceutical compound from the calibration experiment of an instrument. This calibration experiment was conducted on three separate days with three repeated runs at each of the nine standards on each day. For each day we can obtain an estimated standard curve. Hence an estimate of the unknown concentration can be obtained on each day. Although the same unknown concentration was used on each day, estimates of the unknown concentration may be different from day to day, due to the variability of the estimated standard curves between days. Therefore, how to combine standard curves obtained from different days has become an important issue in calibration. In this section we apply the technique of combining data from different random batches for estimating drug shelf life in stability studies (Chow and Shao, 1991; Ho et al., 1992; Shao and Chow, 1994). For simplicity, we consider only the balanced case where the same number of runs are repeated at each of I standards and the same unknown concentration is used on each of the d days. The data can then be described by means of a simple regression model as follows:

$$Y_{hij} = \alpha_h + \beta_h X_i + e_{hij},$$

$$Y_{h0} = \alpha_h + \beta_h X_0 + e_{h0},$$

(2.6.13)

where $h = 1, \ldots, d$, $i = 1, \ldots, I$, $j = 1, \ldots, J$, and $n = IJ$. The primary assumptions for model (2.6.13) are as follows:

1. e_{hij} are i.i.d. normal with mean zero and variance σ^2 for all h, i, and j.
2. e_{h0} are also i.i.d. normal with mean zero and variance σ^2.
3. The vector $(\alpha_h, \beta_h)'$ is i.i.d. bivariate normal with mean vector $\beta = (\alpha, \beta)'$ and covariance matrix Σ_β, which is a 2×2 symmetric positive definite matrix.
4. e_{hij}, e_{h0}, and $(\alpha_h, \beta_h)'$ are mutually independent.
5. $n > 2$.

Define

$$\mathbf{Y}_h = (Y_{h11}, \ldots, Y_{hIJ}), \qquad h = 1, \ldots, d,$$

$$\beta_h = (\alpha_h, \beta_h), \qquad h = 1, \ldots, d,$$

$$\epsilon_h = (e_{h11}, \ldots, e_{hIJ}), \qquad h = 1, \ldots, d,$$

$$\mathbf{Y}_0 = (Y_{10}, \ldots, Y_{d0}),$$

$$\mathbf{X}' = \begin{bmatrix} 1, \ldots, 1 \\ X_1, \ldots, X_I \end{bmatrix}.$$

Then the matrix representation of model (2.6.13) is given by

$$\mathbf{Y}_h = \boldsymbol{\beta}_h X + \boldsymbol{\epsilon}_h, \qquad h = 1, \ldots, d. \tag{2.6.14}$$

Let $\mathbf{b}_h = (a_h, b_h)$ be the ordinary least-squares estimator of $\boldsymbol{\beta}_h$ on day h and

$$\overline{\mathbf{Y}} = \frac{1}{d} \sum_{i=1}^{d} \mathbf{Y}_h \tag{2.6.15}$$

be the average of the response vector.
Then the maximum likelihood estimator of $\boldsymbol{\beta}$ is given by

$$\overline{\mathbf{b}} = \frac{1}{d} \sum_{i=1}^{d} \mathbf{b}_h$$

$$= \frac{1}{d} (\mathbf{X}'\mathbf{X})^{-1}\mathbf{X}'\overline{\mathbf{Y}} \tag{2.6.16}$$

$$= (\overline{a}, \overline{b}),$$

where

$$\overline{a} = \frac{1}{d} \sum_{h=1}^{a} a_h,$$

$$\overline{b} = \frac{1}{d} \sum_{h=1}^{d} b_h. \tag{2.6.17}$$

Therefore, the MLE of $\boldsymbol{\beta}$ is the average of the LSEs of the intercepts and slopes obtained on an individual day. It is an unbiased estimator of $\boldsymbol{\beta}$. In addition, $\overline{\mathbf{b}}$ follows a bivariate normal distribution with mean vector $\boldsymbol{\beta}$ and covariance matrix $\boldsymbol{\Sigma}_b/d$, where

$$\boldsymbol{\Sigma}_b = \boldsymbol{\Sigma}_\beta + \sigma^2 (\mathbf{X}'\mathbf{X})^{-1}. \tag{2.6.18}$$

It can be seen from (2.6.18) that the structure of the covariance matrix for the MLE of $\boldsymbol{\beta}$ consists of the sum of the intraday variability represented by $\sigma^2(\mathbf{X}'\mathbf{X})^{-1}$ and the interday variability represented by $\boldsymbol{\Sigma}_\beta$. It can be verified that unbiased estimators of $\boldsymbol{\Sigma}_b$, σ^2, and $\boldsymbol{\Sigma}_\beta$ are given by

$$S_b = \frac{1}{d-1} \sum_{h=1}^{d} (\mathbf{b}_n - \overline{\mathbf{b}})(\mathbf{b}_n - \overline{\mathbf{b}})',$$

$$\hat{\sigma}^2 = \frac{1}{d(n-2)} \sum_{h=1}^{d} SSE_h, \tag{2.6.19}$$

$$\hat{\boldsymbol{\Sigma}}_\beta = S_b - \hat{\sigma}^2 (\mathbf{X}'\mathbf{X})^{-1},$$

where SSE_h is the sum of squares of residuals obtained from fitting an individual regression line on day h.

It can be seen from (2.6.19) that the unbiased estimator $\hat{\Sigma}_\beta$ is a difference of two matrices. Therefore, it may not be positive definite. In this situation the unbiased estimator suggested by Carter and Yang (1986) might be useful.

For the vector of the unknown concentration $X_0 = (1, X_0)$, the minimum variance unbiased estimator of $X_0'\beta$ is given by X_0' $\overline{b}$, which follows a normal distribution with mean $X_0'\beta = \alpha + \beta X_0$ and variance

$$\frac{1}{d} \sigma_{X_0}^2,$$

where

$$\sigma_{X_0}^2 = X_0' \Sigma_b X_0 + \sigma^2 X_0' (X'X)^{-1} X_0. \tag{2.6.20}$$

Let

$$\overline{Y}_0 = \frac{1}{d} \sum_{i=1}^{h} Y_{h0}.$$

Then $\overline{Y}_0$ also follows a normal distribution with mean $\alpha + \beta X_0$ and variance

$$\frac{1}{d} (X_0' \Sigma_\beta X_0 + \sigma^2).$$

It follows that

$$\overline{Y}_0 - (\overline{a} + \overline{b} X_0) = \overline{Y}_0 - X_0' \overline{b}$$

has a normal distribution with mean zero and variance

$$\sigma_0^2 = \frac{1}{d} \{2X_0' \Sigma_\beta X_0 + \sigma^2 [1 + X_0'(X'X)^{-1} X_0]\}. \tag{2.6.21}$$

Note that σ_0^2 reduces to $\text{var}(Y_0 - a - bX_0)$ given in (2.4.4) when $d = 1$ and $\Sigma_\beta = 0$. An unbiased estimator of σ_0^2 can then be obtained by substituting Σ_β and σ^2 with their respective unbiased estimators given in (2.6.19):

$$\sigma_0^2 = \frac{1}{d} \{2X_0' \hat{\Sigma}_\beta X_0 + \hat{\sigma}^2 [1 + X_0'(X'X)^{-1} X_0]\}. \tag{2.6.22}$$

Then the maximum likelihood estimator of the concentration of the unknown sample is given by

$$\hat{X}_C = \frac{\overline{Y}_0 - \overline{a}}{\overline{b}}. \tag{2.6.23}$$

Define

$$S_b^2 = \frac{1}{d-1} \sum_{i=1}^{d} (b_i - \bar{b})^2,$$

(2.6.24)

$$T_b = \frac{\bar{b}}{S_{\bar{b}}}.$$

Then the null hypothesis of zero slope is rejected at the α level of significance if

$$|T_b| > t(\tfrac{1}{2}\alpha, d - 1).$$

If the slope of the calibration line is statistically different from zero, the lower and upper limits of the $(1 - \alpha) \times 100\%$ confidence interval for X_0 are given by the two roots of the following quadratic equation of X_0:

$$(\bar{Y}_0 - \bar{a} - \bar{b}X_0)^2 = t^2(\tfrac{1}{2}\alpha, d - 1)\,\hat{\sigma}_0^2.$$

(2.6.25)

Example 2.6.3

We use the data set given in Table 2.5.2 to illustrate the methods discussed in this section. Table 2.6.3 gives the results of fitting a simple linear regression model for each day. Figure 2.6.5 plots the data and the estimated regression lines by day. It can be seen from Table 2.6.3 and Fig. 2.6.5 that the slopes are not homogeneous across days. The ANOVA table (Table 2.6.4) gives an F value of 98.84 for day by slope interaction with a p value below 0.0001. We then reject the null hypothesis of homogeneous slopes among days at the 5% level of significance. Consequently, the technique for combining calibration curves discussed in this section, which assumes that the day is a random variable, can be applied.

TABLE 2.6.3   Results of Simple Linear Regression by Day

Day		Intercept	Slope	R^2
1	Estimate	0.0957	0.1264	0.9918
	Standard error	0.0311	0.0023	
	p Value	0.0050	<0.0001	
2	Estimate	−0.0033	0.1071	0.9927
	Standard error	0.0250	0.0018	
	p Value	0.8959	<0.0001	
3	Estimate	0.0169	0.0883	0.9925
	Standard error	0.0208	0.0015	
	p Value	0.4238	<0.0001	

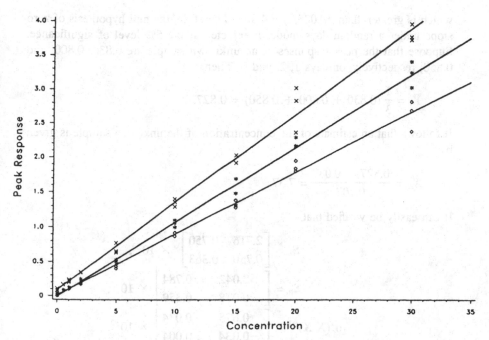

Figure 2.6.5 Regression line by day for data set in Table 2.5.2. X, day 1; star, day 2; diamond, day 3.

The common intercept and slope and their corresponding standard errors (in parentheses) are 0.037 (0.052) and 0.107 (0.019), respectively. It can easily be verified that

$$T_b = \frac{0.107}{0.019} = 5.63,$$

TABLE 2.6.4 ANOVA Table for Homogeneous Slopes

Source of variation	df	Sum of squares	Mean square	F value	p value
Day	2	2.588	1.294	133.53	<0.0001
Slope	1	91.166	91.166	9407.35	<0.0001
Day by slope	2	1.916	0.958	98.84	<0.0001
Error	75	0.727			
Total	80	96.397			

which is greater, than $t(0.025,2) = 4.303$. Therefore, the null hypothesis of zero slope under a random days model is rejected at the 5% level of significance. Suppose that the peak responses of an unknown sample are 0.830, 0.800, and 0.850, respectively, on days 1, 2, and 3. Then

$$\bar{Y}_0 = \frac{1}{3} (0.830 + 0.800 + 0.850) = 0.827.$$

It follows that an estimate of the concentration of the unknown sample is given by

$$\hat{X}_C = \frac{0.827 - 0.037}{0.107} = 7.37.$$

It can easily be verified that

$$S_b = \begin{bmatrix} 2.716 & 0.750 \\ 0.750 & 0.363 \end{bmatrix} \times 10^{-3},$$

$$\hat{\Sigma}_\beta = \begin{bmatrix} 2.042 & 0.784 \\ 0.078 & 0.359 \end{bmatrix} \times 10^{-3},$$

$$\hat{\sigma}^2(X'X)^{-1} = \begin{bmatrix} 0.675 & -0.034 \\ -0.034 & 0.004 \end{bmatrix} \times 10^{-3}.$$

Therefore, the between-day variability accounts for about 99% of the total variability of the estimated common slope. Based on $\hat{\Sigma}_\beta$, $\hat{\sigma}^2 (X'X)^{-1}$, $\bar{Y}_0$, $\bar{a}$, and $\bar{b}$, the 95% confidence interval for an average peak response of 0.827 over 3 days can be obtained, which is given by (5.67,10.01).

3

Assay Validation

3.1. INTRODUCTION

As indicated earlier, during the development of a pharmaceutical compound, there are two different types of validations: assay validation and process validation. *Assay validation* involves the validation of an analytical method or a testing procedure of the active ingredients of the compound. *Process validation* is usually referred to as the validation of a manufacturing process. In this chapter we focus on the assay validation. The process validation is discussed in detail in Chapter 6.

When a pharmaceutical compound is newly discovered, it is necessary to develop an analytical method (or assay method) for the active ingredients of the compound. The assay method should be in compliance with some established specifications. CGMP [21 CFR 211.194(a)] requires that the assay method must meet certain standards of accuracy and reliability. As mentioned in Chapter 1, assays and specifications of the USP/NF constitute the legal standards recognized by the official compendia of the federal Food, Drug and Cosmetic Act. As a result, the CGMP [21 CFR 211.194(a) (2)] indicates that use of assay methods described in the USP/NF is not required to validate accuracy and reliability of analytical procedures. However, any proposed new or revised assay methods for submission to the compendia must be validated and documented with sufficient laboratory data and information according to the requirements stated in the USP/NF. The new or revised assay methods are then reviewed for their relative merits and disadvantages by the members of the USP Committee of Revision.

71

As pharmaceutical products can be either a chemical or a biologic entity, assay methods might employ different techniques, which include chemical methods such as gas chromatography (GC), high-performance liquid chromatography (HPLC), mass spectrometry (MS), or biological assays such as enzyme-linked immunosorbent assay (ELISA) and radioimmunoassay (RIA). However, statistical principles for the validation of any analytical procedures are the same for all methods [see, e.g., Cavenaghi et al. (1987), Brook and Weinfeld (1985), Bohidar and Peace (1988), and Shah et al. (1992)]. For validation of an assay method, the USP/NF requires that a number of validation parameters be examined to evaluate the performance of the assay method. These validation parameters include accuracy, precision, limits of detection and quantitation, selectivity, range, linearity, and ruggedness. Among these parameters, accuracy, precision, linearity, and ruggedness are the primary parameters.

The remainder of this chapter is organized as follows. In the next section we provide a brief description of the key validation parameters stated in the USP/NF. Various statistical methods for evaluation of assay accuracy are outlined in Sec. 3.3. In Sec. 3.4, statistical inference for the assessment of assay precision is discussed. Also included in Secs. 3.3 and 3.4 are the assessment of linearity. In Sec. 3.5 we introduce the concept of assay ruggedness in terms of the repeatability within a laboratory and the reproducibility among laboratories (Mandel, 1972). Statistical methods for evaluation of assay ruggedness are also provided in this section. In Sec. 3.6 some commonly employed statistical designs in assay validation are reviewed. Some basic statistical considerations in assay validation are discussed in Sec. 3.7. At the end of each section, numerical examples are used to illustrate the statistical methods.

3.2. VALIDATION PARAMETERS

When a pharmaceutical compound is discovered, it is of interest to develop an optimal dosage form such that the active ingredients can be delivered to the site of action of the body for the optimal therapeutic effect. However, the dosage form usually consists of active and inactive ingredients. It is therefore very important to develop an assay method to quantify the exact amount of active ingredients in the excipient matrix. To achieve this purpose as indicated in CGMP [21 CFR 211.194(a)], the assay method must be validated and meet required standards of accuracy and reliability.

Basically, there are various definitions for the validation of an analytical method or a testing procedure. For example, Chapman (1983) defined the assay validation as establishing documented evidence that a process does what it purports to do. On the other hand, the USP/NF indicates that the validation of an analytical method is the process by which it is established, by laboratory studies, that the performance characteristics of the method meet the requirements for the intended analytic applications. In this book, unless otherwise stated, the definition of assay validation stated in the USP/NF will be used. For the purpose of illustration of concepts, we focus on the validation of an assay method. The concept and statistical methods introduced in this chapter can be applied similarly to any analytical methods and/or testing procedures.

As indicated by the USP/NF, the performance characteristics of an analytical method or a testing procedure can be assessed through a set of analytical validation parameters. These validation parameters are listed in Table 3.2.1. In the following section we define each validation parameter and its interpretation. More details can be found in the USP/NF, Bohidar (1983), and Bohidar and Peace (1988).

3.2.1. Accuracy and Precision

The accuracy of an assay method is defined as the closeness of the assay result obtained by the assay method to the true value. *Accuracy* means that there is no systematic error in the assay method. Statisticians usually refer to systematic error as *bias*. Accuracy is a parameter that measures the exactness of an assay method. In practice, the accuracy of an assay method is usually determined based on the data obtained from experiments. The assay method is applied to samples or mixtures of excipients. The excipients usually consist of known amounts of analyte which are added both above and below the normal levels expected in the samples. These types of experiments are usually referred to as *recovery studies* (Kohberger, 1988). The assay method employed in a recovery study recovers the active ingredients from the excipients. As a result, the accuracy of an assay method is usually expressed as percent recovery by the assay of known, added amount of active ingredients. The amounts of known analytes added usually vary. In general, the added amounts of active ingredients are expressed as a percentage of the label claim. In addition to the level of 100% label claim, the same number of equally spaced levels are usually added above and below the level of 100% label claim. For example, for the validation of an assay method for tablets, 80%, 100%, and 120% of the label claim may be used.

TABLE 3.2.1 Analytical Validation Parameters in an Assay Validation Program

Accuracy	Selectivity
Precision	Range
Limit of detection	Linearity
Limit of quantitation	Ruggedness

Source: USP/NF (1990).

The *precision* of an assay method is the degree of agreement among individual test results when the procedure is applied repeatedly to multiple sampling of a homogeneous sample. Standard deviation and/or coefficient of variation (CV) or relative standard deviation (RSD) in percent are generally used to represent the precision of an assay method. Precision is an assay parameter that measures the degree of repeatability of the assay method from the same population under a normal operating circumstance. It can be used to measure the variation between two repeated assays within the homogeneous preparations (i.e., same lot or same day). Assays in the context of precision are independent analyses of samples that have been carried through the complete analytical procedure from sample preparation to final test result. The standard deviation and coefficient of variation can also be estimated from the recovery amounts of the recovery study.

In practice, for the evaluation of accuracy and precision of an assay method, the assay method is considered validated if its accuracy and precision are within acceptable limits. For example, for accuracy, if the bias is not significant from zero and is within a specified $|\delta\%|$ of input at each level with 95% assurance, the accuracy of the assay method is considered validated. For precision, if the total variation gives a total of CV less than a specified $\Delta\%$, the precision of the assay method is considered validated. Note that δ and Δ are usually chosen so that the assay method will have the desired accuracy and precision. With 95% assurance, a validated assay method will produce assay results with the desired accuracy and precision.

Bohidar (1983, 1985) indicated that the bias of an assay method is the difference between the average recovered amount and the actual amount added. If both the accuracy and bias are expressed as percent recovery by the known added amount of analyte, the accuracy is equal to 1 minus the bias. Accuracy and precision are the most important validation parameters that an assay method must possess. Figures 3.2.1 through 3.2.4 illustrate the concept of accuracy (unbiasedness) and precision (dispersion). For example, Fig. 3.2.1 shows that not only are the assay results close to the target of 100% (accuracy) but all the results agree with each other (high precision). On the other hand, Fig. 3.2.2 suggests that an assay has high accuracy but low precision. Figure 3.2.3 illustrates the situation where all the assay results are in agreement with each other but off-target. In Secs. 3.3 and 3.4, statistical inferences as to accuracy and precision are provided.

3.2.2. Limits of Detection and Quantitation

The limit of detection is usually referred to as the lowest concentration of analyte in a sample that can be detected, but not necessarily quantitated, under the

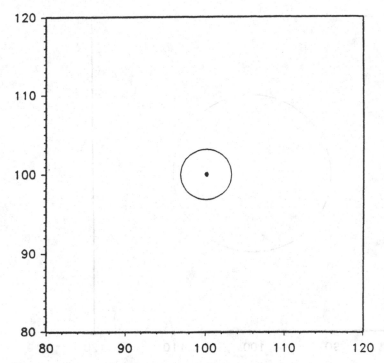

FIGURE 3.2.1 Unbiasedness and high precision.

experimental conditions specified. It is a parameter of limit tests because the limit of detection merely substantiates that analyte concentration is above or below a certain level. The limit of detection is usually expressed as the concentration of analyte in the sample.

The limit of quantitation is the lowest concentration of analyte in a sample that can be determined with acceptable precision and accuracy under the experimental conditions specified. It is a parameter of quantitative assays for low levels of compounds in sample matrices, such as impurities in bulk drug substances and degradation products in finished pharmaceuticals. Similar to the limit of detection, it is often expressed as the concentration of analyte in the sample.

3.2.3. Linearity and Range

The linearity of an assay method is defined as the ability to elicit assay results, such as peak area absorptivity, that are directly, or by a well-defined mathematical transformation, proportional to the concentration of analyte in samples

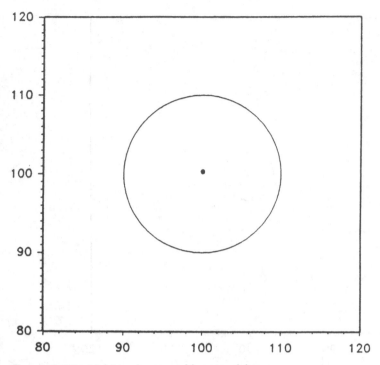

FIGURE 3.2.2 Unbiasedness and low precision.

within a given range. This parameter is also to be used to determine the effect of a nonzero intercept on assay calibration, which assumes a calibration line passing through the origin. The simple linear regression analysis is usually employed to evaluate the linearity over a given range. Statistical analysis may be performed based on the raw measurements of assay and sample concentrations or based on logarithmic transformation of the data. The estimated slope and its estimated variance provide a statistical evaluation of linearity, while the estimated Y intercept can be used to assess the potential bias.

The range of an assay method is the interval between the upper and lower levels (inclusive) of analyte that have been determined with accuracy, precision, and linearity using the method as written. The range is usually expressed in the same unit as assay results obtained by the assay method. Hence the range of the assay method is verified by the fact that the assay method provides acceptable accuracy, precision, and linearity not only to samples within the range but also to samples at the extremes of the range.

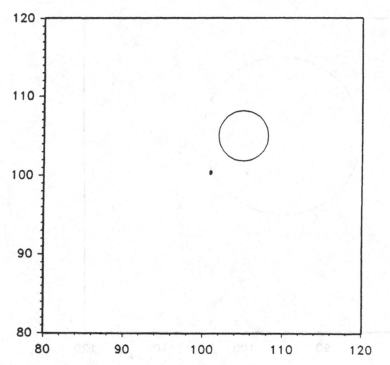

FIGURE 3.2.3 Bias but with high precision.

3.2.4. Selectivity and Ruggedness

The *selectivity* (or *specificity*) is usually referred to as the ability of an assay method to measure the analyte accurately and specifically in the presence of components that may be expected to be present in the sample matrix. Selectivity is often expressed as the difference in assay results obtained by analysis of samples containing added impurities, degradation products, related chemical compounds, or placebo ingredients to those from samples without added substances. Hence selectivity is a measure of the degree of interference in analysis of complex sample matrix. An acceptable assay method should be free of any significant interference by substances known to be present in the drug product.

The *ruggedness* of an assay method is defined as the degree of reproducibility of the assay results obtained by analysis of the same sample under a variety of normal test conditions, such as different laboratories, different analysts, different instruments, different lots of reagents, different assay elapsed times, different assay temperatures, and different days. Ruggedness is a measure of reproducibility of assay results under normal expected operating conditions,

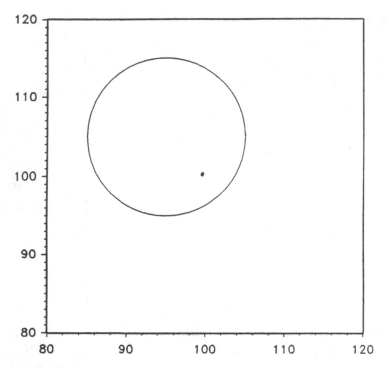

FIGURE 3.2.4   Bias with low precision.

from laboratory to laboratory, from day to day, or from analyst to analyst. Hence the reproducibility is sometimes referred to as the variation among assay results obtained from different environmental settings, such as different days, laboratories, or analysts. Therefore, the technique of variance components is usually employed to identify the source of variation and to estimate the contribution of each source to the total variability.

In the pharmaceutical industry, the development of drug products usually involves many different assay methods. The assay methods, which usually depend on the active ingredients of the drug, may vary from sophisticated exacting analytical determination to very subjective assessment of attribute. In practice, different requirements are posed on different types of assay methods. In general, according to the USP/NF, all assay methods can be classified as one of the following three categories:

Category I: Analytical methods for quantitation of major components of bulk drug substances or active ingredients (including preservatives) in finished pharmaceutical products.

Category II: Analytical methods for determination of impurities in bulk drug substances or degradation compounds in finished pharmaceutical products. These methods include quantitative assays and limit tests.

Category III: Analytical methods for determination of performance characteristics (e.g., dissolution and drug release).

Note that some pharmaceutical companies use the following four categories of assays for which validation data are required:

Category I: Includes methods for quantitation of major components of bulk drug substances, drug products, and other active ingredients (e.g., preservatives and antioxidants).

Category II: Includes methods for quantitative determination of impurities in drug substances or degradation products in drug products.

Category III: These methods include limit tests such as residual solvents and determination of trace contaminants (e.g., organic volatile impurities).

Category IV: Analytical methods for determination of performance characteristics of drug products (e.g., dissolution and drug release).

Table 3.2.2 provides a list of requirements for experimental data for each category of assay methods. It can be seen from Table 3.2.2 that validation parameters of accuracy, precision, linearity, and ruggedness are required for all categories. In the next three sections we discuss statistical methods for the validation of these analytical parameters.

3.3. ASSAY ACCURACY

As mentioned in Sec. 3.2, the accuracy of an assay method is usually assessed using the amount of known added active ingredient recovered from the excipient by the proposed assay method in a recovery study. Since the amount of the added active analytes in a recovery study are known quantities, they are usually assumed fixed. However, the recovered amount by the assay method is a random variable. Let X_i be the amount of the active ingredient added in sample i in a recovery study and Y_i be the corresponding recovered amount, $i = 1, \ldots, n$. Then the percent recovery Z_i, the absolute bias B_i, and percent bias PB_i for sample i are defined, respectively, as

$$Z_i = 100 \left(\frac{Y_i}{X_i}\right) \%,$$

$$B_i = Y_i - X_i, \tag{3.3.1}$$

$$PB_i = 100 \left(\frac{B_i}{X_i}\right) \%,$$

TABLE 3.2.2   Data Elements Required for Assay Validation

(a) Required by USP/NF XXII (p. 1712)

Analytical performance parameters	Assay category I	Assay category II		Assay category III
		Quantitative	Limit tests	
Precision	Yes	Yes	No	Yes
Accuracy	Yes	Yes	—	—
Limit of detection	No	No	Yes	—
Limit of quantitation	No	Yes	No	—
Selectivity	Yes	Yes	Yes	—
Range	Yes	Yes	—	—
Linearity	Yes	Yes	No	—
Ruggedness	Yes	Yes	Yes	Yes

(b) Required by some pharmaceutical companies

Analytical performance parameters	Assay category I	Assay category II	Assay category III	Assay category IV
Selectivity/ specificity	Yes	Yes	Yes	Yes
Linearity/range	Yes	—	—	Yes
Accuracy	Yes	—	—	Yes
System precision	Yes	Yes	Yes	Yes
Method precision	Yes	—	—	Yes
Limit of detection	No	Yes	Yes	—
Limit of quantitation	No	Yes	—	—
Ruggedness	Yes	Yes	Yes	Yes

—: May be required, depending on the nature of the specific test.

where $i = 1, \ldots, n$. It can easily be verified that

$$PB_i = Z_i - 100, \qquad i = 1, \ldots, n. \tag{3.3.2}$$

The percent bias is much more informative than the absolute bias. For example, the absolute bias is a constant across all ranges of the amounts of active ingredients added in a recovery study. On the other hand, the percent bias is larger at lower levels than at the higher levels. As a result, the accuracy of the proposed assay method at lower levels is not as high as at higher levels.

An intuitive approach to quantifying the accuracy and bias is to consider statistical inference for the one-sample problem. Let $\bar{Z}$, $\bar{B}$, and $\overline{PB}$ be the sample means and s_Z^2, s_B^2, and s_{PB}^2 be the sample variances for the samples $\{Z_i, i = 1, \ldots, n\}$, $\{B_i, i = 1, \ldots, n\}$, and $\{PB_i, i = 1, \ldots, n\}$, respectively, where

$$\bar{Z} = \frac{1}{n} \sum_{i=1}^{n} Z_i,$$

$$\bar{B} = \frac{1}{n} \sum_{i=1}^{n} B_i,$$

$$\bar{PB} = \frac{1}{n} \sum_{i=1}^{n} PB_i,$$

and

$$s_Z^2 = \frac{1}{n-1} \sum_{i=1}^{n} (Z_i - \bar{Z})^2,$$

$$s_B^2 = \frac{1}{n-1} \sum_{i=1}^{n} (B_i - \bar{B})^2,$$

$$s_{PB}^2 = \frac{1}{n-1} \sum_{i=1}^{n} (PB_i - \bar{PB})^2.$$

Then $\bar{Z}$, $\bar{B}$, and $\bar{PB}$ can be used to estimate the accuracy, bias, and percent bias, respectively. As a result, their corresponding uncertainties are estimated by s_Z^2, s_B^2, and s_{PB}^2, respectively.

An approach to pooling information of location and dispersion is to construct a $(1 - \alpha) \times 100\%$ confidence interval. The $(1 - \alpha) \times 100\%$ confidence interval for the accuracy, bias, and percent bias can be obtained as follows:

$$U_Z (L_Z) = \bar{Z} \pm s_Z t \left(\tfrac{1}{2}\alpha, n - 1\right),$$

$$U_B (L_B) = \bar{B} \pm S_B t \left(\tfrac{1}{2}\alpha, n - 1\right), \qquad (3.3.3)$$

$$U_{PB} (L_{PB}) = \bar{PB} \pm s_{PB} t \left(\tfrac{1}{2}\alpha, n - 1\right),$$

where $t(\tfrac{1}{2}\alpha, n - 1)$ is the $(\tfrac{1}{2}\alpha)$th upper quantile of a central t distribution with $n - 1$ degrees of freedom. If the $(1 - \alpha) \times 100\%$ confidence interval for accuracy [i.e., (L_Z, U_Z) contains 100], the assay method proposed is considered validated. In other words, it is not biased. On the other hand, if the $(1 - \alpha) \times 100\%$ confidence interval for the percent bias does not include zero, the assay method is not validated in terms of its accuracy. In other words, it is not accurate and biased. Note that the width of the confidence interval also provides useful information regarding precision. For example, in some cases the $(1 - \alpha) \times 100\%$ confidence interval for accuracy may contain 100. However, the width of the confidence interval may be very wide. This indicates that the assay method is accurate but lacks precision, as illustrated in Fig. 3.2.2.

An alternative approach for the assessment of accuracy is simple linear regression analysis (Bohidar, 1983; Kohberger, 1988). Suppose that the empirical relationship between the recovered amount Y_i and the added amount X_i can be described by a simple linear regression model as follows:

$$Y_i = \alpha + \beta X_i + e_i.$$

The rationale behind the application of simple linear regression to the assessment of the accuracy of an assay method is that if $\alpha = 0$ and $\beta = 1$, the expected value of the recovered amount is equal to the amount added. Bohidar (1983) and Kohberger (1988) suggested that the following hypotheses be considered to evaluate the accuracy of an assay method:

$$H_{01}: \beta = 0 \quad \text{vs.} \quad H_{a1}: \beta \neq 0,$$
$$H_{02}: \beta = 1 \quad \text{vs.} \quad H_{a2}: \beta \neq 1, \tag{3.3.4}$$
$$H_{03}: \alpha = 0 \quad \text{vs.} \quad H_{a3}: \alpha \neq 0.$$

The first set of hypotheses is used to quantify a significant linear relationship between recovered (found) and added amounts (input). This is because an assay method cannot be validated if no relationship exists between the recovered and added amounts. The second set of hypotheses is used to verify whether the change in one unit of the added amount will result in the change in one unit of the recovered amount. Theoretically, we do not expect that the assay method will recover any active ingredient if it is not added. This concept is reflected in the third set of hypotheses.

For evaluation of the accuracy of an assay method, statistical inference for the simple linear regression model described in Sec. 2.3 can be applied. Test procedures given in (2.3.20) and (2.3.21) can be applied directly to test H_{01} vs. H_{a1} and H_{03} vs. H_{a3}. The null hypothesis of the slope being equal to 1 is rejected at the α level of significance if

$$|T^*| = \left| \frac{b - 1}{\text{SE}(b)} \right| > t\left(\tfrac{1}{2}\alpha, n - 2\right), \tag{3.3.5}$$

where b is the least-squares estimate of the slope given in (2.3.9) and $\text{SE}(b)$ is the standard error of b provided in (2.3.18). If H_{01} is rejected at the α level of significance and both H_{02} and H_{03} are not rejected at the α level, we may conclude that the accuracy of the assay method is validated.

Bohidar (1983) and Kohberger (1988) also suggested that a multivariate analysis be used to evaluate the accuracy of an assay method by testing the following joint hypotheses:

$$H_0: \alpha = 0 \text{ and } \beta = 1 \quad \text{vs.} \quad H_a: \alpha \neq 0 \text{ and/or } \beta \neq 1. \tag{3.3.6}$$

Let

$$F = \frac{1}{2\hat{\sigma}^2}\left[na^2 + 2a(b-1)\sum_{i=1}^{n} X_i + (b-1)^2 \sum_{i=1}^{n} X_i^2 \right], \tag{3.3.7}$$

where a and b are the least-squares estimates of the intercept and the slope as given in (2.3.9), and $\hat{\sigma}^2$ is the mean-squared error in the ANOVA table given in (2.3.16). The null hypothesis of (3.3.6) is rejected at the α level of significance if

$$F > F\,(\alpha, 2, n-2),$$

where $F\,(\alpha, 2, n-2)$ is the αth upper quantile of a central F distribution with 2 and $n-2$ degrees of freedom. The $(1-\alpha) \times 100\%$ simultaneous confidence region, which is an ellipse, for the intercept and slope can be obtained as follows:

$$n\,(\alpha - a)^2 + 2\,(\alpha - a)\,(\beta - b)\sum_{i=1}^{n} X_i$$

$$+ (\beta - b)^2 \sum_{i=1}^{n} X_i^2 = 2\hat{\sigma}^2\, F(\alpha, 2, n-2). \tag{3.3.8}$$

We fail to reject the null hypothesis of (3.3.6) at the α level of significance if the $(1-\alpha) \times 100\%$ simultaneous confidence ellipse in (3.3.8) contains the point (0,1).

The advantage of the simple linear regression approach for the evaluation of accuracy is that the predicted recovered amount at a particular known added amount of active ingredient within the range of the concentrations used in the recovery studies can be obtained. In addition, the $(1-\alpha) \times 100\%$ confidence interval for the amount recovered can also be obtained. Similarly, the $(1-\alpha) \times 100\%$ confidence interval for the bias over the range can also be obtained. The predicted percent recovery and its corresponding $(1-\alpha) \times 100\%$ confidence interval at a particular known added amount X_i are given, respectively, as

$$\hat{Z}_i = \frac{\hat{Y}_i}{X_i} = 100\left(\frac{a+bX_i}{X_i}\right)\% = 100\left(\frac{a}{X_i}+b\right)\%, \tag{3.3.9}$$

$$U_Z\,(L_Z) = \frac{100}{X_i}\left\{ \hat{Y}_i \pm t\,(\tfrac{1}{2}\alpha, n-2)\hat{\sigma}\left[1 + \frac{1}{n} + \frac{(X_i - \overline{X})^2}{S_{XX}} \right] \right\}, \tag{3.3.10}$$

$$\hat{PB}_i = \hat{Z}_i - 100, \tag{3.3.11}$$

$$U_{PB}(L_{PB}) = U_Z - 100\,(L_Z - 100). \tag{3.3.12}$$

Note that it is recommended that statistical methods described in Sec. 2.6.1 be applied to test the validity of the simple regression model for validation of the assay method. These tests include the test for normality assumptions and the lack-of-fit test. An alternative approach to testing the validity of the simple linear regression model is to fit the following quadratic model:

$$Y_i = \alpha + \beta_1 X_i + \beta_2 X_i^2 + e_i, \qquad i = 1, \ldots, n.$$

Let b_2 and $SE(b_2)$ be the least-squares estimator of β_2 and its estimated standard error, respectively. Then the null hypothesis of $\beta_2 = 0$ is rejected at the α level of significance if

$$|T_2| = \left| \frac{b_2}{SE(b_2)} \right| > t \left(\tfrac{1}{2} \alpha, n - 3 \right).$$

If the null hypothesis H_{01} in (3.3.4) is rejected, the null hypothesis of $\beta_2 = 0$ is not rejected, R^2 is high, and no evidence exists for the departure from normality assumption and the lack of fit, the simple linear regression model may be an adequate model to describe the relationship between the recovered and known added amounts of an active ingredient for evaluation of the accuracy of the assay method.

Example 3.3.1

To illustrate the statistical methods for evaluation of the accuracy of an assay method, consider the data given in Table 3.3.1 from a recovery study that was conducted to quantify the accuracy of the proposed assay method. The data consist of nine determinations of recovery and added amounts of an active ingredient. Table 3.3.1 also provides the percent recovery, absolute bias, and per-

TABLE 3.3.1 Recovered Amounts and Added Amounts of an Active Ingredient from a Recovery Study

Day	Added amount	Recovered amount	Percent recovery	Absolute bias	Percent bias
1	0.128	0.139	108.594	0.011	8.5938
2	0.127	0.132	103.937	0.005	3.9370
3	0.126	0.136	107.937	0.010	7.9365
1	0.383	0.365	95.300	−0.018	−4.7000
2	0.372	0.372	100.000	0.000	0.0000
3	0.376	0.395	105.053	0.019	5.0320
1	0.624	0.625	100.160	0.001	0.1603
2	0.640	0.622	97.188	−0.018	−2.8125
3	0.602	0.628	104.319	0.026	4.3189

cent bias. It can easily be verified that

$$\bar{Z} = 102.45\%, \qquad \bar{B} = 0.004, \qquad \overline{PB} = 2.499\%,$$
$$s_Z^2 = 21.296, \qquad s_B^2 = 2.235 \times 10^{-4}, \qquad s_{PB}^2 = s_Z^2 = 21.296.$$

Hence the 95% confidence interval for percent recovery and percent bias are given by

$$(L_Z, U_Z) = (98.951\%, 106.046\%),$$
$$(L_{PB}, U_{PB}) = (-1.049\%, 6.046\%),$$

respectively. Since the 95% confidence interval for percent recovery contains 100, or equivalently, the 95% confidence interval for percent bias contains 0, the assay method is considered accurate and validated.

Table 3.3.2 summarizes the estimates of the intercept and slope and their estimated standard errors from fitting a simple linear regression model of the recovered amount on the known added amount. The estimated regression line is given by

$$Y = 0.009 + 0.986X.$$

The test statistics for the null hypothesis of zero intercept and zero slope are given by

$$T_a = \frac{0.009}{0.011} = 0.846,$$

$$T_b = \frac{0.986}{0.026} = 32.232,$$

respectively. Since

$$T_a = 0.846 < t(0.025, 7) = 2.365,$$

TABLE 3.3.2 Estimates of the Intercept and Slope for the Recovered Amount in Table 3.3.1

	Intercept	Slope
Estimate	0.009302	0.985875
Standard error	0.010995	0.025787
t statistics	0.846	38.232
p value	0.4255	<0.0001
$\hat{\sigma}^2 = 0.00024$		

we fail to reject the null hypothesis H_{03} of zero intercept at the 5% level. Furthermore, since the corresponding p value of T_b is less than 0.0001, the null hypothesis of zero slope is rejected at the 5% level of significance. However,

$$|T^*| = \left| \frac{0.986 - 1}{0.026} \right| = 0.548,$$

which is less than $t(0.025,7) = 2.365$. Hence we fail to reject the null hypothesis H_{02} of the slope being 1 at the 5% level of significance.

Figure 3.3.1 displays the scatter diagram of the recovered and added amounts, estimated regression line, and the 95% confidence band for the predicted recovered amount. It can be seen from Fig. 3.3.1 that not only a linear regression model provides an adequate fit but also the 95% confidence band is very tight. Since $R^2 = 0.995$ and the null hypothesis of zero coefficient for a quadratic term in the model was not rejected at the 5% level of significance ($T_2 = 0.176$ with a p value of 0.866), the simple linear regression model is an appropriate statistical model.

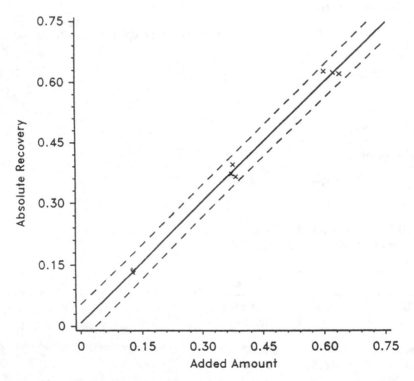

FIGURE 3.3.1   Scatter plot and regression line of data set in Table 3.3.1.

TABLE 3.3.3 Predicted Percent Recovery and Percent Bias by Simple Linear Regression Model

Day	Added amount	Recovered amount	Predicted percent recovery	95% CI recovery	Predicted percent bias	95% CI bias
1	0.128	0.139	105.85	(73.18%, 138.53%)	5.85	(−26.82%, 38.53%)
2	0.127	0.132	105.91	(72.96%, 138.86%)	5.91	(−27.04%, 38.86%)
3	0.126	0.136	105.97	(72.74%, 139.20%)	5.97	(−27.26%, 39.20%)
1	0.383	0.365	101.02	(90.83%, 111.20%)	1.02	(−9.17%, 11.20%)
2	0.372	0.372	101.09	(90.60%, 111.57%)	1.09	(−9.40%, 11.57%)
3	0.376	0.395	101.06	(90.69%, 111.44%)	1.06	(−9.31%, 11.44%)
1	0.624	0.625	100.08	(93.37%, 106.79%)	0.08	(−6.62%, 6.79%)
2	0.640	0.622	100.04	(93.45%, 106.64%)	0.04	(−6.56%, 6.64%)
3	0.602	0.628	100.13	(93.26%, 107.01%)	0.13	(−6.74%, 7.01%)

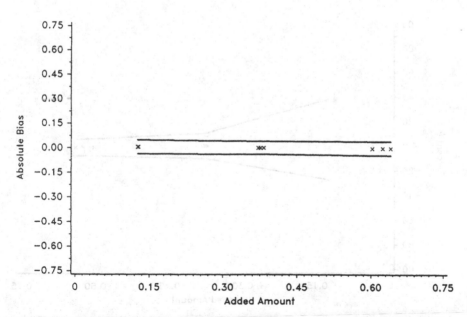

FIGURE 3.3.2 Absolute bias and 95% CI of bias versus input for data set in Table 3.3.1.

Table 3.3.3 gives the predicted percent recoveries, predicted absolute biases, predicted percent biases, and their corresponding 95% confidence intervals. Figure 3.3.2 plots the predicted biases and their corresponding 95% confidence bands, while the predicted percent biases and their corresponding 95% confidence bands are plotted in Fig. 3.3.3. The results given in Table 3.3.3 and Figs. 3.3.2 and 3.3.3 indicate that there are positive predicted bias and percent bias. The magnitudes of biases are large at lower concentrations and small at higher concentrations. The predicted percent bias ranges from 0.04% at the added amount of 0.640 to 5.97% at the added amount of 0.126. The 95% confidence interval for percent bias goes from $(-27.26\%, 39.20\%)$ at 0.126 to $(-6.56\%, 6.64\%)$ at 0.640. Although all of the 95% confidence intervals for percent bias contain zero, the assay method under validation is less precise at lower concentrations than that at higher concentrations. On the other hand, it can be verified that

$$F = 0.45 < F(0.05, 2, 7) = 4.737.$$

Hence we fail to reject the null hypothesis of (3.3.6) at the 5% level of significance. Figure 3.3.4 provides the 95% simultaneous confidence ellipse of intercept and slope. Since the ellipse contains the point (1,0), we reach the same

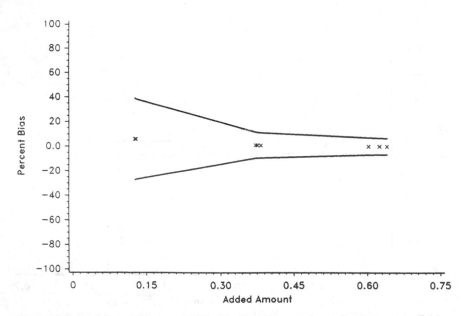

FIGURE 3.3.3 Percent bias and 95% CI of bias versus input for data set in Table 3.2.1.

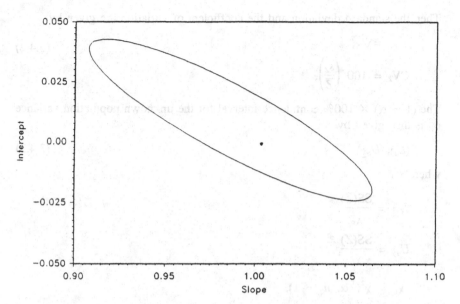

FIGURE 3.3.4 95% joint confidence ellipse of intercept and slope for data set in Table 3.2.1.

conclusion. That is, we fail to reject the null hypothesis of (3.3.6) at the 5% level of significance and conclude that the assay method is accurate and validated.

3.4. ASSAY PRECISION

Similar to the assessment of the accuracy of an assay method, we can also use the percent recovery, Z_i, to quantify the precision of the assay method. Statistical inference for one-sample problem can also be used to assess the precision of an assay method. Let s_Z^2 be the sample variance of the percent recoveries, that is,

$$s_Z^2 = \frac{SS(Z)}{n-1},$$

(3.4.1)

where

$$SS(Z) = \sum_{i=1}^{n} (Z_i - \bar{Z})^2.$$

Then the standard deviation and the coefficient of variation are given by

$$s_Z = \sqrt{s_Z^2},$$ (3.4.2)

$$CV_Z = 100 \left(\frac{s_Z}{\bar{Z}}\right).$$

The $(1 - \alpha) \times 100\%$ confidence interval for the unknown population variance σ_Z^2 is then given by

$$(L_{\sigma_Z^2}, U_{\sigma_Z^2})$$ (3.4.3)

where

$$L_{\sigma_Z^2} = \frac{SS(Z)}{\chi_U^2},$$

$$U_{\sigma_Z^2} = \frac{SS(Z)}{\chi_L^2},$$

$$\chi_U^2 = \chi^2(\tfrac{1}{2}\alpha, n - 1),$$

$$\chi_L^2 = \chi^2(1 - \tfrac{1}{2}\alpha, n - 1),$$

and $\chi^2(\tfrac{1}{2}\alpha, n - 1)$ and $\chi^2(\tfrac{1}{2}\alpha, n - 1)$ are the $(\tfrac{1}{2}\alpha)$th and $(1 - \tfrac{1}{2}\alpha)$th upper quantiles of a central chi-square distribution with $n - 1$ degrees of freedom.

In practice, it is desirable to limit the variability of the assay method within a specified acceptable quantity. If the variability of the assay result obtained from the method is within the acceptable quantity, we consider the assay method is validated. In other words, with certain assurance, the assay method has the targeted precision. Based on this concept, we may evaluate the precision of an assay method by testing the following hypotheses:

$$H_0: \sigma_Z^2 \geq \sigma_0^2 \quad \text{vs.} \quad H_a: \sigma_Z^2 < \sigma_0^2.$$ (3.4.4)

Lehmann (1959) indicated that one may reject the null hypothesis of (3.4.4) at the α level of significance if

$$Q = \frac{SS(Z)}{\sigma_0^2} < \chi^2(1 - \alpha, n - 1).$$ (3.4.5)

Note that test statistic Q is the uniformly most powerful unbiased (UMPU) test for hypotheses (3.4.4).

Example 3.4.1

To illustrate the use of statistical methods for evaluation of the precision of an assay method discussed in this section, we consider the percent recoveries given in Table 3.3.1. From Table 3.3.1 it can be verified that

$$s_Z^2 = 21.296 \quad \text{and} \quad s_Z = 4.615.$$

Hence

$$CV = 100 \left(\frac{s_Z}{\bar{Z}}\right) = 100 \left(\frac{4.615}{102.499}\right) = 4.50\%.$$

Since $\chi^2 (0.975,8) = 2.18$ and $\chi^2 (0.025,8) = 17.53$, the 95% confidence interval for σ_Z^2 is given by

$$L_{\sigma_Z^2} = \frac{170.365}{17.53} = 9.719,$$

$$U_{\sigma_Z^2} = \frac{170.365}{2.18} = 78.149.$$

Suppose that the precision of percent recovery for this type of assay method is considered acceptable if its coefficient of variation is within 10%. This implies that the standard deviation (or variability) of the percent recovery must be less than 10 (or 100), assuming that the true mean is 100. We can then evaluate the precision of the assay method by testing the following hypotheses:

$$H_0: \sigma_Z^2 \geq 100 \quad \text{vs.} \quad H_a: \sigma_Z^2 < 100.$$

Since

$$Q = \frac{170.3651}{100} = 1.704,$$

which is less than $\chi^2(0.95,8) = 2.733$, we reject the null hypothesis at the 5% level of significance and conclude that the assay method is validated in terms of its precision.

3.5. ASSAY RUGGEDNESS

In addition to accuracy and precision, an acceptable assay method should produce similar assay results regardless of any slightly change in environment. In practice, there are many environmental factors that may have a significant impact on the performance of an assay method even assay samples that are from homogeneous lots. These environmental factors include day, laboratory, and analyst. For example, the recovery study discussed in Examples 3.3.1 and 3.4.1 were, in fact, conducted on three different days. It is of interest to examine whether the assay method will produce similar assay results on different days. In other words, statistically, it is desirable to quantify the variation due to day and the proportion of day-to-day variation as compared to the total variation.

In this section, statistical methods for the ANOVA components are applied to evaluate assay ruggedness. For this purpose we introduce two commonly used statistical models, the one-way nested random model and the two-way crossed-classification mixed model. The one-way nested random model is usually employed when the recovery studies are conducted under different levels of one environmental factor with replicates at each level. The two-way crossed-classification mixed model is considered when the recovery studies consist of different levels of potency for the known added active ingredients and one environmental factor.

3.5.1. One-Way Nested Random Model

The one-way nested random model for the percent recovery Z_{ij} with one environmental factor A can be described as follows:

$$Z_{ij} = \mu + A_i + e_{j(i)}, \qquad i = 1, \ldots, I; \quad j = 1, \ldots, J, \tag{3.5.1}$$

where Z_{ij} is the jth percent recovery at the ith level of factor A, μ is the overall mean, A_i is the random effect of the ith level of factor A, and $e_{j(i)}$ is the random error of the jth percent recovery nested within the ith level of factor A.

The usual assumptions for the one-way nested random model are summarized below [see, e.g., Anderson (1982) and Searle et al. (1992)]:

1. A_i are i.i.d. normal with mean zero and variance σ_A^2;
2. $e_{j(i)}$ are i.i.d. normal with mean zero and variance σ^2;
3. A_i and $e_{j(i)}$ are mutually independent for all i and j. $\qquad$ (3.5.2)

Let $\overline{Z}_{i\cdot}$ and $\overline{Z}_{\cdot\cdot}$ be the observed means for the ith level of factor A and the overall mean, respectively. Thus

$$\overline{Z}_{i\cdot} = \frac{1}{J} \sum_{j=1}^{J} Z_{ij},$$

$$\overline{Z}_{\cdot\cdot} = \frac{1}{IJ} \sum_{i=1}^{I} \sum_{j=1}^{J} Z_{ij} = \frac{1}{I} \sum_{i=1}^{I} \overline{Z}_{i\cdot}. \tag{3.5.3}$$

The total corrected sum of squares is given by

$$\mathrm{SST} = \sum_{i=1}^{I} \sum_{j=1}^{J} (Z_{ij} - \overline{Z}_{\cdot\cdot})^2$$

$$= J \sum_{i=1}^{I} (\overline{Z}_{i\cdot} - \overline{Z}_{\cdot\cdot})^2 + \sum_{i=1}^{I} \sum_{j=1}^{J} (Z_{ij} - \overline{Z}_{i\cdot})^2 \tag{3.5.4}$$

$$= \mathrm{SSA} + \mathrm{SSE}.$$

As can be seen from the above, the total sum of squares can be partitioned into the sum of squares of factor A (i.e., SSA) and the sum of squares of errors (i.e., SSE). Table 3.5.1 gives the ANOVA table for the one-way nested random model. Note that in ANOVA table, mean squares are equal to the sum of squares divided by its degrees of freedom.

Under the assumption of (3.5.2), the distributions of SSA and SSE are

$$\text{SSA} \sim (\sigma^2 + J\sigma_A^2) \chi^2 (I - 1), \tag{3.5.5}$$

$$\text{SSE} \sim \sigma^2 \chi^2 [I(J - 1)]. \tag{3.5.6}$$

As a result, the expected values of mean squares for factor A and mean squared error are given by

$$E(\text{MSA}) = \sigma^2 + J\sigma_A^2, \tag{3.5.7}$$

$$E(\text{MSE}) = \sigma^2.$$

Therefore, the analysis of variance estimators of σ_A^2 and σ^2 can be obtained as follows:

$$\hat{\sigma}^2 = \text{MSE}, \tag{3.5.8}$$

$$\hat{\sigma}_A^2 = \frac{\text{MSA} - \text{MSE}}{J}.$$

As can be seen from (3.5.8), $\hat{\sigma}_A^2$ is obtained from the difference between MSA and MSE. Hence it is possible to obtain a negative estimate for σ_A^2. The probability for obtaining a negative estimate of σ_A^2 is given by

$$P\{\hat{\sigma}_A^2 < 0\} = P\{F[I - 1, I(J - 1)] < (F)^{-1}\}, \tag{3.5.9}$$

where $F[I - 1, I(J - 1)]$ is a central F distribution with $I - 1$ and $I(J - 1)$ degrees of freedom and

$$F = \frac{\sigma^2 + J\sigma_A^2}{\sigma^2}. \tag{3.5.10}$$

TABLE 3.5.1 ANOVA Table for One-Way Nested Random Model

Source of variation	df	Sum of squares	Mean square	$E(\text{MS})$	F value
Factor A	$I - 1$	SSA	$\text{MSA} = \text{SSA}/(I - 1)$	$\sigma^2 + J\sigma_A^2$	$F_A = \text{MSA}/\text{MSE}$
Error	$I(J - 1)$	SSE	$\text{MSE} = \text{SSE}/[I(J - 1)]$	σ^2	
Total	$IJ - 1$	SST			

If $\hat{\sigma}_A^2 < 0$, it may suggest that (a) model (3.5.1) is incorrect, (b) $\sigma_A^2 = 0$, or (c) the sample size is too small. In the case where $\sigma_A^2 = 0$, model (3.5.1) reduces to

$$Z_{ij} = \mu + e_{ij}. \qquad (3.5.11)$$

Under model (3.5.11), the ANOVA estimator for σ^2 is given by

$$\hat{\sigma}_{\text{ANOVA}}^2 = \frac{\text{SST}}{IJ - 1}. \qquad (3.5.12)$$

To obtain interval estimates for σ^2 and σ_A^2, define the following quantiles of a central chi-square and a central F distribution:

$$\chi_{Le}^2 = \chi^2(1 - \tfrac{1}{2}\alpha, I(J - 1)),$$

$$\chi_{Ue}^2 = \chi^2(\tfrac{1}{2}\alpha, I(J - 1)),$$

$$\chi_{LA}^2 = \chi^2(1 - \tfrac{1}{2}\alpha, I - 1), \qquad (3.5.13)$$

$$\chi_{UA}^2 = \chi^2(\tfrac{1}{2}\alpha, I - 1),$$

$$F_L = F(1 - \tfrac{1}{2}\alpha, I - 1, I(J - 1)),$$

$$F_U = F(\tfrac{1}{2}\alpha, I - 1, I(J - 1)).$$

The $(1 - \alpha) \times 100\%$ confidence interval for σ^2 is given by (L_e, U_e), where

$$L_e = \frac{\text{SSE}}{\chi_{Ue}^2} \quad \text{and} \quad U_e = \frac{\text{SSE}}{\chi_{Le}^2}. \qquad (3.5.14)$$

Note that there exists no exact $(1 - \alpha) \times 100\%$ confidence interval for σ_A^2. However, Tukey (1951) and Williams (1962) derived a confidence interval with a confidence level between $(1 - 2\alpha) \times 100\%$ and $(1 - \alpha) \times 100\%$. We will refer to this confidence interval as the Williams–Tukey confidence interval, which is given by (L_A, U_A), where

$$L_A = \frac{\text{SSA}\,(1 - F_U/F_A)}{J\chi_{UA}^2},$$

$$\qquad (3.5.15)$$

$$U_A = \frac{\text{SSA}\,(1 - F_L/F_A)}{J\chi_{LA}^2}.$$

One hypothesis of interest is that whether the variation due to factor A is significantly larger than zero:

$$H_0: \sigma_A^2 = 0 \quad \text{vs.} \quad H_a: \sigma_A^2 > 0. \qquad (3.5.16)$$

The null hypothesis of (3.5.16) is rejected at the α level of significance if

$$F_A > F_U = F(\alpha, I - 1, I(J - 1)), \tag{3.5.17}$$

where F_A is defined in Table 3.5.1. The total variation of a single test result and the proportion of the variation due to factor A are defined as follows:

$$\sigma_T^2 = \sigma^2 + \sigma_A^2, \tag{3.5.18}$$

$$\rho_A = \frac{\sigma_A^2}{\sigma_T^2} = \frac{\sigma_A^2}{\sigma^2 + \sigma_A^2}.$$

Searle et al. (1992) suggested the following estimator for σ_T^2:

$$\hat{\sigma}_T^2 = \hat{\sigma}^2 + \hat{\sigma}_A^2. \tag{3.5.19}$$

The estimator for ρ_A and the $(1 - \alpha) \times 100\%$ confidence interval for ρ_A are given by

$$\hat{\rho}_A = \frac{MSA - MSE}{MSA + (J - 1)MSE},$$

$$L_\rho = \frac{F_A/F_U - 1}{J + (F_A/F_U - 1)}, \tag{3.5.20}$$

$$U_\rho = \frac{F_A/F_L - 1}{J + (F_A/F_L - 1)}.$$

Mandel (1972) indicated that the repeatability of an assay method for any two assay results, each based on m replicates at the same level of factor A, can be estimated by

$$\hat{\sigma} \sqrt{\frac{2}{m}}.$$

On the other hand, the reproducibility of the assay method for any two assay results based on m replicates at the two different levels of factor A can be estimated by

$$\sqrt{2\left(\hat{\sigma}_A^2 + \frac{\hat{\sigma}^2}{m}\right)}.$$

Note that to avoid a negative estimate of σ_A^2, Chow and Shao (1988) proposed an alternative approach which is shown to have lower mean-squared error than the customary estimators such as the ANOVA, the maximum likelihood estimator (MLE), and the restricted maximum likelihood (REML) estimator over a large range of the parameter space. For the estimation of total variability, Chow and Tse (1991) proposed a general class of estimators that includes (3.5.19). An optimal estimator in terms of smallest mean-squared error within the general class was derived. An approximate version of this optimal estimator was also provided in Chow and Tse (1991).

Example 3.5.1

Once again we use the percent recoveries data given in Table 3.3.1 to illustrate statistical methods for evaluation of ruggedness described in this section. The ANOVA table is given in Table 3.5.2. It can be seen from the table that

$$SSA = 49.576 \quad \text{and} \quad SSE = 120.789.$$

Hence estimates for σ^2, σ_A^2, σ_T^2, and ρ_A are given by

$$\hat{\sigma}^2 = MSE = 20.131,$$

$$\hat{\sigma}_A^2 = \frac{MSA - MSE}{3} = \frac{24.788 - 20.131}{3} = 1.552,$$

$$\hat{\sigma}_T^2 = \hat{\sigma}^2 + \hat{\sigma}_A^2 = 20.131 + 1.552 = 21.684,$$

$$\hat{\rho}_A = \frac{MSA - MSE}{MSA + (J - 1) MSE} = \frac{24.788 - 20.131}{24.788 + (2)(20.131)} = 0.072.$$

Since $F_A = 1.231$ with a p value of 0.356, we fail to reject the null hypothesis of (3.5.16) at the 5% level of significance.

For construction of 95% confidence intervals, we have

$$\chi^2(0.025,6) = 14.45, \qquad \chi^2(0.975,6) = 1.237,$$
$$\chi^2(0.025,2) = 7.378, \qquad \chi^2(0.975,2) = 0.051,$$
$$F(0.025,2,6) = 7.26, \qquad F(0.975,2,6) = 0.025.$$

It can be verified that

$$L_e = \frac{120.789}{14.45} = 8.359,$$

$$U_e = \frac{120.789}{1.237} = 97.646;$$

$$L_A = \frac{(49.576)(1 - 7.26/1.231)}{(3)(7.378)} = -10.967,$$

$$U_A = \frac{(49.576)(1 - 0.025/1.231)}{(3)(0.051)} = 317.334;$$

$$L_\rho = \frac{(1.231/7.378) - 1}{3 + [(1.231/7.378) - 1]} = -0.383,$$

$$U_\rho = \frac{(1.231/0.025) - 1}{3 + [(1.231/0.025) - 1]} = 0.941.$$

TABLE 3.5.2 ANOVA Table for the Percent Recovery in Table 3.3.1

Source of variation	df	Sum of squares	Mean square	F value	p value
Day	2	49.5764	24.7882	1.2313	0.3564
Error	6	120.7886	20.1314		
Total	8	170.3650			

It should be noted that the probability for obtaining a negative estimate of σ_A^2 is given by

$$P\{\hat{\sigma}_A^2 < 0\} = P\left\{F(2,6) < \frac{1}{1.2312}\right\} = 0.5126,$$

which is not negligible. In practice, if $L_A < 0$ or $L_\rho < 0$, a common approach is to set L_A and L_ρ be equal to 0.

In summary, the proportion of variation explained by day is estimated to be about 7.16%. In addition, the high probability for obtaining a negative day-to-day variation may suggest that there is little day-to-day variation (i.e., $\sigma_A^2 = 0$). Thus we conclude that the assay method is robust against assay results obtained on different days. Note that the repeatability and reproducibility for the assay method based on m replicates can be estimated by $6.345/\sqrt{m}$ and $\sqrt{2(1.522 + 20.131/m)}$, respectively.

3.5.2. Two-Way Crossed-Classification Mixed Model

As indicated earlier, recovery studies for validation of an assay method usually consist of several levels for the known amount of added active ingredient. Several replicates are then obtained at each of several levels of an important environmental factor such as laboratory, day, or analyst. An appropriate statistical model for describing the percent recoveries obtained from a design of this type is the two-way crossed-classification mixed model. In the following we first introduce the two-way crossed-classification mixed model without interaction.

$$Z_{ijk} = \mu + A_i + B_j + e_{ijk}, \qquad i = 1, \ldots, I, \tag{3.5.21}$$
$$j = 1, \ldots, J, \quad k = 1, \ldots, K,$$

where Z_{ijk} denotes the kth percent recovery observed at the ith level of environmental factor A and the jth level of factor B (e.g., potency), μ is the overall mean, A_i is the random effect for the ith level of factor A, B_j is the fixed effect of the jth level of factor B, and e_{ijk} is the random error associated with Z_{ijk}. Note that the assumption for A_i and e_{ijk} are the same as those stated in (3.5.2) for A_i and $e_{j(i)}$ under the one-way nested random model. Factor B, however, is assumed to be fixed.

Define the following sample means and sum of squares:

$$\bar{Z}_{ij\cdot} = \frac{1}{K} \sum_{k=1}^{K} Z_{ijk},$$

$$\bar{Z}_{i\cdot\cdot} = \frac{1}{JK} \sum_{j=1}^{J} \sum_{k=1}^{K} Z_{ijk} = \frac{1}{J} \sum_{j=1}^{J} \bar{Z}_{ij\cdot},$$

$$\bar{Z}_{\cdot j\cdot} = \frac{1}{IK} \sum_{i=1}^{I} \sum_{k=1}^{K} Z_{ijk} = \frac{1}{I} \sum_{i=1}^{I} \bar{Z}_{ij\cdot}, \qquad (3.5.22)$$

$$\bar{Z}_{\cdots} = \frac{1}{IJK} \sum_{i=1}^{I} \sum_{j=1}^{J} \sum_{k=1}^{K} Z_{ijk}$$

$$= \frac{1}{IJ} \sum_{i=1}^{I} \sum_{j=1}^{J} \bar{Z}_{ij\cdot} = \frac{1}{J} \sum_{j=1}^{J} \bar{Z}_{\cdot j\cdot} = \frac{1}{I} \sum_{i=1}^{I} \bar{Z}_{i\cdot\cdot},$$

and

$$\text{SST} = \sum_{i=1}^{I} \sum_{j=1}^{J} \sum_{k=1}^{K} (Z_{ijk} - \bar{Z}_{\cdots})^2,$$

$$\text{SSE} = \sum_{i=1}^{I} \sum_{j=1}^{J} \sum_{k=1}^{K} (Z_{ijk} - \bar{Z}_{i\cdot\cdot} - \bar{Z}_{\cdot j\cdot} + \bar{Z}_{\cdots})^2,$$

$$\qquad (3.5.23)$$

$$\text{SSA} = \sum_{i=1}^{I} JK (\bar{Z}_{i\cdot\cdot} - \bar{Z}_{\cdots})^2,$$

$$\text{SSB} = \sum_{j=1}^{J} IK (\bar{Z}_{\cdot j\cdot} - \bar{Z}_{\cdots})^2.$$

Table 3.5.3 is the ANOVA table with the expected value of mean squares for each source of variation. The ANOVA estimators and $(1 - \alpha) \times 100\%$ confidence intervals for σ^2 and σ_A^2 are summarized in Table 3.5.4. Searle et al. (1992) also provided the maximum likelihood estimators for σ^2 and σ_A^2 for both situations where the MLE of σ_A^2 is either greater or less than zero.

The model for the two-way crossed-classification mixed model with interaction is given by

$$Z_{ijk} = \mu + A_i + B_j + (AB)_{ij} + e_{ijk}, \qquad (3.5.24)$$

where μ, A_i, B_j, and e_{ijk} are as defined in (3.5.21) and $(AB)_{ij}$ denotes the random effect of the interaction between the ith level of factor A and the jth level of factor B. It is assumed that $(AB)_{ij}$ are i.i.d. normal with mean zero and variance

TABLE 3.5.3 ANOVA Table for Two-Way Crossed-Classification Mixed Model Without Interaction

Source of variation	df	Sum of squares	Mean square	E(MS)	F value
Factor A	$I - 1$	SSA	$MSA = SSA/(I - 1)$	$\sigma^2 + JK\sigma_A^2$	$F_A = MSA/MSE$
Factor B	$J - 1$	SSB	$MSB = SSB/(J - 1)$	$\sigma^2 + Q(B)^a$	$F_B = MSB/MSE$
Error	$IJK - I - J + 1$	SSE	$MSE = SSE/(IJK - I - J + 1)$	σ^2	
Total	$IJK - 1$	SST			

$^a Q(B) = [IK/(J - 1)] \Sigma(\beta_j - \bar{\beta})^2.$

TABLE 3.5.4 Point and Interval Estimators for Variance Components Under Two-Way Crossed-Classification Mixed Model Without Interaction

	Variance components[a]	
	σ^2	σ_A^2
Point estimator[b]	MSE	$(MSA - MSE)/JK$
$(1 - \alpha) \times 100\%$ confidence interval		
Lower limit	$SSE/\chi^2(\alpha/2, dfE)$	$[SSA(1 - F_U/F_A)]/JK\chi^2(\alpha/2, dfA)$
Upper limit	$SSE/\chi^2(1 - \alpha/2, dfE)$	$[SSA(1 - F_L/F_A)]/JK\chi^2(1 - \alpha/2, dfA)$

[a] $dfE = IJK - I - J + 1$, $dfA = I - 1$, $F_U = F(\alpha/2, dfA, dfE)$, and $F_L = F(1 - \alpha/2, dfA, dfE)$.
[b] By the method of analysis of variance.

σ_{AB}^2. Define SSA and SSB as given in (3.5.23) and let

$$SSAB = \sum_{I=1}^{I} \sum_{j=1}^{J} K(\overline{Z}_{ij\cdot} - \overline{Z}_{i\cdot\cdot} - \overline{Z}_{\cdot j\cdot} + \overline{Z}_{\cdots})^2,$$

$$SSE = \sum_{i=1}^{I} \sum_{j=1}^{J} \sum_{k=1}^{K} (Z_{ijk} - \overline{Z}_{ij\cdot})^2.$$

(3.5.25)

The ANOVA table with expected mean squares for the two-way crossed-classification mixed model with interaction is given in Table 3.5.5. Table 3.5.6 summarizes ANOVA estimators and $(1 - \alpha) \times 100\%$ confidence intervals for σ^2, σ_{AB}^2, and σ_A^2. Searle et al. (1992) also gave the MLE for the variance components under various conditions for model (3.5.24).

Example 3.5.2

A recovery study was conducted to evaluate an assay method at two different laboratories. At each laboratory three levels of potency were added: 80%, 100%, and 120% of label claim. There were three replicates at each level of potency at each laboratory. The actual recovered amounts in terms of label claim and the percent recovery are given in Table 3.5.7.

Table 3.5.8 gives the ANOVA table for the two-way crossed-classification mixed model with interaction. From Table 3.5.8 it can easily be verified that the ANOVA estimate for σ_{AB}^2 is given by

$$\hat{\sigma}_{AB}^2 = \frac{0.014 - 4.236}{3} = -1.407.$$

According to Searle et al. (1992), the probability of obtaining a negative estimate is estimated by

$$P\{\hat{\sigma}_{AB}^2 < 0\} = P\{F(\mathrm{df}(AB), \mathrm{df}(E)) < (F_{AB})^{-1}\}$$
$$= P\{F(\mathrm{df}(AB), \mathrm{df}(E)) < (0.003)^{-1}\}$$
$$\cong 1,$$

where $\mathrm{df}(AB)$ and $\mathrm{df}(E)$ denote the degrees of freedom associated with factor AB and the error term. In addition, since $F_A = 0.003$, which is less than $F(0.05, 2, 12) = 3.89$, there is little evidence to reject the null hypothesis

$$H_0: \sigma_{AB}^2 = 0$$

at the 5% level of significance. This result suggests a reduced model without interaction be used.

The ANOVA table for the data given in Table 3.5.7 under the two-way crossed-classification mixed model without interaction is given in Table 3.5.9.

TABLE 3.5.5 ANOVA Table for Two-Way Crossed-Classification Mixed Model with Interaction

Source of variation	df	Sum of squares	Mean square	E(MS)	F value
Factor A	$I - 1$	SSA	$MSA = SSA/(I - 1)$	$\sigma^2 + K\sigma_{AB}^2 + JK\sigma_A^2$	$F_A = MSA/MSE$
Factor B	$J - 1$	SSB	$MSB = SSB/(J - 1)$	$\sigma^2 + K\sigma_{AB}^2 + Q(B)^a$	$F_B = MSB/MSAB$
$A \times B$ interaction	$(I - 1)(J - 1)$	SSAB	$MSAB = SSAB/[(I - 1)(J - 1)]$	$\sigma^2 + K\sigma_{AB}^2$	$F_{AB} = MSAB/MSE$
Error	$IJ(K - 1)$	SSE	$MSE = SSE/[IJ(K - 1)]$	σ^2	
Total	$IJK - 1$	SST			

$^a Q(B) = [IK/(J - 1)] \, \Sigma(\beta_j - \bar{\beta})^2$.

TABLE 3.5.6 Point and Interval Estimators for Variance Components Under Two-Way Crossed-Classification Mixed Model With Interaction

	Variance components[a]		
Point estimator[b]	σ^2	σ_{AB}^2	σ_A^2
	MSE	(MSAB − MSE)/K	(MSA − MSAB)/JK
$(1 - \alpha) \times 100\%$ Confidence interval			
Lower limit	SSE/$\chi^2(\alpha/2,\ dfE)$	$[SSAB(1 - F_{UAB}/F_{AB})]/K\chi^2\ (\alpha/2,\ dfAB)$	$[SSA(1 - F_{UA}/F_A)]/JK\chi^2\ (\alpha/2,\ dfA)$
Upper limit	SSE/$\chi^2(1 - \alpha/2,\ dfE)$	$[SSA(1 - F_{LAB}/F_{AB})]/K\chi^2\ (1 - \alpha/2,\ dfAB)$	$[SSA(1 - F_{LA}/F_A)]/JK\chi^2\ (1 - \alpha/2,\ dfA)$

[a] $dfE = IJ(K - 1)$, $dfA = I - 1$, $dfAB = (I - 1)(J - 1)$, $F_{UA} = F(\alpha/2, dfA, dfE)$, and $F_{LA} = F(1 - \alpha/2, dfA, dfE)$, $F_{UAB} = F(\alpha/2, dfAB, dfE)$, and $F_{LAB} = F(1 - \alpha/2, dfAB, dfE)$.

[b] By the method of analysis of variance.

TABLE 3.5.7 Actual (% Label Claim) and Percent Recovery of a Recovery Study

Lab	Day	Sample	Added amount	Recovered amount	Percent recovery
1	1	1	80	80.0	100.0
	2	2	80	80.0	100.0
	3	3	80	82.0	102.5
	1	4	100	101.5	101.5
	2	5	100	101.5	101.5
	3	6	100	103.0	103.0
	1	7	120	122.4	102.0
	2	8	120	118.8	99.0
	3	9	120	126.0	105.0
2	1	1	80	79.6	99.5
	2	2	80	78.0	97.5
	3	3	80	81.2	101.5
	1	4	100	100.0	100.0
	2	5	100	99.0	99.0
	3	6	100	102.5	102.5
	1	7	120	121.2	101.0
	2	8	120	117.6	98.0
	3	9	120	123.6	103.0

It can be seen that the ANOVA estimates for σ^2 and σ_A^2 are given by

$$\hat{\sigma}^2 = \text{MSE} = 3.633,$$

$$\hat{\sigma}_A^2 = \frac{8.681 - 3.633}{9} = 0.561,$$

TABLE 3.5.8 ANOVA Table for the Percent Recovery in Table 3.5.7 with Interaction

Source of variation	df	Sum of squares	Mean square	F value	p value
Lab	1	8.6806	8.6806	624.9532	0.0016
Potency	2	5.0833	2.5417	182.9878	0.0054
Lab-by-potency	2	0.02778	0.01389	0.0033	0.9967
Error	12	50.8333	4.2361		
Total	17	64.6250			

TABLE 3.5.9 ANOVA Table for the Percent Recovery in Table 3.5.7 Without Interaction

Source of variation	df	Sum of squares	Mean square	F value	p value
Lab	1	8.6806	8.6806	2.39	0.1445
Potency	2	5.0833	2.5417	0.70	0.5133
Error	14	50.8611	3.6329		
Total	17	64.6250			

respectively. To obtain 95% confidence intervals for σ^2 and σ_A^2, the following quantiles are needed:

$$\chi^2(0.025,14) = 26.119, \qquad \chi^2(0.975,14) = 5.629,$$
$$\chi^2(0.025,1) = 5.024, \qquad \chi^2(0.975,1) = 0.0098,$$
$$F(0.025,1,14) = 6.298, \qquad F(0.975,1,14) = 0.001.$$

As a result, the 95% confidence interval for σ^2 is given by

$$L_e = \frac{50.861}{26.119} = 1.947,$$

$$U_e = \frac{50.861}{5.629} = 9.036.$$

Since

$$F_A = 2.392 < F(0.05,1,14) = 4.60,$$
$$\chi^2(0.025,1) = 0.0098,$$

the 95% confidence interval for σ_A^2 is given by

$$L_A = \frac{(8.681)(1 - 6.298/2.392)}{(9)(5.024)} = -0.313,$$

$$U_A = \frac{(8.681)(1 - 0.001/2.392)}{(9)(0.0098)} = 983.829.$$

As can be seen, the approximate 95% confidence interval for σ_A^2 is very wide and the lower limit is below zero. Note that since the quantiles of the chi-square in the denominator of L_A and U_A are a function of the degrees of freedom associated with the environmental factor, if the number of levels of the environmental factor is small, we expect to have a wide approximate $(1 - \alpha) \times 100\%$ confidence interval for σ_A^2.

3.6. STATISTICAL DESIGNS

The major objective of the validation of an assay method is to ensure that the assay method can produce unbiased and precise assay results for the active ingredient of a compound. To achieve this objective, the USP/NF indicates that the assay method needs to be validated in terms of the primary validation parameters listed in Table 3.2.1. To meet the USP/NF standards for each of these parameters, an appropriate statistical design is necessarily chosen to provide sound statistical inferences for these parameters and their variances. Bohidar (1983) and Bohidar and Peace (1988) have suggested several designs for validation experiments. In this section we discuss statistical properties of some commonly employed designs in validation experiments.

The most commonly used design in assay validation is probably the randomized block design. Suppose that there are J levels of potency (expressed as percent of label claim) in a recovery study. The number of levels, J, is usually an odd number because additional levels (the same number of equally spaced levels) are usually considered below and above the level of 100% of label claim. For example, the set of {80%, 100%, 120%} or {60%, 80%, 100%, 120%, 140%} is often considered in assay validation experiments. Samples are usually assayed on different days with and/or without the same number of replicates. It should be noted, however, that assays of different levels on the same day are usually performed in sequential order. To avoid the bias that may be introduced by testing order, it is suggested that a Latin square type of design be used to balance the potential bias. In other words, the number of days should be equal to the number of levels of potency. The Latin square design is then applied to the test sequence of the levels of potency. For example, suppose that three levels of percent of label claim (80%, 100%, and 120%) are examined in a recovery study. Denote the three levels by L_1, L_2, and L_3, respectively. The following table gives an example of the application with three levels of potency on three separate days.

	Test sequence		
Day	1	2	3
1	L_1	L_2	L_3
2	L_2	L_3	L_1
3	L_3	L_1	L_2

In recovery studies for assay validation, "day" is usually considered a random effect, while the levels of potency are assumed fixed. Hence the statistical methods described in Sec. 3.5 can be applied directly to this design. Tables 3.5.3 and 3.5.5 give the ANOVA table for this design with and without interaction, respectively. For any recovery study, the statistical methods described in Sec. 3.5 can be applied to examine whether there is a positive relationship between the recovered and added amounts based on the actual recovered amount (not the percent recovery).

In practice, the number of assays performed on each day may not be able to cover all the levels of potency under study, due to financial restrictions and/or limited resources available. In addition, in some cases, the assay can only be conducted on a certain number of days, which is fewer than the number of levels of potency. In these situations, an incomplete block design may be used to randomize test sequences on each day. Bohidar (1983) and Bohidar and Peace (1988) considered use of the following incomplete block design for a recovery study that involves five levels of potency and three days.

| | Test sequence | | | | |
Day	1	2	3	4	5
1	L_3	L_1	L_4	L_2	L_5
2	L_2	L_3	L_1	L_5	L_4
3	L_4	L_5	L_2	L_3	L_1

Note that for the validation of an assay method, recovery studies are used not only to estimate the accuracy, linearity, and precision but also to provide statistical inference on the ruggedness across different days or laboratories. Based on the nature of the various purposes of a recovery study, sample-size determination has become a real challenge to statisticians. For example, we may calculate the required sample size for accuracy based on hypotheses H_{01} given in (3.3.4). However, the precision of the assay method is also needed to be taken into account for sample-size determination for a positive slope which is significantly different from zero. Although the precision is one of the validation parameters that can be estimated from the recovery studies, there is scant literature available on sample-size determination based on the purpose of estimating variance components (Mandel, 1972). In practice, the number of levels for potency, the number of days, and the number of laboratories are usually fixed. Hence sample-size determination can be considered as the problem of estimating the number of replicates for each combination. However, it appears that more research is needed for sample-size determination in validation experiments.

Example 3.6.1

Consider the recovery study discussed in Example 3.5.2. The data for recovered amounts (expressed as percent of label claim) are given in Table 3.5.7. The three replicates in this example actually represent three different days. In addition, the laboratory is considered as a replicate in this example.

Table 3.6.1 provides the ANOVA table with interaction. It can be seen from Table 3.6.1 that there is no significant interaction between day and potency at the 5% level of significance. There is a significant linear relationship between the amount recovered and the levels of the known added active ingredient. However, the departure from linearity is not statistically significant. The variance due to day is significantly greater than zero at the 5% level.

Note that for a given recovery study it is expected that (1) there is no significant day-by-potency interaction, (2) there is a significant linear relationship, (3) the departure from linearity is not statistically significant, and (4) there is a significant random day effect. To evaluate the foregoing properties of a given recovery study, the statistical methods described in Sec. 3.5.2 can be applied to obtain both point and interval estimates for σ^2, σ_{AD}^2, and σ_D^2, where σ_{AD}^2 is the variance component of day-by-potency interaction and σ_D^2 is the variance component of day.

3.7. STATISTICAL CONSIDERATIONS

3.7.1. Assessment of Accuracy

In Sec. 3.3 we summarize the current statistical practice for evaluation of the accuracy of an analytical method. These statistical methods are actually based on the hypotheses of no difference. For example, the accuracy of an assay procedure may be considered validated if the 95% confidence interval for the percent recovery contains 100. However, an assay with a large variability is more likely than an assay with good precision to produce a wider 95% confidence interval. Similarly, the regression technique approach is focused on the concept

TABLE 3.6.1 ANOVA Table for % Label Claim in Table 3.5.7 Under Two-Way Crossed-Classification Mixed Model with Interaction

Source of variation	df	Sum of squares	Mean square	F value	p value
Day	2	0.004603	0.002302	7.84	0.0414
Potency	2	0.5159	0.2580	877.55	<0.0001
Linear	1	0.5158	0.5158	1754.42	<0.0001
Departure from linearity	1	0.00006	0.00006	0.20	0.6749
Day-by-potency	4	0.001174	0.000294	2.38	0.1287
Error	9	0.00111	0.000123		
Total	17	0.5228			

of hypotheses of difference. The inadequacy of such approaches can be demonstrated by the fact that failure to reject H_{02}: $\beta = 1$ does not prove that the slope is 1. Therefore, the interval hypothesis often used in bioequivalence studies (Chow and Liu, 1992) provides a more logical and reasonable approach because it can prove whether the parameter of interest is equivalent to a known quantity.

Let θ be the parameter of interest, such as the unknown average percent recovery, slope, or intercept. An assay is claimed accurate if θ is between θ_L and θ_U, where θ_L and θ_U are specified lower and upper equivalent limits, respectively. For example, we claim that the accuracy of an assay method is validated if the average percent recovery is between 95 and 105%, and/or the slope is between 0.95 and 1.05, and/or the intercept is between -0.05 and 0.05. In general, the interval hypotheses can be formulated as follows:

$$H_0: \theta \geq \theta_U \text{ or } \theta \leq \theta_L \quad \text{vs.} \quad H_a: \theta_L < \theta < \theta_U. \tag{3.7.1}$$

The hypotheses above can be further decomposed into the following two one-sided hypotheses:

$$\begin{aligned} H_{0L}: \theta \leq \theta_L \quad &\text{vs.} \quad H_{aL}: \theta > \theta_L, \\ H_{0U}: \theta \geq \theta_U \quad &\text{vs.} \quad H_{aU}: \theta < \theta_U. \end{aligned} \tag{3.7.2}$$

Let V_θ be an unbiased estimator for θ. V_θ has a normal distribution with mean θ and variance σ_V^2. In addition, s_V^2 is an unbiased estimator of σ_V^2 and $df(s_V^2/\sigma_V^2)$ has a central chi-square distribution with df degrees of freedom. Define

$$T_L = \frac{V_\theta - \theta_L}{s_V} \quad \text{and} \quad T_U = \frac{V_\theta - \theta_U}{s_V}. \tag{3.7.3}$$

The null hypothesis of (3.7.1) is rejected at the α level of significance if

$$T_L > t(\alpha, df) \quad \text{and} \quad T_U < -t(\alpha, df). \tag{3.7.4}$$

Since hypotheses (3.7.2) are two one-sided hypotheses, the foregoing testing procedure is usually referred to as a two one-sided tests procedure (Schuirmann, 1987; Chow and Liu, 1992). The associated $(1 - 2\alpha) \times 100\%$ confidence interval for θ can be obtained as (L_θ, U_θ), where

$$L_\theta = V_\theta - t(\alpha, df)s_V,$$
$$U_\theta = V_\theta + t(\alpha, df)s_V.$$

It can easily be verified that $(L_\theta, U_\theta) \in (\theta_L, \theta_U)$ if and only if (3.7.4) is true. Hence the confidence interval approach is operationally equivalent to the two one-sided tests procedure.

Example 3.7.1

To introduce the concept of interval hypotheses, consider the recovery study described in Example 3.3.1. Suppose that the hypotheses of interest are as follows:

$$H_{01}: \mu_z \leq 95\% \text{ or } \mu_z \geq 105\% \quad \text{vs.} \quad H_{a1}: 95\% < \mu_z < 105\%,$$

$$H_{02}: \beta \leq 0.95 \text{ or } \beta \geq 1.05 \quad \text{vs.} \quad H_{a2}: 0.95 < \beta < 1.05, \qquad (3.7.5)$$

$$H_{03}: \alpha \leq -0.05 \text{ or } \alpha \geq 0.05 \quad \text{vs.} \quad H_{a3}: -0.05 < \alpha < 0.05,$$

where μ_z is the unknown average percent recovery. The first set of hypotheses means that based on percent recovery, the accuracy is considered validated if the average percent recovery is between 95 and 105%. The second set of hypotheses suggests that the slope is equivalent to 1 if it is between 0.95 and 1.05. Finally, the last set of hypotheses indicates that one accepts that the intercept is equivalent to 0 if it is between −0.05 and 0.05.

Table 3.7.1 summarizes the numerical results. It can be seen that for average percent recovery, we fail to reject the null hypothesis at the 2.5% level of significance and the 95% confidence interval is outside (95%, 105%). Thus the accuracy of the assay is not validated at the 2.5% level of significance. Similar results are found for the slope. However, for the intercept, the null hypothesis is rejected at the 2.5% level of significance and the 95% confidence interval (−0.0167, 0.0350) is within (−0.05, 0.05). Therefore, the intercept is equivalent to zero at the 2.5% level of significance with the limit −0.05 and 0.05.

3.7.2. Multiple Validation

Thus far this chapter summarizes statistical methods for evaluation of validation parameters in Table 3.2.1 for a single assay method using the same procedures for the same active ingredients. However, in some cases, an alternative assay method may be developed to save cost and/or time. On the other hand, the technology of an assay method may be transferred from the site where the assay was developed to another site. In these cases the assay method must be validated individually using statistical methods described in this chapter in terms of each validation parameter. In practice, it is imperative to evaluate whether the assay

TABLE 3.7.1   Results of the Two One-Sided Tests Procedure for the Data in Table 3.3.1[a]

	T_L	T_U	95% Confidence interval
Average percent recovery (df = 8)	4.8750	−1.6259	(98.95%,106.05%)
Slope (df = 7)	1.3912	−2.4868	(0.9249,1.0470)
Intercept (df = 7)	5.3935	−3.7015	(−0.01670,0.03530)

[a]$t(0.025,8) = 2.3060$ and $t(0.025,7) = 2.3646$.

results obtained from the alternative method (or new site) are equivalent to those obtained from the original assay method (or site).

To compare two assay methods, the same preparations of active ingredients are usually assayed using the two methods. Two recovered amounts are then obtained on the same preparation by individual method. Similar to a blocking factor for crossover studies in clinical trials, this type of recovery study can be considered as the application of crossover studies to analytical chemistry.

If two methods of analytical procedures are performed at the same time for the same preparation, the test sequence could not be considered as a factor. However, if there is a test sequence, the standard two-sequence, two-period crossover design should be used. In other words, n preparations are randomly assigned to two groups. In the first group, the original assay will be performed first, followed by the alternative method. The test sequence in the second group is reversed. If more than two methods are compared, other crossover designs, such as Williams's design, can be applied (Chow and Liu, 1992). Unlike the crossover studies in clinical trials, there exists no carryover effect for crossover studies in analytical chemistry. Also, the assay methods can be performed simultaneously. Thus the period and sequence effects are not present for most crossover studies in assay validation. As a result, statistical inferences for the paired samples can be applied directly. However, if there is a concern regarding the test sequence, one should apply statistical methods of crossover designs (Jones and Kenward, 1989; Chow and Liu, 1992).

An appropriate statistical model (Kohberger, 1988) for the percent recovery, Z_{ij}, of preparation j assayed by method i is given by

$$Z_{ij} = \mu + \tau_i + S_j + e_{ij}, \quad i = 1,2, \quad j = 1, \ldots, n, \tag{3.7.6}$$

where μ is the overall mean, τ_i is the fixed effect of bias for method i, S_j is the random effect of preparation j, and e_{ij} is the random error associated with Z_{ij}. The primary assumptions for model (3.7.6) are summarized as follows:

1. S_j are i.i.d. normal with mean zero and variance σ_S^2.
2. ϵ_{ij} are independently distributed as a normal random variable with mean zero and variance σ_i^2.
3. S_j and ϵ_{ij} are mutually independent for all i and j.

Note that σ_S^2 is usually referred to as the interassay variability and σ_i^2 denotes the intraassay variability for method i.

The major objective of a crossover study in analytical chemistry is to compare bias and intraassay variability between assay methods. Define the preparation differences as

$$d_j = Z_{1j} - Z_{2j}, \quad j = 1, \ldots, n. \tag{3.7.7}$$

The expected value of d_j is then given by

$$E(d_j) = E(Z_{1j} - Z_{2j})$$
$$= E(Z_{1j}) - E(Z_{2j})$$
$$= (\mu + \tau_1) - (\mu + \tau_2)$$
$$= \tau_1 - \tau_2.$$

Therefore, d_j is an unbiased estimator for the difference in bias between the two methods. The variance of Z_{ij} and the covariance between Z_{1j} and Z_{2j} are given by

$$\mathrm{var}(Z_{ij}) = \sigma_S^2 + \sigma_i^2, \quad i = 1, 2, \quad j = 1, \ldots, n,$$
$$\mathrm{cov}(Z_{1j}, Z_{2j}) = \sigma_S^2, \quad j = 1, \ldots, n.$$

As a result, the variance of d_j is given by

$$\mathrm{var}(d_j) = \sigma_1^2 + \sigma_2^2, \quad j = 1, \ldots, n.$$

Let $\bar{d}$ and s_d^2 be the sample mean and variance of $\{d_j, j = 1, \ldots, n\}$, that is,

$$\bar{d} = \frac{1}{n} \sum_{j=1}^{n} d_j,$$

$$s_d^2 = \frac{1}{n-1} \sum_{j=1}^{n} (d_j - \bar{d})^2.$$

The hypotheses for testing the equality between biases can be formulated as follows:

$$H_0: \tau_1 = \tau_2 \quad \text{vs.} \quad H_a: \tau_1 \neq \tau_2. \tag{3.7.8}$$

The null hypothesis of (3.7.8) is rejected at the α level of significance if

$$|T_d| = \left| \frac{\bar{d}}{s_d \sqrt{n}} \right| > t(\tfrac{1}{2}\alpha, n-1). \tag{3.7.9}$$

Note that when the normality assumptions are not met, the approach based on one-sample t statistics is no longer justified. In this case, however, a nonparametric approach such as the Wilcoxon signed-rank test procedure can be applied directly.

Let R_j be the rank of $|d_j|$, where $d_j \neq 0$, $j = 1, \ldots, n$. Also, let R_d be the sum of ranks, where $d_j > 0$, that is,

$$R_d = \sum_{j=1}^{n} R_j I(d_j > 0), \tag{3.7.10}$$

where

$$I(d_j > 0) = \begin{cases} 1, & \text{if } d_j > 0 \\ 0, & \text{otherwise.} \end{cases}$$

Thus we would reject the null hypothesis of (3.7.8) if

$$R_d > W(\tfrac{1}{2}\alpha) \quad \text{or} \quad R_d < W(1 - \tfrac{1}{2}\alpha),$$

where $W(\tfrac{1}{2}\alpha)$ is the $(\tfrac{1}{2}\alpha)$th upper quantile of the distribution of R_d with n' nonzero d_j and

$$W(\tfrac{1}{2}\alpha) = \frac{n'(n' + 1)}{2} - W(1 - \tfrac{1}{2}\alpha). \tag{3.7.11}$$

It is also of interest to examine whether the intraassay variability is the same for the two methods. We may formulate the hypotheses as follows:

$$H_0: \sigma_1^2 = \sigma_2^2 \quad \text{vs.} \quad H_a: \sigma_1^2 \neq \sigma_2^2, \tag{3.7.12}$$

To derive a test for (3.7.12), consider the preparation sum as

$$V_j = Z_{1j} + Z_{2j}, \quad j = 1, \ldots, n. \tag{3.7.13}$$

The bivariate random vector $\mathbf{b}_j = (d_j, V_j)$ are i.i.d. with mean vector

$$\mu_b = \begin{bmatrix} \tau_1 - \tau_2 \\ 2\mu \end{bmatrix}$$

and covariance matrix

$$\Sigma_b = \begin{bmatrix} \sigma_1^2 + \sigma_2^2 & \sigma_1^2 - \sigma_2^2 \\ \sigma_1^2 - \sigma_2^2 & 4\sigma_S^2 + \sigma_1^2 + \sigma_2^2 \end{bmatrix}.$$

It can be seen from the covariance matrix of $\mathbf{b}_j$ that the covariance between the preparation difference and sum is just the difference in intraassay variability between the two assay methods. Therefore, the null hypothesis of (3.7.12) for the equality between intraassay variabilities is equivalent to the hypothesis for testing the presence of correlation between d_j and V_j, that is,

$$H_0: \rho_{dV} = 0 \quad \text{vs.} \quad H_a: \rho_{dV} \neq 0. \tag{3.7.14}$$

Under model (3.7.6), the Pearson correlation coefficient between d_j and V_j is given by

$$r_{dV} = \frac{s_{dV}}{\sqrt{s_d^2 s_V^2}}, \tag{3.7.15}$$

where

$$s_V^2 = \frac{1}{n-1} \sum_{j=1}^{n} (V_j - \overline{V})^2,$$

$$s_{dV} = \frac{1}{n-1} \sum_{j=1}^{n} (d_j - \overline{d})(V_j - \overline{V}),$$

$$\overline{V} = \frac{1}{n} \sum_{j=1}^{n} V_j.$$

We then reject H_0 in (3.7.12) if

$$|T_{dV}| = \left| \frac{r_{dV}}{\sqrt{(1 - r_{dV}^2)/(n-1)}} \right| > t(\tfrac{1}{2}\alpha, n-1). \tag{3.7.16}$$

The test procedure above is referred to as the Pitman-Morgan test (Chow and Liu, 1992). Similarly, a nonparametric approach for testing hypotheses (3.7.12) is also available when the normality assumptions are not met.

Let $R(d_j)$ and $R(V_j)$ be the ranks of d_j and V_j in the sequence of $\{d_j, j = 1, \ldots, n\}$ and $\{V_j, j = 1, \ldots, n\}$, respectively. The Spearman's rank correlation coefficient r_S can be obtained by replacing d_j and V_j in (3.7.15) with their corresponding ranks $R(d_j)$ and $R(V_j)$, $j = 1, \ldots, n$, that is,

$$r_S = \frac{12 \sum_{j=1}^{n} [R(d_j) - (n+1)/2][R(V_j) - (n+1)/2]}{n(n^2 - 1)}. \tag{3.7.17}$$

We then reject H_0 in (3.7.1) if

$$|r_S| > r_S(\tfrac{1}{2}\alpha, n), \tag{3.7.18}$$

where $r_S(\tfrac{1}{2}\alpha, n)$ is the $(\tfrac{1}{2}\alpha)$th quantile of the distribution of Spearman's rank correlation coefficient based on n observations. For more details regarding ties and large-sample approximation to the Wilcoxon signed-rank test and Pearson's rank correlation coefficient, see Conover (1980).

In some cases it may be of interest to evaluate whether an alternative method is equivalent to the standard assay in terms of bias and intraassay variability. The statistical procedure described in the preceding section can be applied directly to test the equivalence of bias between the two methods with prespecified equivalence limits. For testing the equivalence of intraassay variability, the Pitman–Morgan two one-sided test procedure proposed by Chow and Liu (1992) can be used.

Example 3.7.2

The percent recovery given in Table 3.5.7 is used to illustrate the statistical methods for evaluation of the difference in bias and intraassay variability between two assay methods. For the purpose of illustration, the two different laboratories are treated as two different assay methods; laboratory 1 is considered as the alternative assay method and laboratory 2 is the standard assay. The sample mean and standard deviation of preparation differences are given by

$$\bar{d} = 1.389\% \quad \text{and} \quad s_d = 0.782\%.$$

Hence

$$|T_d| = 5.33 > t(0.025, 8) = 2.306.$$

As a result, the bias between the two assays is statistically significantly different.

Note that there is a positive bias in percent recovery between the alternative assay and the standard assay across all preparations. The sum of the ranks for the positive differences is given by

$$R_d = 45.$$

From Appendix A.1, the 97.5% upper quantile of the Wilcoxon signed-rank statistic for $n = 9$ is 6. Thus the 2.5% upper quantile of the Wilcoxon signed-rank statistic can be obtained as

$$W(0.025) = \frac{9(9 + 1)}{2} - 6 = 39.$$

Since

$$R_d = 45 > W(0.025) = 39,$$

the null hypothesis of (3.7.8) is rejected at the 5% level of significance. We also reach the same conclusion—that the biases of the two assay methods are not the same.

However, an interesting question concerns whether a mean difference of 1.389% in percent recovery really indicates that the two assay methods have different bias. In other words, it is of interest to ask whether the biases of the two assay methods are equivalent. The 95% confidence interval for the difference in bias between the two assay methods is (0.788%, 1.990%). If the limits for equivalence in bias are (−2.0%, 2.0%), the two methods are considered equivalent in bias even though the confidence interval does not contain zero.

From Table 3.5.7 it can be verified that

$$s_d^2 = 0.611, \quad s_V^2 = 13.375, \quad \text{and} \quad s_{dV}^2 = -0.396.$$

This leads to

$$r_{dV} = \frac{-0.396}{\sqrt{(0.611)(13.375)}} = -0.139,$$

$$T_{dV} = \frac{-0.139}{\sqrt{[1 - (0.139)^2]/(9 - 1)}} = -0.396.$$

Since

$$|T_{dV}| = 0.396 < 2.306 = t(0.025, 8),$$

we fail to reject the null hypothesis of equal intraassay variability at the 5% level of significance. It can also easily be verified that Spearman's rank correlation coefficient is given by $r_s = -0.209$ with a p value of 0.589. Similarly, we fail to reject the null hypothesis of no difference in intraassay variability between the two assay methods.

An alternative approach for comparing the two assay methods is based on the linearity. In other words, we may examine the estimated regression lines based on the amount recovered between the two systems. Hence, in essence, we need to test equality of intercepts and slopes as formulated in the following hypotheses:

$$H_{0I}: \alpha_1 = \alpha_2 \quad \text{vs.} \quad H_{aI}: \alpha_1 \neq \alpha_2, \tag{3.7.19}$$

$$H_{0S}: \beta_{11} = \beta_{12} \quad \text{vs.} \quad H_{aS}: \beta_{11} \neq \beta_{12},$$

where α_i and β_{1i} are the intercept and slope for method i, $i = 1,2$. Let a_i and b_{1i} be the least-square estimators of α_i and β_{1i} obtained from fitting a simple linear regression model to recovered amount separately for method i, respectively. Also, let $v(a_i)$ and $v(b_{1i})$ be the estimated variance of a_i and b_{1i}, respectively. Then the null hypothesis of H_{0Z} of (3.7.19) is rejected at the α level of significance if

$$|T_I| = \left| \frac{a_1 - a_2}{\sqrt{v(b_{01}) + v(b_{02})}} \right| > t(\tfrac{1}{2}\alpha, n_1 + n_2 - 4). \tag{3.7.20}$$

Similarly, the null hypothesis of equal slopes in (3.7.19) is rejected at the α level of significance if

$$|T_S| = \left| \frac{b_{11} - b_{12}}{\sqrt{v(b_{11}) + v(b_{12})}} \right| > t(\tfrac{1}{2}\alpha, n_1 + n_2 - 4). \tag{3.7.21}$$

Note that statistical testing procedures for equality between intercepts and slopes can also be obtained from the analysis of covariance (ANOCOV) with the following model:

$$Y_{ij} = \mu + \alpha_i + \beta_1 X_{ij} + (\alpha\beta_1)_i X_{ij} + e_{ij},$$

$$i = 1,2, \quad j = 1, \ldots, n, \quad (3.7.22)$$

where μ is the overall mean, α_i is the fixed effect of method i, β_1 is the common slope, $(\alpha\beta_1)_i$ is the method-by-slope interaction, and e_{ij} is the random error observing Y_{ij}. Thus $\mu + \alpha_i$ represents the intercept α_i of method i and $(\alpha\beta_1)_i$ is the difference in slopes between the two methods.

Model (3.7.22) can be easily be generalized to compare regression lines. The ANOCOV table is given in Table 3.7.2. Note that more details regarding the computations of estimates and various sums of squares can be found in Snedecor and Cochran (1980) and Wang and Chow (1994).

Example 3.7.3

For convenience, once again, we use the recovered amounts given in Table 3.5.7 to illustrate statistical methods for comparing the two regression lines described above. Table 3.7.3 gives least-squares estimates of intercepts and slopes and their corresponding standard errors. It can be seen from Table 3.7.3 that

$$|T_I| = 0.0092 \quad \text{and} \quad |T_S| = 0.220$$

with p values of 0.993 and 0.828, respectively. Therefore, the results indicate that neither intercepts nor slopes are different in the regression model between the two assay methods.

3.7.3. Sample-Size Determination

As mentioned in Sec. 3.6, when a recovery study is conducted to assess the accuracy and precision of an assay at the same time, it is difficult to determine a required sample size for a desired statistical power. However, the sample size for a recovery study can be determined based on the equivalence hypotheses

TABLE 3.7.2 ANOCOV Table for Model In (3.7.20)

Source of variation	df	Test
Method	1 [or $(I - 1)^a$]	Equality of intercepts
Slope	1	Common slope = 0
Method-by-slope interaction	1 [or $(I - 1)^a$]	Equality of slopes
Error	$n - 4$ [or $n - 2I$]	

[a]If there is a total of I methods.

TABLE 3.7.3 Comparison of Regression Line on Recovered Amount in Table 3.5.7

Parameter		Method 1	Method 2	Difference
Intercept	Estimate	−0.02644	−0.02700	−0.00056
	Standard error	0.04319	0.04285	0.06084
	t statistic	−0.612	−0.630	−0.0092
	p value	0.5597	0.5486	0.9928
Slope	Estimate	1.0433	1.0300	0.0133
	Standard error	0.04262	0.04286	0.06044
	t statistic	24.478	24.358	0.2200
	p value	<0.0001	<0.0001	0.8275

given in (3.7.1) for assessment of accuracy provided that there is some prior information regarding the upper bound of the variability.

Let σ^2 be the upper bound of the variance that is obtained from previous experiments. Also, let μ_z and $100 \pm \Delta$ be the true unknown average for percent recovery and lower and upper (symmetric) limits for assessment of accuracy. Then the sample size required for achieving at least $(1 - \beta)$ power at the α level of significance for the equivalence hypotheses is given by

$$
n_0 \geq [t(\alpha, n - 1) + t(\tfrac{1}{2}\beta, n - 1)]^2 \left(\frac{\sigma}{\Delta}\right)^2 \qquad \text{if } \mu_z = 100;
$$

$$
n_I \geq [t(\alpha, n - 1) + t(\beta, n - 1)]^2 \left(\frac{\sigma}{\Delta - \mu_z}\right)^2 \qquad \text{if } \mu \neq 100.
$$

(3.7.23)

Since the degrees of freedom in (3.7.23) is unknown, a numerical iterative procedure is required for obtaining n_0 and n_I.

To illustrate (3.7.23), consider Example 3.3.1. It can be verified from Table 3.3.1 that the estimates of μ_z and σ_z are given by 102.5 and 4.615, respectively. If Δ is chosen to be 5%, it requires 23 preparations to achieve 80% power for the equivalence hypotheses at the 5% level of significance.

In the assessment of accuracy and precision, the added amounts of the active ingredients are assumed known and fixed. In practice, the added amounts of active ingredients might be contaminated with measurement errors. Therefore, strictly speaking, the added amounts should be treated as random variables. In this case, statistical test procedures based on some functional models in measurement error models might be useful (Fuller, 1988). However, it should be noted that most statistical methods for measurement error models are for large samples (e.g., more than 30 preparations per study). For small samples, more research on statistical methods for measurement error models is needed.

4

Scaleup Design and Analysis

4.1. INTRODUCTION

In the pharmaceutical industry it is important to ensure that a production batch can meet the USP/NF standards for the identity, strength, quality, and purity of the drug before a batch of the product is released to the market. Although a number of product tests, such as potency and dissolution testing, may be conducted for this purpose, these tests are usually done based on samples from a laboratory batch or small-scale production batch. In practice it is not clear whether the results from such a laboratory batch or small-scale production batch can be predictive of a regular scale-of-production batch. In this case, a scaleup experiment is usually employed to evaluate the drug product when the batch is scaled up according to a preplanned scaleup program.

The purpose of a scaleup program is not only to identify, evaluate, and optimize critical formulation and/or (manufacturing) process factors of the drug product but also to maximize or minimize excipient ranges. A successful scaleup program can result in an improvement in formulation/process or at least a recommendation on a revised procedure for formulation/process of the drug product. A scaleup program is extremely useful in the development of a formulation or process that helps to reduce the cost within a fixed time frame. It can be applied to various manufacturing processes, such as solid formulation (e.g., tablets, capsules), liquid formulation (e.g., solution), and coating. In addition, a scaleup program can also be applied to evaluate the equipment used in the production line.

To ensure a successful scaleup program, selection of an appropriate scale-up design is essential to achieve the desired objectives. Scaleup designs include screening designs and optimization designs. Different types of designs may be used, depending on whether or not the basic formulation is satisfactory. If the basic formulation is satisfactory, a screening design is usually conducted. The objective of a screening design is not only to study critical process factors but also to determine operating ranges. In many cases it is necessary to test a rather large number of factors that may have important effects on the response variables, especially when little is known about the performance of the factors. In practice, since it is realistic to postulate that only a few of the factors will be of importance, a typical 2^{K-P} fractional factorial design (Box and Hunter, 1961a,b) is usually considered. Other designs, such as the Plackett and Burman design (Plackett and Burman, 1946), factorials in the split-plot design, and the randomized block design (Box et al., 1978) are sometimes considered. When the basic formulation is not all right, it is necessary to conduct an optimization design to estimate the response surface and consequently, to identify levels of formulation and process factors that optimize formulation and process. Typically, a central composite design is employed to achieve these objectives. In some cases, however, factorial designs and Box–Behnken designs (Box and Behnken, 1960) are considered as useful optimization designs.

The remainder of this chapter is organized as follows. In the next section we provide a brief review of some useful experimental designs for scaleup. In Sec. 4.3 we introduce a scaleup program through an example concerning the identification of formulation and process factors in tablet manufacture of a drug product. Also included in this section are applications of some useful screening and optimization designs for a scaleup program. In Sec. 4.4 we discuss statistical methods for analysis of various scaleup designs. In Sec. 4.5 some related statistical issues are discussed briefly.

4.2. EXPERIMENTAL DESIGNS

As indicated earlier, the primary objective of a scaleup program is to identify and evaluate critical factors that optimize formulation and process in drug development and manufacture. To achieve this objective, selection of an appropriate design is critical. In this section we provide a brief review of some useful experimental designs for scaleup. Before we do that, it is helpful to introduce two statistical concepts of the interaction and confounding effects.

4.2.1. Interaction and Confounding Effects

Confounding effects are defined as effects, which are contributed by various factors, that cannot be separated by the design under study. To provide a better idea, consider the following example. Last year, Mrs. Anderson noticed that her winter heating bill was extremely high. Mrs. Anderson suspected that the high heating bill might be caused by the poor insulation of her house and thus decided to upgrade the insulation. As a result, there was a significant decrease in this year's winter heating bill. However, this winter was not as cold as last winter, thus it is not clear whether the reduced heating bill was due to the improved insulation or the warmer winter. As a matter of fact, we are unable to separate the effect due to the improved insulation from the effect due to the warmer winter. In this case, the two effects are said to be confounded (or aliased) with respect to each other. Therefore, to study critical factors that may have an impact on the response, we need to select an appropriate design that can separate the possible confounding effects.

The interaction effect between factors is defined as the joint effect contributed by more than one factor. To introduce the concept of interaction, consider the following example. Suppose that a laboratory analyst was interested in evaluating the function of new equipment as compared to old equipment. An experiment was conducted to test the two types of equipment in both the morning and afternoon. In this experiment we have two factors. One is the equipment and the other is time (morning and afternoon). The results turned out that the new equipment performs better in the morning, whereas the old equipment functions better in the afternoon. It is clear that the difference between the two types of equipment is not consistent across time (morning and afternoon). In this case the two factors are said to have an interaction. It should be noted that when a significant interaction between factors is observed in data analysis, no statistical inference on the main effect can be made.

To illustrate the interaction and confounding effects, it is helpful to consider the following example. Suppose that we have four factors, X_1, X_2, X_3, and X_4, each at two levels, denoted by "-1" and "1," respectively. The arrangement of eight experimental runs is given in Table 4.2.1. To study whether there

TABLE 4.2.1 Factorial Experiment

Run	X_1	X_2	X_3	X_4	X_1X_2	X_3X_4	Response
1	+	+	+	+	+	+	Y_1
2	+	+	−	−	+	+	Y_2
3	+	−	+	−	−	−	Y_3
4	+	−	−	+	−	−	Y_4
5	−	+	+	−	−	−	Y_5
6	−	+	−	+	−	−	Y_6
7	−	−	+	+	+	+	Y_7
8	−	−	−	−	+	+	Y_8

is an interaction between X_1 and X_2, we may rearrange Table 4.2.1 as follows:

		Factor X_2	
		-1	1
Factor X_1	-1	Y_7, Y_8	Y_5, Y_6
	1	Y_3, Y_4	Y_1, Y_2

From the 2×2 table above, the effect of changing X_1 from level -1 to level 1 at level -1 of X_2 can be measured by

$$\frac{Y_3 + Y_4}{2} - \frac{Y_7 + Y_8}{2}.$$

Similarly, the effect of changing X_1 from level -1 to level 1 at level 1 of X_2 can be obtained as

$$\frac{Y_1 + Y_2}{2} - \frac{Y_5 + Y_6}{2}.$$

Therefore, the interaction between X_1 and X_2 can be examined by

$$\left(\frac{Y_1 + Y_2}{2} - \frac{Y_5 + Y_6}{2} \right) - \left(\frac{Y_3 + Y_4}{2} - \frac{Y_7 + Y_8}{2} \right)$$

$$= \tfrac{1}{2} (Y_1 + Y_2 - Y_3 - Y_4 - Y_5 - Y_6 + Y_7 + Y_8). \quad (4.2.1)$$

A large value of (4.2.1) is strong evidence of the presence of an interaction effect between X_1 and X_2. Figure 4.2.1 provides a hypothetical scenario of the interaction effect between X_1 and X_2. For example, if the relationship between X_1 and X_2 is as shown by the dashed line, there is an interaction between X_1 and X_2. On the other hand, if the changes of X_1 from level -1 to level 1 are consistent across the levels of X_2 (as shown by the solid line), there is no interaction. Note that (4.2.1) can also be obtained by taking the sum of the products between the elements of column Y and the corresponding elements of column $X_1 X_2$ in Table 4.2.1 and dividing this sum by 2. We will then use $X_1 X_2$ to denote the interaction between X_1 and X_2.

Similarly, the interaction between X_3 and X_4 can be obtained by means of the following 2×2 table:

		Factor X_4	
		-1	1
Factor X_3	-1	Y_2, Y_8	Y_4, Y_6
	1	Y_3, Y_5	Y_1, Y_7

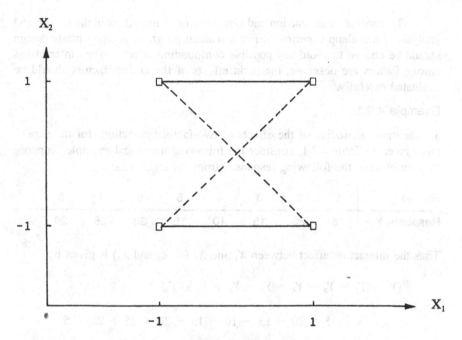

FIGURE 4.2.1 Examination of interaction between X_1 and X_2.

It can be seen from the table above that the changes in X_3 from level -1 to level 1 at levels -1 and 1 of X_4 are given by

$$\left(\frac{Y_3 + Y_5}{2} - \frac{Y_2 + Y_8}{2}\right) \quad \text{and} \quad \left(\frac{Y_1 + Y_7}{2} - \frac{Y_4 + Y_6}{2}\right),$$

respectively. Therefore, the interaction between X_3 and X_4 is given by

$$\left(\frac{Y_1 + Y_7}{2} - \frac{Y_4 + Y_6}{2}\right) - \left(\frac{Y_3 + Y_5}{2} - \frac{Y_2 + Y_8}{2}\right)$$

$$= \tfrac{1}{2}(Y_1 + Y_2 - Y_3 - Y_4 - Y_5 - Y_6 + Y_7 + Y_8). \quad (4.2.2)$$

It is interesting to note that (4.2.1) and (4.2.2) are identical. In this case, interaction between X_1 and X_2 is confounded with the interaction between X_3 and X_4. The existence of the confounding effects between two-factor interactions in the experiment given in Table 4.2.1 is not surprising. It can be seen from Table 4.2.1 that there are only eight observations all together. It is impossible to have independent estimates for four main effects and six two-factor interactions.

The concept of interaction and confounding is important in the design and analysis of a scaleup experiment. For a scaleup program, an appropriate design should be chosen to avoid any possible confounding effects. When interactions among factors are observed, the main effects of the critical factors should be evaluated carefully.

Example 4.2.1

To illustrate calculation of the effects of two-factor interactions for the experiment given in Table 4.2.1, consider the following numerical example. Suppose that we observe the following responses from the eight runs:

Run no.	1	2	3	4	5	6	7	8
Response Y	15	20	15	10	15	30	25	20

Thus the interaction effect between X_1 and X_2 (or X_3 and X_4) is given by

$$\tfrac{1}{2}(Y_1 + Y_2 - Y_3 - Y_4 - Y_5 - Y_6 + Y_7 + Y_8)$$

$$= \tfrac{1}{2}(15 + 20 - 15 - 10 - 15 - 30 + 25 + 20) = 5.$$

As a matter of fact, 5 is an estimate of the sum of the effects of the two interactions (i.e., the interaction between X_1 and X_2 and the interaction between X_3 and X_4). If one interaction is known to be negligible, 5 can be used to estimate the effect of the other interaction alone.

4.2.2. Factorial Designs

A full factorial design is a design that consists of all possible different combinations of one level from each factor. If there are ℓ_k levels for the kth factor X_k, the corresponding full factorial design is called a general $\ell_1\ell_2\cdots\ell_k$ factorial design. When $\ell_i = 2$ (or 3) for all i, the general factorial design is called a 2^K (or 3^K) factorial design. A 2^K (or 3^K) factorial design denotes a full factorial design at two levels (or at three levels). In practice, a factorial design is expressed in terms of a number of arrays (or runs) that indicate the levels of each factor. For example, Table 4.2.2 lists the arrangement of a typical 2^4 factorial design in *standard order*. This means that the first column of the design matrix consists of successive minus ($-$) and plus ($+$) signs, the second column of successive pairs of $-$ and $+$ signs, the third column of four $-$ signs followed by four $+$ signs, and so on. In general, the Kth column consists of 2^{K-1} $-$ signs followed by 2^{K-1} $+$ signs.

In this 2^4 factorial design, there are four factors at two levels, with a total of $N = 2^4 = 16$ runs. The two levels of each factor are conventionally denoted

TABLE 4.2.2 2^4 Factorial Design

	Design matrix				
Run	X_1	X_2	X_3	X_4	Y
1	−	−	−	−	Y_1
2	+	−	−	−	Y_2
3	−	+	−	−	Y_3
4	+	+	−	−	Y_4
5	−	−	+	−	Y_5
6	+	−	+	−	Y_6
7	−	+	+	−	Y_7
8	+	+	+	−	Y_8
9	−	−	−	+	Y_9
10	+	−	−	+	Y_{10}
11	−	+	−	+	Y_{11}
12	+	+	−	+	Y_{12}
13	−	−	+	+	Y_{13}
14	+	−	+	+	Y_{14}
15	−	+	+	+	Y_{15}
16	+	+	+	+	Y_{16}

by + and − (they are sometimes denoted by 1 and −1). If a variable is continuous, the two levels, + and −, denote the high and low levels. If a variable is qualitative, the two levels may denote two different types or the presence and absence of the variable. Each row represents a different combination of one level from each factor. For example, row 3 indicates that the experiment is to be performed at the high level of factor X_2 and at low levels of factors X_1, X_3, and X_4. In this section, unless otherwise stated, we focus on a 2^K factorial design. Other factorial designs, such as the 3^K factorial design, can be treated similarly.

Let $\bar{Y}_i$, $i = 1, \ldots, N$, be the average response obtained from the *ith* run, for a combination of a 2^K factorial design, where $N = 2^K$. A linear contrast for a 2^K factorial design is defined as a linear combination of $\bar{Y}_1, \ldots, \bar{Y}_N$. That is,

$$\ell = \sum_{i=1}^{N} c_i \bar{Y}_i$$
$$= c_1\bar{Y}_1 + \cdots + c_N\bar{Y}_N,$$

where

$$\sum_{i=1}^{N} c_i = 0.$$

Two linear combinations of $\bar{Y}_i$, $i = 1, \ldots, N$, are said to be *orthogonal* to each other if the sum of the cross products of the coefficients of the two contrasts is 0. In other words, let

$$\ell_1 = \sum_{i=1}^{N} c_{1i}\bar{Y}_{1i} \quad \text{and} \quad \ell_2 = \sum_{i=1}^{N} c_{2i}\bar{Y}_{2i}$$

be two contrasts; then ℓ_1 and ℓ_2 are said to be orthogonal if

$$\sum_{i=1}^{N} c_{1i}c_{2i} = 0.$$

The variance of a contrast based on $\bar{Y}_i$ from a 2^K factorial experiment with n runs for each combination is given by

$$\text{var}(\ell) = \frac{\sigma^2}{n} \sum_{i=1}^{N} c_i^2.$$

For a 2^K factorial design, it can be seen from Table 4.2.2 that the design matrix contains K columns and $N = 2^K$ rows. There are a total of $2^K - 1$ effects to be estimated, which are summarized in Table 4.2.3. Under the assumption that the responses Y_i, $i = 1, \ldots, N$, are uncorrelated and have equal variance σ^2, the full 2^K factorial designs provide independent minimum variance unbiased estimates (MVUE) for the $2^K - 1$ effects, which are orthogonal contrasts based

TABLE 4.2.3 Summary of Effects from a 2^4 Factorial Design

Type of effects	Number of effects
Main	K
Two-factor interaction	$\dfrac{K(K-1)}{2}$
Three-factor interaction	$\dfrac{K(K-1)(K-2)}{6}$
.	.
.	.
.	.
h-factor interaction	$\dfrac{K(K-1)(K-2)\cdots(K-h+1)}{h!}$
.	.
.	.
.	.
K-factor interaction	1
Total	$2^K - 1$

on Y_i. For example, we may measure the change in the response from the $-$ (low) to the $+$ (high) of each factor based on Y_i, $i = 1, \ldots, 16$. For the first factor, X_1, the change in response can be measured by individual measures of the effect of changing X_1 from $-$ to $+$ (i.e., $Y_{2i} - Y_i$, $i = 1, \ldots, 8$; $2i = 2, 4, 6, \ldots, 16$). The average of these eight measures, which is given by

$$\frac{1}{8} \sum_{i=1}^{8} (Y_{2i} - Y_i) = \frac{1}{8} \sum_{i=1}^{8} Y_{2i} - \frac{1}{8} \sum_{i=1}^{8} Y_i,$$

is called the main effect of X_1, which measures the average effect of X_1 over all conditions of other factors.

Similar to the example given in Sec. 4.2.1, the effects of two- or three-factor interaction among factors can also be evaluated. For example, the interaction between X_1 and X_2 can be measured by taking the sum of the cross products between the elements of column Y and the corresponding elements of the column X_1 and dividing this sum by $N/2$, where $N = 2^K$. Under the normality assumption, each estimated effect has variance $4\sigma^2/N$, where σ^2 is the variance of the individual observation. Table 4.2.4 lists independent variables, including the two- and three-factor interactions for a 2^4 factorial design.

Note that the complete factorial design provides estimates not only for main effects but also for interactions with maximum precision. The main effects and interaction effects can easily be obtained using a table of contrast coefficients and/or Yates's algorithm, described in Sec. 4.4. The details of analysis of factorial designs can be found in many statistical texts [see, e.g., John (1971), Myers (1976), and Box et al. (1978)].

4.2.3. Fractional Factorial Designs

A fractional factorial design is a design that consists of a fraction of a full factorial experiment. For example, a $(1/2^P$ fraction of a 2^K factorial design is called a 2^{K-P} fractional factorial design. When $P = 1$, a full factorial design reduces to a one-half factorial design.

As discussed in Sec. 4.2.2, for a full 2^4 factorial design there are 16 effects, including the grand average, four main effects, six two-factor interactions, four three-factor interactions, and a single four-factor interaction. The full 2^4 factorial design contains 16 observations, which provide independent estimates for each of these 16 effects. However, if we consider only a one-half fraction (i.e., only eight observations available), due to limited resources available, it is impossible to obtain 16 independent estimates. For a 2^{4-1} fractional factorial design, the eight observations cannot provide independent estimates for the 16 effects alone but for some confounding effects, such as the sum of a main effect and a three-factor interaction that are confounded with each other. In practice, however, the three-factor or higher-factor interactions are usually negligible. In this case a

TABLE 4.2.4   Matrix of Independent Variables for a 2^4 Factorial Design

Run	I	1	2	12	3	13	23	123	4	14	24	124	34	134	234	1234
1	+	−	−	+	−	+	+	−	−	+	+	−	+	−	−	+
2	+	+	−	−	−	−	+	+	−	−	+	+	+	+	−	−
3	+	−	+	−	−	+	−	+	−	+	−	+	+	−	+	−
4	+	+	+	+	−	−	−	−	−	−	−	−	+	+	+	+
5	+	−	−	+	+	−	−	+	−	+	+	−	−	+	+	−
6	+	+	−	−	+	+	−	−	−	−	+	+	−	−	+	+
7	+	−	+	−	+	−	+	−	−	+	−	+	−	+	−	+
8	+	+	+	+	+	+	+	+	−	−	−	−	−	−	−	−
9	+	−	−	+	−	+	+	−	+	−	−	+	−	+	+	−
10	+	+	−	−	−	−	+	+	+	+	−	−	−	−	+	+
11	+	−	+	−	−	+	−	+	+	−	+	−	−	+	−	+
12	+	+	+	+	−	−	−	−	+	+	+	+	−	−	−	−
13	+	−	−	+	+	−	−	+	+	−	−	+	+	−	−	+
14	+	+	−	−	+	+	−	−	+	+	−	−	+	+	−	−
15	+	−	+	−	+	−	+	−	+	−	+	−	+	−	+	−
16	+	+	+	+	+	+	+	+	+	+	+	+	+	+	+	+

fractional factorial design is useful in estimating the main effects. In the following, for simplicity, we introduce how to construct a one-half fraction of a 2^4 factorial design (i.e., a 2^{4-1} fractional factorial design).

Since a full 2^3 factorial design consists of a total of eight runs, we may use these eight runs to construct a one-half 2^4 factorial design that also contains a total of eight runs. The main effect of the fourth factor can be obtained by multiplying the elements of the first three factors. The design matrix of a 2^{4-1} fractional factor design is given in Table 4.2.5. It can be seen from Table 4.2.4 that the combination of observations used to estimate the main effect of X_4 is identical to that used to estimate the three-factor (i.e., $X_1X_2X_3$) interaction. The main effect of X_4 is confounded with the interaction effect of $X_1X_2X_3$. Therefore, the combination of observations for the column of $X_4 = X_1X_2X_3$ really estimates the sum of the effects of X_4 and $X_1X_2X_3$.

From Table 4.2.5 it can easily be verified that each main effect is confounded with a three-factor interaction effect, and each two-factor interaction effect is confounded with another two-factor interaction effect. In summary, for a 2^{4-1} fractional factorial design, we have the following confounding effects:

One-factor vs. three-factor	Two-factor vs. two-factor
$X_1 = X_2X_3X_4$	$X_1X_2 = X_3X_4$
$X_2 = X_1X_3X_4$	$X_1X_3 = X_2X_4$
$X_3 = X_1X_2X_4$	$X_1X_4 = X_2X_3$
$X_4 = X_1X_2X_3$	

Note that Box and Hunter (1961a,b) classified a 2^{4-1} fractional factorial design as a resolution IV design. A design of resolution R is one in which no P-factor

TABLE 4.2.5 Construction of a 2^{4-1} Fractional Factorial Design

Run	Design matrix				
	X_1	X_2	X_3	$X_4 = X_1X_2X_3$	Y
1	−	−	−	−	Y_1
2	+	−	−	+	Y_2
3	−	+	−	+	Y_3
4	+	+	−	−	Y_4
5	−	−	+	+	Y_5
6	+	−	+	−	Y_6
7	−	+	+	−	Y_7
8	+	+	+	+	Y_8

effect is confounded with any other effect containing fewer than $R - P$ factors. For the 2^{4-1} fractional factorial design, no main effect is confounded with any other main effect or two-factor interaction. However, two-factor interactions are confounded with one another. Thus the 2^{4-1} fractional factorial design is of resolution IV. In this case, the 2^{4-1} fractional factorial design is sometimes denoted as 2_{IV}^{4-1}. It can easily be verified that the one-half fraction of 2^3 and 2^5 factorial designs are designs of resolution III and V, that is, 2_{III}^{3-1} and 2_{V}^{5-1}, respectively.

For the construction of a $(1/2)^P$ fractional factorial design, Box and Hunter (1961a,b) suggested using a *defining relation* as a generator of the design. For example, for the construction of the 2^{4-1} fractional factorial design, the design is basically accomplished by inducing the equality

$$X_4 = X_1X_2X_3,$$

where the multiplication product $X_1X_2X_3$ refers to the multiplication of the individual elements in the corresponding columns X_1, X_2, and X_3 given in Table 4.2.5. Multiplying both sides of the equality above by X_4 yields

$$I = X_4X_4 = X_1X_2X_3X_4,$$

where I denotes a column of plus signs. The equality $I = X_1X_2X_3X_4$ is called the *defining relation* of the 2^{4-1} fractional factorial design. Based on this defining relation, all of the confounding effects listed above can be determined. For example, to obtain the confounding effect between the main effect X_1 and the three-factor interaction effect $X_2X_3X_4$, we multiply both sides of the defining relation by X_1. This gives

$$X_1 = X_1^2X_2X_3X_4 = X_2X_3X_4.$$

Note that $X_i^2 = I$ for all i and that each effect times I is equal to itself. Similarly, it can easily be verified that the defining relations for the one-half fraction of 2^3 and 2^5 fractional factorial designs are $I = X_1X_2X_3$ and $I = X_1X_2X_3X_4X_5$, respectively.

As can be seen, a fractional factorial design is useful when there are many factors to be studied. In practice, it is almost impossible to perform a full factorial design even at two levels. For example, if there are five factors, a full 2^5 factorial design requires 32 runs. Instead, only a total of 16 runs is needed if a 2^{5-1} fractional factorial design is considered. However, the fractional factorial design suffers from the confounding effects. In practice, it is then important to evaluate whether the effects of interest are confounded with other effects before a fractional factorial design is conducted. Note that more details regarding the 2^{K-P} fractional factorial design can be found in Box and Hunter (1961a,b) and John (1971).

4.2.4. Central Composite Design

A central composite design is a full factorial design or a fractional factorial design augmented by a $\pm\alpha$ level at each of the K factors and n central points. As an example, Table 4.2.6 gives the design matrix for a central composite design with $K = 3$ and $n = 1$. This central composite design consists of one center point, eight points on the cube (a 2^3 factorial arrangement), and six star points (see also Fig. 4.2.2). Note that a central composite design with $K = 2$, $\alpha = 1$, and $n = 1$ reduces to a 3^2 factorial design.

For a full 2^K factorial design, although the design provides independent estimates for the $2^K - 1$ effects, it does not give an estimate of the experimental error unless some runs are repeated. Unlike the full 2^K factorial design, the central composite design provides an estimate of the experimental error. The experimental error is usually estimated based on n observations at the center point.

A design is said to be *rotatable* if the variance of the predicted response $\hat{Y}$ at some points is a function only of the distance of the point from the design center and not a function of direction [i.e., $\text{var}(\hat{Y})$ is constant on spheres centered at the center of the design]. Therefore, the variance of $\hat{Y}$ of a rotatable design remains unchanged when the design is rotated about the center point. A central composite design can be made rotatable by choosing α to be

$$\alpha = (2^K)^{1/4}.$$

TABLE 4.2.6 Central Composite Design for $K = 3$ and $n = 1$

Run	X_1	X_2	X_3
1	-1	-1	-1
2	1	-1	-1
3	-1	1	-1
4	1	1	-1
5	-1	-1	1
6	1	-1	1
7	-1	1	1
8	1	1	1
9	0	0	0
10	α	0	0
11	$-\alpha$	0	0
12	0	α	0
13	0	$-\alpha$	0
14	0	0	$-\alpha$
15	0	0	$-\alpha$

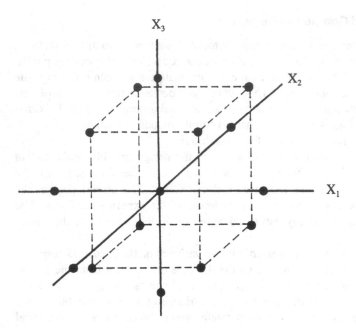

FIGURE 4.2.2   Central composite design for $K = 3$ and $n = 1$.

For example, if $K = 3$, the value of α rotatability is given by

$$\alpha = (2^3)^{1/4} = 1.682.$$

A design is said to be orthogonal if the off-diagonal elements of the sum of the cross products between any two columns of the design matrix is zero. A central composite design can be made orthogonal if α is chosen to be

$$\alpha = \left(\frac{QN}{4}\right)^{1/4},$$

where N is the number of factorial points,

$$Q = [N + T]^{1/2} - N^{1/2}]^2,$$
$$T = 2K + n,$$

which is the number of points added to the factorial. As is clear from the discussion above, the choice of α depends on the property desired, such as orthogonality and/or rotatability, which can be obtained in the design. Table 4.2.7 summarizes various choices of α for central composite designs.

When there are replications at each of the center, factorial, and star points, the central composite design can also be made rotatable or orthogonal by choos-

TABLE 4.2.7 Various Choices of α for
Central Composite Design

	α for:	
K	Orthogonality	Rotatability
2	1.000	1.414
3	1.216	1.682
4	1.414	2.000
5	1.596	2.378
6	1.761	2.828
7	1.910	3.363
8	2.045	3.999

ing appropriate α. Let a and b be the numbers of replicates at factorial and star points. Formulas for α to achieve orthogonal or rotatable composite designs are given by (Draper, 1985)

$$\alpha = \left\{ \frac{[aN(aN + 2bK + n)]^{1/2} - aN}{2b} \right\}^{1/2} \quad \text{(orthogonality)},$$

$$\alpha = \left(\frac{aN}{b} \right)^{1/4} \quad \text{(rotatability)},$$

respectively.

4.2.5. Other Designs

In addition to the factorial design, the fractional factorial design, and the central composite design, other designs, such as the Plackett and Burman design and the factorial or fractional factorial in randomized block design, are also useful in scaleup experiments. These two designs are outlined briefly below.

For a 2^K factorial design or a 2^{K-P} fractional factorial design, the total number of experimental runs is $N = 2^K$ or 2^{K-P}, which is a power of 2. Plackett and Burman (1946) provided a series of two-level fractional factorial designs for examining $N - 1$ factors in N runs where N is a multiple of 4, where $N \leq 100$. The Plackett and Burman designs allow unbiased estimation of all $N - 1$ main effects with the smallest possible variance. Plackett and Burman (1946) also gave design matrices for these designs for 4 up to 100 except for the case of $N = 92$. The design for the case $N = 92$ was given subsequently by Baumert et al. (1962). Box and Hunter (1961a) indicated that Plackett and Burman's design is identical to one of the resolution III designs. In other words, no main effect is confounded with any other main effect, but main effects are confounded with two-factor interactions and two-factor interactions with one another. In recent years, however, the properties of augmenting projected Plackett and Burman designs with a few additional factorial runs have been studied by Draper (1985), Draper and Lin (1990), and Lin and Draper (1992).

In a factorial or fractional factorial experiment, it is desirable to have all of the experiment runs under conditions that are as homogeneous as possible. In practice, however, it may not be possible to generate too many batches using one V-blender, due to the size and capability of the V-blender. Suppose that the V-blender can accommodate half of the batches for the experiment. In this case the experiment is in fact arranged in two blocks (the V-blender is the blocking factor). A design of this kind is called a factorial or fractional factorial in randomized block design. The use of blocks can ensure that the main effects are much more precisely measured because of the homogeneity within blocks. However, the main effects are confounded with the blender effect if the same number of runs are used. In general, we cannot estimate the blocking effect separately from other high-order interactions.

4.3. SCALEUP PROGRAM AND DESIGNS

4.3.1. Scaleup Program

During the development of a drug product, a number of tests are usually performed to ensure the identity, strength, quality, and purity of the drug product. However, these tests are based primarily on a laboratory batch or a small-scale production batch. It is then of particular interest to see whether the results from a laboratory batch or small scale of production batch is predictive of a regular-scale production batch. To ensure that a production batch will maintain the same identity, strength, quality, and purity of the drug product, a scaleup program is necessary.

A scaleup program involves the identification of critical formulation and process factors, evaluation of the equipment involved in the production, and the optimization of response variables. The purposes of a scaleup program are not only to evaluate and optimize critical formulation and process factors of the drug product but also to maximize and minimize excipient ranges. A successful scaleup program can result in an improvement in formulation and process or at least recommendations on a revised procedure for formulation and process.

To provide a better understanding, as an example, consider a scaleup program for the manufacture of tablets of a pharmaceutical compound. Table 4.3.1 lists six possible critical factors that may have an impact on tablet formulation. For example, disintegrant may cause tablets to break apart. To identify and optimize critical factors (or major factors) that affect tablet formulation, appropriate scaleup designs are usually conducted. After the critical formulation fac-

TABLE 4.3.1   Critical Formulation Factors for Tablet Formulation

Formulation factor	Description
Diluent	Bulking agent (lactose)
Binder	"Glues" powder together to form granules (acacia cellulose)
Lubricant	Prevent friction and wear (magnesium stearate)
Glidant	Improve flow (talc)
Antiadherent	Prevent granulations or materials from sticking to faces at punches and die walls (talc)
Disintegrant	Causes tablets to break apart (starch)

tors are identified, we may move on to evaluate and optimize critical process factors. To identify critical process factors for tablet manufacturing, it is helpful to have an understanding of the manufacturing process. The manufacturing process for tablets is described in Fig. 4.3.1. As can be seen from the figure, the process includes wet granulation, slugging, and direct compression of tablets. Studying the process given in Fig. 4.3.1, possible critical process factors are identified which are summarized in Table 4.3.2.

Another primary objective of a scaleup program is to optimize the range of the response with respect to the critical formulation/process factors identified. Table 4.3.3 lists some responses of particular interest in the manufacture of tablets. These responses are to be optimized to meet the USP/NF standards for identity, strength, quality, and purity of the drug product.

To achieve the objectives of a scaleup program, an appropriate scaleup design is critical. Scaleup designs may be classified into two different types of designs: screening designs and optimization designs, depending on the objectives of the design. In the following section these two types of designs are discussed.

4.3.2.   Scaleup Design

In general, the primary objectives of a scaleup design can be summarized as follows:

1. Maximize information with a minimal cost.
2. Determine effects of critical formulation and process factors efficiently.
3. Provide an organized approach.
4. Determine optimum ranges.
5. Answer future questions.

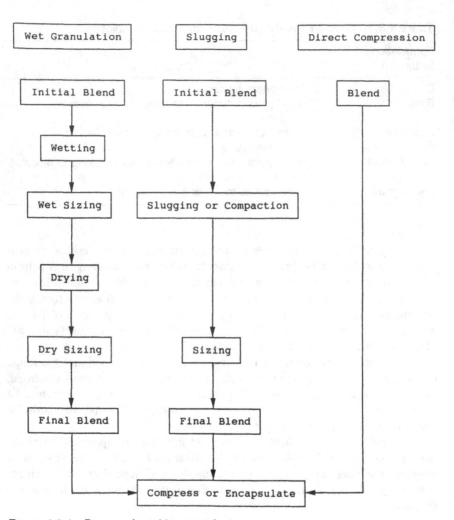

FIGURE 4.3.1   Process for tablet manufacture.

As indicated earlier, when there is little information about the critical formulation and process factors, a large number of formulation and process factors are necessarily tested. In practice, it is too time consuming and/or costly to conduct a large-scale experiment to study all possible critical factors. In addition, the experimenter may not have the capability for a large-scale experiment due to the limited resources available. It is then important to obtain maximum information with minimal cost within a fixed time frame. This objective may be

TABLE 4.3.2 Critical Process
Factors for Tablet Manufacturing

Blender
Use of preblending
Granulating water level
Granulating blending procedure
Granulating blending time
Wet screen size
Drying conditions
Dry screen size
Slug hardness
Roll speed
Degree of compaction
Lubricant blending time

achieved by choosing an appropriate study design. An appropriate design can not only avoid possible interaction and confounding effects but also provide estimates of the effects of critical factors efficiently. Based on estimates of the effects of the critical factors, we can determine the optimal ranges for each factor under the design selected. The information can be used to improve the formulation and process. Moreover, this information is extremely useful in future planning of similar studies.

Scaleup designs include screening designs and optimization designs. Screening designs are usually considered when the basic formulation is satisfactory. When the basic formulation is not all right, optimization designs are employed. In the following we provide some ideas as to what designs are suitable for screening and what designs are useful for optimization. The designs considered here were reviewed in Sec. 4.2.

The objectives of a screening design are not only to study the critical factors but also to determine operating ranges, if possible, provided that the

TABLE 4.3.3 Response Variables of
Tablet Manufacturing

Particle size	Ejection force
Flow	Dissolution
Bulk density	Weight variation
Moisture	Disintegration
Hardness	Friability

basic formulation and process are satisfactory. Typically, a fractional factorial design with two or three levels may be used to achieve these objectives in the following situations (Box and Hunter, 1961a):

1. Where certain interactions can be assumed nonexistent from prior knowledge
2. Where it is expected that the effects of all but a few of the factors under study will be negligible
3. Where groups of experiments are run in sequence and ambiguities remaining at a given stage of experimentation can be resolved by later group of experiments
4. Where certain factors are to be studied simultaneously with other factors whose influence can be described by main effects only

In addition, several other designs, such as the Plackett and Burman design, factorials in the split-plot design, and the randomized block design are also useful for screening in a scaleup program.

When the basic formulation or process is not satisfactory, we may conduct an optimization design to identify critical levels that optimize the formulation or process. For this purpose, central composite designs are useful. Other designs, such as factorial designs and the Box and Behnken design, are sometimes considered. Note that a central composite design with $n > 1$ center points provides an estimate of variance.

Example 4.3.1

A pharmaceutical company is interested in studying the effects of eight process and ingredient factors on various properties of tablets of a drug product. Table 4.3.4 lists these eight process and ingredient factors. Each factor has two levels. A full 2^8 factorial design requires a total of 256 runs. It is almost impossible for a pharmaceutical company to conduct a full 2^8 factorial experiment, due to the limited resources available. Instead of a full 2^8 factorial experiment, a fractional factorial experiment is suggested. It is believed that only three or four factors will have a major impact on the properties of tablets of the drug product and that there are no interactions involving four or more factors based on prior information. This is the basis for a 2^{8-4} fractional factorial experiment.

The 2^{8-4} fractional factorial design, which is a design of resolution IV, can be constructed as follows. We start with the eight 2_{III}^{7-4} design with factors X_1, X_2, X_3, and X_4 through X_7 defined as follows:

$$X_4 = X_1X_2, \quad X_5 = X_1X_3, \quad X_6 = X_2X_3, \quad \text{and} \quad X_7 = X_1X_2X_3.$$

A further variable, denoted by X_8, which consists entirely of plus signs, is added. The remaining eight runs can be obtained by switching all signs in the first set of eight runs. The resultant 2^{8-4} fractional factorial design is given in Table 4.3.5.

TABLE 4.3.4 Process and Ingredient Factors

Factor	Description	Levels	
GBP	Granulation blending procedure	Plows	Plows and choppers
GPT	Granulation paste type	1:1 (vol:vol) MeCl$_2$:EtOH denatured 23A	HPMC + EC dissolved in MeCl$_2$:23A EtOH
GBT	Granulation blend time	1.5 (min)	6 (min)
EC	Ethylcellulose	28 mg/tablet	42 mg/tablet
HPMC	Hydroxypropyl-methylcellulose	112 mg/tablet	168 mg/tablet
MS	Magnesium stearate	3.5 mg/tablet	14.0 mg/tablet
DSP	Dibasic sodium phosphate	35 mg/tablet	140 mg/tablet
LBT	Lubricant blend time	0.5 (min)	5.0 (min)

TABLE 4.3.5 Design Matrix for a 2_{IV}^{8-4} Fractional Factorial Design

Run	X_1	X_2	X_3	X_4 (X_1X_2)	X_5 (X_1X_3)	X_6 (X_2X_3)	X_7 $(X_1X_2X_3)$	X_8
1	−	−	−	+	+	+	−	+
2	+	−	−	−	−	+	+	+
3	−	+	−	−	+	−	+	+
4	+	+	−	+	−	−	−	+
5	−	−	+	+	−	−	+	+
6	+	−	+	−	+	−	−	+
7	−	+	+	−	−	+	−	+
8	+	+	+	+	+	+	+	+
9	+	+	+	−	−	−	+	−
10	−	+	+	+	+	−	−	−
11	+	−	+	+	−	+	−	−
12	−	−	+	−	+	+	+	−
13	+	+	−	−	+	+	−	−
14	−	+	−	+	−	+	+	−
15	+	−	−	+	+	−	+	−
16	−	−	−	−	−	−	−	−

As can be seen, a fractional factorial design is extremely useful for screening in a scaleup program, especially when there are lots of factors and little is known about the factors. The 2^{8-4} fractional factorial design constructed is a design of resolution IV. Thus the main effects do not confound with two-factor interactions. However, two-factor interactions do confound with one another. In practice, the effects of three-factor interactions are usually negligible. Therefore, the 2^{8-4} fractional factorial design provides estimates of the main effects alone if the three-factor interactions are assumed nonexistent.

4.4. SCALEUP ANALYSIS

For the analysis of a full factorial design, a fractional factorial design, or a central composite design, we may consider the following general statistical model:

$$Y = \alpha + \sum_{i=1}^{K} \beta_i X_i + \sum\sum_{i<j} \beta_{ij} X_i X_j + \cdots + e,$$

where α is the overall mean, β_i is the fixed main effect of factor i, β_{ij} is the fixed two-factor interaction between factors i and j, the higher-order interactions are defined similarly, and e is the random error associated with Y.

In practice, since the purpose of a scaleup experiment is to identify the key formulation factors, the general statistical model above is reduced to the following model for the evaluation of main effects.

$$Y = \alpha + \sum_{i=1}^{K} \beta_i X_i + e.$$

For a 2^K factorial design, its design matrix can expressed in the form

$$\mathbf{X} = \begin{array}{ccccc} \alpha & \beta_1 & \beta_2 & \cdots & \beta_K \\ 1 & -1 & -1 & \cdots & -1 \\ 1 & 1 & -1 & \cdots & -1 \\ \cdot & \cdot & \cdot & \cdots & \cdot \\ \cdot & \cdot & \cdot & \cdots & \cdot \\ \cdot & \cdot & \cdot & \cdots & \cdot \\ 1 & -1 & 1 & \cdots & 1 \\ 1 & 1 & 1 & \cdots & 1 \end{array}.$$

It can be verified that the off-diagonal elements of $\mathbf{X}'\mathbf{X}$ are zero. Therefore, the 2^K factorial design is an orthogonal design.

In this section we introduce two quick methods for obtaining estimates of the effects. These methods include the use of a table of contrast coefficients and Yates's algorithm (see, e.g., Box et al., 1978, pp. 322–323).

For the use of a table of contrast coefficients, consider the 2^4 factorial design. The calculations for obtaining various effects (one grand average, four main effects, six two-factor interactions, four three-factor interactions, and a single four-factor interaction) can be characterized by the table of signs given in Table 4.2.3. For example, the estimate of the grand average can be calculated from the first column as follows:

$$\frac{1}{16} \sum_{i=1}^{16} Y_i = \frac{1}{16} (Y_1 + Y_2 + \cdots + Y_{16}).$$

The main effect of the first factor (denoted by 1) is calculated from the second column, that is,

$$\frac{1}{8} \sum_{i=1}^{8} (Y_{2i} - Y_i) = \frac{1}{8} (-Y_1 + Y_2 - \cdots + Y_{16}).$$

The two-, three-, and four-factor interactions can be calculated similarly. It should be noted that the divisor used in the calculation is 2^{K-1} except for the grand average, which is 2^K. Each effect is a contrast and they are mutually orthogonal.

The table-of-contrast method described provides a convenient way of calculating effects from any 2^K factorial design. However, when K is large, calculation of all the effects become tedious. A useful alternative is Yates's algorithm, which is applied to a design matrix of standard order. The design matrix of standard order for the 2^4 factorial design is given in Table 4.2.2. The column of Y represents the response of the experiment. Note that Y could be the average if the run is repeated. We now summarize Yates's algorithm in the following steps. For simplicity, we use the 2^4 factorial design as an example.

Step 1: Consider the responses Y in successive pairs and divide these pairs into two groups of the same number of pairs, [i.e., the first group contains four pairs, $(Y_1, Y_2), \ldots, (Y_7, Y_8)$ and the second group consists of $(Y_9, Y_{10}), \ldots, (Y_{15}, Y_{16})$.

Step 2: Construct a column of 16 entries. The first eight entries are obtained by adding the pairs together. The next eight entries are obtained by subtracting the top number from the bottom number of each pair (see column 1 of Table 4.4.1).

Step 3: Repeat steps 1 and 2 by replacing Y with the column constructed, until there are four (i.e., K) columns are constructed (see columns 2, 3, and 4 of Table 4.4.1).

TABLE 4.4.1 Work Sheet of Yates's Algorithm for a 2^4 Factorial Design

Run	Design matrix X_1	X_2	X_3	X_4	Column 1	Column 2	Column 3
1	−	−	−	−	1 + 2	(1 + 2) + (3 + 4)	(1 + 2) + (3 + 4) + (5 + 6) + (7 + 8)
2	+	−	−	−	3 + 4	(5 + 6) + (7 + 8)	(9 + 10) + (11 + 12) + (13 + 14) + (15 + 16)
3	−	+	−	−	5 + 6	(9 + 10) + (11 + 12)	(2 − 1) + (4 − 3) + (6 − 5) + (8 − 7)
4	+	+	−	−	7 + 8	(13 + 14) + (15 + 16)	(10 − 9) + (12 − 11) + (14 − 13) + (16 − 15)
5	−	−	+	−	9 + 10	(2 − 1) + (4 − 3)	(3 + 4) − (1 + 2) + (7 + 8) − (5 + 6)
6	+	−	+	−	11 + 12	(6 − 5) + (8 − 7)	(11 + 12) − (9 + 10) + (15 + 16) − (13 + 14)
7	−	+	+	−	13 + 14	(10 − 9) + (12 − 11)	(4 − 3) − (2 − 1) + (8 − 7) − (6 − 5)
8	+	+	+	−	15 + 16	(14 − 13) + (16 − 15)	(12 − 11) − (10 − 9) + (16 − 15) − (14 − 13)
9	−	−	−	+	2 − 1	(3 + 4) − (1 + 2)	(5 + 6) + (7 + 8) − (1 + 2) − (3 + 4)
10	+	−	−	+	4 − 3	(7 + 8) − (5 + 6)	(13 + 14) + (15 + 16) − (9 + 10) − (11 + 12)
11	−	+	−	+	6 − 5	(11 + 12) − (9 + 10)	(6 − 5) + (8 − 7) − (2 − 1) − (4 − 3)
12	+	+	−	+	8 − 7	(15 + 16) − (13 + 14)	(14 − 13) + (16 − 15) − (10 − 9) − (12 − 11)
13	−	−	+	+	10 − 9	(4 − 3) − (2 − 1)	(7 + 8) − (5 + 6) − (3 + 4) + (1 + 2)
14	+	−	+	+	12 − 11	(8 − 7) − (6 − 5)	(15 + 16) − (13 + 14) − (11 + 12) + (9 + 10)
15	−	+	+	+	14 − 13	(12 − 11) − (10 − 9)	(8 − 7) − (6 − 5) − (4 − 3) + (2 − 1)
16	+	+	+	+	16 − 15	(16 − 15) − (14 − 13)	(16 − 15) − (14 − 13) − (12 − 11) + (10 − 9)

TABLE 4.4.1 Continued

Run	X₁	X₂	X₃	X₄	Column 4	Effect[a] Average
1	−	−	−	−	(1 + 2) + (3 + 4) + (5 + 6) + (7 + 8) + (9 + 10) + (11 + 12) + (13 + 14) + (15 + 16)	Average
2	+	−	−	−	(2 − 1) + (4 − 3) + (6 − 5) + (8 − 7) + (10 − 9) + (12 − 11) + (14 − 13) + (16 − 15)	1
3	−	+	−	−	(3 + 4) − (1 + 2) + (7 + 8) − (5 + 6) + (11 + 12) − (9 + 10) + (15 + 16) − (13 + 14)	2
4	+	+	−	−	(4 − 3) − (2 − 1) + (8 − 7) − (6 − 5) + (12 − 11) − (10 − 9) + (16 − 15) − (14 − 13)	12
5	−	−	+	−	(5 + 6) + (7 + 8) − (1 + 2) − (3 + 4) + (13 + 14) + (15 + 16) − (9 + 10) − (11 + 12)	3
6	+	−	+	−	(6 − 5) + (8 − 7) − (2 − 1) − (4 − 3) + (14 − 13) + (16 − 15) − (10 − 9) − (12 − 11)	13
7	−	+	+	−	(7 + 8) − (5 + 6) − (3 + 4) + (1 + 2) + (15 + 16) − (13 + 14) − (11 + 12) + (9 + 10)	23
8	+	+	+	−	(8 − 7) − (6 − 5) − (4 − 3) + (2 − 1) + (16 − 15) − (14 − 13) − (12 − 11) + (10 − 9)	123
9	−	−	−	+	(9 + 10) + (11 + 12) + (13 + 14) + (15 + 16) − (1 + 2) − (3 + 4) − (5 + 6) − (7 + 8)	4
10	+	−	−	+	(10 − 9) + (12 − 11) + (14 − 13) + (16 − 15) − (2 − 1) − (4 − 3) − (6 − 5) − (8 − 7)	14
11	−	+	−	+	(11 + 12) − (9 + 10) + (15 + 16) − (13 + 14) − (3 + 4) + (1 + 2) − (7 + 8) + (5 + 6)	24
12	+	+	−	+	(12 − 11) − (10 − 9) + (16 − 15) − (14 − 13) − (4 − 3) + (2 − 1) − (8 − 7) + (6 − 5)	124
13	−	−	+	+	(13 + 14) + (15 + 16) − (9 + 10) − (11 + 12) − (5 + 6) − (7 + 8) + (1 + 2) + (3 + 4)	34
14	+	−	+	+	(14 − 13) + (16 − 15) − (10 − 9) − (12 − 11) − (6 − 5) − (8 − 7) + (2 − 1) + (4 − 3)	134
15	−	+	+	+	(15 + 16) − (13 + 14) − (11 + 12) + (9 + 10) − (7 + 8) + (5 + 6) + (3 + 4) − (1 + 2)	234
16	+	+	+	+	(16 − 15) − (14 − 13) − (12 − 11) + (10 − 9) − (8 − 7) + (6 − 5) + (4 − 3) − (2 − 1)	1234

[a] Divided the first entry by 16 and others by 8.

Step 4: Divide the first entry of column 4 by 16 (i.e., 2^K) and the remaining entries by 8 (i.e., 2^{K-1}). The corresponding entries in column 4 of Table 4.4.1 are the minimum variance unbiased estimates for all $2^K - 1$ effects in standard order (Box et al., 1978). The standard order for all $2^K - 1$ effects is average, 1, 2, (12), 3, (13), (23), (123), 4, (14), (24), (124), (34), (134), (234), and (1234). Readers can verify that the entries for various effects in Table 4.4.1, obtained from Yates's algorithm are exactly the same as those provided in Table 4.2.3.

Note that when the number of factors is getting large, say more than 4, even Yates's algorithm becomes tedious. In this case, however, most commercial statistical packages, such as SAS (SAS, 1990), can provide not only the MVUE of all desirable effects but also the coefficients of linear contrasts corresponding to these effects, provided that the structure of the design matrix of the factorial design is given.

Example 4.4.1

Consider Example 4.3.1 and the design matrix for a 2^{8-4}_{IV} fractional factorial design given in Table 4.3.5. The 16-run fractional factorial experiment was conducted to screen eight process and ingredient factors on various properties in the tablet formulation of a drug product. Based on previous knowledge, granulation paste type (GPT), magnesium stearate (MS), and dibasic sodium phosphate (DSP) are probably the most critical process or ingredient factors. In addition, the lubricant blend time might be an important blocking factor. Therefore, it was decided to start with a 2^{7-4}_{III} fractional factorial design with eight runs using GPT, MS, and DSP as X_1, X_2, and X_3 in Example 4.3.1 by fixing the lubricant blend time at 5 min. Following Example 4.3.1, the columns of the design matrix corresponding to granulation blend time (GBT = X_4), hydroxypropyl methycellulose (MS = X_5), granulation blending procedure (GBP = X_6), and ethylcellulose (EC = X_7) are determined by the following relationship:

$$X_4 = X_1X_2,$$
$$X_5 = X_1X_3,$$
$$X_6 = X_2X_3,$$
$$X_7 = X_1X_2X_3.$$

A 2^{8-4} resolution IV fractional factorial design is then constructed by switching the level (or changing signs, as given in Table 4.3.5). The design layout for the 16 runs is given in Table 4.4.2. The response variables of interest are hardness and ejection force of 3000 and 5000 lb compressive force, respectively, residual methylene chloride level (RMCL), flodex disc width (FDW), and dissolution (percent release) at 2, 4, 6, and 8 h. The results are summarized in Table 4.4.3.

TABLE 4.4.2 2_{IV}^{8-4} Fractional Factorial Experiment

Batch	GPT	MS	DSP	GBT	HPMC	GBP	EC	LBT
1	Low	3.5	35	6	168	P&C	28	5.0
2	High	3.5	35	1.5	112	P&C	42	5.0
3	Low	14	35	1.5	168	P	42	5.0
4	High	14	35	6	112	P	28	5.0
5	Low	3.5	140	6	112	P	42	5.0
6	High	3.5	140	1.5	168	P	28	5.0
7	Low	14	140	1.5	112	P&C	28	5.0
8	High	14	140	6	168	P&C	42	5.0
9	High	14	140	1.5	112	P	42	0.5
10	Low	14	140	6	168	P	28	0.5
11	High	3.5	140	6	112	P&C	28	0.5
12	Low	3.5	140	1.5	168	P&C	42	0.5
13	High	14	35	1.5	168	P&C	28	0.5
14	Low	14	35	6	112	P&C	42	0.5
15	High	3.5	35	6	168	P	42	0.5
16	Low	3.5	35	1.5	112	P	28	0.5

TABLE 4.4.3 Scaleup Experiment Data Display Based on the 2_{IV}^{8-4} Fractional Factorial Design in Table 4.4.2

	Hardness		Ejection force				Etodolac dissolution			
Batch	3000	5000	3000	5000	RMCL	FDW	2	4	6	8
1	12.4	21.3	68	83	349	4	22.5	46.1	71.0	91.5
2	11.5	21.6	108	109	158	5	67.0	81.5	94.5	98.8
3	8.0	13.0	33	40	260	5	20.5	50.2	52.2	70.6
4	9.3	12.8	36	44	235	22	21.4	35.8	50.1	76.1
5	16.3	29.1	80	96	137	10	98.8	103.5	102.7	103.0
6	8.2	17.9	89	107	156	26	28.8	51.5	74.7	95.8
7	9.9	16.2	39	53	172	10	31.4	69.7	100.8	101.8
8	5.6	9.2	31	38	137	5	24.0	41.7	54.7	78.2
9	6.7	10.4	49	59	383	30	27.6	59.3	90.7	99.0
10	5.4	13.5	39	60	300	28	35.8	65.4	90.0	98.9
11	11.8	23.5	84	97	71	9	30.0	89.0	101.5	101.5
12	11.5	24.1	75	86	393	4	31.4	62.7	101.4	101.9
13	11.0	18.8	45	57	339	30	28.7	45.1	59.8	84.4
14	15.7	23.2	39	50	150	26	22.4	40.8	55.8	71.6
15	10.6	18.7	98	113	442	12	30.6	47.3	65.5	88.7
16	13.6	27.7	96	115	157	28	30.8	59.5	78.8	94.6

Since there are a total of 16 runs with no replicates, we can obtain estimates for the 16 effects, which include the overall average, eight main effects, and seven two-factor interactions. Under the assumption that there are no higher than two-factor interactions, we can obtain unbiased estimates for main effects. However, all two-factor interactions are confounded with each other. The confounding patterns are summarized as follows:

$(12) \leftrightarrow (37) \leftrightarrow (48) \leftrightarrow (56)$

$(13) \leftrightarrow (27) \leftrightarrow (46) \leftrightarrow (58)$

$(14) \leftrightarrow (28) \leftrightarrow (36) \leftrightarrow (57)$

$(15) \leftrightarrow (26) \leftrightarrow (38) \leftrightarrow (47)$

$(16) \leftrightarrow (25) \leftrightarrow (34) \leftrightarrow (78)$

$(17) \leftrightarrow (23) \leftrightarrow (68) \leftrightarrow (45)$

$(18) \leftrightarrow (24) \leftrightarrow (35) \leftrightarrow (67)$.

The estimates of average, main effects, and seven two-factor interactions are provided in Table 4.4.4. A linear model that contains only the term of the main effect was used to fit all response variables. This model assumes no interactions among the factors. Therefore, the difference between the total sum of squares (df = 15) and the sum of squares due to the main effects (df = 8) can be used to estimate the random error based on 7 degrees of freedom. Based on the results obtained from the model above, a reduced model is then considered to fit each response variable. The reduced model consists of the factors that are significantly different from zero at the 10% level and the interaction terms, whose estimates are of magnitude similar to that of the significant main effect. The results of statistical tests for zero effect are included in Table 4.4.4. These results indicate that magnesium stearate (MS) is the most critical factor because its effect is significantly different from zero at the 5% level of significance for six of the 10 responses under study. Note that MS is also significant for an etodolac dissolution at 4 hours at the 10% level. Similarly, it can be verified that dibasic sodium phosphate, hydroxpropyl methylcellulose, and type of granulation paste are other important process and ingredient factors. Although there are other sporadic significant results for other factors and interactions, no consistent pattern for these significant results were observed. Therefore, we identify MS, HPMC, DSP, and GPT as the four most critical process and ingredient factors.

4.5. DISCUSSION

To ensure a successful scaleup program, the project statistician needs to consult with scientists in the area of possible critical formulation and process factors and response variables. The design should be chosen to avoid any possible

TABLE 4.4.4   Estimates of the Main Effects and Two-Factor Interactions for the Scaleup Experiment Data Display Based on the 2_{IV}^{8-4} Fractional Factorial Design in Table 4.4.2[a]

Effect	Hardness 3000	Hardness 5000	Ejection force 3000	Ejection force 5000	RMCL	FDW	Etodolac dissolution 2	4	6	8
GPT	-2.26*	-4.40**	8.88*	5.13	0.38	3.00	-4.44	-5.84	-7.65	-1.43
MS	-3.04**	-8.35**	-48.3**	-50.63**	14.13	7.25	-16.01	16.64**	-17.00**	-11.9**
DSP	-2.09	-1.65	-4.63	-1.88	-42.63	-1.25	7.99	17.06*	23.6*	12.98**
GBT	0.84	0.20	-7.38	-5.63	-24.63	-2.75	2.41	-1.24	-7.7	-4.68
HPMC	-2.76**	-3.5*	6.63	-4.88	114.13*	-3.25	-13.39	-16.14*	-13.2*	-4.55
GBP	1.41	1.85	-3.88	-7.63	-37.63	-8.50*	-4.61	-0.51	4.35	0.38
EC	0.54	-0.3	2.13	-3.13	35.13	-7.50	11.61	3.11	-1.15	-4.10
LBT	-0.64	-2.35	-5.13	-8.38	-78.88	-10.00**	9.64	1.36	-5.35	-3.1
GPT × MS	0.66	0.73	-6.13	-6.38	52.63	1.50	2.34	-5.21	-3.23	0.13
GPT × DSP	-0.44	-1.08	-3.88	-3.63	-64.13	1.50	-17.31	-9.11	-10.68	-6.35
GPT × GBT	-0.86	-1.33	-3.13	-4.38	-13.13	-8.0*	-13.94	-4.66	-4.28	-3.70
GPT × HPMC	1.79	2.58	3.13	6.38	-57.38	5.0	4.91	-3.86	-7.33	-2.53
GPT × GBP	-0.14	1.48	2.83	2.13	-90.13	-1.75	14.94	15.34	3.03	0.45
GPT × EC	-2.01	-2.98	5.88	6.63	44.63	-1.25	-1.54	-1.01	5.98	5.83
GPT × LBT	-0.74	-0.13	2.13	1.38	-58.38	4.25	-3.56	-8.91	-5.53	-3.08
Average	10.47	18.81	63.06	75.44	239.94	15.88	34.48	59.32	77.76	91.03

[a]P Values are for the hypothesis of the effect being zero and were based on the reduced models with the effects with p values <0.1: *, $0.05 \leq p$ value <0.1; **, p value <0.05.

confounding effects so that the study objectives can be met. If it is possible, the design should be able to account for any concerns that the scientists may have, such as limited capacity and/or resource availability.

In addition to the statistical methods described above for selection of key critical factors among a large group of factors, several other statistical methods have been suggested in the literature. For example, Bohidar et al. (1979) and Bohidar and Peace (1988) have suggested several procedures for the identification of key critical factors. These procedures include all possible regression (APR) and stepwise regression (SWR), procedures, as well as a combination of APR and SWR procedures (CAS). The idea behind these approaches is to use the minimum central subset, central subset, complementary subset, and interchangeable set, which are generated based on the results of variables selected by APR and SWR, to screen the critical factors for each response variable. In practice, there are many response variables that need to be evaluated in a scaleup program. These response variables usually have an impact on scaleup for the manufacture of a drug product. Bohidar et al. (1975) and Bohidar and Peace (1988) have suggested that a principal components analysis be performed to select critical response variables. The purpose of the principal components analysis is to reduce the dimension of the response measures in the assessment of identity, strength, quality, and purity during the scaleup program for a drug product.

When conducting a scaleup program, some statistical issues may occur during the design phase and/or in data analysis. For example, during the design phase, it is usually desirable to cut down on the number of experimental runs. If a 2^{K-P} fractional design is chosen, it is of interest to determine the largest P that one can be used without losing much information and maintain a desirable precision. In addition, it is of interest to study the relative efficiency for a 2^{K-P} fractional factorial design when P changes from P_1 to P_2. As can be seen, the change from P_1 to P_2 will lead to an increase or decrease in the total of experimental runs by $2^{P_1-P_2}$ in a scaleup program. The objective is to evaluate the relative merits of the change so that we will not lose too much information but gain maximum information within a short period of time and with minimal cost.

Another interesting statistical issue during the design phase is an estimate of the variance of the random error (i.e., σ^2). As indicated earlier, we may not be able to estimate σ^2. In practice, however, we usually assume that there are no high-factor interactions. These interactions are then pooled to estimate σ^2. The estimate can then be used to construct a range or confidence interval for the main effects. Alternatively, one may have some replicates at some factorial points. However, there is no golden rule as to what and how many factorial points should be chosen for replications. Moreover, it is of interest to study the impact of these replications on the rotatability and orthogonality.

In practice, it is always important to justify a minimum sample size that can achieve the targeted objectives. Suppose that we can only perform N experimental runs for a specific design, due to limited capacity and/or resources availability. It is then of interest to (1) allocate these N experimental runs in a factorial of fractional design setting, and (2) provide statistical justification for targeted objectives.

In Sec. 4.4 we have provided several statistical methods, such as the use of a table of contrast and Yates's algorithm for scaleup analysis. These methods, however, are applied to each response variable. In practice, since the critical response variables may be correlated, it may be of interest to see whether a multivariate analysis can be incorporated in a factorial or fractional factorial analysis.

5

USP Tests and Specifications

5.1. INTRODUCTION

To ensure that a drug product will meet the USP/NF (1990) (i.e., USP XXII and NF XVII) standards for the identity, strength, quality, and purity of the drug product, a number of tests, such as potency testing, weight variation testing, content uniformity testing, dissolution testing, and disintegration testing are usually performed at various stages of the manufacturing process of the drug product. The USP/NF provides requirements regarding sampling plan and acceptance criteria for each of these tests. For example, the requirements for disintegration testing, weight variation and content uniformity testing, and dissolution testing can be found in sections [701], [705], and [711] of general chapters of the USP/NF, respectively. The requirements are met if the test results conform to the accompanying acceptance criteria. In this chapter, unless otherwise specified, we refer to these tests as USP tests.

For a given USP test, under the specific sampling plan and acceptance criteria, it is of interest to evaluate the probability of passing the USP test for a given sample. Under underlying distribution assumptions of the test characteristics, the probability of passing a USP test can be evaluated based on the sampling plan and acceptance criteria. The probability of passing a USP test generally depends on the population mean and standard deviation of the test characteristics. In practice, it is desired to obtain acceptance limits which guarantee that future samples will pass the USP test with a high probability. Such acceptance limits are usually constructed based on the sample mean and standard deviation of the test results. For a given sample, the idea is to construct a joint confidence region for the population mean and standard deviation. The probability of passing the USP test for each population mean and standard deviation in the confidence region can then be evaluated. The confidence region is obtained as the set of all possible sample means and standard deviations such that the probability of passing the USP test is greater than a prespecified probability for all points in the confidence region. The confidence region is usually referred to as the acceptance region.

The remainder of this chapter is organized as follows. In the next section, sampling plans and acceptance criteria for potency testing, weight variation testing, content uniformity testing, dissolution testing, and disintegration testing as specified in the USP/NF are described briefly. Lower bounds on the probabilities of passing individual USP tests are derived in Sec. 5.3. Details for constructing acceptance limits for each USP test based on the contour of the lower bounds on the probability of passing the USP test are included in Sec. 5.4. In Sec. 5.5 an example is presented to illustrate how an in-house specifications can be constructed to meet USP or in-house requirements. A brief discussion is given in Sec. 5.6.

5.2. SAMPLING PLAN AND ACCEPTANCE CRITERIA

As indicated in Sec. 5.1, potency testing, weight variation testing, content uniformity testing, dissolution testing, and disintegration testing are usually performed at various stages of the manufacturing process of a drug product to assure that the product meets the USP/NF standards for identity, strength, purity, and quality of the drug product. For this purpose, the USP/NF requires that a specific sampling plan for the individual USP test be employed and that specific acceptance criteria be met in order to pass the test. In the following, sampling plans and acceptance criteria for individual USP tests are described.

5.2.1. Potency Testing

Let Y_i be the assay results of the potency, $i = 1, \ldots, K$. Also, let LPS and UPS denote the lower and the upper product specifications as designated in the USP/NF individual monograph. Then the requirement for potency testing is met if all the individual assay results and the average assay results lie within (LPS, UPS). If the requirement is not met, additional assays may be required.

5.2.2. Weight Variation Testing

The uniformity of dosage units is usually demonstrated either by weight variation testing or content uniformity testing. The USP/NF general chapter [905] describes the requirements for testing the uniformity of dosage units. The requirements apply both to dosage forms containing a single active ingredient and to dosage forms containing two or more active ingredients.

As indicated in the general chapter [905] of the USP/NF, the weight variation requirements may be applied to solid dosage forms that contain no inactive or active added substances, or liquid-filled soft capsule, or the product contains 50 mg or more of an active ingredient comprising 50% or more (by weight) of the dosage unit. More specifically, the weight variation requirements may be applied to uncoated tablets, hard capsules, soft capsules, solids in single-unit containers, and sterile solids for parenteral use.

For the determination of dosage uniformity by weight variation, weigh accurately 10 dosage units individually and calculate the average weight. From the result of the *assay*, as directed in the individual monograph, calculate the content of the active ingredient in each of the 10 units, assuming homogeneous distribution of the active ingredient. The requirements for dosage uniformity are met if the amount of active ingredient in each of the 10 dosage units lies within the range 85 to 115% of label claim and the relative standard deviation (or coefficient of variation) is less than 6.0%. If one unit is outside the range 85 to 115% of label claim and no unit is outside the range 75 to 125% of label claim, or if the relative standard deviation (or coefficient of variation) is greater than 6.0%, or if both conditions prevail, test 20 additional units. The requirements are met if not more than one unit of the 30 is outside the range 85 to 115% of label claim and no unit is outside the range 75 to 125% of label claim and the relative standard deviation of the 30 dosage units does not exceed 7.8%. The acceptance criteria for dosage uniformity by weight variation is summarized in Table 5.2.1. The flowchart of the test procedure for the uniformity of dosage units by weight variation is also given in Fig. 5.2.1.

5.2.3. Content Uniformity Testing

For the determination of dosage uniformity by assay of individual units, the USP/NF general chapter [905] requires that the following be done. First, assay 10 units individually, as directed in the *assay* in the individual monograph, unless specified otherwise in the test for content uniformity. Where a special procedure is specified in the test for content uniformity in the individual monograph, the results should be adjusted based on the following procedure:

1. Prepare a composite specimen of a sufficient number of dosage units to provide the sufficient amount of specimen.
2. Assay separately, accurately measured portions of the composite specimen.
3. Calculate the weight of active ingredient equivalent to one average dosage unit, by (a) using the results obtained by *assay* procedure, and by (b) using the results obtained by the special procedure.

TABLE 5.2.1 Acceptance Criteria for Uniformity of Dosage Units

Stage	Number tested	Pass if:
S_1	10	1. Each of the 10 units lies within the range 85.0 to 115.0% of the label claim. 2. The relative standard deviation is less than or equal to 6.0%.
S_2	20	1. No more than one unit of the 30 units $(S_1 + S_2)$ is outside the range 85.0 to 115.0% of label claim. 2. No unit is outside the range 75.0 to 125% of label claim. 3. The relative standard deviation of the 30 units $(S_1 + S_2)$ does not exceed 7.8%.

4.   Calculate the correction factor, F, by the formula

$$F = \frac{A}{P},$$

in which A is the weight of the active ingredient equivalent to one average dosage unit obtained by the *assay* procedure, and P is the weight of active ingredient equivalent to one average dosage unit obtained by the special procedure. If

$$\frac{100 \, |A - P|}{A} > 10,$$

the use of a correction factor is not valid.
5.   A valid correction may be applied only if F is not less than 1.03 or greater than 1.10, or not less than 0.90 or greater than 0.97. If F is between 0.97 and 1.03, no correction is required.
6.   If F lies between 1.03 and 1.10, or between 0.90 and 0.97, calculate the weight of active ingredient in each dosage unit by multiplying each of the weights found using the special procedure by F.

The requirements for dose uniformity are met if the amount of the active ingredient in each of the 10 dosage units conforms to the acceptance criteria given in Table 5.2.1 (see also Fig. 5.2.1). It should be noted, however, that the acceptance criteria in Table 5.2.1 apply only if the average of the limits specified in the *potency* definition in the individual monograph is 100% or less. If the

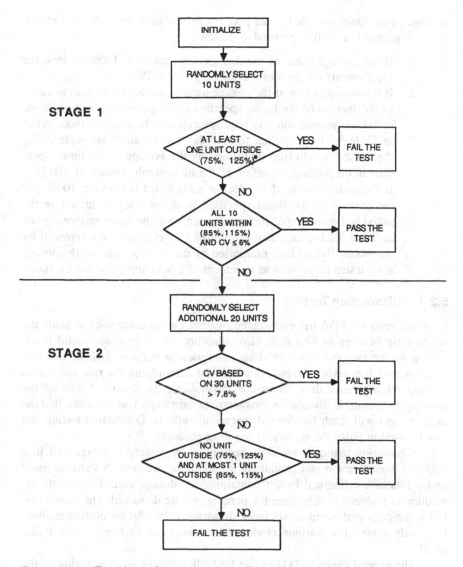

FIGURE 5.2.1 Flowchart of test procedures for uniformity of dosage units. (* = or at least 2 units outside [85%, 115%]).

average of the limits specified in the *potency* definition in the individual monograph is greater than 100%, proceed as follows:

1. If the average value of the dosage units tested is 100% or less, the requirements are the same as those given in Table 5.2.1.

2. If the average value of the dosage units tested is greater than or equal to the average of the limits specified in the *potency* definition in the individual monograph, the requirements are the same as those given in Table 5.2.1 except that the words "label claim" are replaced by the words "label claim multiplied by the average of the limits specified in the *potency* definition in the monograph divided by 100."

3. If the average value of the dosage units tested is between 100% and the average of the limits specified in the *potency* definition in the individual monograph, the requirements are the same as those given in Table 5.2.1 except that the words "label claim" are replaced by the words "label claim multiplied by the average value of the dosage units tested (expressed as a percent of label claim) divided by 100."

5.2.4. Dissolution Testing

In recent years the FDA has encouraged pharmaceutical companies to study the relationship between *in vivo* drug bioavailability, which provides useful information on the rate and extent of drug absorption in humans, and *in vitro* dissolution, which provides a rapid technique for determining the rate and extent of drug release. Since drug absorption depends on the dissolved state of the drug product, suitable dissolution characteristics are important to ensure that the drug product will reach the desired therapeutic effects. Dissolution testing can also be used to judge the quality of the drug product.

Dissolution testing is typically performed by placing a dosage unit in a 1000-mL transparent vessel containing a dissolution medium. A variable-speed motor rotates a cylindrical basket containing the dosage unit. The dissolution medium is analyzed to determine the percent of drug dissolved. The dissolution test is typically performed on six units simultaneously. The dissolution medium is usually sampled at various predetermined intervals to form a dissolution profile.

The general chapter [711] of the USP/NF contains an explanation of the test for acceptability of dissolution rates. The requirements are met if the quantities of active ingredient dissolved from the units conform to the USP/NF acceptance criteria. Let Q be the amount of dissolved active ingredient specified in the individual monograph, which is usually expressed as a percentage of label claim. The USP/NF dissolution acceptance criteria comprise a three-stage sampling plan. For the first stage (S_1), six dosage units are to be tested. The requirement for the first stage is met if each unit is not less than $Q + 5\%$. If the product fails to pass S_1, an additional six units will be tested at the second stage (S_2). The product is considered to have passed if the average of the 12 units from S_1 and S_2 is equal to or greater than Q and if no unit is less than Q − 15%. If the product fails to pass both S_1 and S_2, an additional 12 units will be tested at a third stage (S_3). If the average of all 24 units from S_1, S_2, and S_3 is equal to or greater than Q, no more than two units are less than Q − 15%, and no unit is less than Q − 25%, the product has passed the USP/NF dissolution test. Table 5.2.2 summarizes the acceptance criteria for each stage. The flowchart of the test procedure for dissolution is given in Fig. 5.2.2. Note that we should continue to test through all three stages unless the results conform at S_1 or S_2.

5.2.5. Disintegration Testing

The USP/NF's general chapter [701] requires that a disintegration test be provided to determine compliance with the limits on disintegration as stated in the individual monograph except where the label states that the tablets or capsules are intended for use as troches, are to be chewed, or are designed to liberate the drug content gradually over a period of time or release the drug over two or more separate periods with a distinct interval between periods.

In the first stage (S_1) of disintegration testing, six dosage units are tested. The requirements are met if all six units disintegrate completely. *Complete disintegration* is defined as that state in which any residual of the unit, except fragments of an insoluble coating or capsule shell, that may remain on the test apparatus screen is a soft mass with no palpably firm core. If one or two units fails to disintegrate completely, repeat the test on 12 additional units at the second stage (S_2). The requirements are met if no fewer than 16 units of the total of 18 units tested disintegrate completely. The acceptance criteria for disintegration are given in Table 5.2.3 and the corresponding flowchart is provided

TABLE 5.2.2 Acceptance Criteria for Dissolution

Stage	Number tested	Pass if:
S_1	6	Each unit is not less than Q + 5%.
S_2	6	Average of 12 units $(S_1 + S_2)$ is equal to or greater than Q, and no unit is less than Q − 15%.
S_3	12	Average of 24 units $(S_1 + S_2 + S_3)$ is equal to or greater than Q, no more than two units are less than Q − 15%, and no unit is less than Q − 25%.

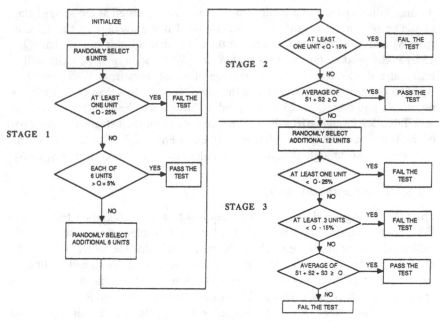

FIGURE 5.2.2 Flowchart of test procedure for dissolution.

TABLE 5.2.3 Acceptance Criteria for Disintegration

Stage	Number tested	Pass if:
S_1	6	All of the units have disintegrated completely.
S_2	12	No less than 16 of the total of 18 units $(S_1 + S_2)$ tested disintegrate completely.

in Fig. 5.2.3. Note that disintegration testing may be applied to uncoated tablets, plain coated tablets, enteric-coated tablets, buccal tablets, sublingual tablets, hard gelatin capsules, and soft gelatin capsules.

5.3. PROBABILITY OF PASSING USP TEST

As discussed earlier, most USP tests are multiple-stage sampling tests. For example, a two-stage sampling test is used for the uniformity of dosage units and disintegration, while dissolution uses a three-stage sampling test. Each stage of

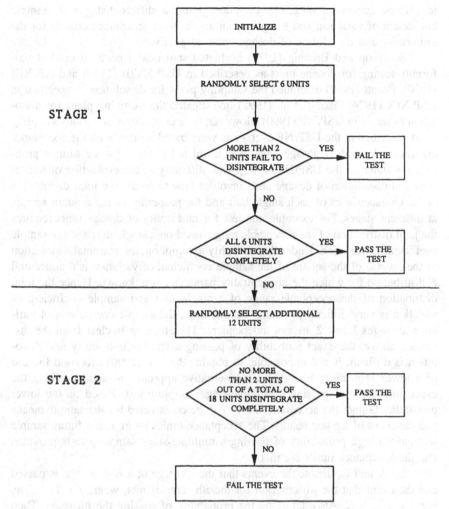

FIGURE 5.2.3 Flowchart of test procedure for disintegration.

sampling tests may have one or more than one acceptance criterion for passing the test. For example, the acceptance criterion for the disintegration test at both stages only involves whether each unit disintegrates completely within the time limit specified in the monograph. However, the acceptance criteria for uniformity and dissolution of dosage units are much more complicated. These criteria contain not only the characteristics of individual dosage units but also involve the properties of the randomly selected sample as a whole. For example, in addition to different acceptable ranges for each dosage unit at different stages, the sample coefficient of variation and sample mean are to meet acceptance criteria for the uniformity and dissolution of dosage units, respectively.

Sampson and Breunig (1971) evaluated statistical aspects of content uniformity testing for dosage units as described in USP XVIII (1970) and NF XIII (1970). Pheatt (1980) examined the sampling plans for dissolution as specified in USP XIX (1974). Tsong et al. (1992) investigated the sampling plans for dissolution as stated in USP/NF (1990). However, their evaluations of various sampling plans described in the USP/NF over years were based primarily on the acceptance criteria for individual dosage units, which did not account for the sample properties as stated in the USP/NF (1990). One difficulty in the evaluation of uniformity and dissolution of dosage units involves how to obtain the joint distribution of the characteristics of each single unit and the properties of the random sample at different stages. For example, the test for uniformity of dosage units requires the joint distribution of the acceptable range based on a single unit and the sample coefficient of variation. Under the normality assumption, the marginal distribution of the inverse of the square of the sample coefficient of variation is a noncentral F distribution for which the noncentrality parameter is unknown. Hence the joint distribution of the acceptable range of a single unit and sample coefficient of variation is very difficult to obtain. Furthermore, the sample coefficients of variation at stages 1 and 2 are not independent. Therefore, as is clear from the discussion above, the exact probability of passing a test for uniformity and dissolution is difficult, if not impossible, to obtain. Bergum (1990) proposed the use of a lower probability bound as a conservative approach to approximating the exact probability of passing a multiple-stage sampling test. Based on the lower probability bound, the acceptance limits can be constructed for the sample means and variances of the test results. The acceptance limits assure that a future sample will have a high probability of passing a multiple-stage sampling tests provided that the acceptance limits are met.

Let S_i and C_{ij} denote the events that the ith stage of a K-stage test is passed and the event that the jth criterion for the ith stage is met, where $j = 1, \ldots, m_i$ and $i = 1, \ldots, K$. Also, let P_i be the probability of passing the ith stage. Then the probability of passing a multiple-stage test is given by

$$
\begin{aligned}
P\{\text{passing a } K\text{-stage test}\} &= P\{S_1 \text{ or } S_2 \text{ or } \cdots \text{ or } S_K\} \\
&= P(S_1) + P(\text{not } S_1)P(S_2 \mid \text{not } S_1) \\
&\quad + \cdots \\
&\quad + P\{\text{not } (S_1, \ldots, S_{K-1})\}P\{S_K \mid \text{not} \\
&\quad (S_1, \cdots, S_{K-1})\} \\
&= P_1 + (1 - P_1)P_2 \\
&\quad + (1 - P_1)(1 - P_2)P_3 + \cdots
\end{aligned}
$$

$$= P_1 + \sum_{i=1}^{K-1} \left\{ \prod_{j=1}^{i} (1 - P_j) \right\} P_{i+1}$$

$$= 1 - \prod_{i=1}^{K} (1 - P_i)$$

$$\geq \max\{P_1, P_2, \ldots, P_K\}. \tag{5.3.1}$$

Furthermore,

$$P_i = P(S_i) = P\{C_{i1} \text{ and } C_{i2} \text{ and } \cdots \text{ and } C_{im_i}\}$$

$$\geq \max\left\{ \sum_{j=1}^{m_i} P(C_{ij}) - (m_i - 1),\, 0 \right\}. \tag{5.3.2}$$

Therefore, a lower bound for passing the multiple K-stage test is given by

$$\max_{1 \leq i \leq K} \left\{ \sum_{j=1}^{m_i} P(C_{ij}) - (m_i - 1),\, 0 \right\}. \tag{5.3.3}$$

In the following we derive lower bounds on the probabilities of passing USP content uniformity testing (which can also be used for weight variation testing), dissolution testing, and disintegration testing, respectively.

5.3.1 Content Uniformity Testing

The probability of passing the USP test for content uniformity, denoted by P_{CU}, is given by

$$
\begin{aligned}
P_{CU} = \; & P\{\text{first 10 units meet USP stage 1 criteria} \\
& \text{or all 30 units meet the USP stage 2 criteria}\} \\
\geq \; & \max\{P\{\text{first 10 units meet USP stage 1 criteria}\}, \\
& P\{\text{all 30 units meet the USP stage 2 criteria}\}\} \\
\geq \; & \max\{P(C_{11}) + P(C_{12}) - 1,\, P(C_{21}) + P(C_{22}) - 1,\, 0\}, \tag{5.3.4}
\end{aligned}
$$

where

$C_{11} = \{$the relative standard deviation is less than 6%$\}$,

$C_{12} = \{$each of the 10 units is within

the range 85 to 115% of the label claim$\}$,

$C_{21} = \{$the relative standard deviation is less than 7.8%$\}$,

$C_{22} = \{$not more than 1 of the 30 units $(S_1 + S_2)$ is outside

the range 85.0 to 115.0% of label claim and no unit is outside

the range 75 to 125% of label claim$\}$.

Therefore, a lower bound (LB) of P_{CU} can be obtained by finding $P(C_{11})$, $P(C_{12})$, $P(C_{21})$, and $P(C_{22})$.

Let Y be the content uniformity assay value, which is usually expressed as a percentage of label claim. Assume that Y follows a normal distribution with mean μ and variance σ^2 [i.e., $Y \sim N(\mu, \sigma^2)$]. The distribution of the inverse of the square of the sample coefficient of variation multiplied by sample size follows a noncentral F distribution. Therefore, given a set of values for μ and σ^2, $P(C_{11})$ and $P(C_{21})$ can be computed by the following probability statements:

$$P(C_{i1}) = P\{W_i < k_i\}, \qquad i = 1, 2, \tag{5.3.5}$$

where $W_i = s_i/\bar{Y}_i$, $\bar{Y}_i$, and s_i are the sample mean and standard deviation for stage i, and $k_1 = 0.06$ and $k_2 = 0.078$. Let

$$F_i = \frac{n_i}{W_i^2} \qquad i = 1, 2,$$

where $n_1 = 10$ and $n_2 = 30$. Then it follows that

$$P(C_{i1}) = P\{W_i < k_i\}$$
$$= P\left\{F_i > \frac{n_i}{k_i^2}\right\}. \tag{5.3.6}$$

It can be verified that $F_i = F_i(1, df_i, \lambda_i)$ follows a noncentral F distribution with 1 and df_i degrees of freedoms and noncentrality parameter

$$\lambda_i = n_i\left(\frac{\mu}{\sigma}\right)^2,$$

where $df_1 = 9$ and $df_2 = 29$.

Although we may use a noncentral F distribution to evaluate the probability $P(C_{i1})$, one of the disadvantages is that it may require a large λ_i to compute $P(C_{i1})$. For example, if the specification of the sample coefficient of variation at stage 1 is the true population coefficient of variation, a noncentral F distribution with a noncentral parameter in the magnitude of 2778 would be required to compute $P(C_{11})$. As an alternative, Bergum (1990) considered the approximation by a central F distribution to evaluate $P(C_{i1})$ based on the following relationship:

$$F(\nu_i, df_i, 0) = \frac{1}{1 + \lambda_i} F(1, df_i, \lambda_i), \tag{5.3.7}$$

where $F(\nu_i, df_i, 0)$ is a central F distribution with ν_i and df_i degrees of freedom, and

$$\nu_i = \frac{(1 + \lambda_i)^2}{1 + 2\lambda_i}. \tag{5.3.8}$$

In addition to the approximation by a central F distribution, a normal approximation to the distribution of the square root of F_i, as suggested by Laubscher (1960), may be useful for the evaluation of $P(C_{i1})$. The method is described as follows. Let

$$g_{1i} = \frac{(2\mathrm{df}_i - 1)F_i}{\mathrm{df}_i}$$

$$g_{2i} = 2(1 + \lambda_i^2) - \frac{1 + 2\lambda_i^2}{1 + \lambda_i^2},$$

$$g_{3i} = \frac{F_i}{\mathrm{df}_i} + \frac{1 + 2\lambda_i^2}{1 + \lambda_i^2}, \qquad\qquad (5.3.9)$$

where $i = 1,2$. Then

$$Z_i = \frac{\sqrt{g_{1i}} - \sqrt{g_{2i}}}{\sqrt{g_{3i}}}, \qquad i = 1,2, \qquad\qquad (5.3.10)$$

follows a standard normal distribution. As a result, $P(C_{i1})$ can be computed by replacing F_i with n_i/k_i^2 for a given set of values of μ and σ^2.

Let p_1 be the probability that an assay result is in the range 85 to 115% of label claim. Then

$$p_1 = P\{85 \leq Y \leq 115\}.$$

Let p_2 be the probability that an assay result is in the range 75 to 85% of label claim or 115 to 125% of label claim. Then

$$p_2 = P\{75 \leq Y \leq 85\} + P\{115 \leq Y \leq 125\}.$$

Therefore, we have

$$P(C_{12}) = P\{\text{all 10 units are between 85 and 115\% of label claim}\}$$
$$= (p_1)^{10},$$

$$P(C_{22}) = P\{\text{all 30 units are between 85 and 115\% of label claim}\}$$
$$+ P\{29 \text{ units are between 85 and 115\% of}$$
$$\text{label claim and 1 unit is between 75 and 85\%}$$
$$\text{of label claim or 115 and 125\% of label claim}\}$$
$$= (p_1)^{30} + 30(p_1)^{29}p_2.$$

Thus, based on (5.3.4), the lower bound (LB) can be calculated for a given set of values of μ and σ. Table 5.3.1 gives the probabilities of passing the USP content uniformity test for various values of μ and σ for LB = 0.5 and LB = 0.95. These probabilities are obtained based on the approximations by a central

TABLE 5.3.1　Probability Contours for Passing the USP
XXII Content Uniformity Test

	σ^a			
	LB = 0.50		LB = 0.95	
μ	F	N	F	N
86	0.67	0.67	0.45	0.44
88	2.01	2.00	1.33	1.33
90	3.33	3.34	2.22	2.21
92	4.39	4.60	3.11	3.10
94	5.60	5.63	3.99	3.99
96	6.44	6.77	4.87	4.87
98	6.92	7.52	5.61	5.64
100	7.12	7.77	5.89	5.96
102	7.06	7.53	5.64	5.64
104	6.63	6.77	4.87	4.87
106	5.64	5.78	3.99	3.99
108	4.54	4.66	3.11	3.10
110	3.34	3.34	2.22	2.21
112	2.01	2.00	1.33	1.33
114	0.67	0.67	0.45	0.44

[a]F, approximation by a central F distribution; N, approximation by a
standard normal distribution.

F distribution and a standard normal distribution. For example, for the normal
approximation, if μ is 94 and σ is less than 3.99, there is at least a 95% chance
of passing the USP test for the uniformity of dosage units. In addition, Table
5.3.1 indicates that the central F approximation is more conservative than the
normal approximation, although both approximations provide essentially the
same set of values of μ and σ when LB = 0.95. Probability contours for LB =
0.5 and LB = 0.95 based on the central F approximation is given in Fig. 5.3.1.

Note that both p_1 and p_2 can be expressed as

$$\sum_{j=1}^{i} p_j = P\{1 - \Delta_i < Y_i < \Delta_i + 1\},$$

where $\Delta_i = 15\%, 25\%$ for $i = 1,2$, respectively. It then follows that

$$\sum_{j=1}^{i} p_j = P\{-\Delta_i < Y_i - 1 < \Delta_i\} = P\left\{\frac{-\Delta_i - \mu}{\sigma} < Z < \frac{\Delta_i - \mu}{\sigma}\right\}.$$

Let $Z(\text{LB})$ be the upper quantile of a standard normal distribution such that the
lower probability bound of passing the USP test is LB. Then it can easily be

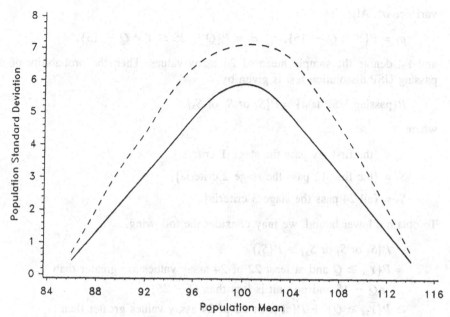

FIGURE 5.3.1   Lower probability bounds for content uniformity. Solid curve, lower probability = 95%; dashed curve, lower probability = 50% [From Bergum (1990).].

shown that

$$\frac{(\Delta_i - \mu)^2}{Z^2(\text{LB})} = \sigma^2.$$

Similarly, it can be verified that $P(C_{i1})$ depends on an unknown noncentrality parameter, which is also a function of the ratio of μ^2 to σ^2. As a result, the contour for μ and σ is a parabola that is symmetric about the population mean μ. Since the contribution of p_2 to the contour of μ and σ is rather small and insignificant, we may focus on the contour of μ and σ only over the range of μ from 85 to 115%. It is interesting to note that for each μ (i.e., $85 < \mu < 115$), as σ decreases to zero, the probability of passing the content uniformity test increases. Thus, for any (μ, σ) below any given LB contour, the probability of passing the content uniformity is greater than LB.

5.3.2.   Dissolution Testing

Let Y be the dissolution assay result, which is usually expressed as a percentage of label claim. Assume that Y follows a normal distribution with mean μ and variance σ^2. Also, let

$$p_1 = P\{Y \geq Q - 15\}, \qquad p_2 = P\{Q - 25 \leq Y < Q - 15\},$$

and $\overline{Y}_{24}$ denote the sample mean of 24 assay values. Then the probability of passing USP dissolution test is given by

$$P\{\text{passing USP test}\} = P\{S_1 \text{ or } S_2 \text{ or } S_3\},$$

where

$S_1 = \{$the first six pass the stage 1 criteria$\}$,

$S_2 = \{$the first 12 pass the stage 2 criteria$\}$,

$S_3 = \{$all 24 pass the stage 3 criteria$\}$.

To obtain a lower bound, we may consider the following.

$$P\{S_1 \text{ or } S_2 \text{ or } S_3\} > P\{S_3\}$$
$$= P\{\overline{Y}_{24} \geq Q \text{ and at least 22 of 24 assay values are greater than}$$
$$Q - 15 \text{ and no unit is less than } Q - 25\}$$
$$\geq P\{\overline{Y}_{24} \geq Q\} + P\{\text{at least 22 of 24 assay values greater than}$$
$$Q - 15 \text{ and no unit is less than } Q - 25\} - 1$$
$$= -P\{\overline{Y}_{24} < Q\} + P\{\text{at least 22 of 24 assay values greater than}$$
$$Q - 15 \text{ and no units is less than } Q - 25\}$$
$$= -P\{Z < (24)^{1/2} \frac{Q - \mu}{\sigma}\}$$
$$+ (276 p_1^{22} p_2^2 + 24 p_1^{23} p_2 + p_1^{24})$$

So a lower bound (LB) for the probability of passing the dissolution test, given μ and σ^2, is given by

$$\text{LB} = -P\left\{Z < (24)^{1/2} \frac{Q - \mu}{\sigma}\right\}$$
$$+ (276 p_1^{22} p_2^2 + 24 p_1^{23} p_2 + p_1^{24}). \quad (5.3.11)$$

It can be seen from (5.3.11) that LB depends on σ^2 and the magnitude of the difference between Q and μ. Let D denote the difference between μ and Q (i.e., $D = \mu - Q$). Figure 5.3.2 plots the (D, σ) combinations such that LB = 0.50 and LB = 0.95. The corresponding values for these contours are given in Table 5.3.2. For example, if D is 10% of label claim and if σ is less than 20.27% of label claim, the lower bound on the probability of passing the USP dissolution test is 50%. Note that for each D (i.e., $D > 0$), as σ decreases to zero, the lower bound on the probability of passing the USP test increases.

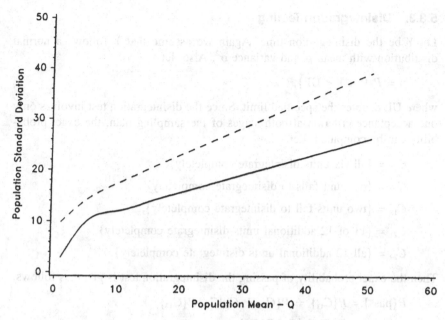

FIGURE 5.3.2 Lower probability bounds for passing dissolution test. Solid curve, lower probability = 95%; dashed curve, lower probability = 50%.

TABLE 5.3.2 Probability Contours for Passing the USP XXII Dissolution Test

	σ	
$D(\mu - Q)$	LB = 0.50	LB = 0.95
1	9.84	2.98
5	14.11	9.94
10	17.40	12.03
15	20.27	13.87
20	23.06	15.67
25	25.81	17.45
30	28.53	19.22
35	31.21	20.97
40	33.87	22.72
45	36.54	24.48
50	39.19	26.22

5.3.3. Disintegration Testing

Let Y be the disintegration time. Again we assume that Y follows a normal distribution with mean μ and variance σ^2. Also, let

$$p = P\{0 < Y < UL\},$$

where UL denotes the specified limit. Since the disintegration test involves only one acceptance criterion at both stages of the sampling plan, the exact probability can be computed. Let

C_{11} = {all six units disintegrate completely},

C_{12} = {one unit fails to disintegrate completely},

C_{13} = {two units fail to disintegrate completely},

C_{21} = {11 of 12 additional units disintegrate completely},

C_{22} = {all 12 additional units disintegrate completely}.

Then the exact probability of passing the disintegration test is given as follows:

$$
\begin{aligned}
P\{\text{pass}\} &= P\{C_{11}\} + P\{C_{21} + C_{22}|C_{12}\}P\{C_{12}\} \\
&\quad + P\{C_{22}|C_{13}\}P\{C_{13}\} \\
&= p^6 + \left\{ \binom{12}{11}p^{11}(1 - p) + p^{12} \right\} \left\{ \binom{6}{1}p^5(1 - p) \right\} \\
&\quad + p^{12} \left\{ \binom{6}{2}p^4(1 - p)^2 \right\} \\
&= p^6 + 6p^{17}(1 - p) + 87p^{16}(1 - p)^2.
\end{aligned}
\tag{5.3.12}
$$

It can easily be verified that if the desired probability of passing the disintegration test is 0.5, p is approximately about 0.831. If, in addition, the specified time limit, UL, is 30 min, it follows that

$$
\begin{aligned}
p &= P\{Y < UL\} \\
&= P\{Y < 30\} \\
&= P\left\{ \frac{Y - \mu}{\sigma} < \frac{30 - \mu}{\sigma} \right\} \\
&= P\{Z < Z(0.169)\} \\
&= 0.831,
\end{aligned}
$$

where Z is a standard normal variable and $Z(0.169)$ is the 16.9% upper quantile of a standard normal distribution. Therefore,

$$\frac{30 - \mu}{\sigma} = Z(0.169) = 0.957.$$

Hence the contour for μ and σ is a linear decreasing function of μ given by

$$0.957\sigma = 30 - \mu, \qquad (5.3.13)$$

where $0.957 = Z(0.169)$. Figure 5.3.3 gives the contours of μ and σ for probabilities of passing the disintegration test being equal to 50% and 95% (i.e., LB = 0.50 and 0.95), respectively. The corresponding values for the contours are provided in Table 5.3.3. It can be seen from Table 5.3.3 that if μ is 13 min and the standard deviation is less than 10.50, there is at least a 95% chance of passing the disintegration test.

Note that the lower bound for the probability of passing USP disintegration test can also be obtained from (5.3.2) as follows:

$P\{$passing USP disintegration test$\}$

$= P\{$first six units meet stage 1 criteria

or all 18 units meet stage 2 criteria$\}$

$\geq P\{$all 18 units meet stage 2 criteria$\}$

$= 153p^{16}(1 - p)^2 + 18p^{17}(1 - p) + p^{18}.$

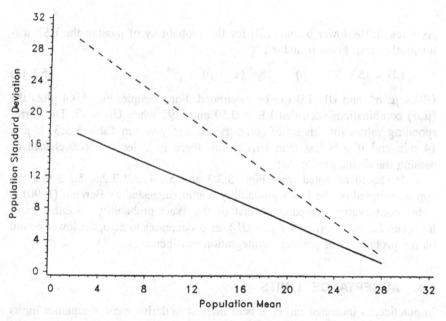

FIGURE 5.3.3 Exact probability bounds for passing disintegration test. Solid curve, lower probability = 95%; dashed curve, lower probability = 50%.

TABLE 5.3.3 Probability Contours for Passing the Disintegration Test

	σ			
	Exact probability		Lower probability bound	
μ	0.50	0.95	0.50	0.95
1	30.29	17.90	27.50	17.32
3	28.20	16.67	25.60	16.12
5	26.11	15.44	23.70	14.93
7	24.03	14.20	21.81	13.73
9	21.94	12.97	19.91	12.54
11	19.85	11.73	18.02	11.35
13	17.76	10.50	16.12	10.15
15	15.67	9.26	14.22	8.96
17	13.58	8.03	12.33	7.76
19	11.49	6.79	10.43	6.57
21	9.40	5.56	8.53	5.37
23	7.31	4.32	6.64	4.18
25	5.22	3.09	4.74	2.99
27	3.13	1.85	2.84	1.79

As a result, the lower bound (LB) for the probability of passing the USP disintegration test, given μ and σ^2, is

$$LB = 153p^{16}(1 - p)^2 + 18p^{17}(1 - p) + p^{18}. \qquad (5.3.14)$$

Given μ, σ^2, and UL, LB can be calculated. For example, Fig. 5.3.4 plots the (μ,σ) combinations such that LB is 0.50 and 0.95 when UL = 30. The corresponding values for this set of contours are also given in Table 5.3.3. If μ is 14 min and if σ is less than 16.12 min, there is at least a 50% chance of passing the disintegration test.

It should be noted from Figs. 5.3.3 and 5.3.4 and Table 5.3.3 that the approach based on the lower probability bound suggested by Bergum (1990) is rather conservative compared to that of the exact probability. In either case, however, for each μ (i.e., $0 < \mu < $ UL), as σ decreases to zero, the lower bound on the probability of passing disintegration test increases.

5.4. ACCEPTANCE LIMITS

In practice, as indicated earlier, it is of interest to derive some acceptance limits which guarantee that future samples will pass the USP tests with a high probability. The acceptance limits are generally used as in-house specifications for

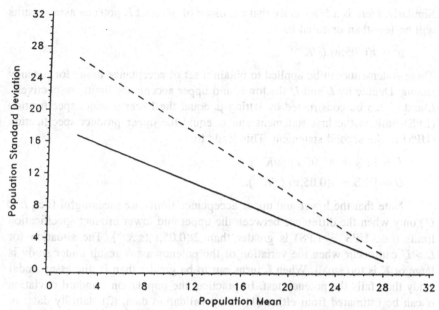

FIGURE 5.3.4 Lower probability bounds for passing disintegration test. Solid curve, lower probability = 95%; dashed curve, lower probability = 50%.

quality assurance of the drug product. The acceptance limits are usually constructed based on the sample mean and standard deviation of test results. For a given sample, the idea is to construct a joint confidence region (or acceptance region) for the population mean and standard deviation. If the sample mean and standard deviation fall inside the acceptance region, there is a high probability of passing the USP test. In this section we derive acceptance limits for potency testing, weight variation testing, content uniformity testing, dissolution testing, and disintegration testing based on the lower bound on the probability of passing the USP test given in Sec. 5.3.

5.4.1. Potency Testing

Let Y be the potency assay result. Assume that Y follows a normal distribution with mean μ and variance σ^2. Let s be an estimate of the standard deviation σ with ν degrees of freedom. Then, there is a 5% chance that the mean of the next K potency assay results will be greater than or equal to

$$\mu + t(0.05,\nu)\,(s/K^{1/2}).$$

Similarly, there is a 5% chance that the mean of the next K potency assay results will be less than or equal to

$$\mu - t(0.05,v) \; (s/K^{1/2}).$$

These statements can be applied to obtain a set of acceptance limits for potency testing. Denote by L and U the lower and upper acceptance limits, respectively. L and U can be constructed by letting μ equal the lower product specification (LPS) limit in the first statement and μ equal the upper product specification (UPS) in the second statement. This leads to

$$L = \text{LPS} + t(0.05,v) \; (s/K^{1/2}),$$
$$U = \text{UPS} - t(0.05,v) \; (s/K^{1/2}).$$

Note that the lower and upper acceptance limits are meaningful (i.e., $L <$ U) only when the difference between the upper and lower product specification limits (i.e., UPS $-$ LPS) is greater than $2t(0.05,v)(s/K^{1/2})$. The situation for $L > U$ can occur when the variation of the potency assay result under study is large or K is too small. When L turns out to be greater than U, the assay under study then fails the potency test. In practice, the population standard deviation σ can be estimated from either (1) assay validation data, (2) stability data, or (3) assay results from released batches. If there is a stability loss, the lower acceptance limit should be adjusted to account for the potential stability loss over drug shelf life.

5.4.2. Weight Variation and Content-Uniformity Testing

Suppose that n content-uniformity assays from each of L locations within a V-blender or transport device (i.e., a total of $N = nL$ assays) are performed. Let Y_{ij} denote the jth assay result from location i, where $j = 1, \cdots, n$, $i = 1, \cdots,$ L. The following one-way random effects model described in Sec. 3.5.1 can be applied directly to obtain the lower probability bound.

$$Y_{ij} = \mu + L_i + e_{ij}, \tag{5.4.1}$$

where L_i are i.i.d. $N(0,\sigma_L^2)$ and e_{ij} are i.i.d. $N(0,\sigma_e^2)$. It is assumed that L_i and e_{ij} are mutually independent. The expected value and variance of Y_{ij} are given by

$$E(Y_{ij}) = \mu,$$
$$\sigma_Y^2 = \text{var}(Y_{ij}) = \sigma_L^2 + \sigma_e^2. \tag{5.4.2}$$

As indicated earlier, LB can be calculated for given values of μ, σ_e^2, and σ_L^2. A joint confidence region for μ and σ_Y can then be derived. In the following we provide confidence regions for each of the following two sampling plans suggested by Bergum (1990):

Plan I: one observation at each location

Plan II: more than one observation at each location

Plan I

Suppose that at each of the L locations there is only one assay performed (i.e., $n = 1$). Hence $N = L$. The sample mean and variance are usually used to estimate μ and $\sigma_Y^2 (= \sigma_L^2 + \sigma_e^2)$, respectively. Under plan I (i.e., $n = 1$) a simultaneous confidence region for μ and σ_Y^2 can be constructed based on the sample mean $\overline{Y}$ and variance s^2 of a given sample as follows [see, e.g., Lindgren (1976)]. Select p and q such that $(1 - 2p)(1 - q) = 1 - \alpha$. Then

$$P\left\{-z(p) < \frac{\overline{Y} - \mu}{\sigma_Y/\sqrt{L}} < z(p) \text{ and } \frac{(L - 1)s^2}{\sigma_Y^2} > \chi^2(q, L - 1)\right\}$$

$$= P\left\{\left(\frac{\overline{Y} - \mu}{\sigma_Y/\sqrt{L}}\right)^2 < z^2(p)\right\} P\left\{\frac{(L - 1)s^2}{\sigma_Y^2} > \chi^2(q, L - 1)\right\}$$

$$= (1 - 2p)(1 - q)$$

$$= 1 - \alpha,$$

where $z(p)$ is the pth upper quantile of a standard normal distribution and $\chi^2(q, L - 1)$ is the qth quantile of a chi-square distribution with $L - 1$ degrees of freedom. Thus the $(1 - \alpha) \times 100\%$ confidence region, which depends on $(\overline{Y}, s^2)$, is defined as the region of (μ, σ_Y^2) that gives a probability of $1 - \alpha$. The shape of the boundary of the confidence region for (μ, σ_Y^2), as shown in Lindgren (1976), is a upside-down cone. For the purpose of illustration and an easy interpretation, in practice, it is always helpful to discuss the confidence region of (μ, σ_Y) rather than the confidence region of (μ, σ_Y^2). An approximate confidence region for (μ, σ_Y) can be obtained by taking the square root of σ_Y^2 from the confidence region of (μ, σ_Y^2). The shape of the approximate confidence region for (μ, σ_Y) then becomes a reverse triangle, as shown in Fig. 5.4.1.

If the confidence region for (μ, σ_Y) is such that all (μ, σ_Y) combinations in the region are below a preselected LB contour, the probability of passing the content uniformity test is greater than LB with the chosen confidence level. For a fixed μ (i.e., $85 < \mu < 115$), the probability of passing the USP test is an decreasing function of σ_Y. Therefore, suppose that $85 < A$ and $B < 115$ in Fig. 5.4.1, and the line segment consists of points resulting in the lowest probability of passing the USP test. Since the LB contours are concave, either point A or point B gives the lowest probability.

For a given sample size, based on the methods described above, the procedure for obtaining the acceptance limits for the sample mean and standard deviation is outlined below. We first choose a lower bound of the probability that would be considered unacceptable (e.g., LB = 0.50). For a fixed value of sample means in the interval [85.0%, 115.0%], we determine the sample stan-

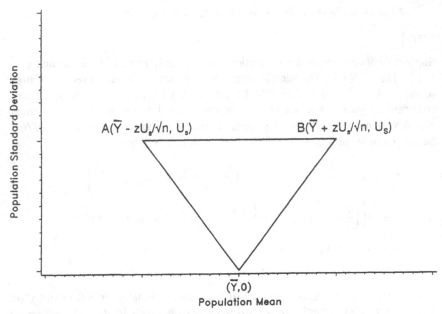

FIGURE 5.4.1   Confidence region for population mean and standard deviation for content uniformity. n, sample size; $\overline{Y}$, sample mean; z, quantile of the standard normal distribution; U_s, upper confidence bound (one-sided) for σ [From Bergum (1990)].

dard deviation such that the point in the resulting confidence region with the lowest probability of passing specification is equal to LB. The standard deviation associated with each mean is the acceptance limit of the standard deviation for that mean. An acceptance region that consists of the set of sample means and standard deviations constructed in this way is then obtained. This acceptance region can be evaluated numerically to determine the probability that a sample mean and standard deviation will fall inside the acceptance region provided that the population mean and standard deviation are given. The sample size can be chosen so that if there is a high probability of meeting the acceptance limits, the probability of passing the USP test is high.

Note that in plan I, since only one assay is performed at each location, the estimates of σ_L^2 and σ_e^2 cannot be obtained. In practice, the total variation can be partitioned into within- and between-location variation if more than one assay is performed at each location.

Plan II

Assume that there are n assays ($n > 1$) performed at each of L locations. A simultaneous confidence region for $(\mu, \sigma_e^2, \sigma_L^2)$ can be constructed based on

$(\bar{Y}, s_e^2, s_L^2)$, where $\bar{Y}$ is the overall mean, s_L^2 is the location mean square, and s_e^2 is the mean-squared error obtained from an ANOVA table under a one-way nested random effects model. For a desired confidence level, say $1 - \alpha$, we choose p and q such that

$$(1 - \alpha) = (1 - 2p)(1 - q)(1 - q).$$

Let $\sigma^2 = \sigma_e^2 + n\sigma_L^2$. Then

$$P\left\{\left\{-Z(p) < \frac{\bar{Y} - \mu}{(\sigma^2/N)^{1/2}} < Z(p)\right\}\right.$$

$$\text{and} \quad \left\{\frac{L(n-1)s_e^2}{\sigma_e^2} > \chi^2(q, L(n-1))\right\}$$

$$\text{and} \quad \left.\left\{\frac{(L-1)s_L^2}{\sigma^2} > \chi^2(q, L-1)\right\}\right\}$$

$$= P\left\{-Z(p) < \frac{\bar{Y} - \mu}{(\sigma^2/N)^{1/2}} < Z(p)\right\}$$

$$\times P\left\{\frac{L(n-1)s_e^2}{\sigma_e^2} > \chi^2(q, L(n-1))\right\}$$

$$\times P\left\{\frac{(L-1)s_L^2}{\sigma^2} > \chi^2(q, L-1)\right\}$$

$$= (1 - 2p)(1 - q)(1 - q) = 1 - \alpha, \quad (5.4.3)$$

where $z(p)$ is the pth upper quantile of a standard normal distribution and $\chi^2(q, L(n-1))$ and $\chi^2(q, L-1)$ are the qth quantiles of chi-square distribution with $L(n-1)$ and $(L-1)$ degrees of freedom, respectively. Bergum (1990) suggested an ad hoc approximate $(1 - \alpha) \times 100\%$ simultaneous confidence region for $(\mu, \sigma_e^2, \sigma_L^2)$ which is given by

$$\bar{Y} - Z(p)\left(\frac{\sigma^2}{N}\right)^{1/2} < \mu < \bar{Y} + Z(p)\left(\frac{\sigma^2}{N}\right)^{1/2},$$

$$0 < \sigma_e^2 < \frac{L(n-1)s_e^2}{\chi^2(q, L(n-1))}, \quad (5.4.4)$$

$$\begin{cases} 0 < \sigma_L^2 < \frac{1}{n}\left[\frac{(L-1)s_L^2}{\chi^2(q, L-1)} - \sigma_e^2\right] & \text{if } \sigma_e^2 \leq \frac{(L-1)s_L^2}{\chi^2(q, L-1)} \\ \sigma_L^2 = 0 & \text{otherwise.} \end{cases} \quad (5.4.5)$$

A value of σ_Y^2 [$= \text{var}(Y_{ij})$] and a range for μ [$= E(Y_{ij})$] can be determined for each σ_e^2 and σ_L^2 contained in the confidence region. If all such (μ, σ_Y) combinations are below the preselected LB contour, the probability of passing the content uniformity test is greater than LB with the chosen level of confidence. However, it is recommended that only two points in the region, which always result in the smallest lower bound for the probability of passing the USP test, be examined. To examine which two points produce the smallest possible probability, we first note from the simultaneous confidence region of $(\mu, \sigma_e^2, \sigma_L^2)$ that each confidence interval for μ is symmetric about the mean. Each set of values of (σ_e^2, σ_L^2) in the confidence region determines a value of σ_Y^2 and consequently determines the width of the confidence interval of μ. If the same value of (σ_e^2, σ_L^2), say σ_0^2, gives the largest value of σ_Y^2 (i.e., the widest confidence interval of μ), the smallest lower bound for the probability of passing the USP is at one of the endpoints of the confidence interval of μ associated with σ_0^2. This is true because the LB contour is concave, and for a given μ, the probability of passing the USP test is an increasing function of the inverse of σ_Y^2.

Denote by U_e and U_L the upper confidence bounds for σ_e^2 and σ^2, respectively. Then we have

$$U_e = \frac{L(n-1)s_e^2}{\chi^2(q, L(n-1))} \quad \text{and} \quad U_L = \frac{(L-1)s_L^2}{\chi^2(q, L-1)}. \tag{5.4.6}$$

Since the confidence region for σ_e^2 and σ_L^2 is independent of μ, it is sufficient to consider the confidence region in the (σ_e^2, σ_L^2) plane. Basically, the magnitude of U_L relative to U_e determines the shape of this confidence region. For example, if U_e is greater than U_L, the confidence region has the shape given in Fig. 5.4.2. If U_e is less than or equal to U_L, the confidence region has the shape shown in Fig. 5.4.3. The largest value of σ_Y^2 can then be determined from Fig. 5.4.2 or 5.4.3 by plotting the line $\sigma_e^2 + \sigma_L^2 = C_0$ ($C_0 \geq 0$), which has a slope of -1. Since the slope of the line connecting $(0, U_L/n)$ to $(U_L, 0)$ is $-1/n$, the (σ_e^2, σ_L^2) contained within the confidence region resulting in the largest C_0 (i.e., the largest σ_Y^2) occurs at

$$\begin{cases} \left(U_e, \dfrac{1}{n}(U_L - U_e) \right) & \text{if } U_e < U_L \\ \\ (U_e, 0) & \text{if } U_e \geq U_L. \end{cases} \tag{5.4.7}$$

Therefore, the upper limit for σ_Y^2 is given by

$$\begin{cases} \left(1 - \dfrac{1}{n} \right) U_e + \dfrac{1}{n} U_L & \text{if } U_e < U_L \\ \\ U_e & \text{if } U_e \geq U_L. \end{cases} \tag{5.4.8}$$

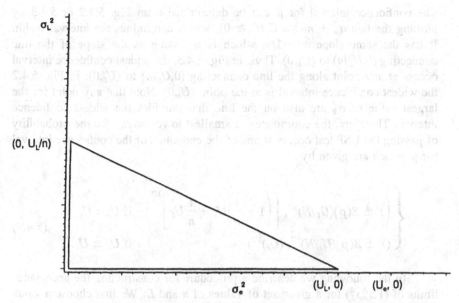

FIGURE 5.4.2 Confidence region for (σ_e^2, σ_L^2) when $U_e > U_L$ [From Bergum (1990)].

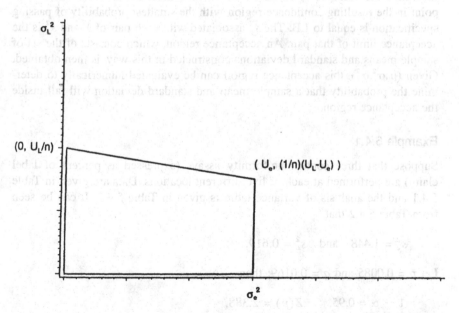

FIGURE 5.4.3 Confidence region for (σ_e^2, σ_L^2) when $U_e \le U_L$ [From Bergum (1990)].

The confidence interval for μ can be determined from Fig. 5.4.2 or 5.4.3 by plotting the line $\sigma_e^2 + n\sigma_L^2 = C$ ($C \geq 0$), which determines the interval width. It has the same slope as $-1/n$, which is the same as the slope of the line connecting $(0, U_L/n)$ to $(U_L, 0)$. Thus, in Fig. 5.4.3, the widest confidence interval occurs at any point along the line connecting $(0, U_L/n)$ to $(U_L, 0)$. In Fig. 5.4.2 the widest confidence interval is at the point $(U_e, 0)$. Note that any point for the largest value of σ_Y^2 are also on the line that provides the widest confidence interval. Therefore, the coordinates of smallest lower bound for the probability of passing the USP test occurs at one of the endpoints of the confidence interval for μ which are given by

$$\begin{cases} \left(\bar{Y} \pm Z(p)(U_L/N)^{1/2}, \left[\left(1 - \frac{1}{n} \right) U_e + \frac{1}{n} U_L \right]^{1/2} \right) & \text{if } U_e < U_L \\ (\bar{Y} \pm Z(p)(U_e/N)^{1/2}, (U_e)^{1/2}) & \text{if } U_e \geq U_L. \end{cases} \qquad (5.4.9)$$

In the following we describe a procedure for constructing the acceptance limits of $(\bar{Y}, s_e^2, s_L^2)$ for a given set of values of n and L. We first choose a value of LB that would be considered unacceptable (e.g., LB = 0.50). Then for each selected value of $\bar{Y}$ in the interval [85.0%, 115.0%], select a value of s_L^2 and determine the value of s_e^2 based on the method described above such that the point in the resulting confidence region with the smallest probability of passing specification is equal to LB. The s_e^2 associated with each pair of $\bar{Y}$ and s_L^2 is the acceptance limit of that pair. An acceptance region, which consists of the set of sample means and standard deviations constructed in this way, is then obtained. Given $(\mu, \sigma_e^2, \sigma_L^2)$, this acceptance region can be evaluated numerically to determine the probability that a sample mean and standard deviation will fall inside the acceptance region.

Example 5.4.1

Suppose that three content uniformity assays (expressed as percent of label claim) are performed at each of five different locations. Data are given in Table 5.4.1 and the analysis of variance table is given in Table 5.4.2. It can be seen from Table 5.4.2 that

$$s_e^2 = 1.448 \quad \text{and} \quad s_L^2 = 0.619.$$

Let $p = 0.0085$ and $q = 0.0169$; then

$$1 - \alpha = 0.95, \qquad Z(p) = 2.388,$$
$$\chi^2(q, 4) = 0.393, \quad \text{and} \quad \chi^2(q, 10) = 2.929.$$

TABLE 5.4.1 Content Uniformity Assay Results, $L = 5$ and $n = 3$

	Location				
	1	2	3	4	5
	98.40	98.68	101.95	100.80	100.45
	99.55	101.21	99.13	99.32	99.32
	100.04	99.93	99.46	98.65	101.64
Mean	99.33	99.94	100.18	99.59	100.47
Variance	0.71	1.60	2.38	1.21	1.35

Therefore, the upper limits of s_e^2 and s_L^2 are given by 4.944 and 6.30, respectively. Since the upper limit of U_e is less than that of U_L, the upper limit for σ_Y^2 is

$$\left(1 - \frac{1}{3}\right)(4.944) + \frac{1}{3}(6.30) = 5.396,$$

and a half of the widest confidence interval width for μ is

$$(2.388)\left(\frac{6.3}{15}\right)^{1/2} = 1.548.$$

The points having the smallest lower bound for the probability of passing the USP test are

$$[99.902 - 1.548, (5.396)^{1/2}] \quad \text{and} \quad [99.902 + 1.548, (5.396)^{1/2}]$$

or

$$(98.354, 2.323) \quad \text{and} \quad (101.45, 2.323).$$

Note that both points are below the LB = 0.95 contour (see Fig. 5.4.1). Therefore, with 95% assurance, at least 95% of all samples will pass the USP content uniformity test.

TABLE 5.4.2 ANOVA Table for the Content Uniformity Data Given in Table 5.4.1

Source	df	Sum of squares	Mean squares	F value
Model	4	2.478	0.619	0.43
Error	10	14.484	1.448	
Total	14	16.962		

Note: The overall mean = 99.902.

5.4.3. Dissolution and Disintegration Testing

A simultaneous confidence region for μ and σ can be constructed similarly based on the sample mean and variance of dissolution testing or disintegration testing using the method described in plan I for weight variation testing and content uniformity testing. However, for dissolution testing, the point that results in the smallest lower bound on probability of passing the USP test is point A on the line segment AB (whenever $A > Q$) in Fig. 5.4.1. On the other hand, for disintegration testing, either point A or B on the line segment (whenever $A > 0$ and $B < UL$) gives the smallest lower bound on the probability of passing the USP test. The acceptance limits for the sample mean and standard deviation for both dissolution testing and disintegration testing can be obtained in a manner similar to that described in Sec. 5.4.2.

5.5. IN-HOUSE SPECIFICATIONS

Specifications are defined as specific intervals that the sample mean and standard deviation must be contained to meet the USP or in-house requirements with a high probability. For example, for a pharmaceutical compound, the dissolution specifications after encapsulation may state that at 4 h the mean percent release of 12 capsules must be between 35% and 60% and the standard deviation must be less than 11%. In this case the specific intervals (35%,60%) and (0%,11%) are the specifications on mean and standard deviation for the dissolution testing at 4 h.

Note that the standard deviation or variance of a test result may consist of several variance components, depending on how the test is conducted. For example, the test may be conducted at different laboratories on different days by different analysts. In addition, the sample may be drawn from different locations of a transport or drum at different stages of a manufacturing process. An appropriate statistical model, which can account for these possible sources of variations, should be fitted to obtain estimates of these variance components and consequently, an estimate of the standard deviation. In practice, estimates of these sources of variations provide valuable information regarding whether the drug product will meet the USP or in-house requirements. The sources of variations of particular interest include laboratory-to-laboratory, day-to-day, analyst-to-analyst, and location-to-location variations.

Applying ideas similar to those described in previous sections, acceptance limits for specifications on the mean and standard deviation can be obtained. Let Y be the assay value which follows a normal distibution with mean μ and variance σ^2. Suppose that a random sample of size N is drawn from this population. Let the specification intervals for the sample mean $\overline{Y}$ and sample variance, s^2 be $[a,b]$ and $[c,d]$, respectively. Since $\overline{Y}$ and s^2 are independent, we have

$$P\{a < \bar{Y} < b \text{ and } c < s^2 < d\}$$
$$= P\{a < \bar{Y} < b\} \cdot P\{c < s^2 < d\}$$
$$= P\{z_L < Z < z_U\} \cdot P\{\chi_L^2 < \chi^2 < \chi_U^2\}, \tag{5.5.1}$$

where

$$Z = \frac{\bar{Y} - \mu}{\sigma/\sqrt{N}}, \quad \chi^2 = \frac{(N-1)s^2}{\sigma^2},$$

$$z_L = \frac{a - \mu}{\sigma/\sqrt{N}}, \quad z_U = \frac{b - \mu}{\sigma/\sqrt{N}},$$

$$\chi_L^2 = \frac{(N-1)c}{\sigma^2} \quad \chi_U^2 = \frac{(N-1)d}{\sigma^2}.$$

Therefore, given μ, σ^2, and N, the probability of a sample passing the specification limits, PL, can be found. For example, Fig. 5.5.1 plots (μ, σ^2) combinations such that PL is 0.50 and 0.95 when $N = 12$, $a = 80$, $b = 120$, $c = 0$, and $d = 16$. The corresponding values for this set of contours are given in Table

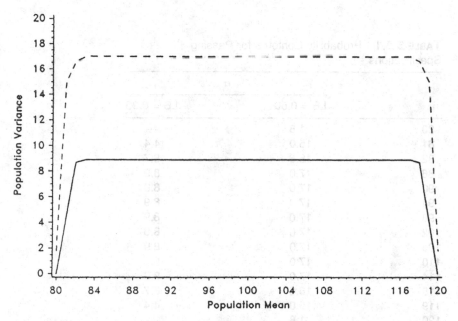

FIGURE 5.5.1 Probability contours for passing specifications on mean and variance. Solid curve, lower probability = 95%; dashed curve, lower probability = 50%.

5.5.1. Thus if μ is 98 and if σ^2 is less than 17.0, there is a 50% chance of passing the specifications. For each μ (i.e., $a < \mu < b$) as σ^2 decreases to zero, the lower bound of the probability for passing specifications increases.

Although one can apply (5.5.1) to obtain the set of values for (μ,σ^2) such that the probability of passing the specifications is greater than a prespecified lower bound, in practice, μ and σ^2 are usually unknown and need to be estimated based on the sample. Furthermore, based on the sample mean and variance (or standard deviation), it is desirable to have some idea with a certainty (i.e., probability) regarding the range where the mean and variance of a future sample. These ranges are referred to as the *prediction intervals* for the sample mean and standard deviation (Hahn, 1970). On the other hand, it is also important to estimate an interval such that $(1 - \gamma) \times 100\%$ of the population lies within the interval with $(1 - \alpha) \times 100\%$ confidence. This interval is known as the *tolerance interval* [see, e.g., Bowker (1947), Hahn (1970), and Graybill (1976)]. In addition, different sources of variation need to be taken into account when constructing the confidence interval for the total variability and the prediction interval for the standard deviation of a future sample. In the following we introduce the concept of the use of the prediction interval and the tolerance interval for the development of an in-house dissolution specification through a real example.

TABLE 5.5.1 Probability Contours for Passing Specifications

	σ	
μ	LB = 0.50	LB = 0.95
80	1.8	—
81	15.0	4.4
82	16.6	8.7
86	17.0	8.9
90	17.0	8.9
94	17.0	8.9
98	17.0	8.9
102	17.0	8.9
106	17.0	8.9
110	17.0	8.9
114	17.0	8.9
118	16.6	8.7
119	15.0	4.4
120	1.8	—

—: less than 1×10^{-8}.

Suppose that an experiment was conducted to develop an in-house dissolution specification for the tablets of a drug product. A total of I batches of granulation were each made into J tablet strengths. K dissolution assays were performed at 2, 4, 8, and 14 h on each of IJ batch-by-strength combinations. The purpose of the study is to recommend in-house specifications for the mean of the percent of the amount of dissolved active ingredient. At a particular time point, a recommended in-house specification can be obtained under the following two-way cross-classification mixed model, described in Sec. 3.5.2:

$$Y_{ijk} = \mu + B_i + S_j + (BS)_{ij} + e_{ijk}, \quad i = 1, \ldots, I, \tag{5.5.2}$$
$$j = 1, \ldots, J, \quad k = 1, \ldots, K,$$

where Y_{ijk} denotes the assay result of the kth tablet in the ith batch for the jth strength, S_j is the fixed effect for the jth strength, B_i is the random effect for the ith batch, $(BS)_{ij}$ is the random effect for the jth strength made from the ith batch, and e_{ijk} is the random error in observing Y_{ijk}. In the model above, it is assumed that B_i's are i.i.d. normal with mean zero and variance σ_B^2 [i.e., $B_i \sim N(0, \sigma_B^2)$], $(BS)_{ij}$'s are i.i.d. normal with mean zero and variance σ_{BS}^2 [i.e., $(BS)_{ij} \sim N(0, \sigma_{BS}^2)$], and e_{ijk}'s are i.i.d. normal with mean zero and variance σ_e^2 [i.e., $e_{ijk} \sim N(0, \sigma_e^2)$].

The ANOVA table with expected mean squares for model (5.5.2) was given in Table 3.5.5, while Table 3.5.6 gives point estimates for σ_e^2, σ_{BS}^2, and σ_B^2, which are

$$\hat{\sigma}_e^2 = \text{MSE},$$

$$\hat{\sigma}_{BS}^2 = \frac{1}{K} [\text{MS(BS)} - \text{MSE}],$$

$$\hat{\sigma}_B^2 = \frac{1}{JK} [\text{MSB} - \text{MS(BS)}], \tag{5.5.3}$$

where MSE, MS(BS), and MSB are the mean squares of errors, mean squares due to batch-by-strength interaction, and mean squares due to batch, respectively. Denote by $\overline{Y}_{ij.}$ the sample mean of assay results of K tablets from the (i, j)th batch-by-strength combination, that is,

$$\overline{Y}_{ij.} = \frac{1}{K} \sum_{k=1}^{K} Y_{ijk}.$$

Then we have

$$E(\overline{Y}_{ij.}) = \mu + S_j, \quad \sigma_{ij}^2 = \text{var}(\overline{Y}_{ij.}) = \frac{1}{K} \sigma_e^2 + \sigma_{BS}^2 + \sigma_B^2. \tag{5.5.4}$$

Hence the sample mean for the jth strength is the average of $\overline{Y}_{ij\cdot}$ over the I batches:

$$\overline{Y}_{\cdot j\cdot} = \frac{1}{I} \sum_{i=1}^{I} \overline{Y}_{ij\cdot}. \qquad (5.5.5)$$

Since batches are independent of one another, $\overline{Y}_{1j\cdot}, \cdots, \overline{Y}_{Ij\cdot}$ are i.i.d. normal with mean $\mu + S_j$ and variance σ_{ij}^2 as given in (5.5.4). Hence the variance of $\overline{Y}_{\cdot j\cdot}$ is given by

$$\mathrm{var}(\overline{Y}_{\cdot j\cdot}) = \frac{1}{I} \left(\frac{1}{K} \sigma_e^2 + \sigma_{BS}^2 + \sigma_B^2 \right)$$

$$= \frac{1}{I} \sigma_{ij}^2. \qquad (5.5.6)$$

An unbiased estimator of the variance of $\overline{Y}_{ij\cdot}$ can be obtained by substituting σ_e^2, σ_{BS}^2, and σ_B^2 with their ANOVA estimates given in (5.5.3), which is

$$\hat{\sigma}_{ij}^2 = \widehat{\mathrm{var}}\,(\overline{Y}_{ij\cdot}) = \left\{ \frac{1}{K}\,\mathrm{MSE} + \frac{1}{K}\,[\mathrm{MS(BS)} - \mathrm{MSE}] \right.$$

$$\left. + \frac{1}{JK}\,[\mathrm{MSB} - \mathrm{MS(BS)}] \right\} \qquad (5.5.7)$$

$$= \left[\frac{J-1}{JK}\,\mathrm{MS(BS)} + \frac{1}{JK}\,\mathrm{MSB} \right].$$

Since SSE/σ_e^2, $\mathrm{SS(BS)}/(\sigma_e^2 + K\sigma_{BS}^2)$, and $\mathrm{SSB}/(\sigma_e^2 + K\sigma_{BS}^2 + JK\sigma_B^2)$ are independent chi-square random variables with $IJ(K-1)$, $(I-1)(J-1)$, and $(I-1)$ degrees of freedom, respectively, the quantity

$$\chi^2 = \frac{\mathrm{df}\,\hat{\sigma}_{ij}^2}{\sigma_{ij}^2}$$

follows an approximately chi-square distribution with df degrees of freedom [see, e.g., Graybill (1976) and Searle et al. (1992)], where df is given by

$$\mathrm{df} = \frac{(\hat{\sigma}_{ij}^2)^2}{d^2}, \qquad (5.5.8)$$

$$d^2 = \frac{1}{(I-1)(J-1)} \left[\frac{(J-1)\,\mathrm{MS(BS)}}{JK} \right]^2 + \frac{1}{I-1} \left(\frac{\mathrm{MSB}}{JK} \right)^2. \qquad (5.5.9)$$

Hence

$$T = \frac{\overline{Y}_{\cdot j\cdot} - (\mu + S_j)}{\sqrt{\sigma_{ij}^2 / I}}$$

is approximately distributed as a central t distribution with df degrees of freedom. Let

$$\overline{W}_{\cdot j\cdot} = \frac{1}{I'} \sum_{i=1}^{I'} \overline{W}_{ij\cdot},$$

where $\overline{W}_{ij\cdot}$ is the sample mean of the assay results of K tablets from a future (i,j) batch-by-strength combination. Then $\overline{W}_{\cdot j\cdot}$ is the average of i.i.d. normal random variables $\overline{W}_{1j\cdot}, \ldots, \overline{W}_{I'j\cdot}$, each with mean $\mu + S_j$ and variance σ_{ij}^2. Hence $\overline{W}_{\cdot j\cdot}$ also follows a normal distribution with mean $\mu + S_j$ and variance σ_{ij}^2/I'. Since $\overline{Y}_{\cdot j\cdot}$ and $\overline{W}_{\cdot j\cdot}$ are obtained from two independent samples, Hahn (1970) indicated that

$$T_d = \frac{\overline{W}_{\cdot j\cdot} - \overline{Y}_{\cdot j\cdot}}{\sqrt{\hat{\sigma}_{ij}^2(1/I + 1/I')}} \tag{5.5.10}$$

is also approximately distributed as a central t distribution with df degrees of freedom. As a result, we have the following probability statement:

$$P\{-t(\tfrac{1}{2}\alpha,\mathrm{df}) < T_d < t(\tfrac{1}{2}\alpha,\mathrm{df})\} \cong 1 - \alpha, \tag{5.5.11}$$

where $t(\alpha/2,\mathrm{df})$ is the $(\alpha/2)$th upper quantile of a central t distribution with df degrees of freedom. A simple algebra shows that

$$P\{L_p < \overline{W}_{\cdot j\cdot} < U_p\} \cong 1 - \alpha, \tag{5.5.12}$$

where

$$U_p(L_p) = \overline{Y}_{\cdot j\cdot} \pm t(\tfrac{1}{2}\alpha,\mathrm{df}) \sqrt{\hat{\sigma}_{ij}^2\left(\frac{1}{I} + \frac{1}{I'}\right)}.$$

Thus a $(1 - \alpha) \times 100\%$ approximate two-sided symmetric prediction interval for any future sample mean of the jth strength over the I' batches at a particular time point is given by (L_p, U_p).

Suppose that $\overline{X}$ and s are the sample mean and standard deviation of the sample $(X_1, \ldots, X_n)$, which are randomly selected from a normal population with mean μ and variance σ^2. A two-sided tolerance interval with a degree of confidence, $1 - \alpha$, and a tolerance proportion, $1 - \gamma$, is defined as (T_L, T_U) such that

$$P\{P\{T_L < X < T_U\} \geq 1 - \gamma\} \geq 1 - \alpha, \tag{5.5.13}$$

where

$$T_U(T_L) = \overline{X} \pm g(\alpha,\gamma,n)s,$$

and $g(\alpha,\gamma,n)$ is the tolerance factor associated with confidence level of $1 - \alpha$, tolerance level of $1 - \gamma$, and sample size n. With the tolerance interval (T_L,T_U), we can assert, with $1 - \alpha$ confidence, that at least $(1 - \gamma) \times 100\%$ of the distribution is within (T_L,T_U). The derivation of the tolerance factor for the symmetrical tolerance interval of a normal distribution can be found in Bowker (1946) and Kendall and Stuart (1961). Bowker (1947) also provided a table of tolerance factors for the symmetrical tolerance interval of a normal population which is given in Appendix A. 7.

Recall that $(\bar{Y}_{1j}., \ldots, \bar{Y}_{Ij}.)$ is a random sample of sizes I chosen from a normal distribution with mean $\mu + S_j$ and variance σ_{ij}^2 which can be estimated unbiasedly by $\bar{Y}_{.j}$ in (5.5.5) and $\hat{\sigma}_{ij}^2$ in (5.5.7), respectively. Therefore, as pointed out by Wallis (1951), an approximate symmetrical tolerance interval with a confidence level of $1 - \alpha$, which contains at least $(1 - \gamma) \times 100\%$ of the sample mean $\bar{Y}_{ij}.$ for the jth strength based on K tablets over a population of I random batches, is given by (T_L,T_U), where

$$T_U(T_L) = \bar{Y}_{.j}. \pm g(\alpha,\gamma,I)\hat{\sigma}_{ij}. \tag{5.5.14}$$

It should be noted that one-sided tolerance limits can also be derived from the construction of a one-sided confidence interval for the quantile of a normal distribution using a noncentral t distribution. Details can be found in Graybill (1976) and Hahn (1970).

At a particular time point the prediction interval for the future overall sample mean and the tolerance interval for the batch means can be derived in a similar manner. Recall that the sample mean for the ith batch is given by

$$\bar{Y}_{i..} = \frac{1}{JK} \sum_{j=1}^{J} \sum_{k=1}^{K} Y_{ijk}. \tag{5.5.15}$$

$\bar{Y}_{i..}$ is an unbiased estimator for μ. The variance of $\bar{Y}_{i..}$ is given by

$$\hat{\sigma}_i^2 = \text{var}(\bar{Y}_{i..}) = \frac{1}{JK} (\sigma_e^2 + K\sigma_{BS}^2 + JK\sigma_B^2), \tag{5.5.16}$$

where $i = 1, \ldots, I$. Therefore, $\bar{Y}_{1..}, \ldots, \bar{Y}_{I..}$ are i.i.d. normal with mean μ and variance σ_i^2. An unbiased estimator of σ_i^2 is given by

$$\sigma_i^2 = \frac{\text{MSB}}{JK}. \tag{5.5.17}$$

Hence a $(1 - \alpha) \times 100\%$ prediction interval for the future mean based on I' batches at a particular time point can be obtained as (L_{TP},U_{TP}), where

$$U_{TP}(L_{TP}) = \bar{Y}_{...} \pm t(\tfrac{1}{2}\alpha, I - 1) \sqrt{\hat{\sigma}_i^2\left(\frac{1}{I} + \frac{1}{I'}\right)}, \tag{5.5.18}$$

where

$$\bar{Y}_{...} = \frac{1}{I} \sum_{i=1}^{I} \bar{Y}_{i..},$$

and $I - 1$ is the degrees of freedom associated with MSB. Furthermore, a symmetrical tolerance interval with confidence level of $1 - \alpha$, which contains at least $(1 - \gamma) \times 100\%$ of the batch means $\bar{Y}_{i..}$ at a particular time point, can be obtained as (T_{TL}, T_{TU}), where

$$T_{TU}(T_{TL}) = \bar{Y}_{...} \pm g(\alpha, \gamma, I) \hat{\sigma}_i. \tag{5.5.19}$$

At a particular time point, the variance of an assay result, Y_{ijk}, of the kth tablet in the ith batch for the jth strength is given by

$$\sigma_Y^2 = \text{var}(Y_{ijk}) = \sigma_e^2 + \sigma_{BS}^2 + \sigma_B^2. \tag{5.5.20}$$

It is clear from (5.5.20) that the variance of Y_{ijk} is the sum of three variance components: one is due to random error, one is due to batch-by-strength interaction, and one is due to batch. An unbiased estimator of σ_Y^2 can be obtained as follows:

$$\hat{\sigma}_Y^2 = \text{MSE} + \frac{1}{K} [\text{MS(BS)} - \text{MSE}] + \frac{1}{JK} [\text{MSB} - \text{MS(BS)}]$$

$$= \frac{K-1}{K} \text{MSE} + \frac{J-1}{JK} \text{MS(BS)} + \frac{1}{JK} \text{MSB}. \tag{5.5.21}$$

The corresponding degrees of freedom associated with σ_Y^2 can also be estimated as

$$df_Y = \frac{(\hat{\sigma}_Y^2)^2}{d_Y^2}, \tag{5.5.22}$$

where

$$d_Y^2 = \frac{1}{IJ(K-1)} \left(\frac{K-1}{K} \text{MSE} \right)^2$$

$$+ \frac{1}{(I-1)(J-1)} \left[\frac{J-1}{JK} \text{MS(BS)} \right]^2 + \frac{1}{I-1} \left(\frac{1}{JK} \text{MSB} \right)^2.$$

Furthermore,

$$\frac{df_Y \hat{\sigma}_y^2}{\sigma_Y^2}$$

is approximately distributed as a chi-square random variable with df_Y degrees of freedom. Therefore, an approximate $(1 - \alpha) \times 100\%$ confidence interval for

σ_Y is given by $(L_{\sigma_y}, U_{\sigma_y})$, where

$$L_{\sigma_Y} = \left[\frac{df_Y \, \hat{\sigma}_Y^2}{\chi^2 \left(\frac{1}{2} \alpha, df_Y \right)} \right]^{1/2},$$

$$U_{\sigma_Y} = \left[\frac{df_Y \, \hat{\sigma}_Y^2}{\chi^2 \left(1 - \frac{1}{2} \alpha, \, df_Y \right)} \right]^{1/2}, \qquad (5.5.23)$$

where $\chi^2(\alpha/2, df_Y)$ is the $(\alpha/2)$th upper quantile of a central chi-square distribution with degrees of freedom df_y.

Suppose that a future experiment is planned with K' tablets for each of a total of J' strengths made from a total of I' batches. Under the same model of (5.5.2), the variance of a single assay from this future experiment is also σ_Y^2, as given in (5.5.20). Let $\hat{\sigma}_Y^{'2}$ be an unbiased estimator of σ_Y^2 obtained based on (5.5.21) from a future experiment. Let df_Y' be the degrees of freedom associated with $\hat{\sigma}_Y^{'2}$. Since

$$\frac{df_Y \, \hat{\sigma}_Y^2}{\sigma_Y^2} \quad \text{and} \quad \frac{df_Y' \, \hat{\sigma}_Y^{'2}}{\sigma_Y^2}$$

are independent and each is approximately distributed as a central chi-square random variable with df_Y and df_Y' degrees of freedom, respectively,

$$F = \frac{\hat{\sigma}_Y^{'2}}{\hat{\sigma}_Y^2} \qquad (5.5.24)$$

follows approximately a central F distribution with df_Y' and df_Y degrees of freedom. As indicated by Hahn (1970), a $(1 - \alpha) \times 100\%$ upper prediction limit for the future standard deviation σ_Y of the assay can be obtained as

$$U_F = [\hat{\sigma}_Y^2 F(\alpha, df_Y', df_Y)]^{1/2}. \qquad (5.5.25)$$

Note that df_Y' in (5.5.25) is usually unknown and needs to be estimated. An ad hoc estimate of df_Y' can be obtained simply by replacing I, J, and K with I', J', and K'. Since the mean squares from the current study are used to estimate the degrees of freedom for the future experiment, strictly speaking, the numerator and denominator in F of (5.5.24) are not truly independent. Further research is necessary in this area.

Example 5.5.1

A pharmaceutical company is interested in conducting an experiment to recommend in-house dissolution specifications for the tablets of a pharmaceutical compound. Three batches of granulation were each made into three tablet strengths (200 mg, 300 mg, and 400 mg). Twelve dissolution assays were performed at 2, 4, 8, and 14 h on each of the nine batches by strength combinations. The results are given in Table 5.5.2. The means and standard deviations for each batch-by-strength combination are given in Tables 5.5.3 and 5.5.4.

Table 5.5.5 provides the ANOVA table with the expected mean squares for model (5.5.2) with batch as a random effect and strength as a fixed effect for $I = 3$, $J = 3$, and $K = 12$. The results of the analysis of variance table for data set given in Table 5.5.2 under model (5.5.2) are summarized in Table 5.5.6 by time point. It can be seen from Table 5.5.6 that there exist significant differences in dissolution among strengths (p values < 0.01). Dissolution decreases as strength increases. Marginal batch-to-batch variability was found at the 2-h point ($p = 0.067$). However, no batch-to-batch variability was found at other time points (p values ≥ 0.14).

Note that although the sample means given in Table 5.5.3 are unbiased estimates of their corresponding population parameter, the pooled standard deviations given in Table 5.5.4 are not the corresponding standard deviations for the pooled means. For example, the overall mean pooled at 2 h is 20.4, which is an unbiased estimate for μ at 2 h. Howver, the corresponding pooled standard deviation at 2 h is 0.76, which is the square root of the mean-squared error (0.5814) of the ANOVA table under model (5.5.2) at 2 h as given in Table 5.5.6. Therefore, the pooled standard deviation at 2 h given in Table 5.5.4 is not the standard deviation associated with the pooled sample mean at 2 h. Similarly, the pooled time point-by-strength standard deviations in Table 5.5.4 are not the standard deviations corresponding to the pooled time point-by-strength means.

At each time point-by-strength combination, two sets of in-house specifications limits were recommended. The first set is constructed using prediction interval. These intervals were computed so that the future time point-by-strength sample mean will be within the limits with 95% assurance. On the other hand, the second set is constructed using a tolerance interval such that each interval will contain 95% of the batch-by-strength sample means based on 12 tablets at a particular time point with 95% assurance. Both sets of in-house specifications were derived based on the corrected standard errors, which account for all sources of variations, such as variations due to random error, batch-by-strength interaction, and batch. Table 5.5.7 gives both sets of specifications limits. Similarly, the recommended in-house specifications for each time point that will cover all three strengths are given in Table 5.5.8. It should be noted that the recommended in-house specifications for time point-by-strength means given in Table 5.5.7 are approximations, while those given in Table 5.5.8 for each time point are exact. The point estimates of σ_Y^2 for each time point and the recommended in-house specifications for σ_Y^2 based on both the 95% confidence interval and the upper 95% prediction limits for $I' = 3$, $J' = 3$, and $K' = 4$ are given in Table 5.5.9.

TABLE 5.5.2 Assay Results (Percent of Claim) for Dissolution

Strength	Batch	Time	1	2	3	4	5	6	7	8	9	10	11	12
200	1	2	22.0	22.9	22.3	22.6	23.5	22.0	23.5	22.3	22.9	22.9	22.6	23.5
		4	43.3	43.3	42.7	44.8	45.1	43.3	43.6	41.3	42.7	43.9	42.7	45.1
		8	77.2	75.5	74.6	79.0	78.7	77.8	77.2	72.9	76.6	76.9	77.2	79.9
		14	101.6	98.4	96.4	98.2	98.8	98.7	99.3	95.8	96.7	97.0	98.7	98.8
	2	2	24.4	23.9	24.1	23.6	23.6	23.0	24.7	22.7	24.1	23.3	23.3	25.0
		4	46.8	45.3	47.3	45.3	44.8	44.8	47.0	42.8	46.2	44.5	42.5	49.3
		8	80.5	80.4	83.0	81.0	80.4	79.3	81.9	78.7	81.6	80.1	78.2	83.3
		14	98.8	96.8	97.4	97.7	97.7	98.5	95.8	100.1	100.2	97.1	99.8	96.4
	3	2	24.8	24.3	24.3	24.8	24.8	23.7	25.4	23.7	25.4	24.8	24.3	25.4
		4	49.5	47.3	47.8	46.2	46.7	45.6	47.9	44.5	47.9	49.0	46.2	49.5
		8	84.7	80.7	81.9	79.6	80.2	80.7	81.3	80.2	95.8	84.7	79.6	85.8
		14	100.7	98.4	99.5	98.4	98.4	98.4	97.9	98.4	99.7	99.0	98.4	98.5
300	1	2	18.0	19.6	17.6	16.2	18.6	19.8	19.8	17.8	19.6	15.8	16.6	16.2
		4	37.1	38.3	35.1	33.6	38.0	41.0	41.6	34.0	41.4	31.8	35.7	33.9
		8	75.3	74.8	73.2	69.9	76.7	78.7	78.7	75.5	79.4	69.3	73.2	71.4
		14	96.9	98.3	99.2	97.2	97.5	96.8	98.2	96.8	98.6	97.8	97.6	97.0
	2	2	19.9	21.8	20.1	22.5	20.6	20.8	21.0	20.1	21.6	20.5	20.5	20.8
		4	38.9	42.1	39.1	43.5	39.1	40.8	39.9	38.9	42.1	39.3	38.2	39.1
		8	74.1	76.6	73.9	82.4	74.9	76.2	76.7	75.6	78.1	73.4	71.7	73.4
		14	96.5	99.0	96.7	102.6	98.0	99.1	101.4	100.4	97.5	98.2	97.6	99.4
	3	2	20.7	21.1	20.3	23.0	21.1	21.4	21.8	21.4	21.4	19.9	20.7	21.4
		4	40.2	41.3	39.4	43.2	39.8	41.7	41.7	40.9	41.3	39.0	40.9	40.9
		8	74.4	76.6	73.2	78.9	75.1	76.2	77.0	75.1	77.0	74.4	74.7	75.5
		14	97.5	100.5	97.1	98.7	97.2	97.9	97.9	97.9	98.3	98.2	99.0	99.0

400												
1	2	16.4	17.6	17.0	17.0	17.3	17.0	18.2	17.3	17.6	16.7	16.1	17.6
	4	34.2	35.1	34.8	35.1	33.7	33.1	36.3	32.5	35.1	35.1	32.8	35.1
	8	66.4	69.9	66.1	68.2	66.4	67.3	71.4	63.8	69.9	68.5	67.3	69.9
	14	89.9	93.1	88.5	92.0	89.6	91.1	94.0	88.2	92.5	89.9	91.1	92.6
2	2	18.6	17.8	18.1	17.2	17.8	17.8	18.3	17.5	17.8	18.1	17.5	18.3
	4	37.4	35.2	35.8	34.1	34.1	34.3	34.9	35.8	34.3	34.9	32.7	37.7
	8	70.3	69.2	69.2	68.3	66.7	68.9	67.5	64.7	67.5	68.6	65.5	72.3
	14	97.0	94.8	95.1	94.0	93.4	95.1	93.7	92.0	93.7	94.0	93.6	96.3
3	2	17.8	17.5	17.8	17.8	17.8	17.5	17.8	17.8	17.8	18.1	17.2	18.3
	4	35.8	33.5	34.1	34.6	33.8	33.2	33.8	34.1	33.5	34.6	31.5	36.6
	8	67.5	65.8	66.1	67.5	66.1	66.4	65.3	65.6	66.4	65.9	61.9	70.0
	14	96.2	93.7	93.4	95.3	95.9	93.9	91.5	92.3	94.2	92.0	88.6	94.8

TABLE 5.5.3   Descriptive Statistics for Means (Percent of Claim)

Time point (h)	Batch	Strength (mg/tablet) 200	300	400	Mean
2	1	22.8	18.0	17.2	19.3
	2	23.8	20.9	17.9	20.9
	3	24.6	21.2	17.8	21.2
	Mean	23.7	20.0	17.6	20.4
4	1	43.5	36.8	34.4	38.2
	2	45.6	40.1	35.1	40.2
	3	47.3	40.9	34.1	40.8
	Mean	45.4	39.2	34.5	39.7
8	1	77.0	74.7	67.9	73.2
	2	80.7	75.6	68.2	74.8
	3	82.9	75.7	66.2	74.9
	Mean	80.2	75.3	67.4	74.3
14	1	98.2	97.7	91.0	95.6
	2	98.0	98.9	94.4	97.1
	3	98.8	98.3	93.5	96.8
	Mean	98.3	98.3	93.0	96.5

TABLE 5.5.4   Descriptive Statistics for Standard Deviations (Percent of Claim)

Time point (h)	Batch	Strength (mg/tablet) 200	300	400	Pooled
2	1	0.55	1.52	0.58	0.99
	2	0.69	0.77	0.40	0.64
	3	0.60	0.78	0.28	0.59
	Pooled	0.62	1.08	0.44	**0.76**
4	1	1.12	3.32	1.15	2.13
	2	1.92	1.66	1.42	1.68
	3.	1.57	1.15	1.28	1.34
	Pooled	1.57	2.24	1.29	**1.75**
8	1	1.93	3.39	2.13	2.57
	2	1.57	2.79	2.06	2.20
	3	4.58	1.54	1.85	2.99
	Pooled	3.01	2.69	2.02	**2.61**
14	1	1.56	0.78	1.85	1.47
	2	1.46	1.86	1.35	1.57
	3	0.79	0.94	2.14	1.42
	Pooled	1.31	1.28	1.81	**1.49**

TABLE 5.5.5   ANOVA Table

Source	df	Expected mean square[a]
S	2	$\sigma_e^2 + 12\sigma_{SB}^2 + Q(S)$
B	2	$\sigma_e^2 + 12\sigma_{SB}^2 + 36\sigma_B^2$
SB	4	$\sigma_e^2 + 12\sigma_{SB}^2$
Error	99	σ_e^2

[a] $Q(S) = 18 \, \Sigma (S_i - \overline{S})^2$.

5.6. DISCUSSION

The results on acceptance limits for uniformity and dissolution of dosage units were derived from the lower probability bound given in (5.3.3), which was proposed by Bergum (1990). This approach is an approximation to the exact probability of passing the USP test. Bergum (1990) also examined the accuracy of the lower probability bound for uniformity of dosage units by the central F approximation through a simulation of 10,000 random samples for several combinations of population means and standard deviations. The results are summarized in Table 5.6.1. Also included in Table 5.6.1 are the results of the normal

TABLE 5.5.6   ANOVA Table by Time Point for the Data Set in Table 5.5.2

Time point (h)	Source of variation	df	Sum of squares	Mean squares	F statistic	P value
2	Strength	2	686.6496	343.3248	52.76	0.0013
	Batch	2	74.4735	37.2368	7.52	0.0671
	Strength by batch	4	26.0270	6.5068	11.19	<0.0001
	Error	99	57.5583	0.5814		
4	Strength	2	2161.9513	1080.9756	55.06	0.0012
	Batch	2	129.2235	64.6118	3.29	0.1429
	Strength by batch	4	78.5237	19.6309	6.43	<0.0001
	Error	99	302.0492	3.0510		
8	Strength	2	2976.5802	1488.2901	32.21	0.0034
	Batch	2	69.6635	34.8318	0.75	0.5275
	Strength by batch	4	184.8398	46.2100	6.81	<0.0001
	Error	99	671.8517	6.7864		
14	Strength	2	682.4280	341.2140	33.54	0.0032
	Batch	2	44.1635	22.0818	2.17	0.2300
	Strength by batch	4	40.6915	10.1729	4.58	0.0020
	Error	99	219.8492	2.2207		

TABLE 5.5.7 Dissolution Specifications Limits for the Time Point-by-Strength Means (Percent of Claim)

Time point (h)	Strength (mg/tablet)	Approximate 95% prediction interval	Approximate tolerance interval[a]
2	200	(20.87,26.59)	(12.01,35.45)
	300	(17.14,22.86)	(8.28,31.72)
	400	(14.75,20.47)	(5.89,29.33)
4	200	(41.73,49.19)	(28.62,62.30)
	300	(35.51,42.97)	(22.40,56.08)
	400	(30.80,38.26)	(17.69,51.37)
8	200	(76.60,83.80)	(62.41,97.99)
	300	(71.71,78.91)	(57.52,93.10)
	400	(63.85,71.05)	(49.66,85.24)
14	200	(90.09,100.60)	(87.58,109.11)
	300	(96.01,100.52)	(87.50,109.03)
	400	(90.72,95.23)	(82.21,103.74)

[a]Tolerance interval = with 95% assurance; 95% of the future batch-by-strength means will lie between the two limits.

approximation. When the standard deviation is small, the lower probability bound by both methods provides an adequate approximation to the simulated exact probability. However, when the standard deviation is 6, the difference between the lower probability bound by approximation and simulated exact probability becomes pronounced. In addition, the difference is in the direction of conservativeness of the lower probability bound in the sense that the probability of passing the test for the simulated exact probability is uniformly larger than that by the lower probability bound. It should be noted, however, that the

TABLE 5.5.8 Recommended Specifications for the Overall Means

Time point (h)	95% Prediction interval	Tolerance interval[a]
2	(16.87,24.02)	(10.36,30.53)
4	(35.04,44.45)	(26.46,53.03)
8	(70.34,78.30)	(63.09,85.54)
14	(93.77,99.27)	(88.76,104.29)

[a]Tolerance interval = with 95% assurance; 95% of the future batch mean will lie between the two limits.

TABLE 5.5.9   Recommended Specifications for Standard Deviation

Time point (h)	Point estimate	Approximate 95% confidence interval	Approximate 95% upper prediction limit[a]
2	2.41	(1.57,5.07)	4.97
4	4.13	(3.08,6.26)	6.72
8	5.32	(4.38,6.78)	7.46
14	3.11	(2.51,4.08)	4.50

[a]For a future experiment with four tablets for each of three batches and three strengths.

normal approximation is less conservative, which provides a better approximation than the central F approximation.

Tsong et al. (1992) investigated the operating characteristic curves of multiple-stage sampling dissolution tests as stated in the USP/NF. They found that these tests are rather liberal in their inability to reject a lot with a high fraction of units dissolved less than Q and with an average amount dissolved just slightly larger than Q. Hence they suggested two alternative multiple-stage sampling tests for dissolution. The first is a modification of the current USP/NF procedure, which changes $Q - 15\%$ at stages 2 and 3 in Table 5.2.2 to a more stringent limit $Q - 5\%$. The second is a three-stage sampling test, which is based primarily on the results of sample mean and sample standard deviation

TABLE 5.6.1   Lower Probability Bound and Simulated Exact Probability for Uniformity of Dosage Units (Percent Passing Test)[a]

		2			4			6	
μ	LB(F)	LB(N)	EP	LB(F)	LB(N)	EP	LB(F)	LB(N)	EP
86	2.5	2.5	2.5	0.0	0.1	0.6	0.0	0.0	0.2
90	98.5	98.5	99.1	26.8	32.5	36.8	0.0	0.9	9.0
94	100.0	100.0	100.0	94.8	94.8	96.8	34.7	39.0	53.7
98	100.0	100.0	100.0	100.0	100.0	100.0	88.4	90.3	92.0
100	100.0	100.0	100.0	100.0	100.0	100.0	93.4	94.6	95.7
102	100.0	100.0	100.0	100.0	100.0	100.0	89.6	90.3	92.9
106	100.0	100.0	100.0	94.8	94.8	97.0	38.8	44.2	55.8
110	98.5	98.5	99.1	32.4	32.7	36.4	0.9	6.4	10.0
114	2.5	2.5	2.5	0.4	0.6	0.5	0.0	0.0	0.3

[a]LB(F), lower probability bound with the approximation by the central F distribution; LB(N), lower probability bound with the approximation by the standard normal distribution; EP, simulated exact probability.

TABLE 5.6.2 Alternative Three-Stage Sampling Test for Dissolution Proposed by Tsong et al. (1992)

Stage	Number tested	Criteria[a]
1	6	Accept if $P\{(\overline{Y}_1 - Q)/s_1 > 0\} > A_1$; reject if $P\{(\overline{Y}_1 - Q)/s_1 > 0\} < B_1$; otherwise, go to stage 2.
2	6	Accept if $P\{(\overline{Y}_2 - Q)/s_2 > 0\} > A_2$; reject if $P\{(\overline{Y}_2 - Q)/s_2 > 0\} < B_2$; otherwise, go to stage 3.
3	12	Accept if $P\{(\overline{Y}_3 - Q)/s_3 > 0\} > A_3$; otherwise, reject.

[a]$\overline{Y}_1$, $\overline{Y}_2$, and $\overline{Y}_3$ and s_1, s_2, and s_3 are the sample means and standard deviations at stages 1, 2, and 3 based on 6, 12, and 24 units, respectively.

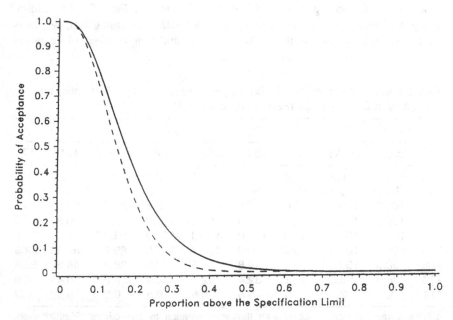

FIGURE 5.6.1 Operating characteristic curves for disintegration test. Solid curve, exact probability; dashed curve, lower probability bound.

and some prespecified limits. This proposed three-stage sampling test is summarized in Table 5.6.2. It can be seen from Table 5.6.2 that the probability of passing the test depends on A_1, A_2, A_3, and B_1 and B_2. It is suggested that $A_1 = A_3 = 0.95$, $A_2 = 0.85$, and $B_1 = B_2 = 0.05$. Tsong et al. (1992) also compared the operating characteristic curves of the three procedures. The USP/NF procedure is the most liberal of the three methods, and their proposed three-stage sampling test is the most conservative; the probability of passing the modified USP/NF test lies between these two procedures. It should be noted that the exact probabilities of these tests are difficult to obtain. More research on the operating characteristics is needed. However, since the disintegration test depends on only a single event, the operating characteristic curves for the exact probability and lower probability bound can easily be obtained using (5.3.12) and (5.3.14), which are plotted in Fig. 5.6.1. It can be seen from the figure that the lower probability bound approach provides an adequate approximation to the exact probability if $P\{0 < Y < \text{UL}\} > 0.9$.

6

Process Validation

6.1. INTRODUCTION

In Chapter 4 we discussed statistical designs and analyses for scaling up a laboratory batch or small-scale production batch to a regular production batch. A scaleup study is conducted to demonstrate that the production batch is equivalent to the laboratory or small-scale production batch often used for product testing prior to manufacture. In Chapter 5 we described requirements for product testing stated in the USP/NF. These requirements are essential to ensure the identity, strength, quality, and purity of the drug product. In this chapter we focus on the validation of a manufacturing process under appropriate statistical designs and analyses according to USP/NF specifications.

A manufacturing process is a continuous process that usually involves a number of stages (see Fig. 6.1.1). As an example, consider the manufacturing process for tablets of a pharmaceutical compound. Table 6.1.1 summarizes the critical stages of the manufacturing process. It can be seen from Table 6.1.1 that the process consists of several critical stages including the active preblending stage, the primary blending stage, the lubricant preblending stage, the final blending stage, and the compression stage. At each critical stage, problems may occur during the process. For example, the ingredients may not be uniformly mixed at the primary blending stage; the segregation may occur at the final blending stage; a significant loss of active ingredient may be encountered during transfer from the V-blender to the transport devices, and the weight of tablets may not be suitably controlled during the compression stage (see also Table

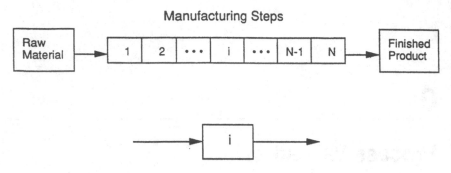

Unit Process Step (i) with Associated Process Characteristics

$$\text{Total Manufacturing Process} \quad = \quad \sum_{i=1}^{N} \quad (\text{Unit Process Step } i)$$

FIGURE 6.1.1   Process decomposition.

6.1.1). When such a problem is encountered at any critical stage of a manufacturing process, the final drug product may not meet the USP/NF specifications for identity, strength, quality, and purity. In practice it is therefore important to evaluate each critical stage of a manufacturing process to ensure that the ingredients are uniformly mixed, segregation does not occur, no significant loss of the active ingredient is encountered, and there is adequate weight control during compression. To achieve these objectives, the in-process and/or processed materials are usually tested for potency, dosage uniformity (i.e., content uniformity or weight variation), dissolution, and disintegration according to sampling plans and acceptance criteria stated in the USP/NF at each critical stage of the manufacturing process. The in-process and/or processed materials at each stage are said to pass the USP/NF tests if the test results meet specifications. A manufacturing process is considered as passing the tests if each critical stage of the manufacturing process and the final drug product meet the required USP/NF specifications for the identity, strength, quality, and purity of the drug product.

TABLE 6.1.1 Schematic of Tablet Manufacturing Process

Stage	USP tests	Test objectives
Active preblending	[a]	[a]
Milling	[a]	[a]
Primary blending	Content uniformity	Uniformity
		Segregation
Lubricant preblending	[b]	[b]
Milling	[b]	[b]
Final blending	Content uniformity	Uniformity
		Segregation
Blending in transports	Potency	Potency loss
	Content uniformity	Uniformity
		Segregation
Compressoin	Potency	Potency loss
	Content uniformity	Uniformity
		Segregation
	Weight variation	Weight control
	Dissolution	Segregation

[a]Not critical stages; content uniformity tested at primary blending stage.
[b]Not critical stages; content uniformity tested at final blending stage.

Since each critical stage of the manufacturing process of a drug product may have a significant impact on the identity, strength, quality, and purity of the drug product, it is important to evaluate the performance of the manufacturing process at each critical stage. For this purpose CGMP indicates that a written procedure be established to document and validate the performance of a manufacturing process. The validation of a manufacturing process assures not only that the process does what it purports to do but also that the drug product will conform to USP/NF specifications (Chapman, 1983; Kohberger, 1988). Basically, a manufacturing process is considered validated if at least three batches (or lots) pass all required USP/NF tests. In practice, for the validation of a manufacturing process, acceptance limits for potency, content uniformity, dissolution, and disintegration are usually constructed according to respective sampling plans and acceptance criteria specified in the USP/NF. These acceptance limits are constructed so that if the validation sample meets the limits, there is high probability that a sample taken for the required USP/NF test will pass the test. These acceptance limits are usually applied to evaluate passage of the critical stages of a manufacturing process.

In the next section we introduce the concept of three approaches to the validation of a manufacturing process: prospective validation, concurrent validation, and retrospective validation. Some basic considerations for the development of a validation protocol are summarized in Sec. 6.3. In Sec. 6.4 the objectives, sampling plans, and testing plans for the critical stages of a manufacturing process are introduced through a real example concerning a manufacturing process for tablets of a drug product. In Sec. 6.5 the construction of acceptance limits for content uniformity testing is outlined briefly. A discussion of process validation is given in Sec. 6.6.

6.2. PROCESS CONTROL AND VALIDATION

6.2.1. Introduction

For the evaluation of a manufacturing process of a drug product, subpart F of part 210 for CGMP in 21 CFR describes the requirements of sampling plans and test procedures for in-process control and process validation. CGMP requires that drug manufacturers establish and follow written procedures for in-process controls and process validations. The in-process controls and process validations should be tested or examined based on appropriate samples drawn from in-process materials of each batch. In practice we may observe some expected or unexpected sources of variabilities in some drug characteristics, such as potency and dissolution. The written procedures for in-process controls and process validation are useful in monitoring the on-line and off-line performance of the manufacturing process and consequently, in validating the manufacturing process. For the establishment of written procedures of in-process controls and process validations, the CGMP indicates that some minimum requirements should be established. These requirements are summarized as follows:

1. Adequacy of mixing to assure uniformity and homogeneity
2. Dissolution time and rate
3. Disintegration time
4. Tablet or capsule weight variation
5. Clarity, completeness, or pH of solution

It should be noted that the USP/NF specifications for content uniformity testing of dosage form, dissolution testing, and disintegration testing described in Chapter 5 satisfy requirements 1 through 3. To ensure the identity, strength, quality, and purity of the drug product, in-process materials as well as the final product must conform to USP/NF specifications. The in-process materials and the final product can be examined by testing their representative samples. Statistical methods are usually applied to determine whether the USP/NF specifications for all drug characteristics are met based on the estimated process average and variability, which may be derived from previously validated or acceptable processes.

The concept of in-process control and process validation is not new, which has been well established in various industries in the United States. The pharmaceutical industry, however, is different from other industries for at least following two aspects. First, drug products are usually administered to human subjects and absorbed into their body system (almost) to relieve a certain illness. It is therefore important to ensure the identity, strength, quality, and purity of drug products. Any derivation from USP/NF specifications for the identity, strength, quality, and purity of the drug products can result not only in not achieving its effectiveness but also cause severe adverse reactions. Second, in the pharmaceutical industry, the size of a batch (e.g., tablets) is usually measured in the unit of millions of tablets. The batch of millions of tablets is either accepted or rejected, depending on the results of a few tablets sampled for the USP/NF tests for potency, content uniformity, dissolution, and disintegration. The rejection of a batch is usually very costly because the batch may have to be destroyed, especially when the active ingredient of the batch cannot be recovered for reuse. In this case the traditional acceptance sampling plan adopted by other industries may not be feasible for drug products. It is then suggested that a well-established control procedure be used to monitor the continuous manufacturing process. When there is a deviation from the established control specifications, the possible causes for deviation must be found and immediate corrective actions taken. CGMP requires that all manufacturers of drug products follow established control procedures for drug products.

6.2.2. Process Validation

A process validation is usually referred to the establishment of documented evidence that a process does what it purports to do (Chapman, 1983). Basically, there are three different types of manufacturing process validations in the pharmaceutical industry: prospective, concurrent, and retrospective (Chapman, 1983; Kohberger, 1988), described below:

1. *Prospective validation*: establishing documented evidence that a process does what it purports to do based on a preplanned protocol
2. *Concurrent validation*: establishing documented evidence that a process does what it purports to do based on information generated during actual implementation of the process
3. *Retrospective validation*: establishing documented evidence that a process does what it purports to do based on review and analysis of historic information

The definitions above indicate that a prospective validation, a concurrent validation, and a retrospective validation may be applied to validate a manufacturing process depending on the timing and manner with which the information for the validation of the manufacturing process is collected.

A prospective validation of a manufacturing process is usually applied when:

1. Historical data are not available or sufficient and in-process and end-product testing data are not adequate. For example, a sterile solution filled by a new piece of equipment needs a media-fill prospective validation.
2. New equipment or components are used.
3. New products, reformulation of an existing product, or significant modifications or changes in the manufacturing process are present.
4. Transferring the manufacturing process from the development laboratory to full-scale production.

In practice, for a prospective validation, since we may not have any prior or very limited information regarding the manufacturing process (e.g., new drug products), a much more tightly controlled environment is usually adopted to ensure that the manufacturing process does what it purports to do. As a result, a prospective validation is usually labor intensive and/or time consuming to establish.

Although the prospective validation requires that three batches be produced and tested and the resulting product may meet its release specifications, the validation may not be tight enough to give the confidence desired. In this case the prospective validation may not be approved until additional validation tests are available. Therefore, current validation can serve as backup prospective validation. A concurrent validation is an option that is often used in the following situations when:

1. A step of a process is modified.
2. The vendor of an inactive ingredient is changed.
3. The product is made infrequently.
4. A process is validated when a coating process or coating solution formula undergoes some changes.
5. A new raw material must be introduced.
6. For established marketed products for which original development data are not sufficient or available.

Therefore, the concurrent validation of a manufacturing process is useful in monitoring whether the manufacturing process has done what it is purported to do up to the point that the manufacturing process is validated. A concurrent validation can generally provide valuable information to modify or correct the manufacturing process when a problem is encountered during the validation. Consequently, a batch itself may be validated concurrently with its manufacture.

It should be noted, however, that FDA feels that a current validation verifies the quality characteristics of a "particular batch" and no high degree of assurance of the same quality will be attained again. Despite the FDA comments, the current validation concept has been widely accepted based on the acceptability of product testing provided in the FDA guideline and incorporated in many validation projects by the pharmaceutical industry.

A retrospective validation is usually considered for drug products currently available in the marketplace. For established products whose manufacturing processes are stable, we may use the large volume of historical data that already exist to demonstrate the validity of the process. It is useful to augment initial premarket prospective validation for a new product or changed process since additional data on production lots can be very useful to support the confidence of the process.

In practice, for a well-established manufacturing process, it may need a revalidation in the following situations when:

1. There are changes in critical components (usually, raw materials).
2. There are changes or replacements in a critical piece of equipment or packing.
3. There are changes in the facility or plant (e.g., location or size).
4. There is a significant increase or decrease in batch size.
5. Sequential lots fail to meet specification limits.

Note that the FDA guideline suggests periodic reevaluation (or revalidation) of the manufacturing process even if no significant process changes are made.

For each type of validation, the USP/NF requires that appropriate representative samples be randomly drawn and statistically analyzed at each critical stage of the manufacturing process to evaluate whether the product conforms to USP/NF specifications. Test results from each critical stage of the manufacturing process provide useful information regarding the performance of the manufacturing process. In addition to product testing for evaluation of the manufacturing process, Chapman (1983) indicated that the following variables are also useful in characterizing the performance of a manufacturing process for drug products:

Control parameters: those operating variables that can be assigned values that are used as control levels
Operating variables: all factors, including control variables, that may potentially affect the process state of control and/or fitness for use of the final product
State of control: a condition in which all operating variables that can affect performance remain within such ranges that the system or process performs consistently and as intended
Edge of failure: a control parameter value that, if exceeded, indicates an adverse effect on the state of control and/or fitness for use of the product

Worst case: the highest or lowest value of a given control parameter actually evaluated in a validation

Installation qualification: documented verification that all key aspects of the installation adhere to appropriate codes and approved design intentions and that the manufacturer's recommendations are suitably considered

Operational qualification: documented verification that a system or subsystem performs as intended throughout all anticipated operating ranges

Validation protocol: a prospective experimental plan that when executed is intended to produce documented evidence that the system has been validated

As an example, Table 6.2.1 provides retrospective validation criteria for some control parameters and operating variables for manufacturing tablets of a pharmaceutical compound.

6.2.3. Prospective Validation

As mentioned earlier, a prospective validation is usually applied to the manufacturing process for new drug products. Typically, fewer batches, which may be obtained at the early stage of drug development, are available for statistical evaluations. A prospective validation generally requires that at least three batches be evaluated. For each batch, data are usually collected at each critical stage of the manufacturing process according to a validation protocol. Figure 6.2.1 is a flowchart of a prospective validation. A commonly adopted prospective validation usually consists of the following steps:

1. Qualification of systems and subsystems, such as installation qualification, operational qualification, and calibration
2. Approval of the validation protocol

TABLE 6.2.1 Retrospective Validation Criteria

Criteria	Statistical test
1. High percentage of batches meet specifications	Determine that probability batch meets specifications: a. Binomial confidence limits b. Statistical tolerance limits c. Individual test determination
2. Process meets target value	Confidence limits on process average
3. Lack of trends in key parameters	Trend tests, such as mean-squared successive difference test (Nelson, 1980)

Source: Kohberger (1988).

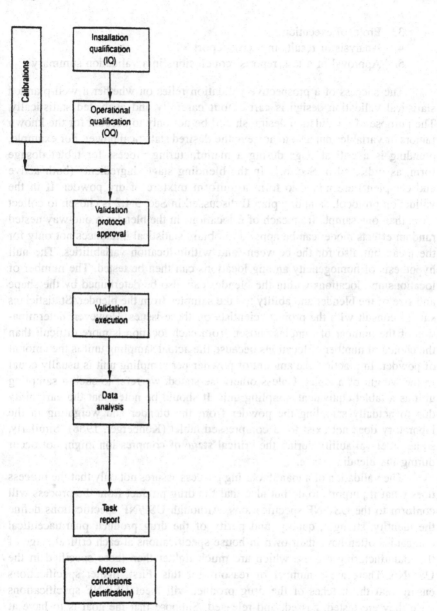

FIGURE 6.2.1 Prospective process validation. [From Chapman (1983).]

3. Protocol execution
4. Analysis of results in a task report
5. Approval of a task reports' conclusions in a validation summary

The success of a prospective validation relies on whether a well-planned statistical validation design is carried out carefully and evaluated statistically. The purpose of a validation design should be not only to account for the known factors or variables but also to achieve the desired statistical power. For example, blending is a critical stage during a manufacturing process for tablet dosage form, as indicated in Sec. 6.1. In the blending stage, ingredients (both active and excipient) are mixed to form a uniform mixture of dry powder. If in the validation protocol, sampling plan II discussed in Sec. 5.4.2 is chosen to collect more than one sample from each of L locations in the blender, a one-way nested random effects model can be applied to obtain statistical inferences not only for the mean but also for the between- and within-location variabilities. The null hypothesis of homogeneity among locations can then be tested. The number of locations and locations within the blender can also be determined by the shape and size of the blender and ability to take samples from the blender. Statisticians should consult with the project scientists on these issues. However, determination of the number of samples chosen from each location is more difficult than the choice of number of locations because the actual sampling unit is the amount of powder. In practice, the amount of powder per sampling unit is usually equal to the weight of a tablet. Unless otherwise stated, we refer to such a sampling unit as a tablet equivalent sampling unit. It should be noted that the variability due to actually sampling the powder from the blender and weighting in the laboratory does not exist for a compressed tablet (Kohberger, 1988). Similarly, some other variability during the critical stage of compression might not occur during the blending stage.

The validation of a manufacturing process assures not only that the process does what it purports to do but also that the drug product from the process will conform to the USP/NF specifications. Although USP/NF specifications define the identity, strength, quality, and purity of the drug product, pharmaceutical companies often have their own in-house specifications at each critical stage of the manufacturing process which are much tighter than those specified in the USP/NF. There are a number of reasons for this. First, tighter specifications ensure that the batches of the drug product will meet USP/NF specifications once they are tested, passed, and released. Suppose that the goal is to have at least 95% of batches from the manufacturing process pass USP/NF specifications. Suppose that there are three critical stages in this manufacturing process. Furthermore, the in-house specifications at each critical stage are selected to have about 95% of incoming materials meet USP/NF specifications. Thus it is easy to see that only $(0.95)^3 = 85.7\%$ of batches of the final product will meet

USP/NF specifications. To achieve the goal of 95% for the final product, stringent in-house specifications are necessarily chosen so that at least 98.3% of incoming materials will meet USP/NF specifications at each stage. However, if in-house specifications are too strict, not many batches will pass the tests. Therefore, a proper balance between the goal for the final product and stringency in in-house specifications should be reached. In addition to the fact that a manufacturing process is a multiple-stage process, the characteristics of the drug product for evaluating the performance of a manufacturing process is also multivariate (see Table 4.3.3). Hence there is an urgent need for research to take into account both the multistage process and multidimensionality in design and analysis for validation of the manufacturing process of a drug product.

6.2.4. Retrospective Validation

For a retrospective validation, data from manufacturing batch records, in-process testing for content uniformity, dissolution, disintegration, and other USP/NF criteria, and stability testing are compiled, reviewed, and analyzed statistically to reconfirm that control parameter ranges are in fact validated. Revelation of worst-case conditions and the edges of failure can also be achieved through a review of process waiers, results from quality assurance investigation, and final product or in-process rejection. Retrospective validation, in general, does not require a validation protocol. However, it is necessary to obtain appropriate formal approvals of the final results from upper management. The flowchart of a retrospective validation is given in Fig. 6.2.2 (Chapman, 1983). Table 6.2.1 provides a list of the common criteria used in retrospective validations for a manufacturing process for drug products (Kohberger, 1988)

Since a retrospective validation is based on the history of a manufacturing process, it is usually evaluated based on a large number of batches over an extended period of time. However, the information for each batch is sometimes limited, due to the fact that only a few random samples are taken from a batch for determining the acceptability for release. The approach of binomial confidence limits as indicated in Table 6.2.1 has very limited applications. This is because almost all the USP/NF specifications involve multiple-stage sampling plans. In addition, other environmental factors, such as batches or location, should also be taken into account for determining the probability that a batch will pass the specifications. Based on a large number of batches, in addition to the process average, the within-batch and between-batch variabilities can also be estimated. Nelson (1980) indicated that a trend analysis may be performed to check whether a significant trend exists among batches over a given period of time. In summary, as suggested by Kohberger (1988), a retrospective validation may be the most conclusive proof that a manufacturing process produces the drug product that it purports to produce.

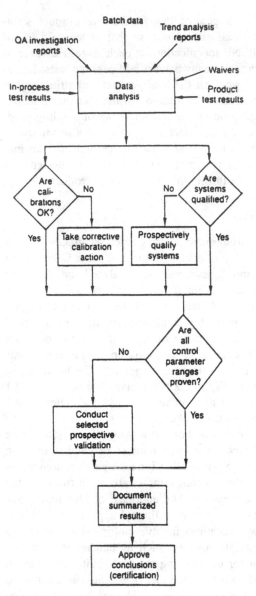

FIGURE 6.2.2   Retrospective process validation. [From Chapman (1983).]

Since a prospective validation executes a preplanned experiment through a validation design, statistical inference regarding the performance of a manufacturing process can be assessed without bias. In the next few sections we focus on prospective validations. Details such as basic statistical considerations, sampling and testing plans at each critical stage during a manufacturing process, and the construction of specifications in the form of acceptance limits for content uniformity are given.

6.3. BASIC CONSIDERATIONS

6.3.1. Introduction

As indicated earlier, the primary objective of process validation is to provide documented evidence that a manufacturing process does reliably what it purports to do. To accomplish this prospectively, a validation protocol is usually developed. A validation protocol should include the formulation of the drug, the manufacturing procedure, and objectives, sampling plans, testing plans, and acceptance criteria for each USP test to be performed at each critical stage of the manufacturing process. The statistically based sampling plans, testing plans, and acceptance criteria ensure, with a high degree of confidence, that the manufacturing process does what it purports to do.

Since manufacturing procedures vary from drug product to drug product and/or from site to site during the development of a validation protocol of a manufacturing process, it is important to discuss the following issues with project scientists to acquire a good understanding of the manufacturing process:

1. Critical stages
2. Equipment to be used at each critical stage
3. Possible problems
4. USP tests to be performed
5. Sampling plans
6. Testing plans
7. Acceptance criteria
8. Pertinent information
9. Test or specification to be used as reference
10. Validation summary

When a problem is observed in a manufacturing process, it is crucial to locate at which stage the problem occurred so that it can be corrected and the manufacturing process can do what it purports to do. As indicated earlier, in practice, the manufacturing process is usually evaluated by constant monitoring of its critical stages. Therefore, for the validation of a manufacturing process, it is recommended that project scientists be consulted to identify the critical stages of the manufacturing process. At each stage of the manufacturing process, it is also helpful to have knowledge of the equipment to be used and its components. The equipment may affect the conformance with compendial specifications for product quality. For example, at the blending stage, a V-blender with an intensifier bar is often used. The size of the blender may have an impact on the degree of segregation that may occur during blending. In addition, when blending is complete, the material may be transferred to either transports or drums, which may cause a certain degree of segregation or potency loss.

For a different manufacturing process, different problems may be encountered. For example, for the tablet manufacturing process described in Table 6.1.1, since no granulating or drying stages are involved, the major concerns of the manufacturing process are that (1) the active ingredients and excipients are uniformly mixed, (2) segregation does not occur at later stages in the process; (3) no significant losses of active ingredients are encountered, and (4) there is suitable weight control during compression. An understanding of potential problems that may occur at each critical stage of a manufacturing process is crucial in the validation and quality assurance of the manufacturing process.

After having understood the problems that may occur at each critical stage of a manufacturing process, appropriate USP tests should be performed to evaluate whether the problems have occurred. For this purpose, the validation protocol should establish statistically based sampling plans, testing plans, and acceptance criteria. Sampling plans and acceptance criteria are usually chosen such that:

1. There is a high probability of meeting the acceptance criteria if the batch at a given stage is "acceptable." This probability is 1 minus the *producer's risk* (i.e., probability of type I error).
2. There is a low probability of meeting the acceptance criteria if the batch at a given stage is "unacceptable." This is the *consumer's risk*, (i.e., probability of type II error).

Next, we look at situations in which a batch is considered acceptable or unacceptable with respect to potency and content uniformity.

6.3.2. Potency

Suppose that potency is to be tested at the blending stage in transport devices and that the potency specifications for finished tablets is between 90 and 110% of the label claim. Since there is no specification for potency in transport devices, the potency specifications for the finished tablets could be used as a reference for the transport sample. If the sample were taken from finished tablets, the reference would be the product specifications. Once the reference specification is chosen, the acceptable–unacceptable situations can be determined. For example, the transport might be considered acceptable if the true mean is 100% of label claim and the only variation encountered is assay variation. On the other hand, the transport might be considered unacceptable if the true mean is at the specification limit and the only variation observed is assay variation. The risk probabilities (i.e., the probability of not meeting acceptance limits given that the batch is acceptable or the probability of meeting acceptance limits given that the batch is not acceptable) might be chosen as follows.

If potency testing at the transport of the blending stage is acceptable (i.e., the true mean is 100% of the label claim with only assay variability), the probability of not meeting the acceptance limits must be at most 0.05. If the transport is unacceptable (i.e., the true mean at the specification limit with only assay variability), the probability of meeting the acceptance limits must be at most 0.05. In this case, both risk probabilities are chosen to be 0.05. Note that the definitions of acceptable and unacceptable situations may differ between products or between stages. It is possible that for some products at one stage, 95% of label claim may be considered acceptable, whereas in other products at other stages, 95% of claim may be considered unacceptable even though the specifications are 90% and 110% of label claim.

6.3.3. Content Uniformity

Suppose that the samples are taken from various locations in transport devices to evaluate dosage uniformity at the blending stage in transport. Also, suppose that the specification for finished tablets is to pass the USP/NF content uniformity. Since there is no specification for content uniformity for samples from the transport devices, the USP/NF test could be that the true mean at the blending stage in the transport is 100% of the label claim and that the only variability is assay variability. Another acceptable situation might be that the smallest probability that a sample taken from the transport will pass the USP test is at least 0.99. An unacceptable situation might be that the smallest probability that a sample taken from the transport will pass the USP test is at most 50%. The risk probability or confidence level might be chosen as follows.

If the content uniformity test at the blending stage in the transport device is acceptable (as defined by either of the two methods noted above), the probability of not meeting the acceptance limits is at most 0.05. However, if the smallest probability that another sample will pass the USP test cannot be guaranteed with 95% assurance greater than 50%, the validation sample will not meet the acceptance limits. In this case the risk probability of not meeting the acceptance limits when the transport is acceptable is 0.05. The confidence level that another sample will pass the USP test at least 50% of the time is 95%.

Since acceptance limits may be obtained based on data from various sources, such as specification sheets, precision studies, scaleup data, statistical control charts, stability data, and assay validations, it is helpful to obtain such pertinent information during the development of a validation protocol. The project scientists should also be consulted for test or specifications to be used as the reference to ensure that the active ingredients and excipients conform with the compendial specifications.

In addition, statistical properties regarding the acceptance limits that will meet USP/NF requirements should be examined. These properties include confidence levels and/or risk probabilities. Sampling plans and acceptance limits should be determined to have these properties. Furthermore, it is helpful to assess the acceptance limits to determine if they are reasonable using available data and to discuss acceptance limits with project scientists and/or quality assurance personnel.

Finally, it is important to provide a validation summary for project scientists following validation of the manufacturing process. The scientists should be consulted regarding necessary information to be included in the validation summary. Typically, a validation summary includes descriptive statistics, acceptance limits, the evaluation of results against limits, the indication of passage, or failure to meet limits.

6.4. SAMPLING AND TESTING PLANS

As indicated in Sec. 6.3, the validation of a manufacturing process requires satisfactory results at each critical stage during a manufacturing process for three batches. For each batch, however, sampling plan, test procedure, and acceptance limits may be different from stage to stage. To provide a better understanding, consider the manufacture of tablets of a drug product with a weight of 5 g per tablet which contains two active ingredients and other excipients. The drug product is manufactured using a direct compression processing method. Suppose that the theoretical batch size is 12 million tablets. We summarize the manufacturing procedure below.

Primary Blending Stage

> *Step 1*: Blend two active ingredients and other inactive ingredients in a 150-ft^3 V-blender for 5 min with the intensifier running. Pass the blend through a Fitzpatrick comminuting mill (model U-12 or U-6) using a number 16 mesh screen, operating at high speed with the impact forward.
>
> *Step 2*: Blend the material from step 1 and other excipients, such as talc triturate and lactose (NF), in the V-blender for 1 h with the intensifier bar running.

Final Blending Stage

> *Step 3*: Blend the stearic acid (NF) and magnesium stearate (NF) with a portion of the blend from step 2 and pass through a Fitzpatrick comminuting mill using a number 2A plate, operating at medium speed with the knives forward.
>
> *Step 4*: Add the blend from step 3 to step 2 and blend for 2 min with the intensifier bar running.

Blending in Transports Stage

> *Step 5*: Discharge the developed in step 4 from the V-blender into conical transport devices.

Compression Stage

> *Step 6*: Compress the blend from step 5 on a hexagonal 21/64-in. flat to flat, with a hardness of 6 to 8 scu (Erweka hardness tester) or 5 to 7 scu (Schleuniger hardness tester) and a thickness of 0.147 to 0.157 in. (process guides).

Clearly, this process involves several critical stages, including the primary blending stage (i.e., steps 1 and 2), the final blending stage (i.e., steps 3 and 4), the blending stage during transport (i.e., step 5), and the compression stage (i.e., step 6). Since no granulating or drying steps are involved, the major concerns of the manufacturing process are to establish that all ingredients are uniformity mixed, that segregation does not occur at later steps in the process, and that no significant losses of active ingredient are encountered.

The objective of the primary blending stage is to ensure that a 60-min blending time with the intensifier bar running produces a uniform dry blend and that uniformity is still acceptable at intervals on either side of the time selected (50, 60, and 70 min for initial batch and 60 min for subsequent batches). For the final blending stage, the purpose is to guarantee that addition of the lubricant to the dry blend does not affect uniformity adversely. For blending during transport, it is important to ensure that the transfer from the V-blender to the transport devices is accomplished without causing significant classification or potency loss. It is critical to ensure that the tablets compressed from the blend during transport conform to specified criteria for content uniformity, weight variation, potency, and dissolution throughout the compression run.

To evaluate potency, content uniformity, weight variation, and dissolution at each critical stage of the manufacturing process, the active ingredients and excipients are tested for conformance with compendial specifications. Objectives, sampling plans, and test plans at each stage are summarized below according to sampling plan I described in Chapter 5. Note that the dissolution and disintegration tests cannot be performed at all stages described above except for the compression stage, because they involve only powder. The sampling unit at these stages is a tablet equivalent to 5 g of sampling powder.

Primary Blending Stage

Objective. Perform a content uniformity test to demonstrate that a 60-min blend time with the intensifier bar running produces a uniformity dry blend and that uniformity is still acceptable at intervals on either side of the time selected.

Sampling plan. Twelve 5-g samples are drawn, one each from the top, middle, and bottom of the front and back from the right and left sides of the V-blender after blending for 50, 60, and 70 min with the intensifier bar running (see Fig. 1.4.1).

Testing plan. For the first batch, 36 samples are used, testing one tablet equivalent per 5-g sample (12 samples per blending time × 3 blending times). For the second and third batches, 12 samples (from each batch) are used to test one tablet equivalent per 5-g sample. Thus a total of 60 samples are tested for three batches.

Final Blending Stage

Objective. Perform a content uniformity test to demonstrate that the addition of lubricant to the dry blend does not adversely affect dose uniformity.

Sampling plan. Twelve 5-g samples are drawn, two each (front and back) from the top, middle, and bottom of the right and left sides of the V-blender after blending for 2 min with the intensifier bar running (see Fig. 1.4.1).

Testing plan. Twelve samples are used to test one tablet equivalent per 5-g sample. A total of 36 samples for three batches are tested.

Blend in Transports Stage

Objective. Perform potency and content uniformity tests to demonstrate that transfer from the blender to the transport devices is accomplished without causing significant potency loss.

Sampling plan. For potency, one 100-g composite sample taken with a grain thief from each transport device (see Fig. 1.4.2). For content uniformity, twelve 5-g samples, one from each quadrant of the filling port from the top, middle, and bottom of each transport (see Fig. 1.4.3).

Testing plan. For potency, one per transport device; sufficient granulation to perform assay. For content uniformity, 12 samples testing one tablet equivalent per 5-g sample. Total number of samples for three batches are 24 for potency and 288 for content uniformity.

Compression Stage

Objective. Perform potency, content uniformity, weight variation, and dissolution tests to demonstrate that the tablets compressed from blend in transports conform to the USP/NF specifications.

Sampling plan. 200 tablets are removed at the beginning and after each one-ninth by weight of the contents of the transport device as compressed for the first, fourth (middle), and last transport devices emptied from the V-blender.

Testing plan. For potency, 15 assays (one from the beginning and from the 2/9, 4/9, 2/3, and end sample from each of three transport devices sampled); sufficient granulation to perform assay. For content uniformity, 120 tablets (40 tablets from each point in the sampling plan). For weight variation, 600 tablets (200 tablets from each of three transport devices sampled; 20 tablets from each point in the sampling plan). For dissolution, 18 tablets (6 tablets from each of three transport devices sampled; 3 tablets each from the beginning and end of each transport device).

At each critical stage, the sampling plan and test plan provide statistical evaluation of the manufacturing process which guarantees that the manufacturing process does what it purpurts to do with a desired level of confidence.

6.5. ACCEPTANCE LIMITS FOR PROCESS VALIDATION

Acceptance limits for the validation of a manufacturing process are usually designed to be more stringent to assure that the final product will pass USP/NF specifications. Acceptance limits are defined in Sec. 5.4 as a set of sample statistics from which a joint confidence region for the corresponding parameters is constructed to meet a prespecified lower probability bound for passing a particular USP test. In this section we illustrate, through a real example, the construction of acceptance limits. Since the concept for construction of acceptance limits is the same for all USP tests, the content uniformity of dosage units is used to demonstrate the procedure. The acceptance limits for dissolution and disintegration testing can be constructed similarly.

For the purpose of illustration, we first consider sampling plan II discussed in Sec. 5.4.2. In sampling plan II, an equal number of n ($n > 1$) assays is performed for samples collected from each of L locations within the V-blender or transport device for each combination of strength and batch. Denote as $\bar{Y}$, s_e^2, and s_L^2 the overall sample mean, the mean-squared error, and the location mean square, respectively, which are obtained from the ANOVA table under the one-way nested random effects model given in (5.4.1), where

$$\bar{Y} = \frac{1}{nL} \sum_{i=1}^{L} \sum_{j=1}^{n} Y_{ij} = \frac{1}{L} \sum_{i=1}^{L} \bar{Y}_{i \cdot},$$

$$s_e^2 = \frac{1}{L(n-1)} \sum_{i=1}^{L} \sum_{j=1}^{n} (Y_{ij} - \bar{Y}_{i \cdot})^2,$$

$$s_L^2 = \frac{n}{L-1} \sum_{i=1}^{L} (\bar{Y}_{i \cdot} - \bar{Y}_{\cdot \cdot})^2,$$

$$\bar{Y}_{i \cdot} = \frac{1}{n} \sum_{j=1}^{n} Y_{ij}.$$

The acceptance limits for content uniformity under sampling plan II can be expressed as follows:

$$[(\bar{Y}_L, \bar{Y}_U), s_e, s_M],$$

where s_M is the between-location standard deviation, that is,

$$s_M = \sqrt{\frac{s_L^2}{n}}.$$

Then each point of the $(1 - 2p) \times 100\%$ confidence interval for μ constructed from $(\bar{Y}, s_e, s_L)$ will result in a probability of passing the content uniformity testing equal to a prespecified lower bound, where

$$\bar{Y} \in (\bar{Y}_L, \bar{Y}_U),$$

and p is as defined in Sec. 5.4.2. For evaluation of the probability of passing the content uniformity testing, not only are the lower and upper limits of the $(1 - 2p) \times 100\%$ confidence interval for μ required but the $(1 - q) \times 100\%$ upper limits for the variance of $\bar{Y}$ and σ_Y^2 are also needed. It should be noted that

$$\left(1 - \frac{1}{n}\right) U_e + \frac{1}{n} U_L,$$

given in (5.4.9), strictly speaking, is not a $(1 - q) \times 100\%$ upper confidence limit for σ_Y^2. An unbiased estimator of σ_Y^2 is given as

$$\hat{\sigma}_Y^2 = \left(1 - \frac{1}{n}\right) s_e^2 + \frac{1}{n} s_L^2. \tag{6.5.1}$$

Thus an $(1 - q) \times 100\%$ approximate upper limit for σ_Y^2 can be constructed based on $\hat{\sigma}_Y^2$ as follows:

$$U_Y^2 = \frac{(\mathrm{df}_Y \, \hat{\sigma}_Y^2)^2}{\chi^2(q, \mathrm{df}_Y)}, \tag{6.5.2}$$

where

$$df_Y = \frac{(\hat{\sigma}_Y^2)^2}{d_Y^2},$$

$$d_Y = \frac{[1 - 1/n)s_e^2]^2}{L(n - 1)} + \frac{[1/n)s_L^2]^2}{L - 1},$$

and $\chi^2(q,df)$ is the qth quantile of a central chi-square distribution with df_Y degrees of freedom. In what follows we provide a step-by-step summary for construction of acceptance limits for content uniformity testing. For a given set of s_e and s_M obtained from a content uniformity testing, suppose that the desired lower probability bound for passing the test is LB. Then the procedure can be summarized as follows.

Step 1: Select approximate values of p and q to reflect the desirable confidence levels on μ, σ_e^2, and σ^2 ($= \sigma_e^2 + n\sigma_L^2$), respectively, so that the confidence level for the joint confidence region for μ, σ_e^2, and σ^2 is at least $(1 - \alpha) \times 100\%$. In the case of equal confidence levels for each parameter, we may choose q as

$$q = 1 - (1 - \alpha)^{1/3}, \tag{6.5.3}$$

where $q = 2p$.

Step 2: Calculate the $(1 - q) \times 100\%$ upper limits for σ^2 based on U_L as given in (5.4.6) and for σ_Y^2 based on U_Y^2 as given in (6.5.2), respectively.

Step 3: Choose an initial value of $\bar{Y}_L$ and calculate the lower limit of the $(1 - 2p) \times 100\%$ confidence interval by

$$\mu_L = \bar{Y}_L - z(p)\left(\frac{U_L}{N}\right)^{1/2}, \tag{6.5.4}$$

where $N = nL$ and $z(p)$ is the pth upper quantile of a standard normal distribution.

Step 4: Use μ_L and U_Y to evaluate P_{CU} through $P(C_{11})$, $P(C_{12})$, $P(C_{21})$, and $P(C_{22})$ as discussed in Sec. 5.3.1.

Step 5: Let δ be a prespecified convergence criterion. If the absolute value of the difference between P_{CU} and LB is less than δ, stop. If the difference between P_{CU} and LB is either less than $-\delta$ or greater than δ, update the new value of $\bar{Y}_L$ by some numerical method such as the method of successive bisection (Kellison, 1975) and repeat steps 3 to 5 until it converges.

Note that for the upper limit $\overline{Y}_U$, we may replace (6.5.4) with

$$\mu_U = \overline{Y}_U + z(p)\left(\frac{U_L}{N}\right)^{1/2}, \tag{6.5.5}$$

and repeat steps 3 to 5. Given a pair of s_e and s_L, for any value of $\overline{Y} \in$ $(\overline{Y}_L, \overline{Y}_U)$ with $(1 - \alpha) \times 100\%$ assurance, there is at least an LB chance that the sample taken for the USP content uniformity test will pass the test. A SAS program for computing the acceptance limits for the USP content uniformity, that is,

$$[(\overline{Y}_L, \overline{Y}_U), s_e, s_M]$$

with LB = 50% and 95% is included in Appendix B. Table 6.5.1 gives $(\overline{Y}_L, \overline{Y}_U)$ for $n = 4$, $L = 10$ with s_e and s_M ranging from 0.1 to 3.5 and 0.1 to 2.4 for LB = 50% and 95%, respectively.

Suppose that there is only one assay performed at each of L locations. Then $N = L$ and between-location and within-location variance components cannot be estimated separately. However,

$$\sigma_Y^2 = \text{var}(Y_i) = \sigma_e^2 + \sigma_L^2,$$

$$\text{var}(\overline{Y}) = \frac{\sigma_Y^2}{L}.$$

The $(1 - q) \times 100\%$ upper limit for σ_Y^2 is given as

$$U_Y^2 = \frac{(L - 1)s^2}{\chi^2(q, L - 1)}, \tag{6.5.6}$$

where

$$(L - 1)s^2 = \sum_{i=1}^{L} (Y_i - \overline{Y})^2,$$

and $\chi^2(q, L - 1)$ is the qth quantile of a central chi-square distribution with $L - 1$ degrees of freedom. Thus the acceptance limits for content uniformity testing when $n = 1$ can also be constructed from steps 1 to 5 with the following minor modifications in steps 1, 2, and 3:

Step 1: Replace (6.5.3) with

$$q = 1 - (1 - \alpha)^{1/2} \tag{6.5.7}$$

Step 2: Calculate the $(1 - q) \times 100\%$ upper limit for σ_Y^2 based on U_Y^2 as given in (6.5.6).

Step 3: Substitute U_Y for U_L in the calculation of μ_L in (6.5.4) and μ_U in (6.5.5).

TABLE 6.5.1a Acceptance Limits for Content Uniformity for 50% Lower Probability Bound for Passing (Dosage Form: Tablet)[a]

SE[b]	SM[c] 0.1		0.2		0.3		0.4		0.5		0.6		0.7		0.8	
	LL	UL	LL	UL	LL	UL	LL	UL	LL	UL	LL	UL	LL	UL	LL	UL
0.1	85.43	114.57	85.85	114.15	86.28	113.72	86.72	113.27	87.15	112.83	87.61	112.39	88.04	111.95	88.48	111.55
0.2	85.54	114.46	85.86	114.14	86.26	113.74	86.69	113.30	87.14	112.86	87.56	112.44	88.02	112.00	88.45	111.55
0.3	85.70	114.30	85.95	114.06	86.30	113.72	86.69	113.31	87.12	112.90	87.54	112.46	87.97	112.03	88.42	111.60
0.4	85.87	114.13	86.08	113.93	86.37	113.63	86.72	113.28	87.12	112.88	87.53	112.46	87.95	112.03	88.39	111.60
0.5	86.04	113.96	86.23	113.76	86.48	113.52	86.79	113.22	87.15	112.85	87.55	112.46	87.95	112.05	88.38	111.60
0.6	86.22	113.78	86.40	113.61	86.61	113.39	86.90	113.10	87.22	112.79	87.59	112.42	87.97	112.03	88.38	111.60
0.7	86.39	113.61	86.57	113.43	86.76	113.24	87.02	112.97	87.31	112.67	87.65	112.35	88.02	111.98	88.41	111.60
0.8	86.58	113.44	86.75	113.25	86.93	113.06	87.15	112.83	87.43	112.59	87.74	112.27	88.08	111.92	88.44	111.55
0.9	86.75	113.26	86.92	113.07	87.10	112.92	87.31	112.68	87.56	112.43	87.83	112.18	88.15	111.85	88.51	111.49
1.0	86.92	113.08	87.09	112.90	87.27	112.72	87.47	112.54	87.70	112.29	87.97	112.02	88.25	111.76	88.59	111.43
1.1	87.11	112.91	87.27	112.72	87.44	112.55	87.64	112.39	87.84	112.14	88.10	111.92	88.36	111.65	88.68	111.33
1.2	87.28	112.73	87.45	112.54	87.62	112.41	87.80	112.23	88.00	111.98	88.24	111.75	88.49	111.48	88.78	111.23
1.3	87.45	112.56	87.62	112.40	87.79	112.21	87.97	112.06	88.16	111.82	88.39	111.59	88.64	111.39	88.90	111.11
1.4	87.64	112.38	87.80	112.22	87.97	112.03	88.13	111.89	88.32	111.67	88.55	111.44	88.76	111.21	89.03	110.99
1.5	87.81	112.20	87.98	112.04	88.14	111.85	88.30	111.72	88.50	111.48	88.70	111.28	88.93	111.10	89.16	110.86
1.6	87.98	112.03	88.16	111.86	88.32	111.72	88.47	111.55	88.66	111.33	88.87	111.12	89.06	110.90	89.30	110.66
1.7	88.17	111.84	88.34	111.68	88.49	111.52	88.64	111.37	88.84	111.14	89.03	110.96	89.24	110.79	89.45	110.56
1.8	88.34	111.67	88.52	111.50	88.67	111.32	88.81	111.20	89.00	110.99	89.20	110.78	89.41	110.59	89.63	110.36
1.9	88.51	111.50	88.69	111.32	88.85	111.14	88.99	111.03	89.18	110.80	89.37	110.62	89.57	110.41	89.75	110.25
2.0	88.70	111.33	88.87	111.14	89.03	111.01	89.16	110.85	89.36	110.62	89.53	110.44	89.74	110.31	89.94	110.04
2.1	88.87	111.14	89.05	110.96	89.21	110.82	89.34	110.68	89.52	110.46	89.71	110.27	89.90	110.09	90.07	109.94
2.2	89.04	110.97	89.23	110.78	89.38	110.62	89.51	110.50	89.70	110.28	89.88	110.10	90.07	109.91	90.27	109.71
2.3	89.23	110.79	89.40	110.60	89.56	110.42	89.69	110.33	89.88	110.10	90.06	109.92	90.24	109.81	90.40	109.61
2.4	89.40	110.62	89.58	110.47	89.74	110.31	89.87	110.16	90.04	109.92	90.23	109.75	90.41	109.59	90.60	109.38
2.5	89.58	110.44	89.76	110.29	89.92	110.12	90.04	109.91	90.22	109.76	90.40	109.57	90.59	109.40	90.73	109.29
2.6	89.76	110.26	89.94	110.11	90.10	109.92	90.22	109.77	90.40	109.58	90.58	109.40	90.76	109.30	90.94	109.04
2.7	89.93	110.09	90.12	109.93	90.23	109.72	90.39	109.62	90.59	109.40	90.75	109.23	90.93	109.04	91.07	108.95
2.8	90.11	109.92	90.26	109.75	90.43	109.61	90.57	109.46	90.77	109.21	90.92	109.05	91.10	108.95	91.29	108.70
2.9	90.29	109.73	90.44	109.57	90.63	109.42	90.74	109.19	90.93	109.03	91.10	108.86	91.28	108.70	91.41	108.61
3.0	90.46	109.56	90.62	109.39	90.81	109.22	90.92	109.05	91.11	108.85	91.29	108.69	91.46	108.61	91.63	108.36
3.1	90.65	109.39	90.80	109.22	90.99	109.02	91.09	108.90	91.29	108.69	91.46	108.52	91.64	108.36	91.76	108.26
3.2	90.82	109.20	90.98	109.04	91.12	108.83	91.28	108.76	91.47	108.51	91.64	108.34	91.81	108.27	91.98	108.01
3.3	91.01	109.03	91.16	108.86	91.32	108.72	91.46	108.49	91.66	108.33	91.83	108.17	91.99	108.01	92.11	107.92
3.4	91.19	108.86	91.34	108.68	91.51	108.52	91.64	108.35	91.84	108.15	92.00	107.98	92.18	107.92	92.34	107.67
3.5	91.38	108.68	91.52	108.50	91.71	108.32	91.82	108.20	92.02	107.96	92.19	107.91	92.36	107.67	92.48	107.58

TABLE 6.5.1a Continued

	SM^c 0.9		1.0		1.1		1.2		1.3		1.4		1.5		1.6	
SE^b	LL	UL	LL	UL	LL	UL	LL	UL	LL	UL	LL	UL	LL	UL	LL	UL
0.1	88.90	111.12	89.33	110.68	89.78	110.20	90.20	109.82	90.64	109.32	91.10	108.95	91.51	108.49	91.95	107.65
0.2	88.88	111.12	89.33	110.68	89.76	110.25	90.20	109.82	90.64	109.37	91.08	108.95	91.51	108.49	91.95	107.65
0.3	88.85	111.15	89.29	110.72	89.72	110.25	90.15	109.82	90.61	109.37	91.05	108.95	91.48	108.49	91.92	107.65
0.4	88.82	111.19	89.25	110.72	89.70	110.33	90.15	109.86	90.57	109.42	91.00	108.95	91.45	108.55	91.89	107.65
0.5	88.80	111.19	89.23	110.79	89.68	110.33	90.11	109.86	90.54	109.47	91.00	109.01	91.43	108.55	91.86	107.72
0.6	88.80	111.19	89.22	110.79	89.64	110.33	90.08	109.91	90.52	109.47	90.94	109.06	91.40	108.61	91.84	107.72
0.7	88.80	111.19	89.22	110.79	89.64	110.37	90.06	109.91	90.50	109.52	90.94	109.06	91.37	108.61	91.81	107.72
0.8	88.83	111.19	89.23	110.79	89.64	110.37	90.06	109.91	90.50	109.52	90.92	109.06	91.34	108.67	91.78	107.78
0.9	88.87	111.12	89.27	110.72	89.66	110.37	90.06	109.91	90.50	109.52	90.92	109.06	91.34	108.67	91.78	107.78
1.0	88.93	111.05	89.31	110.72	89.70	110.29	90.08	109.91	90.50	109.52	90.92	109.06	91.34	108.67	91.75	107.78
1.1	89.01	110.99	89.37	110.64	89.74	110.29	90.13	109.91	90.52	109.47	90.92	109.06	91.34	108.67	91.75	107.85
1.2	89.11	110.89	89.44	110.57	89.80	110.21	90.18	109.82	90.57	109.47	90.94	109.06	91.34	108.61	91.75	107.85
1.3	89.21	110.80	89.52	110.50	89.88	110.13	90.22	109.78	90.59	109.37	91.00	109.01	91.37	108.61	91.78	107.85
1.4	89.32	110.70	89.62	110.39	89.96	110.05	90.31	109.69	90.64	109.37	91.02	109.01	91.43	108.61	91.81	107.78
1.5	89.44	110.58	89.73	110.28	90.04	109.97	90.40	109.60	90.74	109.28	91.08	108.90	91.46	108.50	91.84	107.78
1.6	89.56	110.46	89.84	110.18	90.16	109.85	90.48	109.51	90.81	109.18	91.16	108.85	91.51	108.50	91.90	107.72
1.7	89.70	110.32	89.97	110.05	90.28	109.73	90.57	109.43	90.91	109.09	91.24	108.75	91.57	108.39	91.96	107.72
1.8	89.84	110.18	90.09	109.92	90.40	109.61	90.70	109.34	91.00	109.00	91.34	108.65	91.68	108.33	92.02	107.59
1.9	89.99	110.03	90.23	109.78	90.52	109.49	90.79	109.21	91.10	108.90	91.42	108.55	91.74	108.22	92.08	107.59
2.0	90.14	109.81	90.38	109.64	90.64	109.38	90.92	109.08	91.21	108.81	91.52	108.44	91.85	108.17	92.20	107.47
2.1	90.29	109.72	90.53	109.50	90.78	109.24	91.05	108.95	91.35	108.67	91.63	108.34	91.96	108.06	92.26	107.40
2.2	90.45	109.58	90.68	109.35	90.92	109.10	91.18	108.82	91.44	108.57	91.73	108.24	92.06	107.95	92.37	107.28
2.3	90.60	109.34	90.83	109.20	91.06	108.95	91.30	108.69	91.58	108.43	91.88	108.14	92.17	107.84	92.49	107.22
2.4	90.77	109.24	90.98	109.04	91.21	108.81	91.46	108.57	91.72	108.29	91.98	108.04	92.28	107.73	92.58	107.09
2.5	90.97	109.01	91.14	108.88	91.37	108.66	91.61	108.41	91.86	108.15	92.13	107.88	92.39	107.62	92.70	106.97
2.6	91.10	108.91	91.30	108.72	91.52	108.50	91.76	108.26	92.00	108.01	92.28	107.78	92.55	107.51	92.82	106.84
2.7	91.26	108.67	91.46	108.47	91.68	108.35	91.92	108.13	92.14	107.87	92.38	107.63	92.66	107.35	92.93	106.72
2.8	91.47	108.58	91.62	108.40	91.83	108.19	92.07	107.98	92.28	107.73	92.54	107.48	92.82	107.24	93.05	106.60
2.9	91.60	108.33	91.79	108.14	92.00	108.03	92.22	107.81	92.45	107.59	92.69	107.33	92.93	107.08	93.22	106.47
3.0	91.81	108.23	91.96	108.07	92.16	107.86	92.38	107.65	92.62	107.43	92.84	107.18	93.10	106.97	93.34	106.35
3.1	91.94	107.99	92.13	107.81	92.33	107.71	92.53	107.50	92.75	107.29	92.99	107.03	93.26	106.81	93.51	106.23
3.2	92.17	107.92	92.30	107.73	92.50	107.54	92.70	107.33	92.92	107.12	93.14	106.88	93.42	106.65	93.63	106.10
3.3	92.29	107.66	92.47	107.46	92.67	107.38	92.87	107.18	93.09	106.95	93.32	106.73	93.58	106.48	93.80	105.98
3.4	92.52	107.56	92.71	107.39	92.84	107.21	93.05	107.01	93.25	106.79	93.50	106.58	93.74	106.32	93.97	105.85
3.5	92.66	107.30	92.83	107.11	93.02	106.92	93.22	106.84	93.44	106.65	93.65	106.43	93.90	106.21	94.14	105.73

SE[b]	SM[c] 1.7		1.8		1.9		2.0		2.1		2.2		2.3		2.4	
	LL	UL	LL	UL	LL	UL	LL	UL	LL	UL	LL	UL	LL	UL	LL	UL
0.1	92.39	107.65	92.80	107.21	93.25	106.70	93.71	106.28	94.14	105.84	94.62	105.38	95.04	105.06	95.53	104.59
0.2	92.39	107.65	92.80	107.21	93.25	106.70	93.71	106.28	94.14	105.84	94.58	105.46	95.04	105.06	95.53	104.59
0.3	92.36	107.65	92.80	107.21	93.25	106.77	93.68	106.28	94.14	105.92	94.54	105.46	95.04	105.06	95.53	104.59
0.4	92.33	107.65	92.77	107.21	93.18	106.77	93.64	106.36	94.11	105.92	94.54	105.46	95.00	105.06	95.48	104.59
0.5	92.30	107.72	92.74	107.28	93.18	106.77	93.64	106.36	94.07	105.92	94.54	105.46	95.00	105.06	95.48	104.59
0.6	92.27	107.72	92.71	107.28	93.15	106.85	93.56	106.43	94.03	106.00	94.46	105.54	94.96	105.06	95.44	104.68
0.7	92.24	107.72	92.67	107.28	93.11	106.85	93.56	106.43	93.99	106.00	94.46	105.54	94.92	105.14	95.40	104.68
0.8	92.21	107.78	92.64	107.35	93.08	106.92	93.53	106.43	93.99	106.00	94.42	105.54	94.88	105.14	95.36	104.68
0.9	92.21	107.78	92.64	107.35	93.08	106.92	93.49	106.51	93.91	106.08	94.42	105.63	94.84	105.14	95.31	104.77
1.0	92.18	107.78	92.61	107.35	93.05	106.92	93.49	106.51	93.91	106.08	94.33	105.63	94.84	105.23	95.31	104.77
1.1	92.18	107.85	92.61	107.42	93.05	106.99	93.46	106.51	93.91	106.08	94.33	105.63	94.80	105.23	95.27	104.77
1.2	92.18	107.85	92.61	107.42	93.01	106.99	93.46	106.51	93.87	106.08	94.33	105.71	94.80	105.23	95.23	104.77
1.3	92.18	107.85	92.61	107.42	93.01	106.99	93.46	106.59	93.87	106.16	94.29	105.71	94.75	105.32	95.23	104.86
1.4	92.21	107.78	92.61	107.35	93.01	106.99	93.46	106.59	93.87	106.16	94.29	105.71	94.75	105.32	95.18	104.86
1.5	92.24	107.78	92.61	107.35	93.05	106.99	93.46	106.59	93.87	106.16	94.29	105.71	94.75	105.32	95.18	104.86
1.6	92.27	107.72	92.68	107.35	93.05	106.92	93.46	106.59	93.87	106.16	94.29	105.71	94.75	105.32	95.18	104.86
1.7	92.34	107.72	92.71	107.28	93.12	106.92	93.49	106.51	93.91	106.16	94.29	105.71	94.75	105.32	95.18	104.86
1.8	92.40	107.59	92.74	107.28	93.12	106.85	93.53	106.51	93.91	106.08	94.33	105.63	94.75	105.23	95.18	104.86
1.9	92.47	107.59	92.81	107.15	93.19	106.85	93.56	106.43	93.95	106.08	94.37	105.63	94.75	105.23	95.23	104.86
2.0	92.53	107.47	92.88	107.15	93.26	106.71	93.64	106.43	94.03	106.00	94.41	105.63	94.84	105.23	95.27	104.77
2.1	92.60	107.40	92.95	107.02	93.30	106.71	93.68	106.29	94.03	106.00	94.45	105.47	94.93	105.14	95.31	104.77
2.2	92.70	107.28	93.02	107.02	93.37	106.57	93.75	106.29	94.11	105.84	94.49	105.47	94.93	105.14	95.36	104.77
2.3	92.79	107.22	93.12	106.89	93.44	106.57	93.83	106.14	94.19	105.84	94.57	105.47	95.02	104.98	95.45	104.60
2.4	92.89	107.09	93.19	106.75	93.55	106.43	93.90	106.14	94.27	105.76	94.66	105.38	95.11	104.98	95.49	104.60
2.5	93.02	106.97	93.32	106.69	93.63	106.36	93.98	106.00	94.35	105.68	94.70	105.22	95.19	104.89	95.58	104.60
2.6	93.12	106.84	93.43	106.55	93.76	106.22	94.06	106.00	94.43	105.60	94.78	105.22	95.28	104.89	95.67	104.42
2.7	93.24	106.72	93.56	106.42	93.84	106.22	94.20	105.85	94.51	105.52	94.87	105.06	95.37	104.72	95.76	104.42
2.8	93.36	106.60	93.63	106.35	93.98	106.08	94.28	105.71	94.63	105.37	94.95	105.06	95.46	104.72	95.86	104.25
2.9	93.49	106.47	93.76	106.22	94.09	105.94	94.42	105.63	94.71	105.37	95.11	104.98	95.54	104.55	95.95	104.25
3.0	93.61	106.35	93.89	106.09	94.22	105.81	94.50	105.48	94.87	105.22	95.19	104.89	95.71	104.47	96.04	104.07
3.1	93.80	106.23	94.02	105.96	94.36	105.67	94.65	105.41	94.95	105.06	95.35	104.73	95.80	104.30	96.21	104.07
3.2	93.92	106.10	94.21	105.83	94.50	105.53	94.79	105.26	95.10	104.98	95.44	104.73	95.97	104.30	96.31	103.90
3.3	94.04	105.98	94.35	105.70	94.64	105.39	94.94	105.12	95.25	104.83	95.60	104.57	96.10	104.13	96.48	103.72
3.4	94.23	105.85	94.48	105.57	94.78	105.25	95.08	104.97	95.41	104.68	95.76	104.41	96.27	103.96	96.66	103.72
3.5	94.41	105.73	94.67	105.44	94.98	105.11	95.23	104.89	95.56	104.68	95.92	104.25	96.27	103.96	96.66	103.72

[a]Table entries are the 95% lower (LL) and upper (UL) limits based on the mean of 40 assays, 4 tablets at each of 10 different locations. Model, one-way nested random effect model with location as random effect;
[b]SE is the pooled standard deviation across locations (square root of the mean-squared error);
[c]SM is the standard deviation of location means (square root of the mean square for location divided by the number of assays per location).

TABLE 6.5.1b Acceptance Limits for Content Uniformity for 95% Lower Probability Bound for Passing (Dosage Form: Tablet)[a]

SE[b]	SM[c] 0.1		0.2		0.3		0.4		0.5		0.6		0.7		0.8	
	LL	UL	LL	UL	LL	UL	LL	UL	LL	UL	LL	UL	LL	UL	LL	UL
0.1	85.57	114.43	86.12	113.87	86.71	113.27	87.29	112.68	87.87	112.10	88.49	111.54	89.05	110.92	89.62	110.37
0.2	85.73	114.27	86.15	113.86	86.68	113.29	87.26	112.71	87.83	112.13	88.45	111.54	89.00	110.97	89.62	110.37
0.3	85.98	114.03	86.28	113.73	86.72	113.29	87.26	112.74	87.79	112.17	88.40	111.58	89.00	110.97	89.57	110.43
0.4	86.23	113.78	86.47	113.50	86.84	113.18	87.29	112.71	87.83	112.17	88.36	111.58	88.95	111.02	89.51	110.43
0.5	86.49	113.52	86.72	113.28	87.02	112.99	87.42	112.57	87.87	112.13	88.40	111.58	88.95	111.02	89.51	110.49
0.6	86.75	113.26	86.94	113.06	87.22	112.79	87.56	112.42	88.00	111.99	88.45	111.58	88.95	111.02	89.51	110.49
0.7	87.02	113.00	87.20	112.80	87.43	112.52	87.73	112.28	88.14	111.84	88.53	111.41	89.02	111.02	89.51	110.49
0.8	87.28	112.74	87.46	112.55	87.70	112.32	87.98	112.01	88.29	111.66	88.70	111.36	89.10	110.82	89.59	110.43
0.9	87.55	112.47	87.72	112.29	87.91	112.05	88.16	111.85	88.48	111.48	88.86	111.14	89.27	110.77	89.68	110.35
1.0	87.81	112.21	87.97	112.03	88.18	111.86	88.42	111.59	88.68	111.30	89.04	110.93	89.37	110.55	89.78	110.11
1.1	88.07	111.95	88.26	111.77	88.45	111.59	88.68	111.32	88.89	111.11	89.23	110.74	89.59	110.47	89.99	110.06
1.2	88.34	111.69	88.52	111.51	88.72	111.32	88.93	111.06	89.18	110.79	89.44	110.52	89.79	110.22	90.09	109.80
1.3	88.61	111.42	88.78	111.26	88.99	111.05	89.19	110.80	89.36	110.60	89.66	110.30	89.99	109.96	90.33	109.74
1.4	88.87	111.16	89.04	111.00	89.26	110.78	89.46	110.54	89.67	110.42	89.88	110.08	90.21	109.89	90.53	109.45
1.5	89.14	110.90	89.30	110.74	89.53	110.51	89.72	110.39	89.86	110.09	90.10	109.86	90.43	109.63	90.73	109.37
1.6	89.40	110.63	89.59	110.45	89.73	110.31	89.98	110.13	90.18	109.91	90.35	109.64	90.65	109.38	90.95	109.08
1.7	89.67	110.37	89.84	110.19	90.00	110.04	90.24	109.87	90.37	109.58	90.60	109.42	90.91	109.12	91.17	108.78
1.8	89.94	110.11	90.10	109.94	90.27	109.77	90.51	109.60	90.70	109.40	90.84	109.21	91.13	108.87	91.40	108.73
1.9	90.20	109.85	90.36	109.68	90.54	109.50	90.77	109.34	90.88	109.07	91.09	108.81	91.38	108.61	91.63	108.43
2.0	90.46	109.58	90.62	109.42	90.81	109.23	91.03	109.08	91.21	108.89	91.34	108.59	91.64	108.36	91.89	108.14
2.1	90.73	109.32	90.91	109.16	91.07	108.96	91.29	108.82	91.39	108.56	91.59	108.38	91.89	108.10	92.12	107.85
2.2	90.99	109.05	91.16	108.90	91.34	108.70	91.56	108.55	91.72	108.38	91.85	108.16	92.15	107.85	92.37	107.56
2.3	91.26	108.79	91.42	108.61	91.61	108.43	91.82	108.29	91.92	108.05	92.10	107.94	92.40	107.59	92.62	107.50
2.4	91.53	108.53	91.68	108.36	91.88	108.16	92.08	108.03	92.25	107.87	92.47	107.54	92.66	107.34	92.88	107.21
2.5	91.79	108.26	91.97	108.10	92.15	107.96	92.34	107.77	92.43	107.54	92.69	107.33	92.91	107.08	93.13	106.92
2.6	92.05	108.01	92.23	107.84	92.42	107.69	92.60	107.51	92.76	107.36	92.91	107.11	93.17	106.83	93.38	106.63
2.7	92.33	107.74	92.49	107.58	92.69	107.42	92.87	107.24	93.09	107.03	93.15	106.89	93.42	106.57	93.63	106.34
2.8	92.59	107.48	92.74	107.33	92.96	107.15	93.13	106.98	93.27	106.71	93.40	106.67	93.68	106.32	93.89	106.04
2.9	92.85	107.21	93.00	107.04	93.16	106.88	93.39	106.72	93.60	106.52	93.68	106.28	93.93	106.06	94.18	105.75
3.0	93.12	106.95	93.23	106.78	93.43	106.61	93.65	106.46	93.78	106.20	94.01	106.06	94.19	105.81	94.44	105.75
3.1	93.38	106.69	93.55	106.52	93.70	106.34	93.92	106.19	94.11	106.01	94.23	105.84	94.44	105.55	94.68	105.46
3.2	93.65	106.42	93.81	106.26	93.97	106.07	94.18	105.93	94.29	105.69	94.45	105.62	94.70	105.30	94.94	105.17
3.3	93.92	106.16	94.07	106.00	94.24	105.80	94.44	105.67	94.62	105.50	94.85	105.23	94.95	105.04	95.23	104.88
3.4	94.18	105.89	94.36	105.75	94.51	105.53	94.70	105.41	94.95	105.18	95.06	105.01	95.21	104.79	95.48	104.59
3.5	94.44	105.63	94.61	105.46	94.78	105.26	94.97	105.14	95.13	104.99	95.28	104.79	95.46	104.53	95.73	104.30

SE[b]	SM[c] 0.9		1.0		1.1		1.2		1.3		1.4		1.5		1.6	
	LL	UL	LL	UL	LL	UL	LL	UL	LL	UL	LL	UL	LL	UL	LL	UL
0.1	90.26	109.74	90.77	109.20	91.35	103.56	91.93	108.11	92.50	107.49	93.16	106.85	93.66	106.17	94.34	105.20
0.2	90.19	109.74	90.77	109.20	91.35	103.56	9 .93	108.11	92.50	107.49	93.16	106.85	93.66	106.28	94.34	105.20
0.3	90.12	109.81	90.77	109.20	91.35	103.64	9 .93	108.11	92.50	107.49	93.06	106.85	93.66	106.28	94.23	105.20
0.4	90.12	109.87	90.69	109.27	91.27	108.64	91.84	108.11	92.41	107.49	93.06	106.85	93.66	106.28	94.23	105.20
0.5	90.06	109.87	90.62	109.27	91.27	108.72	91.84	108.11	92.41	107.49	92.96	106.95	93.55	106.39	94.11	105.20
0.6	90.06	109.87	90.62	109.34	91.19	108.72	91.75	108.20	92.31	107.59	92.96	106.95	93.55	106.39	94.11	105.20
0.7	90.06	109.87	90.62	109.34	91.19	108.80	91.75	108.20	92.31	107.59	92.96	107.06	93.44	106.50	94.11	105.32
0.8	90.12	109.87	90.62	109.34	91.19	108.80	91.75	108.20	92.31	107.59	92.86	107.06	93.44	106.50	93.99	105.32
0.9	90.19	109.87	90.69	109.34	91.19	108.80	91.75	108.20	92.31	107.59	92.86	107.06	93.44	106.50	93.99	105.32
1.0	90.26	109.77	90.77	109.27	91.27	108.80	91.75	108.20	92.31	107.59	92.86	107.06	93.44	106.50	93.99	105.32
1.1	90.35	109.68	90.84	109.20	91.35	108.72	91.84	108.20	92.31	107.59	92.86	107.06	93.44	106.50	93.99	105.32
1.2	90.49	109.39	90.95	109.12	91.43	108.64	91.93	108.11	92.41	107.59	92.96	107.06	93.44	106.50	93.99	105.32
1.3	90.72	109.39	91.05	108.83	91.51	108.56	92.01	108.02	92.50	107.59	92.96	107.06	93.44	106.50	93.99	105.32
1.4	90.81	109.07	91.20	108.83	91.63	108.42	92.10	107.94	92.60	107.49	93.06	106.95	93.55	106.50	94.11	105.32
1.5	91.07	109.00	91.35	108.52	91.77	108.10	92.19	107.85	92.69	107.40	93.06	106.95	93.66	106.39	94.11	105.32
1.6	91.19	108.67	91.62	108.45	91.91	108.10	92.32	107.72	92.79	107.30	93.16	106.85	93.66	106.39	94.23	105.32
1.7	91.47	108.61	91.72	108.13	92.07	107.78	92.47	107.37	92.88	107.16	93.26	106.75	93.77	106.28	94.23	105.32
1.8	91.60	108.28	92.01	108.13	92.36	107.78	92.62	107.37	93.02	107.02	93.47	106.60	93.88	106.17	94.34	105.20
1.9	91.89	108.21	92.12	107.77	92.48	107.38	92.80	107.24	93.19	106.65	93.62	106.45	94.04	106.06	94.46	105.07
2.0	92.15	107.89	92.44	107.69	92.65	107.38	92.98	106.87	93.35	106.65	93.77	106.30	94.15	105.90	94.58	104.95
2.1	92.38	107.56	92.56	107.33	92.96	106.98	93.29	106.87	93.54	106.51	93.92	106.15	94.31	105.74	94.75	104.82
2.2	92.63	107.49	92.88	107.26	93.08	106.98	93.38	106.43	93.72	106.10	94.07	105.74	94.47	105.57	94.86	104.70
2.3	92.76	107.16	93.01	106.89	93.40	106.58	93.71	106.43	93.90	106.10	94.25	105.74	94.63	105.41	95.04	104.58
2.4	93.08	106.84	93.32	106.82	93.52	106.50	93.83	105.99	94.24	105.69	94.45	105.59	94.80	105.25	95.21	104.45
2.5	93.37	106.77	93.60	106.45	93.87	106.10	94.15	105.99	94.33	105.69	94.64	105.15	94.99	105.09	95.38	104.33
2.6	93.61	106.44	93.72	106.09	93.98	106.02	94.28	105.55	94.67	105.28	94.84	105.15	95.18	104.62	95.55	104.15
2.7	93.87	106.11	94.09	106.09	94.33	105.62	94.61	105.55	94.77	105.28	95.05	105.00	95.37	104.62	95.72	103.96
2.8	93.99	105.79	94.22	105.73	94.45	105.62	94.74	105.12	95.12	104.80	95.42	104.49	95.58	104.46	95.93	103.78
2.9	94.32	105.79	94.58	105.36	94.80	105.22	95.08	105.12	95.22	104.80	95.52	104.49	95.79	103.98	96.10	103.60
3.0	94.64	105.46	94.71	105.36	94.94	105.14	95.17	104.68	95.59	104.33	95.72	104.05	96.01	103.98	96.31	103.42
3.1	94.91	105.13	95.07	105.00	95.34	104.73	95.55	104.59	95.69	104.33	96.10	104.05	96.22	103.82	96.53	103.23
3.2	95.00	104.80	95.36	104.63	95.46	104.33	95.58	104.15	96.06	103.86	96.20	103.60	96.61	103.35	96.74	102.70
3.3	95.33	104.80	95.47	104.27	95.80	104.33	96.06	104.15	96.16	103.86	96.40	103.60	96.72	103.55	96.96	102.70
3.4	95.66	104.48	95.83	104.27	95.92	103.93	96.15	103.72	96.54	103.38	96.81	103.09	96.91	102.87	97.19	102.57
3.5	95.94	104.15	96.15	103.90	96.32	103.85	96.52	103.63	96.63	103.38	96.91	103.09	97.31	102.87	97.41	102.04

TABLE 6.5.1b Continued

SE[b]	SM[c] 1.7 LL	UL	1.8 LL	UL	1.9 LL	UL	2.0 LL	UL	2.1 LL	UL	2.2 LL	UL	2.3 LL	UL	2.4 LL	UL
0.1	94.85	105.20	95.51	104.54	95.97	103.88	96.56	103.50	97.24	102.82	97.86	102.13	98.29	101.44	98.95	101.11
0.2	94.85	105.20	95.51	104.54	95.97	103.88	96.56	103.50	97.24	102.82	97.86	102.13	98.29	101.44	98.95	101.11
0.3	94.85	105.20	95.38	104.54	95.97	103.88	96.56	103.50	97.24	102.82	97.70	102.13	98.29	101.61	98.95	101.11
0.4	94.85	105.20	95.38	104.54	95.97	103.88	96.56	103.50	97.09	102.82	97.70	102.13	98.29	101.61	98.95	101.11
0.5	94.73	105.20	95.38	104.54	95.97	104.02	96.56	103.50	97.09	102.82	97.70	102.13	98.29	101.61	98.78	101.11
0.6	94.73	105.20	95.24	104.67	95.83	104.02	96.42	103.50	97.09	102.82	97.70	102.29	98.29	101.61	98.78	101.11
0.7	94.61	105.32	95.24	104.67	95.83	104.02	96.42	103.50	96.93	102.82	97.54	102.29	98.12	101.78	98.78	101.11
0.8	94.61	105.32	95.24	104.67	95.83	104.16	96.42	103.50	96.93	102.82	97.54	102.29	98.12	101.78	98.78	101.11
0.9	94.61	105.32	95.11	104.81	95.69	104.16	96.27	103.65	96.93	102.98	97.54	102.45	98.12	101.78	98.60	101.29
1.0	94.61	105.32	95.11	104.81	95.69	104.16	96.27	103.65	96.93	102.98	97.38	102.45	98.12	101.94	98.60	101.29
1.1	94.61	105.32	95.11	104.81	95.69	104.16	96.27	103.65	96.78	103.13	97.38	102.45	97.95	101.94	98.60	101.29
1.2	94.61	105.32	95.11	104.81	95.69	104.30	96.27	103.65	96.78	103.13	97.38	102.45	97.95	101.94	98.60	101.29
1.3	94.61	105.32	95.11	104.81	95.69	104.30	96.27	103.65	96.78	103.13	97.38	102.61	97.95	101.94	98.60	101.29
1.4	94.61	105.32	95.11	104.81	95.69	104.30	96.27	103.65	96.78	103.13	97.38	102.61	97.95	101.94	98.43	101.46
1.5	94.61	105.32	95.11	104.81	95.69	104.30	96.27	103.65	96.78	103.13	97.38	102.61	97.95	101.94	98.43	101.46
1.6	94.73	105.32	95.24	104.81	95.69	104.30	96.27	103.65	96.78	103.13	97.38	102.61	97.95	101.94	98.43	101.46
1.7	94.73	105.32	95.24	104.81	95.83	104.30	96.27	103.65	96.78	103.13	97.38	102.61	97.95	101.94	98.43	101.46
1.8	94.85	105.20	95.38	104.67	95.83	104.16	96.42	103.65	96.93	103.13	97.38	102.61	97.95	101.94	98.43	101.46
1.9	94.98	105.07	95.38	104.67	95.97	104.16	96.42	103.65	96.93	103.13	97.38	102.61	97.95	101.94	98.60	101.46
2.0	95.10	104.95	95.51	104.54	95.97	104.02	95.56	103.65	96.93	103.13	97.54	102.61	97.95	101.94	98.60	101.46
2.1	95.23	104.82	95.64	104.41	96.11	104.02	96.56	103.50	97.09	102.98	97.54	102.45	98.12	101.94	98.60	101.46
2.2	95.35	104.70	95.77	104.28	96.24	103.88	96.71	103.35	97.09	102.98	97.70	102.45	98.12	101.94	98.60	101.46
2.3	95.47	104.58	95.90	104.15	96.38	103.74	96.85	103.35	97.24	102.82	97.70	102.29	98.29	101.94	98.78	101.29
2.4	95.60	104.45	96.03	104.02	96.52	103.61	96.85	103.21	97.39	102.67	97.86	102.29	98.29	101.78	98.78	101.29
2.5	95.72	104.33	96.16	103.89	96.66	103.47	97.00	103.06	97.54	102.67	97.86	102.13	98.46	101.61	98.95	101.29
2.6	95.90	104.15	96.29	103.76	96.80	103.33	97.14	102.92	97.54	102.52	98.02	101.97	98.46	101.61	98.95	101.11
2.7	96.09	103.96	96.49	103.62	96.94	103.19	97.29	102.77	97.70	102.36	98.18	101.97	98.62	101.44	99.13	100.94
2.8	96.27	103.78	96.62	103.43	97.08	103.05	97.44	102.63	97.85	102.21	98.34	101.81	98.79	101.27	99.13	100.94
2.9	96.45	103.60	96.81	103.24	97.21	102.91	97.58	102.48	98.00	102.06	98.50	101.65	98.96	101.27	99.30	100.76
3.0	96.63	103.42	97.01	103.11	97.35	102.71	97.73	102.33	98.16	101.91	98.66	101.49	98.96	101.11	99.48	100.59
3.1	96.85	103.23	97.20	102.91	97.56	102.51	97.94	102.19	98.31	101.75	98.66	101.33	99.13	100.94	99.65	100.59
3.2	97.07	102.70	97.39	102.34	97.76	102.37	98.09	101.97	98.46	101.60	98.82	101.17	99.29	100.77	99.65	100.41
3.3	97.25	102.70	97.59	102.34	97.90	102.16	98.30	101.83	98.62	101.45	99.05	101.01	99.46	100.60	99.83	100.24
3.4	97.47	102.57	97.78	102.21	98.10	101.96	98.45	101.61	98.84	101.29	99.21	100.85	99.63	100.44	100.00	100.00
3.5	97.69	102.04	98.01	102.08	98.31	101.75	98.66	101.40	98.99	101.07	99.38	100.69	99.80	100.27	100.00	100.06

[a] Table entries are the 95% lower (LL) and upper (UL) limits based on the mean of 40 assays, 4 tablets at each of 10 different locations. Model, one-way nested random effect model with location as random effect;

[b] SE is the pooled standard deviation across locations (square root of the mean-squared error);

[c] SM is the standard deviation of location means (square root of the mean square for location divided by the number of assays per location).

Note that acceptance limits for dissolution and distintegration testing can be obtained similarly from computation of the probability of passing in step 4. Uses (5.3.11) for dissolution and (5.3.12) for disintegration, respectively.

Example 6.5.1

For the validation of tablet manufacturing, content uniformity tests are usually performed at final blending, final blending in transports, compressed cores, and coating stages. In this example, for simplicity, we consider validation at the compression stage. Since there are two strengths for the drug product (10 mg and 25 mg), six batches (three batches each) are used for the validation. For each batch, four tablets were taken from each of 10 locations throughout the compression run. The results (in mg/tablet) are given in Table 6.5.2.

Table 6.5.3 provides an overall evaluation for test results of content uniformity testing for each combination of strength, batch, and transport at the compressed stage. The overall evaluation include the overall mean, between-location standard deviation s_M, and the within-location standard deviation s_e, where $s_M = \sqrt{s_L^2/n}$. Based on each pair of (s_e, s_M), the 95% acceptance limits $(\overline{Y}_L, \overline{Y}_U)$ are computed and are presented in Table 6.5.3 for LB = 50% and in Table 6.5.4 for LB = 95%. From Table 6.5.3 the overall means of all combinations are within their respective acceptance limits $(\overline{Y}_L, \overline{Y}_U)$ for LB = 50%. Consequently, if the lower probability bound is chosen to be 50%, all batches at both transport devices passed the USP/NF content uniformity test. When LB is chosen to be 95%, Table 6.5.4 indicates that batch B003 at transport device 1 did not meet the acceptance limits and hence fails to pass the test.

Although for LB = 50%, the manufacturing process for strength 10 mg and 25 mg can be considered validated at the compressed stage, the within-location variability for batches B001, B002, and B003 used for strength 10 mg is generally larger than that of the batches for 25 mg. Tables 6.5.3 and 6.5.4 also indicate that the null hypothesis of homogeneity among locations is rejected at the 5% level of significance for 7 of 12 combinations of strength, batch, and transport. Therefore, heterogeneous mixtures at different transport locations exist even though they all pass the USP content uniformity test.

6.6. DISCUSSION

Chapman (1983) indicated that each of the three validation approaches—prospective, concurrent, and retrospective—are useful in providing documented evidence for validating a manufacturing process to ensure that it does what it purports to do. However, each approach has its own merits and limitations and therefore may not be able to provide sufficient evidence for the validation of a manufacturing process if the approach is used alone to validate the manufacturing process. For example, at the primary blending stage, one may apply a

TABLE 6.5.2　Content Uniformity of Compressed Tablet Data Display

Strength (mg)	Batch	Transport	Location	Left side	Left side	Right side	Right side
10	B001	1	1	10.7817	10.4724	10.1410	10.2957
	B001	1	2	10.2073	10.0968	10.2515	10.2736
	B001	1	3	10.2957	9.9864	10.2073	10.0305
	B001	1	4	10.1189	10.1631	10.3178	10.4061
	B001	1	5	10.4724	10.2957	10.2515	10.4061
	B001	1	6	10.3620	10.2736	10.3178	10.2957
	B001	1	7	10.2515	10.2957	10.2294	10.2294
	B001	1	8	10.2736	10.2294	10.1410	10.2515
	B001	1	9	10.1189	10.0526	10.4282	10.2073
	B001	1	10	10.4724	10.1189	10.0968	10.3840
	B001	2	1	10.0995	9.8790	9.9892	9.9231
	B001	2	2	10.2318	9.9672	10.0113	10.2318
	B001	2	3	10.0775	10.2318	10.4303	10.1657
	B001	2	4	10.2318	10.1877	10.2318	10.2759
	B001	2	5	10.1216	10.0333	10.0995	10.0554
	B001	2	6	10.0113	10.1436	10.2980	10.0995
	B001	2	7	10.1877	10.0333	10.0995	10.1877
	B001	2	8	10.1657	10.2098	10.1436	10.2098
	B001	2	9	10.1657	10.1877	10.0995	10.0333
	B001	2	10	10.1436	10.0995	10.2980	10.3421
	B002	1	1	10.2647	10.2647	10.1695	10.4552
	B002	1	2	10.1659	10.0266	10.3124	10.2647
	B002	1	3	9.9075	9.9551	10.0266	10.0742
	B002	1	4	9.9075	9.8837	10.2885	10.2409
	B002	1	5	9.7884	10.0504	9.9789	10.3124
	B002	1	6	9.7646	9.8360	10.3362	9.9789
	B002	1	7	9.7170	9.6455	10.2171	10.0266
	B002	1	8	9.6217	9.6931	9.8598	10.0266
	B002	1	9	9.8122	9.7408	10.1933	10.2171
	B002	1	10	9.9313	9.4073	10.3124	10.0980
	B002	2	1	10.1687	9.9790	10.2840	10.0976
	B002	2	2	10.0264	10.0027	9.9553	10.0739
	B002	2	3	10.1450	10.0502	10.0264	10.0502
	B002	2	4	10.2161	9.9790	10.3346	10.1213
	B002	2	5	10.0264	10.0739	9.9553	10.0027
	B002	2	6	10.0264	10.0502	10.0502	9.9842
	B002	2	7	10.1450	9.8368	9.8131	10.1450
	B002	2	8	9.9079	10.0264	9.9553	10.0502
	B002	2	9	9.6709	9.8842	10.2635	10.1450
	B002	2	10	10.1924	10.5005	10.9035	10.0976

TABLE 6.5.2 Continued

Strength (mg)	Batch	Transport	Location	Left side	Left side	Right side	Right side
10	B003	1	1	10.8964	10.5113	10.7605	10.7832
	B003	1	2	10.1942	10.3528	9.6052	10.0356
	B003	1	3	10.2168	10.3754	10.0356	10.1489
	B003	1	4	10.2621	10.1262	10.2621	9.8997
	B003	1	5	10.0809	9.3091	10.4207	9.9903
	B003	1	6	9.6731	9.9450	10.2168	10.2168
	B003	1	7	9.9450	10.3981	9.9676	10.1715
	B003	1	8	8.9935	10.4887	10.3074	9.8544
	B003	1	9	9.8091	10.0356	10.2395	10.1036
	B003	1	10	10.0809	10.5793	10.3754	10.3528
	B003	2	1	10.2429	10.2663	10.1474	10.0996
	B003	2	2	10.1951	10.4578	10.1474	10.5772
	B003	2	3	10.2429	10.1236	10.1713	10.3145
	B003	2	4	10.6483	10.3145	10.2907	9.9303
	B003	2	5	10.5294	10.0996	10.3862	10.1474
	B003	2	6	10.1713	10.1474	10.4578	10.3145
	B003	2	7	10.3384	10.4339	10.4578	10.1235
	B003	2	8	10.3862	10.0519	9.9803	10.4578
	B003	2	9	10.2663	10.0260	10.2907	10.3145
	B003	2	10	10.8876	10.4578	10.0758	10.4339
25	B004	1	1	23.5538	23.9087	24.4409	24.0417
	B004	1	2	23.6369	23.9974	23.9530	23.7312
	B004	1	3	25.1063	25.3725	25.3735	25.1507
	B004	1	4	25.6627	24.7514	25.0176	25.3281
	B004	1	5	25.5055	24.9732	24.6627	25.2394
	B004	1	6	25.4612	25.0620	25.5499	25.1063
	B004	1	7	25.9491	25.5942	25.1507	25.5499
	B004	1	8	25.5499	25.5281	24.7514	25.0176
	B004	1	9	25.3725	24.9289	25.5499	24.9732
	B004	1	10	25.5449	25.0176	24.9289	25.2837
	B004	2	1	25.1190	25.0307	25.0748	24.8541
	B004	2	2	24.7658	24.5892	25.1190	24.9865
	B004	2	3	24.8100	24.5892	25.4721	25.4721
	B004	2	4	24.6334	24.7217	25.1190	24.8983
	B004	2	5	25.5604	25.6487	25.2073	25.1631
	B004	2	6	25.0748	25.5604	24.9865	25.4280
	B004	2	7	24.7217	25.4280	25.3839	25.5163
	B004	2	8	24.8893	25.2514	25.4280	25.3397
	B004	2	9	25.8839	25.6487	25.4280	25.2514
	B004	2	10	26.4875	26.0902	25.2956	25.3839

TABLE 6.5.2   Continued

Strength (mg)	Batch	Transport	Location	Left side	Left side	Right side	Right side
25	B005	1	1	24.8037	24.8037	25.8744	25.4729
	B005	1	2	24.9821	24.8929	25.6959	25.3390
	B005	1	3	25.9636	25.4729	26.1420	24.9821
	B005	1	4	25.2052	24.9821	27.7145	25.8744
	B005	1	5	25.5175	25.4282	25.6513	25.5175
	B005	1	6	25.6067	25.2498	24.8929	25.1606
	B005	1	7	25.7851	25.0714	26.0082	25.2052
	B005	1	8	24.8929	25.1606	25.5175	26.3205
	B005	1	9	25.2498	25.7405	25.6959	24.4282
	B005	1	10	25.4282	25.6959	24.9821	25.7851
	B005	2	1	24.6704	24.8040	24.8931	24.8931
	B005	2	2	25.3829	25.2048	25.2048	25.6056
	B005	2	3	25.3384	23.4681	25.2939	25.4275
	B005	2	4	25.2939	25.1603	25.6056	25.0712
	B005	2	5	25.4720	26.1845	25.1603	25.6946
	B005	2	6	25.8282	25.1603	25.4275	25.2493
	B005	2	7	25.3384	25.6501	25.8728	25.3384
	B005	2	8	25.4720	25.4275	26.0954	25.1603
	B005	2	9	25.2939	25.4720	25.8728	25.6946
	B005	2	10	25.3384	26.0064	26.1845	25.4275
	B006	1	1	24.6039	23.9608	24.6819	24.8363
	B006	1	2	24.4216	24.6059	24.4676	24.5698
	B006	1	3	24.7902	24.6059	24.3755	24.8823
	B006	1	4	24.5137	24.3755	24.5598	24.7902
	B006	1	5	25.1127	23.2970	24.5589	24.4676
	B006	1	6	24.8823	25.2510	24.5598	24.5137
	B006	1	7	25.2043	25.0203	25.3431	25.0206
	B006	1	8	24.6059	24.4678	25.1588	25.1588
	B006	1	9	25.4814	26.0804	25.2049	26.3569
	B006	1	10	25.2049	25.3802	25.2970	25.1127
	B006	2	1	24.9543	24.4041	24.3578	24.6420
	B006	2	2	25.6081	25.0061	24.9598	25.2840
	B006	2	3	25.0524	24.5894	25.0061	24.7283
	B006	2	4	24.7283	25.4229	24.4041	24.9598
	B006	2	5	25.1914	25.3303	24.7746	25.1451
	B006	2	6	25.0524	25.3766	25.1451	25.3766
	B006	2	7	25.6544	25.1451	25.0524	25.0988
	B006	2	8	24.7283	25.4692	24.9135	24.9135
	B006	2	9	25.6081	25.1914	24.9598	24.3578
	B006	2	10	24.9135	25.1914	24.8672	24.4505

TABLE 6.5.3 Overall Evaluation for Test Results of Content Uniformity of Compressed Tablets with 50% Lower Probability Bound for Passing

Strength (mg)	Batch	Transport	Mean	s_M	s_e	Acceptance limits	Evaluation
10	B001	1	102.63	0.84	1.41	(89.2,110.9)	Pass
		2	101.41	0.80[a]	0.97	(88.6,111.5)	Pass
	B002	1	100.19	1.41	2.26	(91.8,108.2)	Pass
		2	100.80	1.35[a]	1.70	(91.1,108.9)	Pass
	B003	1	103.51	2.41[a]	3.21	(96.3,104.0)	Pass
		2	102.85	0.82	2.03	(90.0,110.0)	Pass
25	B004	1	99.93	2.32[a]	1.24	(94.8,105.2)	Pass
		2	100.93	1.21[a]	1.29	(90.3,109.7)	Pass
	B005	1	101.52	0.65	1.84	(89.4,110.6)	Pass
		2	101.51	1.24[a]	1.66	(90.7,109.3)	Pass
	B006	1	99.38	1.74[a]	1.49	(92.4,107.7)	Pass
		2	100.00	0.84	1.28	(89.0,111.0)	Pass

[a]The hypothesis of homogeneity among locations is rejected at the 5% level of significance.

TABLE 6.5.4 Overall Evaluation for Test Results of Content Uniformity of Compressed Tablets with 95% Lower Probability Bound for Passing

Strength (mg)	Batch	Transport	Mean	s_M	s_e	Acceptance limits	Evaluation
10	B001	1	102.63	0.84	1.41	(90.6,109.4)	Pass
		2	101.41	0.80[a]	0.97	(89.8,110.3)	Pass
	B002	1	100.19	1.41	2.26	(94.3,105.9)	Pass
		2	100.80	1.35[a]	1.70	(93.2,107.0)	Pass
	B003	1	103.51	2.41[a]	3.21	(99.8,100.4)	No
		2	102.85	0.82	2.03	(92.0,108.1)	Pass
25	B004	1	99.93	2.32[a]	1.24	(98.1,102.1)	Pass
		2	100.93	1.21[a]	1.29	(92.0,107.9)	Pass
	B005	1	101.52	0.65	1.84	(91.1,109.0)	Pass
		2	101.51	1.24[a]	1.66	(92.6,107.4)	Pass
	B006	1	99.38	1.74[a]	1.49	(94.8,105.3)	Pass
		2	100.00	0.84	1.28	(90.4,109.6)	Pass

[a]The hypothesis of homogeneity among locations is rejected at the 5% level of significance.

prospective approach to control a known major source of variation such as the between-location variability. However, it can hardly be utilized to document batch-to-batch homogeneity because only three batches are generally used in a prospective validation. Furthermore, it should be noted that blending is a very complicated process which often consists of many components of formulation and process factors, such as the size and shape of the blender, blending time, rotational speed, particle size, specific volume, hygroscopicity, residual solvent, moisture, and others stated in Tables 4.3.1 and 4.3.2. It is hence very inappropriate and unlikely to use a prospective validation to control all of these factors for each of multicomponents in the primary blending stage of a manufacturing process for a tablet dosage form. Instead, either a concurrent or retrospective validation approach may be applied to verify batch-to-batch homogeneity.

In practice, at the early stage of the development of a manufacturing process for a new pharmaceutical compound, initial batches are produced on a very small scale. Before the batch is scaled up to a production batch, a validation protocol is usually designed to obtain, prospectively, crucial developmental information at every stage of the manufacturing process. As the new drug and manufacturing process are developed, information on each lot accumulated is reviewed and analyzed retrospectively. Finally, when the development of the manufacturing process reaches the stage of commercial production, its validation also approaches completion in both retrospective and prospective manners. Once the entire manufacturing process is validated, it is said to be in a state of control. The process is in its validated status as long as all control parameters and the characteristics of the drug product remain within USP/NF specifications. It is very important to monitor the process constantly so that any significant changes are found before or at the time they occur and corrective action can be taken immediately to preserve the state of control.

As indicated earlier, the efficacy and safety of a drug product are usually demonstrated based on a laboratory batch or small-scale production batch prior to FDA approval. It is therefore crucial to validate the manufacturing process to ensure that the commercial production batch will maintain the same identity, strength, quality and purity of the drug product after approval, especially when the size of the batch is scaled up to a regular commercial production batch and/ or the techniques are transferred from one site to another. It should be noted, however, that two manufacturing processes at different sites may not be equivalent even though both meet USP standards.

As can be seen, dosage uniformity can be assessed either by weight variation or content uniformity test, as stated in USP/NF specifications. In practice, the sampling plan and acceptance criteria for weight variation specified in USP XIX (1974) can be used to evaluate weight variation during process validation. The acceptance criteria are described below.

First weigh the number of tablets equivalent to one rotation of the tablet press. The weight variation test is passed if both of the following conditions are true:

1. Not more than 10% of the tablet weights are outside the range $T + dT$, where T is the theoretical tablet weight (mg/tablet) and d is a function of T as follows:
   (a) If $T \leq 130$, then $d = 0.100$.
   (b) If $130 < T < 324$, then $d = 0.075$.
   (c) If $324 < T$, then $d = 0.050$.
2. No tablet is outside $T + 2dT$.

For more details on statistical evaluation for weight variation, readers may refer to Roberts (1969).

For the validation of a manufacturing process, at least three batches or lots must be evaluated. If all three batches or lots pass USP tests, the manufacturing process is considered validated. In practice, however, one of the three batches may fail USP tests at critical stages of the manufacturing process. In this case the possible causes for the failure should be investigated. An additional batch or lot should be tested after the problem is identified and corrected.

7

Quality Assurance

7.1. INTRODUCTION

In Chapter 6 we addressed the importance of the validation of manufacturing processes for drug products. A validated manufacturing process can guarantee the identity, strength, quality, and purity of the drug product with certain assurance. However, since a manufacturing process is a continuous process that usually involves a number of critical stages, if anything goes wrong at any stage of the process, it can certainly have a negative impact on the identity, strength, quality, and purity of the final product. Therefore, it is necessary to monitor the performance of the manufacturing process closely at each critical stage. As indicated in Sec. 1.4, CGMP recommends that there be a quality control unit within the pharmaceutical companies to approve or reject all procedures or specifications that may have an impact on the identity, strength, quality, and purity of the drug product. The decision is usually made based on USP tests on certain drug characteristics of interest, such as potency, content uniformity, and dissolution. Any raw materials, in-process materials, and lot or batch of the final product that meets USP/NF specifications may be either approved for further use or released for sale. Any raw materials, in-process materials, and lot or batch of the final product that does not meet such specifications will be rejected.

For monitoring the performance of the manufacturing process, the CGMP requires that a well-written procedure for in-process controls be established and followed. The in-process controls should be examined based on appropriate samples drawn from each batch. Appropriate samples are usually referred to as representative samples drawn from respective raw materials, in-process materials, and lot or batch of the final product according to sampling plans as specified in CGMP or USP/NF. The objective of in-process controls is to control expected and/or unexpected sources of variabilities that may occur during the manufacturing process. When there is a deviation from established control specifications, the possible causes for deviation must be found and immediate corrective actions taken. In this chapter we focus on in-process controls for quality assurance of a manufacturing process. Unless otherwise specified, in-process controls are referred to as raw materials inspection, in-process materials quality assurance, and final product quality control and release targets.

For quality assurance of a manufacturing process, CGMP requires that the number of samples to be tested be chosen based on appropriate statistical criteria for variability, confidence levels, and degree of precision desired. Acceptance criteria for the sampling and testing should be chosen so that the drug product meets established in-house statistical quality control criteria in compliance with USP/NF specifications during the expiration dating period. If test results of the drug meet all of the in-house acceptance criteria, the quality control unit may approve and release the drug for sale. A drug product that fails to meet USP/NF specifications during the expiration dating period of the drug product is subject to recall even if it meets the in-house acceptance criteria. In-process controls are important for quality assurance of drug products, to ensure the identity, strength, quality, and purity of the drug products. A successful quality assurance program can guarantee that if a batch meets prespecified in-house quality assurance criteria, a sample taken from the batch will have a high chance of meeting USP/NF specifications before the expiration dating period with a high level of assurance.

Quality assurance generally starts with raw material inspection. All the raw materials must be tested for their identity, strength, quality, and purity prior to being used for manufacturing. Unacceptable raw materials can certainly lead to unacceptable products. For example, suppose that the desired strength of a particular drug product is 10 mg. If the raw materials are of strength much lower than 10 mg, the final product may not be able to achieve the desired strength. Therefore, before the manufacturing process is initiated, it is crucial to inspect all of the raw materials to make sure that they meet the identity, strength, quality, and purity of the active ingredient of the dug product. For the inspection of raw materials, the quality control unit usually perform USP/NF tests for drug characteristics such as potency based on samples drawn from the raw materials that are usually stored in drums. Based on test results, the quality control unit can determine whether the raw materials should be approved for future use or be rejected. Once the raw materials pass the inspection, they can be used for manufacturing. During each stage of manufacturing, a commonly used approach for in-process quality control is to construct statistical control charts, such as an $\overline{X}$

chart, a range chart (or R chart), an acceptance control chart, and a cumulative sum (CUSUM) chart over a fixed time period. These control charts are useful in identifying a potential problem that may occur during the process of manufacturing. If a problem is identified, the quality control unit is to issue a warning and action must be taken to investigate and correct the possible causes of the problem. For quality assurance of the final product, the concept of acceptance limits introduced in Chapter 6 can be used to serve as in-house acceptance criteria, known as *release targets*. It should be noted, however, that these release targets do not take into account the manufacturer's profit and risk. To account for the manufacturer's expected gain or loss, alternatively, Shao and Chow (1991) proposed a Bayesian decision theory approach for construction of release targets for final product. The proposed release targets are obtained by minimizing the manufacturer's expected loss (or maximizing its expected gain).

In the next section, a commonly used sampling plan for raw materials inspection is introduced. Some statistical issues regarding raw materials quality assurance are also addressed. Some useful statistical control charts for in-process controls are reviewed in Sec. 7.3. In Sec. 7.4 we outline a Bayesian decision theory approach proposed by Shao and Chow (1991) for construction of release targets of final drug products. In Sec. 7.5 an example from a pharmaceutical company concerning quality assurance of a batch of a drug product is presented. Sec. 7.6 provides a brief discussion for the chapter.

7.2. RAW MATERIALS INSPECTION

When a pharmaceutical company receives the raw materials of the active ingredients of a drug product, its quality control unit usually performs USP/NF tests on drug characteristics such as potency to determine whether the raw materials meet USP/NF specifications for the identity, strength, quality, and purity of the drug product. The quality control unit will accept or reject the raw materials, depending on whether the raw materials meet USP/NF specifications. Since the raw materials are usually stored in drums, a two-stage sampling technique is usually performed for inspection. For the first stage of sampling, one selects a number of drums at random. A conventional ad hoc approach is to select the square root of the total number of drums. For example, if there are 10 drums, $\sqrt{10} \approx 3$ drums will be selected for inspection. For each sampled drum, CGMP suggests that random samples be drawn from the top, middle, and bottom parts of the drum with a grain thief, which consists of three (top, middle, and bottom) compartments. Based on test results, the quality control unit is able to determine whether the raw materials pass the inspection. If the raw materials pass quality control inspection, they are accepted and considered ready for future use in manufacturing. If the raw materials fail to pass inspection, the raw materials are to be rejected.

In practice, the strengths of the raw materials stored in the drums, which had passed quality control inspection, may differ from drum to drum due to the possible segregation of the materials. Typically, the quality control unit will test the raw materials in each drum to determine its strength based on appropriate samples drawn from each drum. The strength of each drum will be labeled based on test results obtained from that drum. Prior to manufacturing, it is important to determine the amount of materials to be used for mixing from each drum so that the mixed raw materials will achieve the desired strength. For example, suppose that there are five drums of the same size with the following labeled strengths:

Drum no.	1	2	3	4	5
Strength (mg)	8.0	15.0	7.0	12.0	8.0

Also, suppose that the desired strength of the drug product is 10 mg. Then we may achieve the desired strength of 10 mg by mixing all the drums. However, suppose that due to the size and/or capacity of the V-blender, the blender can handle no more than two drums at a time. In this case we may achieve the desired strength of 10 mg by mixing the materials in drums 4 and 5 at 1:1 ratio. The strength may be too potent if we mix drums 2 and 4, while the strength may be less potent if we mix drums 1 and 3. Therefore, how to mix the raw materials from each drum uniformly so that the mixed materials can achieve the targeted strength becomes an important issue.

However, each drum may have a different volume of materials toward mixing to achieve the targeted strength. Therefore, prior to manufacturing, it is necessary for the quality control unit to select the number of drums and the corresponding volumes of materials for mixing so that the capacity of the blend is fully utilized and the mixed raw materials will achieve the targeted strength. To assure that the mixed raw materials will achieve the targeted strength, the quality control unit usually establishes quality assurance (QA) limits to accept or reject the mixed materials. In the following, we introduce an ad hoc procedure for construction of QA limits.

Let X_{ij} be the potency assay result of the jth sample drawn from the ith drum, where $j = 1$ (top), 2 (middle), and 3 (bottom) and $i = 1,2,\ldots,K$ (drums). Assume that X_{ij} follows a distribution with mean μ_i and variance σ_i^2, which can be estimated by within-drum sample mean and variance. That is,

$$\overline{X}_{i.} = \frac{1}{3}\sum_{j=1}^{3} X_{ij} \quad \text{and} \quad s_i^2 = \frac{1}{2}\sum_{j=1}^{3}(X_{ij} - \overline{X}_{i.})^2$$

can be used to estimate μ_i and σ_i^2. Note that $\overline{X}_{i.}$ are usually used as the labeled strength for the ith drum. To construct a set of QA limits for the mixed materials, we may consider the following limits:

$$\mu \pm \delta = (L, U),$$

where μ is the prespecified (or target) strength and L and U are the lower and upper QA limits. In practice, we may consider to choose the following δ as a conservative approach:

$$\delta = 2 \max\{s_i, i = 1, \ldots, K\}.$$

The QA limits are constructed so that there is a high probability that a future sample from the mixed materials will fall within the QA limits (L, U) with (at least) 95% assurance. It should be noted, however, that if the QA limits constructed are too wide, we may pass too many "bad" mixed materials. As a result, the decision increases the customer's risk (i.e., probability of type II error). On the other hand, if the constructed QA limits are too narrow, we may reject too many "good" mixed materials. Consequently, the decision increases the manufacturer's risk (i.e., probability of type I error). Therefore, the selection of δ for QA limits depends on a proper balance between customer's risk and manufacturer's risk.

After the materials of the selected drums are mixed, the quality control unit may draw samples and test to see whether the mixed materials meet the desired strength according to the established QA limits. Let V_i be the volume of the ith drum to be used for mixing. Let Y be a sample unit (e.g., a tablet equivalent) drawn from the mixed materials and W_i be the mixing ratio for the ith drum, where

$$W_i = \frac{V_i}{\sum_{i=1}^{K} V_i}.$$

Then Y follows a distribution with mean μ^* and variance σ^{*2}, which are given by

$$\mu^* = E(Y) = \sum_{i=1}^{K} W_i \mu_i \approx \mu,$$

$$\sigma^{*2} = \text{var}(Y) = \sum_{i=1}^{K} W_i^2 \sigma_i^2,$$

respectively. Note that μ^* is not necessarily equal to the target strength μ. One primary objective for quality assurance of the raw materials prior to manufacturing is to select appropriate W_i so that μ^* is as close to μ as possible. In practice, the selection of W_i is usually based on the experience of technicians and hence lacks statistical justification.

As indicated in Sec. 1.4, for a V-blender, CGMP suggests that 12 samples be drawn for testing from the top, middle, and bottom, front and back, of the right and left sides of the blender after blending for a certain period with the intensifier bar running (see Fig. 1.4.1). Therefore, we have Y_i, $i = 1, \ldots, 12$ potency assay results. Based on these assay results, a 95% confidence interval for the mean, μ^*, can be constructed, say (L^*, U^*). The purpose of raw materials quality assurance is to have a high probability that (L^*, U^*) is within the QA limits (L, U) with certain assurance. It should be noted that under normality assumptions, to maximize the probability

$$P\{(L^*, U^*) \subset (L, U)\}$$

is equivalent to minimizing the variance

$$\sum_{i=1}^{K} W_i^2 \, \sigma_i^2$$

under the constraint that

$$\sum_{i=1}^{K} W_i = 1$$

provided that

$$\mu^* = \mu, \quad \text{i.e.,} \quad \sum_{i=1}^{K} W_i \mu_i = \mu.$$

This can be viewed as a linear programming problem. Hence techniques such as the simplex method (Dantzig, 1963) can be applied to this problem. Depending on the values of μ_i and σ_i^2, the solution might not even exist or there may be more than one solution.

7.3. IN-PROCESS CONTROLS

7.3.1. Introduction

As indicated in Sec. 1.4, the in-process materials include any material fabricated, compounded, blended, or derived by chemical reaction that is produced for, and used in preparation of the drug product. At each stage of manufacture the in-process materials should be tested to control the expected and unexpected sources of variations. As an example, consider the example of tablet manufacturing of a drug product. The major concerns regarding quality assurance of manufacturing are to ensure that the ingredients are uniformly mixed, that segregation does not occur in the blending, and that significant losses of active ingredients are not encountered. When blending is complete, the material is transferred to conical transport devices. At each blending and blending-in-transport stage, the quality control unit should evaluate potency and content uniformity and establish acceptance limits that will ensure statistically that tablets within the batch meet USP/NF specifications for dose uniformity.

For in-process materials testing, at the primary and final blending stages, CGMP recommends that 12 samples be drawn for content uniformity testing from the top, middle, and bottom, front and back, of the right and left sides of the V-blender after blending for a certain period with the intensifier bar running. The specific locations for sampling are indicated in Fig. 1.4.1. For blending during transport, a composite sample should be taken with a grain thief from each transport device for potency testing. Figure 1.4.2 indicates the respective sampling locations. On the other hand, CGMP suggests that 12 samples be drawn from each quadrant of the filling port from the top, middle, and bottom of each transport device (see Fig. 1.4.3) for content uniformity testing.

Since the manufacturing process of a drug product is a continuous process, at each critical stage, the characteristics of a finished drug product may fluctuate from time to time during the process. Some fluctuations may be explained by the inherent variability of the process. This type of variability, known as the *noise* of the process, is due to normal variation and cannot economically be eliminated or reduced. Other fluctuations may be due to variation from identifiable sources. This type of variability is usually referred to as *signals*. The identifiable sources, also known as *assignable causes*, of variabilities usually can be found during the process. The quality control unit is to remove this type of variability to ensure the identity, strength, quality, and purity of the drug product.

During the manufacturing process, statistical control charts are often employed as useful graphical devices to monitor whether the variabilities of some drug characteristics of particular interest are within acceptable limits. The most commonly used statistical control chart is the Shewhart control chart, invented in 1924 at the Bell Telephone Laboratories by W. A. Shewhart (1891–1967). In early 1930, as a result of Shewhart's concept for quality control, a foundation for statistical quality control was formed (Shewhart, 1931). The Shewhart control charts provide a useful graphical presentation regarding the information of time-by-statistics sequences. This information allows us not only to detect a unnatural pattern that may exist in the process but also to identify the time at which the unnatural pattern occurs. In addition, we may obtain information regarding the short-term variability of some population measures using a sequence of small samples over a relatively short period from the established control charts based on the current behavior of the process. The sample size used to construct a control chart ranges from 2 to 12. Samples of size 4 or 5 are probably the most commonly used for Shewhart control charts. It should be noted that the determination of sample size requires a clear understanding of the manufacturing process. Knowledge of specific drug characteristics is extremely useful and can certainly maximize the chance for identifying any unnatural patterns and locating the time of occurrence of problems during the process. On the other hand, long-term variability can also be assessed by examining historical patterns of the process based on sample-to-sample changes in some measures of location.

The basic idea of Shewhart control charts for monitoring a manufacturing process is first to remove any assignable causes of variations whenever possible based on an estimated short-term variability. After the assignable causes of variations have been identified and removed, the estimated variability can be used to establish control limits for evaluation of long-term variability. To ensure that the manufacturing process will reach the state of statistical control, it is important that any changes in location and variation at any time during the manufacturing process will remain within the expected limits which would be predicted from statistical theory. Shewhart recommended that the sample mean and sample range be used to capture any changes in location and variability in the control charts. The reason for using the sample range rather than sample standard deviation may be due to the simplicity of computation in small samples. However, for sample sizes between 2 and 12, the decrease in relative efficiency for using the sample range for variation instead of sample standard deviation is negligible. It should be noted that Shewhart control charts based on the sample standard deviation as well as its nonparametric version based on the median are also available [see, e.g., Ott and Schilling (1990)].

As indicated earlier, the concept of Shewhart control charts for quality assurance can be applied to monitor the performance of a manufacturing process in terms of some drug characteristics, such as potency, tablet weight variation, content uniformity, and dissolution. These drug characteristics, however, are continuous variables. In some cases we may be interested in discrete variables (e.g., binary responses) such as detective versus nondetective or disintegrated versus nondisintegrated. In this case, Shewhart control charts can also be applied with minor modification. For simplicity, we will denote Shewhart control charts for location, range, and proportion as $\bar{X}$ charts, R charts, and $\bar{P}$ charts, respectively. In the next section, the Shewhart $\bar{X}$ chart for location, R chart for variation, and $\bar{P}$ chart for binary data are discussed.

Basically, the Shewhart $\bar{X}$ chart considers only a single acceptable process level (APL), which is the arithmetic average of sample means. However, in general, acceptance process levels for a drug product depend on USP/NF specifications, which are usually expressed in terms of an interval. Freund (1957) introduced the concept of acceptance control chart, which combines the Shewhart control chart with an acceptance sampling plan. In Sec. 7.3.3 we describe the construction of such an acceptance control chart. One disadvantage of Shewhart control charts is that they are relatively insensitive and slow in detecting small-to-moderate fluctuations. To overcome this drawback, a cumulative sum (CUSUM) control chart, first developed by Page (1954), is useful. The use of

CUSUM control charts has been studied extensively [see, e.g., Barnard (1959), Ewan (1963), and Johnson and Leone (1962a,b)]. The construction of CUSUM chart is described in Sec. 7.3.4.

7.3.2. Shewhart $\overline{X}$, R, and $\overline{P}$ Charts

The primary objective of Shewhart control charts is not only to detect and identify the possible causes of any unusual fluctuations in a process but also to locate the time at which the unusual fluctuation occurs. An unusual (or significant) fluctuation in Shewhart control charts is defined as an observation that deviates from its designated population measure by at least three standard deviations. For example, for population location, the control limits are usually selected as three standard deviations below and above the population mean μ; that is, the control limits are set at $\mu \pm 3\sigma$, where μ and σ are population mean and population standard deviation, respectively. If an observation is outside the control limits, we claim that a significant fluctuation has occurred. In practice, μ and σ are usually unknown and have to be estimated from samples. Similarly, for range and standard deviation, the corresponding control limits for Shewhart control charts can also be constructed as three standard deviations below and above the mean of their corresponding measures. In what follows we provide some details for construction of Shewhart control charts.

Let X_{ij} be the jth observation in the sample collected at the ith time period during a manufacturing process, where $j = 1, \ldots, n$, and $i = 1, \ldots, I$. Also, let

$$X_{i(1)} < \cdots < X_{i(j)} < \cdots < X_{i(n)}$$

be the order statistics for the sample $\{X_{i1}, \ldots, X_{in}\}$. Define the sample mean, sample variance, and sample range for the ith sample as follows:

$$\overline{X}_{i\cdot} = \frac{1}{n} \sum_{j=1}^{n} X_{ij},$$

$$S_i^2 = \frac{1}{n-1} \sum_{j=1}^{n} (X_{ij} - \overline{X}_{i\cdot})^2,$$

$$R_i = X_{i(n)} - X_{i(1)}, \tag{7.3.1}$$

where $i = 1, \ldots, I$. Thus the arithmetic averages of $\overline{X}_{i\cdot}$, S_i, and R_i can be obtained as

$$\overline{\overline{X}} = \frac{1}{I} \sum_{i=1}^{I} \overline{X}_{i\cdot} = \frac{1}{In} \sum_{i=1}^{I} \sum_{j=1}^{n} X_{ij},$$

$$\overline{S} = \frac{1}{I} \sum_{i=1}^{I} S_i,$$

$$\overline{R} = \frac{1}{I} \sum_{i=1}^{I} R_i = \frac{1}{I} \sum_{i=1}^{I} [X_{i(n)} - X_{i(1)}]. \tag{7.3.2}$$

Based on the information above, a Shewhart control chart can be constructed. Typically, a control chart consists of three parts: the central line and two control limits (i.e., the lower and upper control limits).

We first introduce the construction of Shewhart control chart for variability based on sample range R. Let R_C, R_L, and R_U be the central line and the lower and upper control limits of the control chart, respectively. Then R_C, R_L, and R_U are given by

$$R_C = \bar{R},$$
$$R_L = D_1\bar{R},$$
$$R_U = D_2\bar{R}, \tag{7.3.3}$$

where D_1 and D_2 are the scaling factors for the lower and upper control limits. The values of D_1 and D_2 for various sample sizes ranging from $n = 2$ to $n = 15$ are given in Table 7.3.1.

Similarly, we may construct a Shewhart control chart for variability based on sample standard deviation. Let S_C, S_L, and S_U be the central line and the lower and upper limits of the control chart, respectively. Then S_C, S_L, and S_U can be obtained as follows:

$$S_C = \bar{S},$$
$$S_L = B_1\bar{S},$$
$$S_U = B_2\bar{S}, \tag{7.3.4}$$

where B_1 and B_2 are the scaling factors for the lower and upper control limits. The values of B_1 and B_2 for various sample sizes ranging from $n = 2$ to $n = 15$ are also given in Table 7.3.1. From (7.3.3) and (7.3.4) it can be seen that the Shewhart control chart for the location of a process can be constructed based on either sample range or sample standard deviation.

Let X_C, X_L, and X_U denote the central line and the lower and upper control limits of the control chart, respectively. The central line for both $\bar{X}$ charts (i.e., one based on the sample range and the other based on the sample standard deviation) is the same as the arithmetic average of sample means, that is,

$$X_C = \bar{\bar{X}}. \tag{7.3.5}$$

The lower and upper control limits for the $\bar{X}$ chart based on sample range are given by

$$X_L = \bar{\bar{X}} - A_1\bar{R},$$
$$X_U = \bar{\bar{X}} + A_1\bar{R}, \tag{7.3.6}$$

where A_1 is the scaling factor of the lower and upper control limits of the $\bar{X}$ chart based on sample range. The values of A_1 for various sample sizes are also

TABLE 7.3.1 Factors for Limits on Shewhart Control Charts

Sample size (n)	Mean		Range		Standard deviation	
	A_1	A_2	D_1	D_2	B_1	B_2
2	1.880	2.659	0.000	3.267	0.000	3.267
3	1.023	1.954	0.000	2.575	0.000	2.568
4	0.729	1.625	0.000	2.282	0.000	2.266
5	0.577	1.427	0.000	2.115	0.000	2.089
6	0.483	1.287	0.000	2.004	0.030	1.970
7	0.419	1.182	0.076	1.924	0.118	1.882
8	0.373	1.099	0.136	1.864	0.185	1.815
9	0.337	1.032	0.184	1.816	0.239	1.761
10	0.308	0.975	0.223	1.777	0.284	1.716
11	0.285	0.927	0.256	1.744	0.321	1.679
12	0.266	0.886	0.284	1.716	0.354	1.646
13	0.249	0.850	0.308	1.692	0.382	1.618
14	0.235	0.817	0.329	1.672	0.406	1.594
15	0.223	0.789	0.348	1.652	0.428	1.572

Source: Schilling (1982).

given in Table 7.3.1. Similarly, let A_2 be the scaling factor for the lower and upper control limits of the $\overline{X}$ chart based on the standard deviation. Then the lower and upper control limits of the $\overline{X}$ chart based on sample standard deviation can be obtained as follows:

$$X_{LS} = \overline{X} - A_2\overline{S},$$
$$X_{US} = \overline{\overline{X}} + A_2\overline{S}. \qquad (7.3.7)$$

Note that all of the scaling factors A_1, A_2, B_1, B_2, D_1, and D_2 are multiplying constants which are used to ensure that the resulting lower and upper control limits are unbiased estimates for three population standard deviations below and above their respective population measures. A summary of control limits for these Shewhart control charts is provided in Table 7.3.2.

It is also interesting to note that the control limits for the R chart and standard deviation are not symmetrical about the central line $\overline{R}$ or $\overline{S}$. Under normality assumption, the expected value and standard deviation of sample range are given by, respectively,

$$E(R_i) = c_1\sigma,$$
$$SD(R_i) = c_2\sigma, \qquad (7.3.8)$$

TABLE 7.3.2 Summary of Control Limits for Shewhart Control Chart

Statistic	Central line	Control limits
Mean $\bar{X}$	$\bar{\bar{X}}$	$\bar{X}_U(\bar{X}_L) = \bar{\bar{X}} \pm A_1 \bar{R}$
		$\bar{X}_{US}(\bar{X}_{LS}) = \bar{\bar{X}} \pm A_2 \bar{R}$
Range	$\bar{R}$	$R_L = D_1 \bar{R}$
		$R_U = D_2 \bar{R}$
Standard	$\bar{S}$	$S_L = B_1 \bar{S}$
deviation S		$S_U = B_2 \bar{S}$

where c_1 and c_2 are given in Table 7.3.3. As a result,

$$E(\bar{R}) = c_1 \sigma.$$

Since the control limits of Shewhart $\bar{X}$ chart lie within three standard deviations below and above the population mean, based on $\bar{\bar{X}}$ and $\bar{R}$, we need to find an unbiased estimator for

$$\mu \pm \frac{3}{\sqrt{n}} \sigma.$$

Obviously, $\bar{\bar{X}}$ is an unbiased estimator of μ. From (7.3.8), an unbiased estimator of σ based on sample range can be obtained as

$$\frac{\bar{R}}{c_1}.$$

TABLE 7.3.3 Factors c_1 and c_2 and Relative Efficiency

Sample size	c_1	c_2	Relative efficiency[a]
2	1.128	0.853	1.000
3	1.693	0.888	0.992
4	2.059	0.880	0.975
5	2.326	0.864	0.955
6	2.534	0.848	0.933
7	2.704	0.833	0.911
8	2.847	0.820	0.890
10	3.078	0.787	0.850
12	3.258	0.778	0.814
15	3.472	0.756	0.766

[a]Relative efficiency to minimum variance unbiased estimator for population standard deviation.

Hence

$$\overline{\overline{X}} \pm \frac{3\overline{R}}{c_1 \sqrt{n}}.$$ (7.3.9)

As mentioned earlier, the reason for Shewhart to choose the sample range instead of the sample standard deviation for construction of the $\overline{X}$ chart is probably due to the simplicity of the computation. However, it should be noted that the relative efficiency for using the sample range as an estimator for population standard deviation compared to the minimum variance unbiased estimator is at least 91% for a sample size of less than 7. As a matter of fact, the sample range is more robust than the sample standard deviation for small samples from nonnormal populations.

Although the Shewhart $\overline{X}$ chart and R chart can be used to detect and identify any unusual fluctuations or patterns of variability from a manufacturing process, in practice, however, it still requires a lot of exercises, and hands-on experiences distinguish a unnatural pattern from natural ones. In the following we provide some general rules that may be useful in identifying a unnatural pattern when it does occur. More details for detection of unnatural patterns and/ or troubleshooting can be found in Ott and Schilling (1990) and Gitlow et al. (1989). The primary properties of a natural pattern for the $\overline{X}$ chart is that sample means fluctuate at random within the control limits that would be expected from a normal distribution. The characteristics of a natural pattern for a manufacturing process can then be summarized as follows:

1. Most sample means are scattered at random around the central line $\overline{\overline{X}}$.
2. A few sample means spread out and are close to either the lower or upper control limit.
3. No sample mean is outside the control limits.
4. No recognized pattern of the distribution of sample means is observed.

Figure 7.3.1 illustrates a typical natural pattern for the $\overline{X}$ chart of a manufacturing process. The unnatural patterns can be detected by adding *wanning limits* at $\pm 2\sigma_{\overline{x}}$ to the control chart. The warning limits cannot only improve the sensitivity of the $\overline{X}$ chart but also to help the identification of an unnatural pattern. The following are some examples for unnatural patterns:

1. A sample mean is outside the control limits ($\pm 3\sigma_{\overline{x}}$). The probability of this event under normality assumption is about 0.0027. In general, from Chebyshev's inequality, there is a probability of 0.11 that a sample mean is outside the three standard deviation control limits (or action limits).

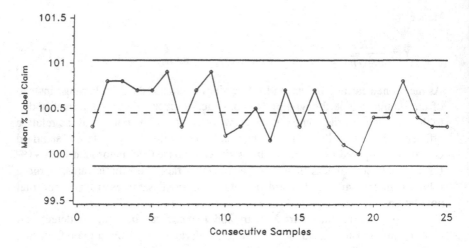

FIGURE 7.3.1 Shewhart control chart of means for a natural pattern. Dashed line, grand sample mean; solid line, action limits = 3 standard deviations.

2. Two out of three consecutive sample means are outside the two standard deviation warning limits. Under normality assumption, the probability of this event can be calculated as

$$\binom{3}{2}(0.05)^2(0.95) = 0.007125.$$

3. Eight consecutive sample means are on the same side of the central line. The probability of this event for any distribution symmetrical about the population mean is

$$2(0.5)^8 = 0.00078.$$

4. Sometimes, it is also worthwhile noticing that four of five successive sample means are outside the one standard deviation limits because that probability of this event under the normality assumption is given by

$$\binom{5}{4}(0.3174)^4(0.6826) = 0.0346.$$

5. In many cases, samples collected from two or more underlying distributions are combined together for construction of control chart. An unnatural pattern of all sample means scattering around the central line with unnaturally small fluctuations will occur. This type of control

charts is invalid because samples from different distributions have been combined. This phenomenon is referred to as *stratification*. An example of stratification for an $\overline{X}$ chart is given in Fig. 7.3.2.

6. If half the samples come from one distribution and the other half come from another distribution, the sample means will scatter within the control limits rather than concentrate on the central line. This phenomenon is called *mixture*. Figure 7.3.3 provides an illustration of an $\overline{X}$ chart with a stable mixture.

7. The existence of a trend for a manufacturing process can be identified by the following unnatural patterns:
   (a) One sample mean outside the control limits on one side is followed by the next consecutive sample mean, which is outside the control limits on the other side.
   (b) There are at least six consecutive sample means, one of which is greater (or lower) than the previous one.

8. The presence of a systematic variable in the process is suggested if at least eight consecutive sample means alternate large, small, large, and small without interruption. This pattern may occur when samples are selected alternately from different operators or machines.

The natural and unnatural patterns for the $\overline{X}$ chart described above can also be applied to the R chart. However, probabilities for the occurrence of certain unnatural patterns for the R chart are different from those for the $\overline{X}$ chart.

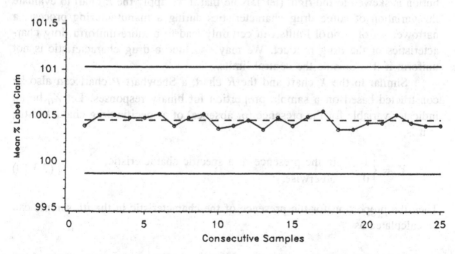

FIGURE 7.3.2 Shewhart control chart of means for a stratification pattern. Dashed line, grand sample mean; solid line, action limits = 3 standard deviations.

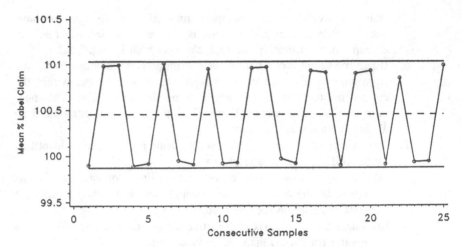

FIGURE 7.3.3 Shewhart control chart of means for a mixture pattern. Dashed line, grand sample mean; solid line, action limits = 3 standard deviations.

In general, the pattern of scattering of sample means on the $\overline{X}$ chart should have no correlation with the pattern of distribution of sample ranges on the R chart. However, if sample means go up (down) and the corresponding sample range goes up (down) at the same time, this may indicate that the underlying distribution is skewed to the right (left). Note that if we apply the R chart to evaluate the variation of some drug characteristics during a manufacturing process, a narrower set of control limits can certainly lead to a more uniform drug characteristics of the drug product. We may conclude a drug characteristic is not uniform if it is outside the control limits.

Similar to the $\overline{X}$ chart and the R chart, a Shewhart $\overline{P}$ chart can also be constructed based on a sample proportion for binary responses. Let X_{ij} be an indicator variable for the presence (or absence) of a specific drug characteristic, that is,

$$X_{ij} = \begin{cases} 1 & \text{in the presence of a specific characteristic,} \\ 0 & \text{otherwise.} \end{cases} \tag{7.3.10}$$

Then the proportion for the presence of the characteristic in the ith sample can be calculated as

$$P_i = \frac{1}{n} \sum_{i=1}^{I} X_{ij}.$$

Let $\bar{P}$, P_L, and P_U be the central line and the lower and upper control limits for the Shewhart $\bar{P}$ chart, respectively. Then $\bar{P}$, P_L, and P_U are given by

$$\bar{P} = \frac{1}{I} \sum_{i=1}^{I} P_i = \frac{1}{nI} \sum_{i=1}^{I} \sum_{j=1}^{n} \frac{\{\text{no. presence of characteristics}\}}{nI},$$

$$P_L = \bar{P} - 3 \sqrt{\frac{\bar{P}(1 - \bar{P})}{n}},$$

$$P_U = \bar{P} + 3 \sqrt{\frac{\bar{P}(1 - \bar{P})}{n}}, \qquad (7.3.11)$$

Similar techniques for detection of unnatural patterns described above for the $\bar{X}$ chart and R chart can also be applied to the $\bar{P}$ chart.

7.3.3 Acceptance Control Chart

During a manufacturing process, since the characteristics of a drug product may vary from time to time, we may classify the characteristics as either at an acceptable process level (APL) or a rejectable process level (RPL). APL is defined as a process level at which it is acceptable and should be accepted most of the time (Freund, 1957). On the other hand, RPL is a process level at which it is rejectable and should be rejected most of the time. When we classify the characteristics into either APL or RPL, two types of errors have occurred. Type I error is the error by rejecting an acceptable process. The probability associated with type I error is called producer's risk. Type II error is referred to as the error by accepting a rejectable process. The probability corresponding to type II error is known as consumer's risk. For convenience's sake, we use the traditional α and β to denote the probabilities of type I and type II errors.

As can be seen, the Shewhart $\bar{X}$ chart is applied to a single acceptable process level which is the arithmetic average of sample means $\bar{\bar{X}}$. In practice, as indicated earlier, the acceptance process level for drug characteristics according to USP/NF specifications is usually an interval. In this case the Shewhart $\bar{X}$ chart may not be appropriate. As an alternative, the acceptance control charts developed by Freund (1957) may be useful. An acceptance control chart can be used to determine whether a process should be accepted or rejected based on whether the drug product meets USP/NF specifications according to the predetermined producer's risk for APL and consumer's risk for RPL. Acceptance control charts are usually applied when the variability of a manufacturing process is stable and in the statistical control state. In practice, acceptance control charts are generally used in conjunction with the R chart or a control chart for S to ensure the stability of the process in terms of its process variability.

In what follows we introduce how to construct an acceptance control chart. For simplicity, we assume that the population standard deviation of the process σ is known. If σ is not known or cannot be obtained from the past experience, it can be replaced by the sample standard deviation. In this case we simply replace all quantiles of a standard normal distribution with those of a central t distribution with $n - 1$ degrees of freedom. The first step for construction of a two-sided acceptance control chart is to determine the sample size as follows:

$$n = \frac{\sigma^2}{(\text{RPL} - \text{APL})^2} \left[Z(\tfrac{1}{2}\alpha) + Z(\beta) \right]^2, \qquad (7.3.12)$$

where $Z(1/2\ \alpha)$ and $Z(\beta)$ are the $(1/2\alpha)$th and βth quantiles of a standard normal distribution. Suppose that there are lower and upper APL, denoted as $\text{APL}(L)$ and $\text{APL}(U)$, respectively. Then the lower and upper acceptance control limits (ACL) are given by

$$\text{ACL}(L) = \text{APL}(L) - \frac{Z(\alpha)\sigma}{\sqrt{n}},$$

$$\text{ACL}(U) = \text{APL}(U) + \frac{Z(\alpha)\sigma}{\sqrt{n}}, \qquad (7.3.13)$$

respectively. On the other hand, if the lower and upper rejectable process levels are used, the lower and upper acceptance control limits are given by

$$\text{ACL}(L) = \text{RPL}(L) + \frac{Z(\beta)\sigma}{\sqrt{n}},$$

$$\text{ACL}(U) = \text{RPL}(U) - \frac{Z(\beta)\sigma}{\sqrt{n}}, \qquad (7.3.14)$$

respectively.

On a two-sided acceptance control chart, the central line is usually drawn as the average of lower and upper acceptance control limits. In practice, the relative importance of producer's risk to consumer's risk determines the probabilities of type I and type II errors. Then, based on APL and RPL, the sample size is determined and both of (7.3.13) and (7.3.14) can be applied to determine the acceptance control limits.

7.3.4. Cumulative Sum Control Chart

Shewhart control charts are based on a one-point rule which declares that a manufacturing process is out of the state of statistical control if the last sample mean is beyond the control limits. These procedures are graphic presentations of results from the repeated hypothesis testing based on the fixed sample size. As indicated earlier, Shewhart control charts are easy to implement and are able to detect large fluctuations effectively. However, Shewhart control charts are not efficient in identifying small-to-moderate deviations. To overcome this drawback, Page (1954) developed a procedure for control charts based on the sum of observations. Each point on this type of control charts contains information on all previous points, including itself. In other words, Page's proposed control chart utilizes all cumulative historical data up to the present time. Page's proposed control chart was shown to be able to detect any changes rapidly. Page's proposes control chart has been studied and improved extensively, and is later known as the cumulative sum (CUSUM) control chart. In this section we introduce the CUSUM control chart suggested by Barnard (1959).

Let μ_0 be the acceptance process level for a manufacturing process. Then the cumulative sum of deviation of $\overline{X}_i$ from μ_0 is given by

$$Y_i = \sum_{h=1}^{i} (\overline{X}_h - \mu_0), \qquad i = 1, \ldots, I. \tag{7.3.15}$$

The CUSUM control chart is constructed by plotting Y_i against the time point i. The idea behind the CUSUM control chart for detecting small-to-moderate shifts is that if the process is in the state of statistical control, its process average should be at μ_0 and each point on the CUSUM control chart should not deviate too far from the horizontal line of zero. Barnard (1959) suggested using a V-mask at point $(I + d, Y_I)$ with a lead distance d from the last point (I,Y_I). If only symmetric deviations from μ_0 are considered, the V-mask should be symmetric about Y_I with a half-angle θ. Let μ_1 be the rejectable process level, α and β be the probabilities of type I and type II errors defined in Sec. 7.3.3, and D be the absolute value of the change in process to be detected:

$$D = |\mu_1 - \mu_0|. \tag{7.3.16}$$

Then the lead distance d is given as

$$d = \frac{2}{\delta^2} \ln \frac{1 - \beta}{\alpha/2}, \tag{7.3.17}$$

where δ is the standardized change to be detected, which is given by

$$\delta = \frac{|D|}{\sigma/\sqrt{n}}. \tag{7.3.18}$$

The half-angle θ can be obtained from the following formula:

$$\tan \theta = \frac{D}{2w} = \frac{\delta(\sigma/\sqrt{n})}{2w},$$

where w is the scaling factor for the ratio of the plotting scales for Y_I and I.

Note that a w of $2\sigma/\sqrt{n}$ is usually recommended because a shift of the size of $2\sigma/\sqrt{n}$ in a sample mean will change the slope of a V-mask from 0 to 45 degrees. If the lower arm of the V-mask obscures any previous plotted Y_i, a positive change in the process mean is indicated. On the other hand, if any previous plotted points are obscured by the upper arm of the V-mask, it indicates a negative shift occurring in the process.

7.4. RELEASE TARGETS

As indicated earlier, before the quality control unit can release a batch for sale, the batch needs to be tested for potency, content uniformity, dissolution, weight variation, and disintegration time to assure that the batch conforms with USP/NF specifications. Such tests are usually referred to as release testing. A common approach to release testing is to obtain a single sample and test the characteristic of interest. If the specification for the tested characteristic is met, the batch is released. For each test the quality control unit may construct release targets based on other experiments such as assay validation and stability study. The constructed release targets guarantee that future samples from a batch meet a given product specification a given percentage of the time. For example, for potency testing, the USP/NF requires that the average drug potency of a batch be within an interval (L,U), where $0 < L < U$ represents USP/NF specification limits. Since the average potency is unknown, the release test is based on a potency assay result of a sample (or the average potency results of n samples) from the batch. A batch might be released for sale if its potency assay result is within (L,U). However, a batch released according to such a test criterion could have average potency outside (L,U) with a high probability. A batch having average potency outside the USP/NF specifications before the expiration dating period is subject to recall. To have a certain degree of assurance that the average potency of a batch is within (L,U), the quality control unit usually selects in-house release targets (a,b) as a guide for releasing a batch.

In this section we focus on the construction of release targets for final products. The idea can be applied similarly to any critical stage of the manufacturing process. For illustration purpose, we focus on the construction of release targets for potency.

Let a and b denote the release targets, which may be constructed based on data from experiments such as assay validation and stability studies before the drug product is manufactured. After a batch of drug has been manufactured, the batch is released for sale if its potency assay result is within (a,b). Assuming that the potency assay result is normally distributed, a commonly used set of release targets is

$$(L + 1.645\hat{\sigma} + \hat{s}, \ U - 1.645\hat{\sigma}), \tag{7.4.1}$$

where $\hat{s}$ is the estimated stability loss in potency over the entire expiration period and $\hat{\sigma}$ is the estimated variability of an assay. Both $\hat{s}$ and $\hat{\sigma}$ are obtained from experimental data. The idea behind release targets (7.4.1) is that if all future batches have the same average potency, release targets guarantee that among all the future batches released, 90% have average potency within (L,U). (a,b) should, however, be considered as random variables (Chow and Shao, 1989). Furthermore, the use of release targets (7.4.1) does not take into account the manufacturer's costs and/or profits. The interval given in (7.4.1) could be too narrow and the chance of passing is extremely low (i.e., only a few batches can be released). Also, even if one has 90% assurance that the average potency is within (L,U), with a 10% chance of the true average potency being outside (L,U), the cost for a recall and possible penalty could be a disaster for the manufacturer.

As an alternative to (7.4.1), Shao and Chow (1991) proposed a Bayesian decision theory approach to construct release targets for drug characteristics such as potency, dissolution, and disintegration by minimizing the manufacturer's expected loss (or maximizing the expected gain). In their approach, release targets (a,b) are viewed as the manufacturer's action (decision). Let μ be a vector of average of k drug characteristics for a batch and Y be the vector of corresponding k assay results of a sample from the batch. Note that Y may be the average of n assay results. Y is observed after release targets are established. Thus Y is a future observation at the stage of constructing release targets.

Let $f(Y|\mu,\nu)$ be the density of Y, where ν is a vector of q nuisance parameters. In practice, we assume that $f(Y|\mu,\nu)$ follows a normal distribution. Note that μ is considered to be random when there is batch-to-batch variation. Let $p(\mu,\nu)$ be the believed joint density of μ and ν at the time of decision making. Note that the release targets a and b and the USP/NF specification limits L and U are k-vectors. Denote the ith component of a (b, L, or U) by a_i (b_i, L_i, or U_i). The pair $d = (a,b)$ is called an action or a decision of the manufacturer. d will be chosen from the following collection (or action space):

$$\mathcal{D} = \{d: L_i \leq a_i \leq b_i \leq U_i \text{ for all } i\}.$$

For a given future batch, the batch is released if

$$a_i \leq Y_i \leq b_i \qquad \text{for all } i, \tag{7.4.2}$$

where Y_i is the ith component of Y. Otherwise, the batch has to be disposed of or recovered for future reuse. Thus it can be seen that the utility and the loss of the manufacturer depends on μ, Y, and the action d.

Now, let $\ell(\mu,Y,d)$ be the loss of the manufacturer if the action d is taken and μ turns out to be the true average of the drug characteristics of the batch. The function $\ell(\mu,Y,d)$ is usually determined through a utility analysis. Since Y and μ are unobserved at the stage of constructing release targets and the release targets are to be used for all future batches, we may consider the average over all the future batch loss of the manufacturer when the action **d** is taken, which is given by

$$\rho(\mathbf{d}) = E^{(\mu, Y)} \{\ell(\mu, \mathbf{Y}, \mathbf{d})\},$$

where $E^{(\mu, Y)}$ is the expected value taken under the joint distribution of μ and $\mathbf{Y}$. Thus

$$\rho(\mathbf{d}) = \int \int \int \ell(\mu, \mathbf{Y}, \mathbf{d}) f(\mathbf{Y}|\mu, \nu) p(\mu, \nu) \, d\mathbf{Y} \, d\mu \, d\nu.$$

Note that ρ (**d**) is often referred to in the literature as the expected loss. Then an optimal action is an action $\mathbf{d}^* \in \mathcal{D}$ such that

$$\rho(\mathbf{d}^*) = \min\{\rho(\mathbf{d}): \mathbf{d} \in \mathcal{D}\}. \tag{7.4.3}$$

In practice, although $L(\mu, \nu, \mathbf{d}) = \int \ell(\mu, \mathbf{Y}, \mathbf{d}) f(\mathbf{Y}|\mu, \nu) \, d\mathbf{Y}$ may have an explicit form, $\rho(\mathbf{d})$ usually does not. Therefore, a numerical method is required to obtain a solution for (7.4.3). Shao (1989) proposed the following Monte Carlo method to approximate the optimal action $\mathbf{d}^*$. He suggested generating i.i.d. random $(k + q)$-vectors

$$\{(\mu^{(j)}, \nu^{(j)}, \quad j = 1, \ldots, m\}$$

from a density $h(\mu, \nu)$ which has the same support as $p(\mu, \nu)$. Then approximate ρ (**d**) by

$$\rho_m(\mathbf{d}) = \frac{\sum_{j=1}^{m} L(\mu^{(j)}, \nu^{(j)}, \mathbf{d}) \, p(\mu^{(j)}, \nu^{(j)})/h(\mu^{(j)}, \nu^{(j)})}{\sum_{j=1}^{m} p(\mu^{(j)}, \nu^{(j)})/h(\mu^{(j)}, \nu^{(j)})}$$

and $\mathbf{d}^*$ by $\mathbf{d}_m^*$, which satisfies

$$\rho_m(\mathbf{d}_m^*) = \min\{\rho_m(\mathbf{d}): \mathbf{d} \in \mathcal{D}\}. \tag{7.4.4}$$

Shao (1989) indicated that $\mathbf{d}_m^*$ converges to $\mathbf{d}^*$ as m tends to infinity. As a result, we may use $\mathbf{d}_m^* = (\mathbf{a}_m^*, \mathbf{b}_m^*)$ as an optimal action.

In practice, one may wish to take into account potential stability loss over the expiration period. In this case, s is an additional vector of parameters and the loss function will also depend on s, say $\ell(\mathbf{s}, \mu, \mathbf{Y}, \mathbf{d})$. Furthermore, if different batches have different stability losses, s is random and the expected loss is

$$\rho(\mathbf{d}) = E^{(\mathbf{s}, \mu, Y)} \{\ell(\mathbf{s}, \mu, \mathbf{Y}, \mathbf{d})\}, \tag{7.4.5}$$

where $E^{(\mathbf{s}, \mu, Y)}$ is the expected value taken under the joint distribution of s, μ, and $\mathbf{Y}$. Suppose that the data collected are of the form

$$X_{it}, \quad i = 1, \ldots, n, \quad t = 0, t_1, \ldots, t_T,$$

where X_{it} is the ith replicates of a sample batch after t months from the production data. For given μ and s, X_{it} are independently distributed with mean $\mu - (t/t_T)s$. Typically, the conditional distribution of X_{it} is normal. Let $\Pi(s,\mu,\nu)$ be a prior density, say informative prior, if no past information is available. Also, let $g(x|s,\mu,\nu)$ be the joint distribution of X_{it} for given μ, ν, and s. Then the posterior distribution of μ, ν, and s is given by

$$p(s,\mu,\nu) = \frac{g(x|s,\mu,\nu)\Pi(s,\mu,\nu)}{m(x)}, \tag{7.4.6}$$

where

$$m(x) = \int \int \int g(x|s,\mu,\nu)\Pi(s,\mu,\nu) \, ds \, d\mu \, d\nu.$$

We then use $p(s,\mu,\nu)$ for calculating $\rho(d)$ in (7.4.5).

7.5. EXAMPLES

In this section we provide two examples to illustrate the use of Shewhart control charts, acceptance control charts, and CUSUM control charts for quality assurance of in-process materials and release targets for quality assurance of final drug products.

7.5.1. In-process Controls

A pharmaceutical company would like to evaluate a manufacturing process for tablets of a new pharmaceutical entity. Suppose that the primary drug characteristic of interest is content uniformity of tablets which are usually expressed as percent of label claim. Table 7.5.1 displays assay results of individual tablets from 25 consecutive samples of 10 tablets each as well as sample descriptive statistics sample mean, median, standard deviation, and sample range for each sample. A sample size of 10 tablets is chosen because the first sample stage of content uniformity testing stated in the USP/NF requires 10 tablets. Readers can easily verify that the arithmetic means of sample means and sample ranges are

$$\overline{\overline{X}} = 100.473 \quad \text{and} \quad \overline{R} = 17.702.$$

From Table 7.3.1, when $n = 10$, $D_1 = 0.223$, $D_2 = 1.777$, and $A_1 = 0.308$. Hence the lower and upper control limits for the $\overline{X}$ chart and R chart are given by

$$R_L = (0.223)(17.702) = 3.947,$$

$$R_U = (1.777)(17.702) = 31.456,$$

$$\overline{X}_L = 100.473 - (0.308)(17.702) = 95.021,$$

$$\overline{X}_U = 100.473 + (0.308)(17.702) = 105.925,$$

TABLE 7.5.1 Assay Results (Percent of Label Claim) of 25 Consecutive Samples of 10 Tablets for Content Uniformity

Sample	Assay results										Mean	Median	Standard deviation	Range
1	99.2	106.7	101.5	99.8	101.8	90.1	98.8	95.7	107.9	95.7	99.7	99.5	5.3	17.8
2	102.9	98.7	98.7	95.3	93.8	97.5	101.9	100.2	94.9	95.6	97.9	98.1	3.1	9.1
3	101.7	97.7	104.6	95.8	107.5	96.5	104.2	104.4	103.4	94.5	101.0	102.5	4.5	13.0
4	101.2	103.1	98.4	101.5	99.1	95.7	112.9	106.2	91.6	96.9	100.7	100.1	5.9	21.4
5	98.3	105.4	94.2	103.9	106.4	99.9	103.2	113.0	109.7	94.7	102.9	103.6	6.2	18.8
6	100.3	104.1	91.7	93.9	101.1	104.2	96.3	99.2	93.8	90.5	97.5	97.7	5.0	13.7
7	105.8	98.9	108.9	101.6	109.6	101.9	95.2	107.0	107.0	103.1	103.9	104.5	4.6	14.3
8	100.5	88.6	96.1	96.0	95.7	94.1	86.9	96.5	100.2	106.6	96.1	96.0	5.7	19.7
9	105.5	103.2	106.9	102.6	85.7	90.4	86.3	106.5	109.5	107.8	100.4	104.4	9.2	23.7
10	110.5	102.1	101.8	104.2	97.4	105.8	100.4	106.0	100.6	105.0	103.4	103.2	3.7	13.1
11	100.5	96.5	93.8	94.0	106.4	96.8	106.7	109.6	99.3	99.0	100.3	99.2	5.5	15.8
12	100.7	111.6	102.9	104.5	96.4	103.0	96.5	101.0	100.0	97.8	101.5	100.9	4.5	15.3
13	109.0	96.4	106.2	107.5	103.2	102.2	99.0	99.1	90.4	106.1	101.9	102.7	5.8	18.6
14	91.9	106.0	103.5	102.4	100.3	113.5	102.0	91.6	91.6	97.5	100.0	101.1	7.1	21.9
15	91.4	100.8	86.3	102.7	109.8	90.4	102.7	97.9	105.8	101.3	98.9	101.0	7.4	23.5
16	91.3	98.3	102.5	108.7	103.5	96.9	104.0	99.9	87.3	101.2	99.4	100.6	6.3	21.4
17	102.0	97.2	91.1	106.4	96.2	99.9	100.2	91.1	102.1	106.8	99.3	100.1	5.5	15.6
18	105.6	94.1	96.2	94.9	104.5	96.5	105.6	100.6	102.8	102.7	100.4	101.7	4.5	11.5
19	108.0	93.6	101.8	113.8	105.7	87.2	104.4	97.0	102.2	99.4	101.3	102.0	7.5	26.6
20	105.7	104.7	106.8	104.1	106.3	100.5	98.1	95.4	108.3	102.8	103.3	104.4	4.1	12.9
21	103.5	104.1	88.7	105.3	97.9	102.0	99.6	106.4	107.6	99.6	101.5	102.8	5.5	19.0
22	107.2	100.6	111.6	108.6	94.7	106.8	89.6	106.2	98.8	102.4	102.6	104.3	6.8	22.0
23	100.7	98.1	86.0	97.3	98.4	104.9	93.3	103.3	100.9	89.7	97.2	98.2	6.0	18.9
24	103.7	100.6	96.8	92.3	104.8	102.9	99.1	101.2	108.6	98.1	100.8	100.9	4.6	16.2
25	100.7	92.1	110.7	100.8	97.0	102.2	99.8	103.0	93.9	99.2	99.9	100.3	5.1	18.6

respectively. The values of c_1 in Table 7.3.3 and (7.3.8) can be used to calculate the warning limits at two standard deviations as follows:

$$\bar{\bar{X}} \pm \frac{2\bar{R}}{c_1 \sqrt{n}} = 100.473 \pm \frac{2(17.702)}{(3.078) \sqrt{10}}$$

$$= 100.473 \pm 3.637$$

$$= (96.835, 104.111).$$

The $\bar{X}$ chart and the R chart are given in Figs. 7.5.1 and 7.5.2, respectively. From the R chart, it indicates that variability of the process is quite stable. Figure 7.5.1 shows that there is one sample mean (sample 8) outside the warning limits of two standard deviations. However, the sample mean is still within the control limits. It should be noted that the previous sample mean (sample 9) almost reached the warning limits at the opposite direction. In addition, five consecutive sample means from sample 14 to sample 18 are below the central line.

Suppose that the company sets its in-house specifications for tablets to be between 97 and 103%, with an allowance of 2.25% above and below these specifications. From past experience the standard deviation σ is known to be around 5.5. The probabilities of type I and type II errors are assigned to be 5% and 20%, respectively. From this information, the lower and upper APL and RPL can be obtained as follows:

APL(L) = 97,

APL(U) = 103,

RPL(L) = 97(1 − 0.0225) = 94.818,

RPL(U) = 103(1 + 0.0225) = 105.318.

The sample size for the lower and upper acceptance control limits can also be calculated by (7.3.12):

$$n_L = \frac{(1.96 + 0.845)^2}{(94.818 - 97)^2} (5.5)^2 = 50.0,$$

$$n_U = \frac{(1.96 + 0.845)^2}{(105.318 - 103)^2} (5.5)^2 = 44.2.$$

Hence a sample size of 50 is chosen to calculate the ACL. The lower and upper ACLs based on RPLs are given by

$$\text{ACL}(L) = 94.818 + 0.845 \frac{5.5}{\sqrt{50}} = 95.475,$$

$$\text{ACL}(U) = 105.318 - 0.845 \frac{5.5}{\sqrt{50}} = 104.661.$$

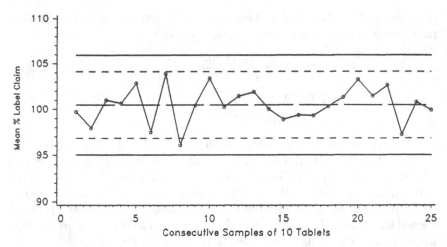

FIGURE 7.5.1 Shewhart control chart of means for percent label claim of content uniformity test. Long-dashed line, grand sample mean; solid line, action limits = 3 standard deviations; short-dashed line, warning limits = 2 standard deviations.

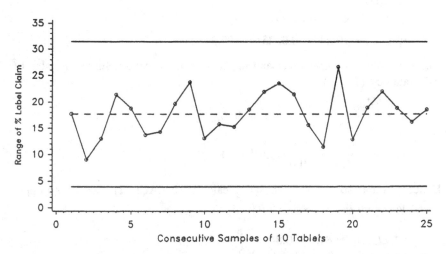

FIGURE 7.5.2 Shewhart control chart of ranges for percent label claim of content uniformity test. Dashed line, mean of ranges; solid line, action limits = 3 standard deviations.

The central line is the average of ACL(*L*) and ACL(*U*), which turns out to be 100.07. The resulting acceptance control chart is plotted in Fig. 7.5.3. Each point on the figure is the sample mean of the assay of 50 tablets. No sample mean is outside both ACLs. Therefore, the tablets manufactured from this process is accepted according to the in-house specifications.

From the experience of construction of acceptance control limits obtained above, the company revised its in-house specifications such that the target value is 100% of label claim and the lower and upper RPLs are 95% and 105%, respectively. With these new specifications, an updated standard deviation of 5.96, the same probability of type I error of 5% but a small probability of type II error of 10%, a CUSUM control chart can be constructed for the first 20 samples of 10 tablets each. From the information above, it can be seen that

$$\mu_0 = APL = 100,$$

$$D = |105 - 100| = |95 - 100| = 5,$$

$$\delta = \frac{5}{5.96/\sqrt{10}} = 2.653,$$

and the lead distance *d* is given by

$$d = \frac{z}{(2.653)^2} \ln \frac{1 - 0.1}{0.025} = 1.018.$$

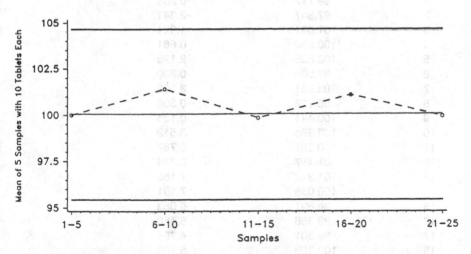

FIGURE 7.5.3 Acceptance control chart for percent label claim of content uniformity test. Dashed line, mean of five samples with 10 Tablets Each; solid line, lower and upper limits.

If the scaling factor w is chosen to be $\sigma / \sqrt{n}$, the half-angle θ is given as

$$\theta = \tan^{-1} \frac{2.653}{2} = 52.988°.$$

Table 7.5.2 provides the cumulative sum of deviations for the first 20 samples while the CUSUM control chart with a V-mask is given in Fig. 7.5.4. Since Fig. 7.5.4 shows that the lower arm of the V-mask obscures Y_i at time points 18 and 19, the process is considered as having a positive shift in the process mean at time point 20.

7.5.2. Final Product Release Targets

To illustrate the procedure for release targets introduced in Sec. 7.4 for simplicity, we consider only the construction of the release targets for the potency of a drug product. In this case $s = s$, $\mu = \mu$, and $v = v$ are scale parameters rather than vectors. Suppose that the USP/NF specification limits for the drug product

TABLE 7.5.2 Cumulative Sum of Deviations from 100% for Data in Table 7.5.1

Sample	Sample mean	Cumulative sum of deviations
1	99.712	−0.288
2	97.947	−2.341
3	101.021	−1.321
4	100.660	0.661
5	102.859	2.198
6	97.502	−0.300
7	103.881	3.582
8	96.112	−0.306
9	100.441	0.135
10	103.385	3.519
11	100.267	3.787
12	101.457	5.244
13	101.912	7.155
14	100.036	7.191
15	98.891	6.083
16	99.366	5.450
17	99.301	4.751
18	100.359	5.109
19	101.326	5.435
20	103.266	9.701

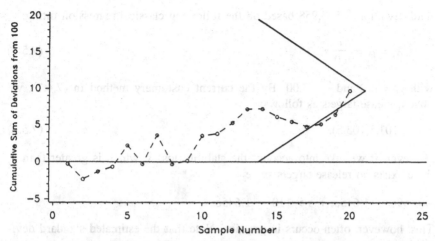

FIGURE 7.5.4 Cumulative sum chart of deviations for percent label claim of content uniformity test. Dashed line; cumulative sum of deviations from 100; solid line, boundary of V-mask.

are $L = 90$ and $U = 110$. The quality assurance personnel would like to construct a set of release targets a and b ($90 \le a < b \le 110$) to account for the stability loss over the shelf-life period. For this purpose, information regarding assay variability and stability loss may be obtained from other experiments, such as assay validation and stability study, and is needed for the construction of release targets. Suppose that the following potency assay results (percent of label claim) of a batch of the drug product were collected from a stability study, which included a preapproval (or NDA) stability (0 to 24 months) and a postapproval (or marketing) stability (36 to 60 months).

t (months)	0	6	12	24	36	60
X_t	104.0	104.9	100.5	92.2	99.2	94.4

Note that the preapproval stability study was conducted to establish a labeled shelf life that is required for FDA new drug application submission, while the postapproval stability study was performed to monitor the stability of the drug product until the end of its labeled shelf life. More detailed information regarding designs and analyses of stability studies will be given in the remaining chapters of this book.

We first consider the classical method for construction of release targets. Note that the stability data above exhibit a large variability. The estimated standard deviation $\hat{\sigma}$ is 3.958 based on the following classical regression fitting:

$$X_t = \hat{\mu} - \frac{t}{60}\hat{s} \tag{7.5.1}$$

with $\hat{\mu} = 102$ and $\hat{s} = 5.00$. By the current customary method in (7.4.1), we obtain release targets as follows:

$$(101.5, 103.5). \tag{7.5.2}$$

However, if we take into account the stability loss $\hat{s}$, which is greater than 7, there exists no release targets since

$$90 + 1.645\hat{\sigma} + \hat{s} > 110 - 1.645\hat{\sigma}.$$

This, however, often occurs in practice. Note that the estimated standard deviation of $\hat{s}$ is 4.771, which is too large to draw a useful conclusion. One solution to this problem is to conduct more experiments for a more accurate analysis. However, this is usually too time consuming and/or costly. Another disadvantage of the classical method is that it does not account for the manufacturer's profit and loss.

For the Bayesian decision theory approach proposed by Shao and Chow (1991), to account for the stability loss, for given μ and s, we have

$$X_t = \mu - \frac{t}{60}s + e_t, \quad t = 0, 6, 12, 24, 36, \text{ and } 60,$$

where e_t are i.i.d. normal with mean zero and variance σ^2, which is a nuisance parameter. Assume that for given σ^2 the prior of μ and s is a bivariate normal distribution with mean $(100, 100r)$ and covariance matrix $\sigma^2 G$, where

$$G = \begin{bmatrix} 10 & 10r \\ 10r & 1 \end{bmatrix},$$

where $r = 0.05$ is the expected percentage of stability loss. For given μ and σ^2, $E(s|\mu, \sigma^2) = r\mu$. We choose this prior because for this type of drug the stability loss is generally about 5% of the average potency μ, and the variability of stability loss over the variability of average potency is about 10%. The prior for σ^2 chosen to be a noninformative prior with $\Pi(\sigma^2) = \sigma^{-2}$. Let $\nu = \sigma^{-2}$, $\eta = (10, 0)'$, $\xi = (\Sigma_t X_t, \Sigma_t t x_t/60)'$, and

$$M = \begin{bmatrix} 6 & -\sum_t t/60 \\ -\sum_t t/60 & \sum_t t^2/3600 \end{bmatrix}.$$

Then the posterior $p(s,\mu,\nu)$ given in (7.4.6) is equal to

$$p_1(s,\mu|\nu)p_2(\nu),$$

where $p_2(\nu)$ is the density of a gamma distribution with shape parameter equal to 3 and scale parameter equal to

$$2\left\{\sum_t x_t^2 - (\xi + \eta)(\mathbf{M} + \mathbf{G}^{-1})^{-1}(\xi + \eta) + 1000\right\}^{-1},$$

and $p_1(s,\mu|\nu)$ is the density of a bivariate normal with mean $(\mathbf{M} + \mathbf{G}^{-1})^{-1}$ $(\xi + \eta)$ and covariance matrix $\nu^{-1}(\mathbf{M} + \mathbf{G}^{-1})^{-1}$.

Another crucial step is to construct an appropriate loss function, which can be done by an analysis of the manufacturer's profits and costs. Typically, the manufacturer's costs include the fixed cost and costs associated with the decision as to when the batch is released. Let C_0 be the total fixed costs, which include the production and laboratory testing costs; C_1 be the sum of the packaging cost, the distribution cost, and the storage cost; C be the cost of a batch due to disposal or recovery when the batch fails to pass the release test; B be the manufacturer's profit; and D be the cost and/or penalty of a recall. These costs are summarized in Table 7.5.3. It can be seen that the manufacturer's cost is C_1 if a released batch has μ within the USP/NF specification limits and is $C_1 + D$ otherwise. In practice, D is difficult to predict, so we may consider a reasonable range, say $D_1 \leq D \leq D_2$. Thus the loss function of the manufacturer can be formulated as follows:

$$
\begin{aligned}
\ell(s,\mu,\mathbf{Y},\mathbf{d}) = \; & C_0 + C(1 - I_{(a<Y<b)}) \\
& + (C_1 + D)I_{(a<Y<b)}(1 - I_{(90+s<\mu<110)}) \\
& + (C_1 - B)I_{(a<Y<b)}I_{(90+s<\mu<110)},
\end{aligned}
\tag{7.5.3}
$$

TABLE 7.5.3 List of Costs, Profit, and Penalty

Parameter	Description	Amount[a] ($)
C_0	Total fixed costs	2000
C_1	Packaging, distribution and storage costs	1000
C	Disposal or recovery cost	c
B	Profit	$3c$
D	Cost and penalty of a recall	$(40–150)c$

[a] c is a fixed constant.

where I_A is the indicator function of the set A. Note that **Y** has the same distribution as x_0. Thus the expected loss function is given by

$$\rho(\mathbf{d}) = C_0 + C\{1 - E^{(\mu,\nu)}(p)\}$$
$$+ (C_1 + D)E^{(s,\mu,\nu)}\{p(1 - I_{(90+s<\mu<110)})\}$$
$$+ (C_1 - B)E^{(s,\mu,\nu)}(pI_{(90+s<\mu<110)}), \quad\quad (7.5.4)$$

where

$$p = P\{a < Y < b\} = \Phi\left(\frac{b - \mu}{\sigma}\right) - \Phi\left(\frac{a - \mu}{\sigma}\right)$$

and Φ is the standard normal distribution function. It should be noted that (7.5.3) and (7.5.4) can easily be modified for a more general case when there are K drug characteristics as follows:

$$\ell(s,\mu,\mathbf{Y},\mathbf{d}) = C_0 + C\left(1 - \prod_{i=1}^{K} I_i\right)$$
$$+ (C_1 + D)\prod_{i=1}^{K} I_i \left(1 - \prod_{i=1}^{K} J_i\right)$$
$$+ (C_1 - B)\prod_{i=1}^{K} I_i J_i,$$

where

$$I_i = I_{(a_i<Y_i<b_i)}, \quad J_i = I_{(L_i+s_i<\mu_i<U_i)}, \quad \text{and}$$

$$\rho(\mathbf{d}) = C_0 + C\left[1 - \prod_{i=1}^{K} E^{(\mu,\nu)}(p_i)\right]$$
$$+ (C_1 + D)\prod_{i=1}^{K} E^{(s,\mu,\nu)}\left[p_i\left(1 - \prod_{i=1}^{K} J_i\right)\right]$$
$$+ (C_1 - B)\prod_{i=1}^{K} E^{(s,\mu,\nu)}(p_i J_i).$$

Finally, since $p_1(s,\mu|\nu)$ and p_2 have known forms, we approximate $\rho(\mathbf{d})$ by means of a Monte Carlo simulation with 20,000 samples $(s^{(j)},\mu^{(j)},\nu^{(j)})$ from $p_1(s,\mu|\nu)p_2(\nu)$. The release targets a and b are obtained by minimizing $\rho(\mathbf{d})$ over

$$\mathbf{d} = (a,b) \in \{90 \leq a < b \leq 110\}.$$

In practice, since the value of D may vary, release targets are constructed for various D values ranging from $40c$ to $150c$, where c is a fixed constant. The

TABLE 7.5.4 Release Targets for Various D/C Ratios[a]

a	b	D/C
90.0	110.0	40
92.6	110.0	60
94.3	110.0	80
94.7	109.8	85
95.0	109.5	90
95.4	109.1	95
95.7	108.8	100
96.0	108.5	105
96.2	108.3	110
96.5	108.0	115
96.8	107.7	120
97.0	107.5	125
97.3	107.2	130
97.5	106.9	135
97.8	106.7	140
98.0	106.4	145
98.3	106.2	150
98.5	105.9	155

[a]a, Lower release target; b, upper release target; C, disposal or recovery cost; D, cost and penalty of a recall.

results are given in Table 7.5.4 and Fig. 7.5.5. Table 7.5.4 and Fig. 7.5.5 are useful in determining the release targets if the ratio D/C can be determined approximately. In some situations the recommendation of a set of suitable release targets is not made by the project statistician but by high-level management personnel. In this case it is helpful for the project statistician to report the results given in Table 7.5.4 and Fig. 7.5.5 with various D/C ratios within a reasonable range. It should also be noted that Table 7.5.4 and Fig. 7.5.5 can also be used after the future assay result Y has been observed in the following way. Suppose that we observe $Y = 98$. From Table 7.5.4 or Fig. 7.5.1, if $D/C \geq 145$, the corresponding $a \geq 98$ and therefore the batch cannot be released. However, if $D/C < 145$, then $a < 98$ and the batch will be released. Thus 145 can be viewed as a tolerance (or critical) value of the costs ratio D/C. If the value D/C is difficult to measure when making the decision whether or not a batch of the drug product should be released, a prior value may be useful for the decision maker.

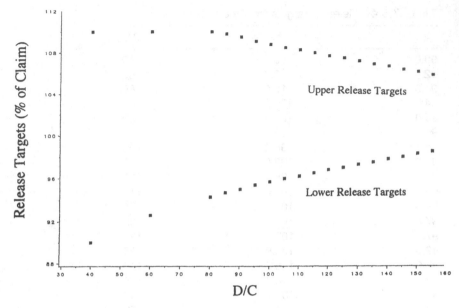

FIGURE 7.5.5   Plot of release targets versus D/C ratios.

7.6. DISCUSSION

For quality assurance of raw materials, it should be noted that the capacity of a V-blender usually has an impact on the selection of W_i. Moreover, since three samples are drawn from the top, middle, and bottom of each drum, it is possible that the materials in each part of the drum have different strengths due to the possible segregation. In this case μ_i is in fact a vector of μ_{ij}, $j = 1$, 2, and 3. If we are to account for the fact that the materials in each drum may have different strength depending on the location and the capacity limitation of the blender, the ad hoc procedure for selection of W_i is much more complicated. In this case the objective function and the corresponding constraints should be carefully laid out when applying the simplex method.

As can be seen from Sec. 7.3, the construction of Shewhart control charts and CUSUM control charts are based on the normality assumption for measurements of characteristics of drug products. Burr (1967) indicated that the $\bar{X}$ chart and the R chart are quite robust against moderate deviation from normality. However, it should be noted that serial correlations among observations have substantial impact on both Shewhart and CUSUM control charts [see, e.g., Goldsmith and Whitfield (1961), and Vasilopoulos and Stamboulis (1978)]. Bissell (1969) showed that except for extreme cases, skewness of the underlying distribution has a minimal effect on CUSUM charts. In general, CUSUM control charts are more effective than Shewhart control charts for small probabilities of type I error. Furthermore, Ewan (1963) pointed out that the CUSUM control chart is the most effective control chart for detecting a mean shift of a process in the range between $\frac{1}{2}$ and 2 standard deviations from APL. The designs for CUSUM control charts have been studied extensively [see, e.g., Taylor (1968), Goel and Wu (1973), and Duncan (1971)]. A commonly adopted method for construction of a CUSUM control chart is to apply certain criteria to select values of parameters such as sample size n, lead distance d, and half-angle θ to obtain desirable APL and RPL. Since a CUSUM control chart can be considered as a sequential sampling procedure in reverse (Johnson and Leone, 1962a,b), another method for designing a CUSUM is to use this property to obtain the values of parameters that satisfy the probabilities of type I and type II errors.

Since a manufacturing process being in control does not necessarily imply that the final products will meet USP/NF specifications, acceptance control charts are usually considered to combine the concept of control chart with an acceptance sampling plan. Schilling (1982) gave a detailed summarization of acceptance sampling and quality control. However, as mentioned in Chapter 5, the USP/NF testing plans are multistage-dependent mixed sampling plans (Schilling, 1982) which involve not only discrete random variables for attributes but also sample statistics computed from continuous random variables. In addition, the decision of acceptance or rejection of the lots is based on the combined samples of different stages according to criteria that differ from stage to stage. For example, in content uniformity testing, the acceptance process level for each tablet is between 85 and 115%. However, the rejectable process level for each tablet is either below 75% or above 125%. Although the rejectable process level is not stated explicitly at the first stage, it is clear that occurrence of two tablets with content outside the rejectable process level will reject the entire lot at the first stage. However, the testing plan of content uniformity allows occurrence of one tablet with content between APL and RPL. But APL and RPL in content uniformity testing plan is used to classify the tablets as detective and nondetective, so that it is a multiple-stage attributes sampling plan. On the other hand, acceptance or rejection of a lot also depends on the magnitude of the sample coefficient of variation. Therefore, it is also a multiple-stage variables sampling plan (Schilling, 1982). The criteria based on sample CV are 6% for the first stage and 7.8% based on the combined sample for the second stage. Although from the discussion above it is clear that the USP/NF test plan is very complicated, more research is urgently needed to develop acceptance control charts that combine the Shewhart control charts and USP/NF testing plan.

For the construction of release targets described in Sec. 7.4 it is also possible to make the decision to release a batch after the assay result $\mathbf{Y}$ of the batch has been observed; that is, we may minimize $E^{\mu}\{\ell(\mu,\mathbf{Y},\delta)\}$ conditionally on **Y**, where $\delta = 1$ if the batch is released and $\delta = 0$ otherwise, and $\ell(\mu,\mathbf{Y},\delta)$ is the loss function. This approach is known as the *conditional approach* (Shao and Chow, 1991). The approach described in Sec. 7.4 is, in fact, an unconditional approach since it uses an average loss over all future observations **Y**. In practice, the conditional approach is statistically more sound. However, it is not widely accepted because (1) different groups are often involved in product testing and/or the construction of release targets, and (2) the conditional approach requires the computation of $E^\mu\{\ell(\mu,\mathbf{Y},\delta)\}$ for every batch. It may not be of practical interest to compute $E^\mu\{\ell(\mu,\mathbf{Y},\delta)\}$ for every batch not only because that there are usually a number of batches manufactured but also because it requires a huge amount of computation. In the unconditional approach, the information provided by **Y** is not fully used. It is difficult (or impossible) to update the posterior $p(s,\mu,\nu)$ after the assay result of each new batch of the product is obtained. Shao and Chow (1991) suggested that the posterior and corresponding release targets be updated within a reasonable time period, say every 3 months, by using **Y** as part of X_{it}. Shao and Chow (1991) have indicated that a frequently updated posterior can provide a more accurate and robust result because the posterior is less dependent on the prior when n is large.

In Sec. 7.4 we have discussed release targets for quality assurance of some drug characteristics, such as potency according to USP/NF specifications. In addition, it is also important to evaluate other components related to the drug product such as the package of the drug product. As an example, consider the evaluation of drug package for birth control pills. For this type of drug, several tablets of the same drug but with different strengths are often packed in a specific order in the same package. The efficacy or safety of the medication with time depends on strict adherence to specific dose schedules. Thus it is important to ensure that the tablets within the package are each of the correct strength before the quality control unit releases a batch of the drug for sale. For quality assurance, Shao and Chow (1993) proposed a two-stage sampling, testing procedure, and set of acceptance criteria to evaluate whether the tablets are packed in the correct positions. The proposed procedure minimizes the expected squared volume (or the generalized variance) of the confidence region related to the test.

8

Stability Studies

8.1. INTRODUCTION

For every drug product on the market, it is required by the FDA that an expiration dating period be indicated on the immediate container label. The expiration date provides the consumer with the confidence that the drug product will retain its identity, strength, quality, and purity throughout the expiration period. To provide such assurance, the pharmaceutical companies find it necessary to collect, analyze, and interpret data on the stability of their drug products throughout the expiration period. If the drug product fails to remain within the approved USP/NF specifications for the identity, strength, quality, and purity of the drug product, the drug product is considered unsafe and should not be used. The FDA has the authority to issue recalls for drug products that fail to meet USP/NF specifications for the identity, strength, quality, and purity of the drug products prior to the expiration date. Note that the cost for a recall and possible penalty could be a disaster for the pharmaceutical company. Therefore, it is important to conduct a study not only to investigate the stability of a drug product but also to establish an accurate and reliable expiration dating period for the product. In this chapter we refer to such a study as a *stability study*.

The definition of *stability* has evolved over time with different meanings by different organizations. For example, the stability in the context of dispensing for pharmacists is defined differently (USP/NF, 1990) from that in the context of pharmaceutical dosage forms for manufacturer. Carstensen (1990) gave the following definition: ''The term *pharmaceutical stability* could imply several things. First of all, it is applied to chemical stability of a drug substance in a dosage form, and this is the most common interpretation. However, the performance of a drug when given as a tablet . . . depends also on its pharmaceuticas properties (dissolution, hardness, etc.). All of these aspects must, therefore, be a part of the stability program.'' In the 1987 FDA guideline for the stability of human drugs and biologics (FDA, 1987), *stability* is defined as ''the capacity of a drug product to remain within specifications established to ensure its identity, strength, quality, and purity.''

Most recently, a guideline issued by the International Conference on Harmonization (ICH, 1993) indicates that the purpose of stability testing is to provide evidence on how the quality of a drug substance or drug product varies with time under the influence of a variety of environmental factors, such as temperature, humidity, and light, and enables recommended storage conditions, retest periods, and shelf lives to be established (ICH, 1993). In this book, unless otherwise stated, we adopt the definition given in the 1987 FDA stability guideline. Note that the FDA guideline indicates that manufacturers should establish stability not only for drug products but also for bulk drug substances. Note that the FDA 1987 stability and ICH guidelines are included in Appendix C of this book.

The purpose of a stability study is not only to characterize the degradation of a drug product but also to establish an expiration dating period or shelf life applicable to all future batches of the drug product. In early 1970, although some drug products such as penicillin are known to be unstable, there are no requirements in regulations regarding drug stability. Since then it has become a concern that an unstable drug product may not be able to maintain its identity, strength, quality, and purity after being stored over a period of time, especially when the drug product is expected to degrade over time. To assure the identity, strength, quality, and purity of drug products, in 1975 the USP included a clause regarding the drug expiration dating period. In 1984 the FDA issued the first stability guideline. However, specific requirements on statistical design and analysis of stability studies for human drugs and biologics were not available until the current FDA guideline issued in 1987. Some statistical concerns and/or issues concerning the design and analysis of stability studies stated in the guideline have become popular topics in the pharmaceutical industry. These concerns and/ or issues include the use of a significance level of 0.25 for data pooling and the number of batches to be tested. The FDA guideline is being revised in 1994 to account for these concerns and/or issues. It should be noted that the European Community (EC, 1987) and Japan (MHW, 1991) have similar but slightly different requirements on stability in their respective guidelines (Helboe, 1992). In 1993 the International Conference on Harmonization issued a guideline on stability based on a strong industrial interest in international harmonization of requirements for marketing in the European Community (EC), Japan, and the

United States (ICH, 1993). Note that the World Health Organization (WHO, 1993) also published a draft guideline for stability in 1993.

Basically, there are two different types of stability studies: short-term and long-term studies. A typical short-term stability study is an accelerated stability testing study under stressed storage conditions. The purpose of an accelerated stability testing study is not only to determine the rate of chemical and physical reactions but also to predict a tentative expiration dating period under ambient marketing storage conditions. Information regarding the rate of degradation and tentative expiration dating period are vital and useful for designing long-term stability studies. Long-term studies, which include both preapproval and post-approval stability studies, are usually conducted under ambient conditions. A preapproval stability study is also known as an NDA stability study, while a postapproval stability is usually referred to as a marketing stability study. The purpose of an NDA stability study is to determine (estimate) a drug expiration dating period applicable to all future batches. The objective of a marketing stability study is to make sure that the drug product currently on the market can meet the USP/NF specifications up to the end of the expiration dating period.

In the next section important statistical requirements and issues stated in the FDA guideline are outlined briefly. Also included in this section is a brief review of the ICH guideline. In Sec. 8.3 we describe an approach, which is acceptable to the FDA, for determination of a drug expiration dating period. The concept of adding an overage to account for stability loss over time is also introduced in Sec. 8.3. Accelerated stability testing studies under stressed storage conditions and long-term stability studies under ambient conditions are introduced in Sec. 8.4. In Sec. 8.5 we include some important statistical issues that may occur in the design and analysis of stability studies.

8.2. REGULATORY REQUIREMENTS

As indicated earlier, the EC, Japan, and the United States have similar but slightly different requirements as to stability. In this section we first summarize some key requirements for the design and analysis of stability studies stated in the current FDA guideline (FDA, 1987). The discrepancies among the EC, Japan, and the United States in the requirements are then described. In addition, we provide a brief review of the guideline issued recently by the ICH (ICH, 1993).

8.2.1. FDA Guideline

In 1987, under 21 CFR 10.9, the FDA issued a guideline for the stability of human drugs and biologics. The purpose of the guideline is twofold. One objective is to provide recommendations for the design and analysis of stability studies to establish an appropriate expiration dating period and product requirements. The other objective is to provide recommendations for the submission of stability information and data to the FDA for investigational and new drug applications and product license applications.

The guideline indicates that a stability protocol must describe not only how the stability study is to be designed and carried out, but also the statistical methods to be used for analysis of the data. As pointed out by the FDA guideline, the design of a stability protocol is intended to establish an expiration dating period applicable to all future batches of the drug product manufactured under similar circumstances. Therefore, as indicated in the FDA guideline, the design of a stability study should be able to take into consideration the following variabilities: (1) individual dosage units, (2) containers within a batch, and (3) batches. The purpose is to ensure that the resulting data for each batch are truly representative of the batch as a whole and to quantify the variability from batch to batch. In addition, the FDA guideline provides a number of requirements for conducting a stability study for determination of an expiration dating period for drug products. Some of these requirements are summarized below.

Batch Sampling Consideration

The FDA guideline indicates that at least three batches and preferably more should be tested to allow for some estimate of batch-to-batch variability and to test the hypothesis that a single expiration dating period for all batches is justifiable. It is a concern that testing a single batch does not permit assessment of batch-to-batch variability and that testing of two batches may not provide a reliable estimate. It should be noted that the specification of at least three batches being tested is a minimum requirement. In general, more precise estimates can be obtained from more batches.

Container (Closure) and Drug Product Sampling

To ensure that the samples chosen for stability study can represent the batch as a whole, the FDA guideline suggests that selection of such containers as bottles, packages, and vials from the batches be included in the stability study. Therefore, it is recommended that at least as many containers be sampled as the number of sampling times in the stability study. In any case, sampling of at least two containers for each sampling time is encouraged.

Sampling-Time Considerations

The FDA guideline suggests that stability testing be done at 3-month intervals during the first year, 6-month intervals during the second year, and annually thereafter. In other words, it is suggested that stability testing be performed at 0, 3, 6, 9, 12, 18, 24, 36, and 48 months for the 4-year duration of a stability study. However, if the drug product is expected to degrade rapidly, more frequent sampling is necessary.

8.2.2. International Harmonization of Requirements

As indicated earlier, there are different requirements as to stability among the EC, Japan, and the United States. Based on different requirements, pharmaceutical companies may have to conduct stability studies repeatedly for different markets. Therefore, there is a strong industrial and regulatory interest and need in international harmonization of requirements on stability so that if information generated in any of the three areas of the EC, Japan, and the United States would be acceptable to the other two areas.

In the following we briefly summarize the differences in requirements regarding stability aspects among the EC, Japan, and the United States, which were discussed in a workshop on stability testing in *International Conference on Harmonization* held in Brussels, Belgium, November 5–7, 1991. In addition, we provide some statistical justifications for the differences whenever it is suitable.

Minimum Duration of Stability Testing

In the EC it is required to file an application based on the results of stability tests performed after at least six months of storage. In the United States, however, the FDA requires that a minimum of 12 months of stability data be provided. The Japanese government also requires 12 months.

Statistically, it is undesirable to extrapolate a drug shelf life too far beyond the sampling intervals under study. Therefore, as a rule of thumb, it is suggested that stability extrapolation not extend beyond six months. Stability data should be obtained to cover up to six months prior to the desired expiration dating period. In other words, if a desired shelf life is 18 months, stability testing should cover at least a one-year period. However, as indicated in the FDA guideline, although a tentative shelf life may be granted based on a short-term stability study, the pharmaceutical companies are expected to have a commitment to obtain complete data that cover the full expiration dating period.

Minimum Number of Batches Required for Stability Testing

Under the current stability guideline, the FDA requires at least three batches, and preferably more should be tested to allow a reasonable estimation of batch-to-batch variability and to test the hypothesis that a single expiration period for all future batches is justifiable. However, the EC requires only that stability data on two batches of the active drug substances be submitted for the evaluation of a drug expiration period. For the number of batches required in stability testing, the Japan government's requirement is consistent with the United States.

The FDA guideline provides some justification for the use of a minimum number of three batches for stability testing. The FDA guideline indicates that a single batch does not permit assessment of batch-to-batch variability, and testing of two batches provides an unreliable estimate. To provide a more precise estimate of drug shelf life, it is preferred to have stability testing on more batches. However, there are some practical considerations, such as the cost, resources, and capacity, which may prevent the collection of data from more batches. As a result, the specification that at least three batches be tested has become a minimum requirement representing a compromise between statistical considerations and actually practice.

Definition of Room Temperature

According to the USP/NF, the definition of room temperature is between 15 and 30°C. However, in the EC, the room temperature is defined as being 15 to 25°C, while in Japan it is defined as being 1 to 30°C.

If the drug product is sensitive to the temperature range 0 to 30°C, degradation of the drug product may vary from one temperature to another within the range. Therefore, it is important to investigate the stability of the drug product at different range of temperatures if the drug product is to be marketed in different countries. In this case, harmonization of the definition of room temperatures may not be useful. However, if the drug product is not sensitive to this range of temperatures, harmonization of the definition of room temperatures may be needed, so that similar stability testing need not be conducted repeatedly to fulfill different requirements.

Extension of Shelf Life

In practice, when an NDA submission is filed, there are usually limited data available on the stability of the drug product. In the United States, it is a common practice for the FDA to grant tentatively marketing authorization of the drug product based on limited stability data. However, it is required by the FDA that a pharmaceutical company must submit the results of stability studies obtained up to the expiration date granted. However, the EC does not accept an extension of shelf life beyond real-time data submitted.

Least Stable Batch

When there is a batch-to-batch variation, or the batches are not equivalent, the European Health Authorities expect the pharmaceutical industry to consider the least stable batch for the determination of shelf life and to refrain from averaging the values statistically. When there is batch-to-batch variation, the FDA guideline suggests considering the minimum of individual shelf lives.

Note that use of the least stable batch for determination of shelf life is conservative, yet lacks statistical justification (Chow and Shao, 1991). However, in their recent paper, Shao and Chow (1994) provided statistical justification for use of the least stable batch.

Least Protective Packaging

The Japanese Health Authorities prefer to determine the drug shelf life based on the results of stability tests using the least stable packaging material instead of testing the product in all packages. The FDA guideline, however, encourages sampling of at least two containers of each packaging material for each sampling time in all cases.

The idea of testing the least stable packaging material is well taken. However, how to identify the least stable packaging material is an interesting statistical question. To identify the least stable packaging material, a pilot study may be required. As a result, a fractional factorial design described in Chapter 4 may be applied. However, it should be noted that the chosen pilot design should be able to avoid any possible confounding and interaction effects.

Replicates

In Japan each test must be repeated three times without provision for scientific and statistical justification. However, the FDA guideline encourages testing an increased number of replicates at later sampling times, particularly the latest sampling time. The reason for doing this is that it will increase the precision on the estimation for the desired expiration dating period, which occurs more often at later sampling time points than at earlier time points for long-term stability studies.

Although the accuracy and precision of the estimated shelf life based on replicates of test results will be improved, it is not clear how much improvement the test replicates will achieve. Replications at each sampling time point not only increase the precision on the estimation for shelf life but also provide data on the lack-of-fit test for fitting individual simple linear regressions to each batch. However, it is of interest to investigate the impact of replicates at each sampling time point on the accuracy and precision of shelf-life estimation.

8.2.3. ICH Guideline for Stability

In the interest of having international harmonization of stability testing requirements for a registration application within the three areas of the EC, Japan, and the United States, a tripartite guideline for the stability testing of new drug substances and products was developed by the Expert Working Group (EWG) of the ICH in 1993. The ICH guideline (ICH, 1993) provides a general indication of the requirements for stability testing but leaves sufficient flexibility to encompass the variety of practical situations required for specific scientific situations and characteristics of the materials being evaluated. The ICH guideline establishes the principle that information on stability generated in any of the three areas of the EC, Japan, and the United States would be mutually acceptable in both of the other two areas provided that it meets the appropriate requirements of the guideline and the labeling is in accordance with national and regional requirements. It should be noted that the choice of test conditions defined in the ICH guideline is based on an analysis of the effects of climatic conditions in the three areas of the EC, Japan, and the United States. Therefore, the mean kinetic temperature in any region of the world can be derived from climatic data.

Basically, the ICH guideline is similar to the current FDA guidelines. For example, the ICH guideline suggests that testing under the defined long-term conditions normally be done every three months over the first year, every six months over the second year, and then annually. It requires that the container to be used in the long-term real-time stability evaluation be the same as or simulate the actual packaging used for storage and distribution. For the selection of batches it requires that stability information from accelerated and long-term testing be provided on at least three batches and the long-term testing should cover a minimum of 12 months' duration on at least three batches at the time of submission. For the drug product it is required that the three batches be of the same formulation and dosage form in the containers and closure proposed for marketing. Two of the three batches should be at least pilot scale. The third batch may be smaller (e.g., 25,000 to 50,000 tablets or capsules for solid oral dosage forms). However, the ICH guideline also requires that the first three production batches of drug substance or drug product manufactured post-approval, if not submitted in the original registration application, be placed on long-term stability studies using the same stability protocol as in the approved drug application. For storage conditions the ICH guideline requires that accelerated testing be carried out at a temperature at least 15°C above the designated long-term storage temperature in conjunction with the appropriate relative humidity conditions for that temperature. The designated long-term testing conditions will be reflected in the labeling and retest date. The retest date are referred to the date when samples of the drug substance should be reexamined to ensure that material is still suitable for use. The ICH guideline also indicates that where significant change occurs during six months of storage under conditions of accelerated testing at 40 ± 2°C/75 ± 5% relative humidity, additional testing at an intermediate condition (such as 30 ± 2°C/60 ± 5% relative humidity) should be conducted for drug substances to be used in the manufacture of dosage forms tested long term at 25°C/60% relative humidity. Note that a significant change at 40°C/75% relative humidity or 30°C/60% relative humidity is considered failure to meet the specification.

For the evaluation of stability data, the ICH guideline indicates that statistical methods should be employed to test the goodness of fit of the data on all batches and combined batches (where appropriate) to the assumed degradation line or curve. If it is inappropriate to combine data from several batches, the overall retest period may depend on the minimum time a batch may be expected to remain within acceptable and justified limits. A retest period is defined as the period of time during which the drug substance or drug product can be considered to remain within specifications and therefore acceptable for use in the manufacture of a given drug product provided that it has been stored under the defined conditions.

Finally, it should be noted that the EC, the Ministry of Health and Welfare (MHW) of Japan, and the FDA representatives at the recent EWG meeting held in Washington, D.C., recommended that a three-year phase-in period be allowed once the ICH guideline is adopted by the three authorities. Thus the requirements of the harmonized guideline would have to be met at the time of submission of applications by January 1997.

8.3. STABILITY LOSS, OVERAGE, AND SHELF LIFE

As indicated earlier, the primary objective of a stability study is not only to characterize the degradation of a drug product over time but also to establish an expiration dating period for the drug product. According to the FDA guideline, the expiration dating period or shelf life is defined as the interval that a drug product is expected to remain within the approved USP/NF specifications after manufacture. The shelf life is used to establish the expiration dates for individual batches. The shelf life should be applicable to all future batches produced by the manufacturing process for the drug product.

For a single batch, the FDA guideline indicates that an acceptable approach for drug characteristics (e.g., potency) that are expected to decrease with time is to determine the time at which the 95% one-sided lower confidence limit (or 95% lower confidence bound) for the mean degradation curve intersects the acceptable lower specification limit (Fig. 8.3.1). The degradation of the strength for a drug product over time can be described by the following equation:

$$E(Y_j) = \alpha + \beta X_j, \qquad j = 1, \ldots, n, \tag{8.3.1}$$

where $E(Y_j)$ is the expected strength at time X_j, α is the batch effect and β is the degradation rate of that batch. Note that as indicated in the FDA guideline, the variable of interest is the percent of label claim, not the percent of initial average value. Since the slope β is the rate of degradation over time, stability loss over time period x is defined as βx. Easterling (1969) also provided an interpretation based on hypothesis testing for estimation of an expiration dating period using the mean degradation curve. Carstensen and Nelson (1976) proposed that the shelf life be determined based on the prediction limit, which is considered equally acceptable to the FDA. More details on the estimation of an

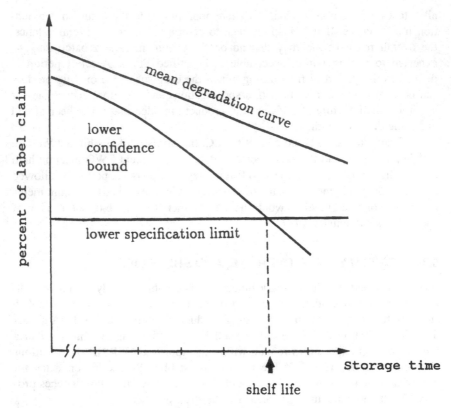

FIGURE 8.3.1 Determination of drug shelf life.

expiration dating period based on (8.3.1) for long-term stability studies will be given in Chapters 11 and 12.

In practice, an additional amount of active ingredients is sometimes added to account for the possible stability loss over a desired expiration period provided that the resulting initial value is within the USP/NF upper specification limit. The additional amount of active ingredient is called an *overage* of the drug product. For example, suppose that the desired shelf life of a drug product is 36 months, the expected stability loss over 36 months is 15% of label claim, and USP/NF specifications limits are (90%, 110%) of label claim. Then the pharmaceutical company may consider adding an overage of 5% of the label claim to the drug product to ensure that the drug product will remain within (90%, 110%) specification limits by the end of shelf life. The overage of 5% may result in an average potency of 105%, which is still within USP/NF specification limits. However, it should be noted that adding an overage of 5% may increase the manufacturing cost and/or the chance of causing a potential safety problem.

In this section we assume that the drug characteristics are expected to decrease with time. For drug product characteristics expected to increase with time, the shelf life can be determined similarly based on the 95% one-sided upper confidence limit for the mean. In some cases the drug characteristics of interest may be concentration of unchanged active ingredient for a solution. Chemical degradation of the active ingredient would decrease the concentration. On the other hand, evaporation of the solvent would increase the concentration. In this case, to allow both possibilities (i.e., decrease and increase in concentration over time), the FDA guideline recommends that two-sided confidence limits be used.

8.4. SHORT-TERM AND LONG-TERM STABILITY STUDIES

As indicated earlier, stability studies include short-term and long-term studies. A typical short-term stability study is an accelerated stability testing study under stressed conditions. Long-term stability studies, which are usually conducted under ambient conditions, include NDA stability studies and marketing stability studies. The purpose of a stability study is not only to characterize degradation of the drug product but also to establish drug shelf life.

In practice, since it may take a long time to observe the degradation of a drug product at the ambient storage conditions in the market place, at the early stage of product development, pharmaceutial companies are usually interested in conducting a short-term stability study such as an accelerated stability testing study under stressed storage conditions to accelerate the rate of chemical or physical degradation of the drug product. The purpose of accelerated stability testing is to estimate essential kinetic parameters and to establish a tentative drug shelf life for preparation of the design of a long-term stability study. As indicated in the FDA guideline, stressed conditions ordinarily include temperature (e.g., 5, 50, and 75°C), relative humidity (e.g., 75% or greater), and exposure to various wavelengths of electromagnetic radiation [e.g., 190 to 780 nanometers (i.e., ultraviolet and visible range)]. The FDA guideline emphasizes that a tentative shelf life may be granted if a commitment to obtain complete data is made when available data do not cover the full expiration dating period for the drug product provided that there are sufficient supporting data to predict a favorable outcome with a high degree of confidence. A commitment usually constitutes an agreement to:

1. Conduct or complete the desired studies.
2. Submit results periodically.

3. Withdraw from the market any lots found to fall outside the approved specifications for the drug product.

Note that in addition to the determination of a tentative shelf life, an accelerated stability testing is frequently used to identify potential problems that may be encountered during storage and transportation.

For an accelerated testing, one needs to determine the order of a reaction to estimate the rate of chemical or physical degradation and consequently, to provide a prediction of a tentative expiration dating period. A commonly used reaction equation is either a zero-order or first-order equation. A zero-order equation describes a linear relationship between the drug characteristics and time, and a first-order equation indicates that a logarithmic transformation of the drug characteristic is a linear function of time. Once the order of the reaction is empirically determined, the relationship between the rate of degradation and the temperature can then be characterized through the *Arrhenius equation*, which describes the linear relationship between the log-degradation and the reciprocal of the absolute temperature. A prediction of a tentative expiration dating period can then be obtained. For the analysis of an accelerated stability testing, Davies and Hudson (1981) suggested that a standard nonlinear regression procedure be used, while Bohidar and Peace (1988) recommended that the weighted least-squares procedure be considered. In either case it should be noted that assumption of the Arrhenius equation be verified using a standard lack-of-fit test. More details regarding accelerated testing (or stressed testing) are provided in Chapter 9.

Based on a tentative shelf life established from accelerated stability under stressed conditions, a long-term stability study can then be conducted under some ambient conditions to support the claimed shelf life. The FDA guideline recommends that a long-term stability study be conducted to generate stability data on the drug product stored in the proposed container closures for marketing under storage conditions that support the proposed drug shelf life. Stability data obtained from a long-term stability study are usually referred to as the primary stability data. The data obtained from an accelerated testing are classified as the supportive stability data.

After the drug is approved and after a labeled shelf life is granted by the FDA and manufactured, it is important to ensure that the product in the market can meet the approved specifications and its expiration dating period. In other words, it is important to ensure that the true shelf life of the product is longer than the labeled shelf life. For this purpose a marketing stability study is usually conducted to monitor the product over the labeled shelf-life period by testing some batches in the market at fewer sampling-time intervals. The true shelf life is estimated based on these test results. Chow and Shao (1991) indicated that a marketing stability study can generally achieve the following objectives:

1. If the estimated shelf life from the marketing stability study is not longer than the labeled shelf life with 95% assurance, the product in

the market cannot meet the approved specifications at the end of the labeled shelf life, and therefore the product has to be recalled.

2. When the estimated shelf life appears to be shorter than the labeled shelf life, it may indicate that the manufacturing process for the drug product has changed or is out of control. An action for finding the possible causes should be taken to improve the manufacturing quality.

3. If the estimated shelf life from the marketing stability appears to be much longer than the labeled shelf life, a change in labeled shelf life for the product may be applied.

8.5. STATISTICAL CONSIDERATIONS

When conducting a stability study, the FDA guideline requires that a detailed plan be described in an approved study protocol and be applied to generate and analyze acceptable stability data in support of the expiration dating period. As indicated in the guidelines, a stability study protocol must describe not only how the stability study is to be designed and carried out, but also the statistical methods to be used in analyzing the data. Some requirements regarding the design of a stability study were given in Sec. 8.2. In Sec. 8.3 we introduced an approach for determination of drug shelf life which is acceptable to the FDA. In this section we provide some insight to some statistical issues which often occurs in the design and analysis of stability studies.

8.5.1. Batch Similarity

In previous sections we focus on the determination of drug shelf life for a single batch. As indicated in the FDA guidelines, a minimum requirement for a stability study is to test at least three batches. If batch-to-batch variability is small, it would be advantageous to combine the data into one overall estimate with high precision and a large degree of freedom for mean-squared error. As indicated in the guideline, combining the data should be supported by preliminary testing of batch similarity. The similarity of the degradation curves for each batch tested should be assessed by applying statistical tests of the *equality* of slopes and of zero-time intercepts. Chow and Shao (1989) proposed several tests for batch-to-batch variability under a normality assumption. Note that the test suggested in the FDA guideline is the one for detecting the difference of slopes and intercepts among batches to be performed at a significance level of $\alpha = 0.25$ (Bancroft, 1964). If tests for equality of slopes and for equality of intercepts do not result in rejection at the 25% level of significance, the data from the batches would be pooled. However, if tests resuled in p values less than 0.25, a judgment would be made by the FDA reviewers as to whether pooling would be permitted.

It should be noted, however, that there are some criticisms regarding use of a significance level of 0.25. Among these criticisms, the following are probably the most common:

1. Acceptance or rejection of the null hypothesis of no difference in slopes among batches does not guarantee that the batches have similar degradation rates. This is because the problem of similarity is incorrectly formulated by the wrong hypothesis of difference.
2. It is not a common practice to increase test power by increasing the level of significance.

As an alternative, the concept of the interval hypotheses for bioequivalence problem (Schuirmann, 1987; Chow and Liu, 1992) can be applied to test batch similarity. Under the assumption that the batch effect is fixed, the concept of the interval hypotheses is to claim similarity if the intercepts and slopes of the degradation curves for each batch are within an acceptable *equivalent* limits. If tests for equivalence of slopes and for equivalence of intercepts do not result in rejection at the 5% level of significance, the data from the batches would be pooled for determination of drug shelf life.

The FDA guideline indicates that the design of a stability study is intended to establish, based on testing a limited number of (at least three) batches of a drug product, an expiration dating period applicable to all *future* batches of the drug product manufactured under similar circumstances. In practice, there may be slight or moderate variation among batches, and therefore the degradation curves have different intercepts and/or slopes from batch to batch. According to the FDA guideline, if there is batch-to-batch variation (i.e., we reject the null hypothesis of batch similarity), the data cannot be pooled for determination of an expiration dating period. A method suggested in the guideline is to consider the minimum of individual shelf lives, where each shelf life is obtained by fitting an ordinary linear regression within a batch. The minimum of individual shelf lives is then used to reflect the shelf life of all future batches of the drug product. The minimum approach, however, appears to be conservative and lacks statistical justification (Chow and Shao, 1991). Note that if the batch is assumed random, the shelf life can be estimated without the preliminary test for batch similarity. However, estimation of drug shelf life under the assumption of random batches requires more than three batches, which are specified in the FDA guideline.

Recently, several methods for combining information from different batches have been proposed. Under assumption of the fixed batch effect, Ruberg and Hsu (1992) proposed the use of a multiple comparison technique for pooling with the worst batch. Estimation procedures for shelf life under assumption of a random batch effect can be found in Murphy and Weisman (1990), Chow and Shao (1991), and Shao and Chow (1994). Ho et al. (1992) conducted a Monte

Carlo simulation study to compare various methods, including the approach proposed by the FDA under either fixed or random batch effects. Morris (1992) also examined the consequences of drug shelf-life estimation when an incorrect linear model is used for the true exponential model.

8.5.2. Sampling-Time Considerations

The FDA guideline indicates that sampling times be chosen so that any degradation can be adequately characterized (i.e., at a sufficient frequency to determine with reasonable assurance the nature of the degradation curve). Usually, the relationship can be represented adequately by a linear, quadratic, or cubic function on an arithmetic or logarithmic scale of the percent of label claim. As a rule of thumb, more frequent sampling should be taken at which a curvature of the degradation curve is expected to occur in order to adequately characterize degradation of the drug product. In addition, the FDA guideline also encourages testing an increased number of replicates at later sampling times, particularly the latest sampling time, because this will increase the average sampling time toward the desired expiration dating period.

Assuming that the drug characteristic is expected to decrease with time, for long-term stability studies under ambient conditions such as NDA stability studies, the FDA guideline suggests that stability testing be done at 3-month intervals during the first year, 6-month intervals during the second year, and annually thereafter. However, for drug products predicted to degrade rapidly, more frequent sampling is necessary. For marketing stability studies, less frequent sampling is usually considered on more batches. The purposes of a stability study are to characterize the degradation of the drug product and consequently, to establish drug shelf life. For these purposes, the following statistical issues are of concern:

1. How can the number and allocation of time points be selected such that the degradation of ingredients of a drug product will be adequately characterized?
2. How frequently is sampling necessary to have a desired degree of accuracy and precision for the estimated shelf life?
3. Is is reliable to predict drug shelf life beyond the time interval under study?
4. Is it necessary to have replicates at each sampling time point?
5. How can the number of assays at each sampling time point be allocated efficiently if a fixed number of assays are to be done?

Mathematically, if the degradation curve is linear, it can be determined uniquely by two time points. One may consider having stability testing at the initial (i.e., the time at which the batch is manufactured) and latest sampling time points. However, it should be noted that, statistically, there are no degrees of freedom for the error term if only two sampling time points are considered. However, the pharmaceutical companies are usually interested in acquiring stability information regarding the drug product within a short period of time after the drug product is manufactured. However, if only two time points are employed in a long-term stability study, no information about degradation can be obtained between these two points. In addition, if the latest sampling time point is too close to the initial point, the fitted degradation line may not be reliable for establishing an expiration dating period beyond the time interval under study.

It is therefore of interest to study the impact of the frequency of sampling on the characterization of the degradation curve and the determination of drug shelf life. Moreover, the 95% confidence interval for mean degradation at points such as the initial and final time points, which is further away from the middle of the range of time points, could be very wide. Consequently, the estimated shelf life may not be reliable. Study of the reliability of an estimated drug shelf life beyond the time interval under study is then an interesting and important topic in stability analysis.

In the current guideline, the FDA does not require that stability testing be done repeatedly at each time point. Replicates at each time point certainly enable us to estimate the degradation curve more precisely in terms of the width of the confidence intervals about the estimated curve around the average of the sampling times included in the study. As a result, replicates improve the accuracy and precision of the estimated shelf life. In addition, the information from replicates can be used to perform a goodness-of-fit test for the fitted degradation curve. The discussion above may provide some justification as to why it is required that each test be repeated three times in Japan. When the pharmaceutial company can perform only a fixed number of assays, due to the limited resources available, it is important to allocate the number of assays efficiently at each sampling time point included in the study. As indicated earlier, we may consider either placing more assays at the latest sampling time point and the time point at which the curvature is expected to occur or to place equal number of assays at each time point. However, there is little or no literature available for selection of sampling time points and/or allocation of number of assays at each time point. The problem is worthy of further investigation.

8.5.3. Interval Estimate for Shelf Life

As suggested by the FDA guideline, drug shelf life can be determined as the time at which the 95% one-sided lower confidence limit for the mean degradation curve intersects the approved specification limit, which is often used as the labeled shelf life. The labeled shelf life provides the consumer with confidence that the drug product will retain its identity, strength, quality, and purity throughout the expiry period. Although there is no assurance that the drug product will retain its identity, strength, quality, and purity or that the drug product will be safe beyond the expiration period, the expired drug product may still be used by the consumer. It should be noted, however, that point estimates of shelf life may overestimate or underestimate the true shelf life. If the labeled shelf life underestimates the true shelf life, the drug product will retain its identity, strength, quality, and purity beond the expiration period. On the other hand, if the labeled shelf life overestimates the true shelf life, the expired drug product is no longer safe.

In general, it is believed that the drug product beyond the expiry period will maintain its identity, strength, quality, and purity within a short period of time. The pharmaceutical companies often receive queries regarding the safety of newly expired drug products. It is a common practice for the pharmaceutical companies to suggest that the consumer not to take any expired drug products. However, it may be of interest for the pharmaceutical companies to establish an interval estimate rather than a point estimate for the drug shelf life. An interval estimate may provide useful information regarding drug safety beyond labeled shelf life.

8.5.4. Drug Characteristics

Generally, there are different criteria for acceptable levels of stability with respect to chemical, physical, microbiological, therapeutic, and toxicological characteristics of drug products (USP/NF, 1990). The requirements of stability on these five characteristics are also different from dosage form to dosage form. Table 8.5.1 lists drug characteristics for different dosage forms which should be evaluated in a stability study. As indicated earlier, the objective of stability studies is to characterize the degradation of drug products in terms of some essential drug characteristics and consequently, to establish an expiration dating period. The approach suggested in the FDA guideline for determination of drug shelf life is based primarily on a single drug characteristic such as strength. The strength of a drug product is defined as either (1) the concentration of the drug substance or (2) the potency, that is, the therapeutic activity of the drug product, which can be determined by an appropriate laboratory test or by adequately developed and controlled clinical data. However, in the FDA guideline, the strength of a drug product is interpreted as a quantitative measure of the active ingredient of a drug product as well as other ingredients requiring quantitation, such as alcohol and preservatives. For an analysis of stability data, the FDA requires that percent of label claim, not percent of initial average value, be used as the primary variable for strength. Furthermore, the stability of the characteristics of a drug product for a particular dosage form may be influenced by storage conditions, such as temperature, humidity, light, or air and by package types, such as high-density polyethylene (HDPE).

TABLE 8.5.1 Drug Characteristics for Different Dosage Forms

Dosage form	Drug characteristics
Tablets	Appearance, friability, hardness, color, odor, moisture, strength, dissolution
Capsules	Strength, moisture, color, appearance, shape, brittleness, dissolution
Emulsions	Appearance, color, odor, pH, viscosity, strength
Oral solution and suspensions	Appearance, strength, pH, color, odor, redispersibility, dissolution, clarity
Oral powder	Appearance, pH, dispersibility, strength
MDI aerosols	Strength, delivered dose per actuation, number of metered doses, color, clarity, particle size, loss of propellant, pressure, valve corrosion, spray pattern
Topical and ophthalmic preparations	Appearance, clarity, color, homogeneity, odor, pH, resuspendibility, consistency, particle-size distribution, strength, weight loss
Small-volume parenterals	Strength, appearance, color, particulate matter, pH, sterility, pyrogenicity
Large-volume parenterals	Strength, appearance, color, clarity, particulate matter, pH, volume, extractables, sterility, pyrogenicity
Suppositories	Strength, softening range, appearance, dissolution

For any drug product that is intended for use as an additive to another drug product, the possibility of incompatibilities may exist. In such cases, the FDA guideline requires that a drug product labeled to be administered by addition to another drug product (e.g., parenterals or aerosols) be studied for stability and compatability in a mixture with the other product. A suggested stability protocol should provide for tests to be conducted at 0-, 6-, to 8-, and 24-h intervals, or as appropriate over the intended period of use. These tests should include assay of the drug product and additive, pH (especially for unbuffered large-volume parenterals), color, clarity, particulate matter, and interaction with the container.

As indicated in Table 8.5.1, for a given dosage form, the FDA guideline requires that a number of drug characteristics be evaluated for determination of drug shelf life. However, in most stability studies, shelf life is usually based on the primary drug characteristics of interest, such as the strength (or potency) of the drug product rather than all the drug characteristics. On the other hand, a drug product may have more than one active ingredients. In practice, to fulfill the FDA requirements, we may determine shelf lives for each drug characteristic of each active ingredient and consider the minimum shelf life if different drug characteristics among different active ingredients have different shelf lives of the drug product.

8.5.5. Frozen Drug Products

Unlike most drug products, some are stored at several temperatures such as −20, 5, and 25°C (room temperature). We will refer to drug products of this type as frozen drug products. For frozen drug products, a typical shelf life statement for drug products of this kind is different. For example, it may require (1) 24 months at −20°C followed by either 1 month at 5°C *or* 2 days at 25°C, or (2) 24 months at −20°C followed by 2 weeks at 5°C *and* 1 day at 25°C. The drug shelf life is determined based on a two-phase stability study. The first-phase stability study is to determine drug shelf life under frozen storage conditions such as −20°C, while the second-phase stability study is to estimate drug shelf life under re-frigerated or ambient conditions. A first-phase study is usually referred to as a frozen study, and a second-phase study is known as a thawed study. Determi-nation of the shelf life for frozen drug products involves a two-phase linear regression. Mellon (1991) suggested that stability data from the frozen study and the thawed study be analyzed separately to obtain a combined shelf life for the drug product. Figure 8.5.1 shows a two-phase degradation of the drug prod-uct. Concerns in the design and analysis of stability studies for frozen drug products are as follows:

1. When are the best times to assay?
2. How many assays should be made?
3. Does frozen time affect thawed degradation?
4. Does concentration level at time points during the frozen state (i.e., strength) affect degradation during the thawed state?
5. Do different lots affect degradation?

Mellon (1991) also provided a number of approaches that may be used for the analysis of frozen drug products:

1. Cell means model
2. Estimation of trends separately for each lot and temperature
3. One grand regression, including lot and temperature
4. Regression of frozen and thawed data separately

With separate analyses for frozen and thawed studies, Mellon (1991) sug-gested that the following approximate confidence intervals be obtained:

1. Bonferroni intervals
2. Asymptotic theory

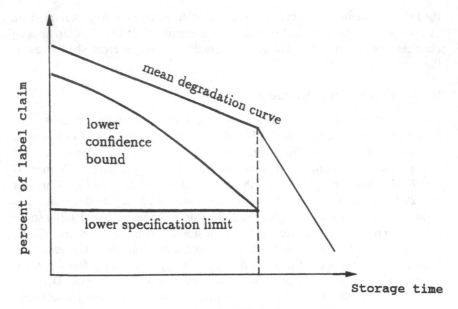

FIGURE 8.5.1   Determination of drug shelf life for frozen products.

3.   Bootstrap
4.   Satterthwaite approximation

However, the most important issue for determination of shelf lives for frozen drug products is that the same acceptable lower specification limit cannot be used for both frozen and thawed studies. The strength of a frozen drug product at the time it is to be administered at room temperature (25°C) is very likely to be below the acceptable lower specification limit if it is used to establish the shelf life for the frozen product. Second, determination of the shelf life for refrigerated and ambient conditions should be analyzed separately from that for frozen conditions. The shelf life for frozen conditions, measured in months, is usually much longer than those under refrigerated or ambient conditions, measured in either weeks or days. Therefore, the design for the thawed study should have different measures for time points than the frozen study. Note that if one uses only one regression model to fit the data from both states, the resulting estimated shelf lives under refrigerated and ambient conditions may not be reliable, due to rapid degradation and a much shorter time interval for the thawed study.

Since the determination of shelf life for frozen drug products involves a two-phase linear regression, instead of analyzing the data separately, we may consider this a well-known changing-point problem in two-phase regression (Shaban, 1980). The changing point, usually unknown, occurs at the time point at which the 95% lower confidence limit of the mean degradation curve at the first phase intersects the approved lower specification limit. Therefore, an estimate of the changing point can be used as the shelf life of the drug product under frozen storage conditions. Some details for estimating the changing point in two-phase regression can be found in Hinkley (1969, 1971).

It should be noted that no specific requirements regarding frozen drug products are stated in the guidelines. However, it is suggested that the statistical model selected for the analysis be verified. For sample-size determination (i.e., number of lots, number of frozen intervals, and number of replicates per sampling intervals), Mellon (1991) suggested that the portable power approach proposed by Wheeler (1974, 1975) be used to iterate the appropriate sample size.

8.5.6. Design Issues

Since the primary objective of a stability study is to characterize the degradation of a drug product and consequently, to establish an expiration dating period for the product, a stability design should be chosen to achieve these objectives. First, an appropriate stability design should be able to characterize the degradation of the drug product. For this purpose, the selection of sampling-time intervals is important. If the drug product is expected to degrade linearly over time, the sampling-time intervals suggested in the FDA guidelines should be used. However, if the drug product is expected to degrade in a quadratic fashion, it is suggested that more sampling be taken at the time at which the curvature is expected to occur. Furthermore, since it is of interest to establish a single shelf life for the drug product regardless of the strength and package type, an appropriate design should be chosen to avoid possible confounding and interaction effects. If there is interaction between strength and package type, the stability of the drug product should be evaluated at each combination of strength and package type. A significant interaction between strength and package type indicates that stability loss between strengths are not consistent across different package types. A typical stability design to achieve these objectives is a full factorial design.

However, in many cases, most pharmaceutical companies are unable to conduct a full factorial design with sampling-time intervals suggested by the FDA due to limited resources. To achieve a certain degree of precision without losing much information, a fractional factorial design with fewer sampling time points is usually considered as an alternative. Nordbrock (1992) evaluated a number of stability designs commonly used in the assessment of drug shelf life. These designs are discussed further in Chapter 10.

It should be noted that the selection of an appropriate stability design depends on the criteria used. Nordbrock (1992) compared several commonly used stability designs in terms of their statistical powers for detection of a significant difference in slope (or the rate of stability loss). Chow (1992), however, indicated that the criteria for selection of an appropriate design should be based on the precision of the estimated drug shelf life obtained under the design. These issues are discussed further in Chapter 10.

8.6. DISCUSSION

For determination of drug shelf life, the FDA guideline recommends that model (8.3.1) be used. In (8.3.1), the response variable Y is assumed to be a continuous variable. Under normality assumptions, the shelf life can be determined. In practice, however, some drug characteristics, such as particle size, are discrete rather than continuous variables. For discrete variables, although a similar concept for determination of drug shelf life may be applied, thus far there is little or no literature available for determination of drug shelf life based on discrete or categorical variables. In addition, how to determine drug shelf life based on two drug characteristics (one continuous and the other one discrete) is an interesting research topic. A typical example is stability testing for capsules. We may want to determine the shelf life of the capsules based on strength and particle size. In this case, two different types of drug characteristics are involved.

In Sec. 8.3, model (8.3.1) is used to determine drug shelf life based on the method of ordinary least squares. Basically, we assume that the degradation curve is linear as follows:

$$E(Y) = E(Y_0) - \beta x, \tag{8.6.1}$$

where $E(Y_0)$ represents the expected initial strength and βx is the expected stability loss overtime, $t = x$, and Y is the expected strength at time $t = x$. Equation (8.6.1) is usually referred to as a zero-order equation. In practice, however, the degradation curve may not be linear. In this case a commonly used approach is to consider the following degradation curve:

$$E[\ln(Y)] = E[\ln(Y_0)] - \beta x, \tag{8.6.2}$$

where $E[\ln(Y_0)]$ is the log-transformed expected initial strength and $E[\ln(Y)]$ is the log-transformed expected strength at time $t = x$. Equation (8.6.2) is known as a first-order equation. It should be noted that a first-order model occurs much more frequently in practice than a zero-order model.

As indicated in the FDA guideline, the estimated shelf life of a drug product, denoted by $t = x_L$, can be obtained at the time point at which the 95% one-sided lower confidence limit for the mean degradation curve intersects the acceptable lower specification limit. In practice, it is of interest to study the biasedness of the estimated shelf life [i.e., bias(x_L)]. If the bias is positive, x_L overestimates the true shelf life. On the other hand, if there is a downward bias, the estimated shelf life is said to underestimate the true shelf life. In the interest of the safety of the drug product, the FDA might prefer a conservative approach, which is to underestimate rather than overestimate the true shelf life.

For the study of drug stability, the FDA guideline requires that all drug characteristics be evaluated (see Table 8.5.1). In most drug products we obtain an estimated drug shelf life based primarily on the study of the stability of the strength of the active ingredient. However, some drug products may contain more than one active ingredient. For example, Premarin (conjugated estrogens, USP) contains three active ingredients: estrone, equilin, and 17α-dihydroequilin. The specification limits for each component are different. To ensure identity, strength, quality, and purity, it is suggested that each component be evaluated separately for determination of drug shelf life. In this case, although a similar concept can be applied, the method suggested in the FDA guideline is necessarily modified. It should be noted that the assay values observed from each component may not add up to a fixed total, which is due to the possible assay variability for each component. The modified model should be able to account for these sources of variations.

In Sec. 8.3 we mentioned that an additional overage may be added to account for some stability loss over time to ensure that the drug product maintain its strength throughout the expiry period. It should be noted, however, that an overage may cause a safety problem at the time the drug product is manufactured. For example, suppose that the target label of claim for a drug product is 100%. If the drug product is expected to have 15% stability loss over a desired 3-year shelf life, the pharmaceutical company may consider adding 5% overage to account for 5% stability loss, so that the drug product will retain the USP/NF approved specification limits of 90% and 110%. Therefore, the expected label of claim is 105% at the time when the drug product is manufactured. If we take into consideration possible expected and unexpected sources of variabilities, the true strength at the time the drug product is manufactured may exceed the upper approved specification limit of 110%. Thus when an overage is to be added to account for the possible stability loss over the desired shelf life, it is suggested that all possible sources of variability be taken into account for determination of drug shelf life.

9

Accelerated Testing

9.1. INTRODUCTION

As defined in the FDA guideline, the expiration dating period or shelf life of a drug product is the time interval that the drug product is expected to remain within specifications after manufacture. The shelf life of a drug product is usually established based on the primary stability data. The primary stability data are obtained from long-term stability studies conducted under an approved stability protocol with ambient storage conditions. Drug products under ambient storage conditions in long-term stability studies, however, usually degrade very slowly. Therefore, for most drug products, it may take more than a year to observe significant degradation.

As is well known, the development of a drug product is a lengthy process that usually involves many stages. The goals and meanings of drug stability functions may be different from stage to stage. For example, the purpose of stability studies before filing an IND is twofold. First, it is to verify that the stability of the drug product will be maintained within specifications for animal studies such as toxicological trials. Second, it is to provide useful stability information for modification of the formulation of the drug product. At the very early stage of drug development, however, the primary goal of stability functions is to determine the rates of chemical and physical reactions and their relationships with storage conditions such as temperature, moisture, light, and others. To achieve this goal, accelerated stability testing is usually conducted. As defined in the FDA guideline, an accelerated stability test is a short-term stability

295

study conducted under exaggerated (or stressed) conditions to increase the rate of chemical or physical degradation of a drug substance or drug product. Accelerated testing is also known as stressed testing. As stated in the FDA guideline, exaggerated storage conditions may include temperature (e.g., 5, 50, or 75°C), humidity of 75% or greater, and exposure to various wavelengths of electromagnetic radiation, and storage in an open container. The use of exaggerated storage conditions is to accelerate the reaction rate so that significant degradation of the drug product can be observed in a relatively short period of time (e.g., a few months). Based on the degradation data observed, the kinetic parameters of the reaction rate can be estimated. A predicted shelf life under marketplace storage conditions can then be obtained by extrapolation. Note that extrapolation from stressed testing conditions to ambient conditions is usually done based on established relationships between the kinetic parameters and storage conditions. In the pharmaceutical industry, the Arrhenius equation is often employed to relate the degradation reaction rate and the corresponding temperature. Other models, such as the Eyring equation (Kirkwood, 1977), can also be used. In this chapter, however, we focus on application of the Arrhenius equation to the prediction of drug product shelf life.

For a given drug product, the estimated shelf life based on the data obtained from accelerated stability testing is usually referred to as the tentative expiration dating period. As indicated by the FDA stability guideline, this period is a provisional expiration dating period determined by projecting results from less-than-full-term data using the drug product to be marketed in its proposed container closure. Therefore, the FDA guideline indicates that the results obtained from accelerated testing can be used only as supportive stability data. However, accelerated testing is useful in the following ways: (1) the results provide estimates of the kinetic parameters for the rates of reactions; (2) the results can be used to characterize the relationship between degradation and storage conditions; and (3) the results supply critical information in the design and analysis of long-term stability studies under ambient conditions at the planning stage.

In this chapter our efforts are directed to a discussion of accelerated stability testing in terms of application of the Arrhenius equation for the relationship between degradation and temperature. In Sec. 9.2 we describe briefly some deterministic chemical kinetic models. The Arrhenius equation is also described in Sec. 9.2. Applications of statistical methods to estimation of kinetic parameters and a tentative expiration period using the Arrhenius equation are given in Sec. 9.3. Section 9.4 covers determination of the order of a reaction by selection of adequate models. Also included in this section are issues that often occur in the design of accelerated stability testing. A numerical example using the data set given in Carstensen (1990) is given in Sec. 9.5. A brief discussion regarding other methods and possible future research topics can be found in Sec. 9.6.

9.2. CHEMICAL KINETIC REACTION

In this section we describe some functional relationships of chemical kinetic reactions. Unless otherwise stated, all quantities and equations considered in this chapter will be deterministic. In other words, there are no random error terms. Carstensen (1990) indicated that if in a reaction with two entities A and B

$$A + B \rightarrow C$$

the reaction rate is given by

$$\frac{dY(t)}{dt} = -K_{(r_A + r_B)} [A]^{r_A} [B]^{r_B}, \qquad (9.2.1)$$

the reaction is said to be of order $r_A + r_B$, where $dY(t)/dt$ is a differential quotient between concentration and time, $Y(t)$ is the concentration of the species being studied at time t, [A] and [B] represent the concentrations of A and B, and K is a rate constant. Note that in the pharmaceutical industry, we are only interested in the integer orders of reaction (e.g., 0, 1, and 2). The differential equation for a zero-order reaction is given by

$$\frac{dY(t)}{dt} = -K_0 \qquad (9.2.2)$$

where K_0 is the zero-order rate constant, which is expressed as concentration unit per time unit. Integrating both sides of (9.2.2) with respect to time gives

$$\int \frac{dY(t)}{dt} = -\int K_0 \, dt$$

or

$$Y(t) = C_0 - K_0 t, \qquad (9.2.3)$$

where C_0 is a constant.

Let $Y(0)$ be the initial concentration at time 0. Then (9.2.3) becomes

$$Y(t) = Y(0) - K_0 t$$

or

$$Y(t) - Y(0) = -K_0 t. \qquad (9.2.4)$$

It can be seen from (9.2.4) that a drug product based on the zero-order reaction degrades at a constant rate over time which is independent of both concentrations at the initial and at time t.

On the other hand, for the first-order reaction, since the amount of degradation is proportional to the concentration at time t, the corresponding differential equation is given by

$$\frac{dY(t)}{dt} = -K_1 Y(t), \tag{9.2.5}$$

where K_1 is the first-order rate constant. Equation (9.2.5) can be rewritten as

$$\frac{dY(t)}{dt} / Y(t) = -K_1. \tag{9.2.6}$$

Similarly, integrating both sides of (9.2.6) with respect to time yields

$$\int \frac{dY(t)}{Y(t)} dt = -\int K_1 dt,$$

or

$$\ln Y(t) = C_1 - K_1 t, \tag{9.2.7}$$

where ln denotes the natural logarithm and C_1 is a constant. If the initial concentration at time 0 is $Y(0)$, it can be shown that

$$\ln Y(t) = \ln Y(0) - K_1 t$$

or

$$\ln Y(t) - \ln Y(0) = -K_1 t \tag{9.2.8}$$

or

$$\ln \frac{Y(t)}{Y(0)} = -K_1 t.$$

Hence it can be seen from (9.2.8) that the degradation of a drug product described by a first-order reaction can be characterized by a rate constant for the logarithm of concentrations.

For the second-order reaction, since it proceeds at a constant rate that is proportional to the square of concentration, that is,

$$\frac{dY(t)}{dt} = -K_2 Y^2 (t) \tag{9.2.9}$$

or

$$\frac{dY(t)}{dt} / Y^2 (t) = -K_2,$$

we have

$$\int \frac{dY(t)}{Y^2(t)} dt = -\int K_2 dt$$

$$\frac{1}{Y(t)} = \frac{1}{Y(0)} - K_2 t. \qquad (9.2.10)$$

As a result, the second-order reaction describes a degradation characterized a rate constant for the inverse of concentration.

In the pharmaceutical industry, the first-order reaction is probably the most commonly employed model for describing the decomposition and the degradation of active ingredients of a drug product. The zero-order reaction is used occasionally, but the second-order reaction is rarely adopted. It should be noted, however, that the discussion above is made based on the assumption that there is only one decomposed end chemical entity for each active ingredient contained in the drug product. In many situations the active ingredient of a drug product may be decomposed into more than one end chemical entity. The description and determination of orders for such a reaction are usually very complicated. In this chapter, for simplicity, we focus on the zero- and first-order reactions for a single end chemical entity decomposed from one active ingredient of a drug product.

For thermal stability accelerated testing, samples of drug products are usually stored over time at different temperatures, (e.g., 5, 50, or 75°C). There are, in general, two methods for determination of the strength (i.e., concentration or potency) of a sample that has been stored over time t at temperature T (Davies and Hudson, 1981). The time is usually expressed in terms of either days or months. Absolute temperature is used for the study of the relationship between rate constant and temperature. For the first method, each sample stored at an elevated temperature over time t is assayed side by side with a sample stored for the same period of time but at a lower temperature in which no appreciable degradation can occur. Then the strength of the sample stored at the elevated temperature is expressed as a percentage of the sample at the lower temperature. The second method assays the sample stored at temperature T and time t and a sample prior to storage together against an independent standard. The strength of the sample at temperature T and time t is scaled to that of the sample prior to storage, which is made to be 100.

The difference between these two methods is the determination of the strength for the sample at time 0. The strength at time 0 obtained by the second method is an observation subject to random error. On the other hand, the first method provides an initial strength by definition exactly to 100 without error. Because of this advantage for determination of initial strength at time 0, the first method has become a popular method in practice. Therefore, in this chapter, we focus on the projection of a tentative expiration dating period based on the data obtained from the first method. It should be noted that there are other sources of variations in the first method which are not discussed in this chapter. For more details, see Davies (1980).

Based on the first method, since the initial strength at time 0 is 100% of label claim without error [i.e., $Y(0) = 100$], the equations for the zero- and first-order reactions given in (9.2.4) and (9.2.8) become

$$Y(t) = 100 - K_0 t, \tag{9.2.11}$$

$$\ln[Y(t)] = \ln(100) - K_1 t, \tag{9.2.12}$$

respectively. At the early stage of drug development, it is necessary to project the degradation rate at marketing storage temperature based on the data collected from thermal stability accelerated testing at elevated temperatures. To achieve this goal, we first need to establish the relationship between rate constant and temperature. The relationship between the rate constant (or reaction rate) and absolute temperature can be expressed by the following Arrhenius equation [see, e.g., Bohidar and Peace (1988), Davies and Hudson (1981), and Carstensen (1990)]:

$$\frac{d \ln K}{dT} = \frac{E}{RT^2}, \tag{9.2.13}$$

where T is the absolute temperature, E is the activation energy, and R is the gas constant. Integrating both sides of (9.2.13) gives

$$\ln K = -\frac{E}{R} \cdot \frac{1}{T} + \ln A,$$

or

$$K = A \exp\left(-\frac{E}{RT}\right), \tag{9.2.14}$$

where A is a frequency factor. Substituting (9.2.14) into (9.2.11) and (9.2.12) yields the following equations:

$$Y(t) = 100 - A \exp\left(-\frac{E}{RT}\right)t, \tag{9.2.15}$$

$$\ln[Y(t)] = \ln(100) - A \exp\left(-\frac{E}{RT}\right)t. \tag{9.2.16}$$

Rearranging the terms in (9.2.15) and (9.2.16) gives

$$\frac{Y(t) - 100}{t} = -A \exp\left(-\frac{E}{RT}\right), \tag{9.2.17}$$

$$\frac{\ln[Y(t)/100]}{t} = -A \exp\left(-\frac{E}{RT}\right). \tag{9.2.18}$$

The quantities on the left-hand side of (9.2.17) and (9.2.18) are, in fact, the degradation per time unit based on either the original scale of the strength for the zero-order reaction or the log scale of the strength for the first-order reaction. As a matter of fact, $(Y(t) - 100)/t$ or $\ln(Y(t)/100)/t$ can be interpreted as the observed reaction rates that can be used for estimation of the unknown parameters A and $-E/R$ in (9.2.14). For the purpose of estimating the parameters A and $-E/R$, it is preferable to use the following negative observed reaction rates:

$$\frac{100 - Y(t)}{t} = A \exp\left(-\frac{E}{RT}\right), \tag{9.2.19}$$

$$\frac{\ln[100/Y(t)]}{t} = A \exp\left(-\frac{E}{RT}\right). \tag{9.2.20}$$

The estimates obtained from (9.2.19) and (9.2.20) are the same as those from (9.2.17) and (9.2.18).

9.3. STATISTICAL ANALYSIS AND PREDICTION

Let Y_{ij} be the strength of a sample stored after time t_j at temperature T_i, where $l = 1, 2, \ldots, I$, $j = 1, 2, \ldots, J$. Since the first method for determination of the strength is used throughout the rest of this chapter, Y_{ij} will not represent the initial strength at time 0, which is 100 without error, and all Y_{ij} are expressed in terms of percentage. Define the degradation for the zero- and first-order reactions, respectively, as

$$D_{ij}(0) = Y_{ij} - 100,$$

$$D_{ij}(1) = \ln(Y_{ij}/100)$$

$$= \ln(Y_{ij}) - \ln(100), \tag{9.3.1}$$

where $i = 1, 2, \ldots, I$ and $j = 1, 2, \ldots, J$. The negative reaction rates or the negative degradation rates per time unit are given, respectively, as follows:

$$K_{ij}(0) = -\frac{D_{ij}(0)}{t_j} = \frac{100 - Y_{ij}}{t_j},$$

$$K_{ij}(1) = -\frac{D_{ij}(1)}{t_j} = \frac{\ln(100/Y_{ij})}{t_j}, \tag{9.3.2}$$

where $i = 1, 2, \ldots, I$ and $j = 1, 2, \ldots, J$.

In this section we illustrate the application of some well-established statistical methods for the estimation of rate constants and the unknown parameters in the Arrhenius equation. Based on estimates of the unknown parameters and their estimated standard deviations and covariance, a projected tentative expiration dating period can be obtained using the relationships given in (9.2.15) and (9.2.16). From (9.2.4) and (9.2.8), the degradation at time t_j can be expressed by the following linear regression model through the origin:

$$D_{ij}(h) = \beta_i(h)t_j + e_{ij}, \qquad i = 1, \ldots, I, \quad j = 1, \ldots, J, \tag{9.3.3}$$

where

$$\beta_i(h) = -K_{hi},$$

$$h = \begin{cases} 0 & \text{for the zero-order reaction} \\ 1 & \text{for the first-order reaction.} \end{cases}$$

It is assumed that random errors e_{ij} in (9.3.3) follow a normal distribution with mean 0 and variance $\sigma_i^2(h)$. The least-squares estimator for $\beta_i(h)$ is then given by (Draper and Smith, 1981)

$$b_i(h) = \frac{\displaystyle\sum_{j=1}^{J} t_j D_{ij}(h)}{\displaystyle\sum_{j=1}^{J} t_j^2}. \tag{9.3.4}$$

Note that the foregoing estimator is not the same as that obtained from the linear regression model with intercept given in Sec. 2.3. However, they are expressed in a similar form. Under the normality assumption, $b_i(h)$ is the minimum variance unbiased estimator (MVUE) for $-K_{hi}$. An unbiased estimator for the error variance can also be obtained as

$$\hat{\sigma}_i^2(h) = \frac{\text{SSE}_i(h)}{J - 1}, \qquad i = 1, 2, \ldots, I \quad h = 0, 1, \tag{9.3.5}$$

where $\text{SSE}_i(h)$ is the sum of squares of residuals for the hth order of reaction at temperature i, that is,

$$\text{SSE}_i(h) = \text{SST}_i(h) - \text{SSR}_i(h), \tag{9.3.6}$$

where $\text{SST}_i(h)$ and $\text{SSR}_i(h)$ are the total uncorrected sum of squares and the sum of squares due to regression, that is,

$$\text{SST}_i(h) = \sum_{j=1}^{J} D_{ij}^2(h), \tag{9.3.7}$$

$$SSR_i(h) = \frac{\left[\sum_{j=1}^{J} D_{ij}(h) t_j\right]^2}{\sum_{j=1}^{J} t_j^2}. \tag{9.3.8}$$

The corresponding degrees of freedom for $SST_i(h)$, $SSR_i(h)$, and $SSE_i(h)$ are J, 1, and $J - 1$, respectively. The relationship among the total uncorrected sum of squares, the sum of squares due to regression, and the sum of squares of residuals is the same as that for the linear regression model with intercept. This relationship is summarized in the ANOVA table in Table 9.3.1.

The variance of $b_i(h)$ can be estimated by

$$\widehat{var}[b_i(h)] = \frac{\hat{\sigma}_i^2(h)}{\sum_{j=1}^{J} t_j^2}, \qquad i = 1,2,\ldots,I, \quad h = 0,1. \tag{9.3.9}$$

Thus the standard error of $b_i(h)$, denoted by $SE[b_i(h)]$, is given by

$$SE[b_i(h)] = \sqrt{\widehat{var}[b_i(h)]}. \tag{9.3.10}$$

Under the hypothesis that $\beta_i(h) = 0$, the statistic

$$T_b = \frac{b_i(h)}{SE[b_i(h)]} \tag{9.3.11}$$

TABLE 9.3.1 ANOVA Table for Simple Linear Regression Without Intercept

Source of variation	df	Sum of Squares[a]	Mean squares	F value
Regression	1	$SSR_i(h)$	$MSR_i(h) = SSR_i(h)$	$F = \dfrac{MSR_i(h)}{MSE_i(h)}$
Residual	$J - 1$	$SSE_i(h)$	$MSE_i(h) = SSE_i(h)/(J - 1)$	
Total	J	$SST_i(h)$		

$$^aSSR_i(h) = \frac{\left[\sum D_{ij}(h)t_j\right]^2}{\sum t_j^2}$$

$$SSE_i(h) = \sum D_{ij}^2(h) - \frac{\left[\sum D_{ij}(h)t_j\right]^2}{\sum t_j^2}$$

$$SST_i(h) = D_{ij}^2(h).$$

follows a central t distribution with $J - 1$ degrees of freedom. Based on (9.3.11), a $(1 - \alpha) \times 100\%$ confidence interval for $\beta_i(h)$ can be obtained as follows:

$$b_i(h) \pm t(\alpha/2, J - 1)SE[b_i(h)], \tag{9.3.12}$$

where $t\alpha/2, J - 1)$ is the $(\alpha/2)$th upper quantile of a central t distribution with $J - 1$ degrees of freedom. To test for a negative reaction after time t_j at temperature T_i, we may consider the following hypotheses:

$$H_0: \beta_i(h) = 0 \quad \text{vs.} \quad H_a: \beta_i(h) < 0. \tag{9.3.13}$$

The null hypothesis of (9.3.13) is rejected at the α level of significance if

$$T_b < -t(\alpha, J - 1), \tag{9.3.14}$$

where $t(\alpha, J - 1)$ is the αth upper quantile of a central t distribution with $J - 1$ degrees of freedom. On the other hand, if one is interested in examining whether the reaction rate is different from zero, the following hypotheses should be tested.

$$H_0: \beta_i(h) = 0 \quad \text{vs.} \quad H_a: \beta_i(h) \neq 0. \tag{9.3.15}$$

The null hypothesis of zero reaction rate above is rejected at the level of significance if

$$F_i = \frac{MSR_i(h)}{MSE_i(h)} > F(\alpha, 1, J - 1), \tag{9.3.16}$$

where $F(\alpha, 1, J - 1)$ is the αth upper quantile of a central F distribution with 1 and $J - 1$ degrees of freedom.

We have illustrated the application of a simple linear regression model without intercept through the least-squares method for the estimation of a rate constant for each combination of time points and temperature. At the early stage of drug development, however, data of strength are usually available at only a few time points for each elevated temperature. In this case the estimates of error variances may not be reliable due to insufficient degrees of freedom. To enhance the precision of the estimates of error variances, we may consider the following regression model:

$$D_{ij}(h) = \sum_{i=1}^{I} \beta_i(h)X_{ij}(h) + e_{ij}, \tag{9.3.17}$$

where $i = 1, \ldots, I, j = 1, \ldots, J, h = 0,1$, and the value of $X_{ij}(h)$ for $D_{ij}(h)$ is t_j if the temperature is T_i, and is zero, otherwise, that is,

$$X_{i'j}(h) = \begin{cases} t_j & \text{if } i = i' \text{ for } D_{ij}(h) \\ 0 & \text{otherwise.} \end{cases} \tag{9.3.18}$$

If the random errors e_{ij} in model (9.3.17) are independently identically distributed as a normal distribution with mean zero and variance σ^2, then $b_i(h)$, given in (9.3.4), is also the MVUE of $\beta_i(h)$ in model (9.3.17). The total uncorrected sum of squares, sum of squares due to regression, and sum of squares of residuals under model (9.3.17) are given, respectively, as

$$\text{SST}(h) = \sum_{i=1}^{I} \text{SST}_i(h) = \sum_{i=1}^{I} \sum_{j=1}^{J} D_{ij}^2(h),$$

$$\text{SSR}(h) = \sum_{i=1}^{I} \text{SSR}_i(h)$$

$$= \sum_{i=1}^{I} \left\{ \frac{\left[\sum_{j=1}^{J} t_j D_{ij}(h)\right]^2}{\sum_{j=1}^{J} t_j^2} \right\},$$

$$\text{SSE}(h) = \sum_{i=1}^{I} \text{SSE}_i(h), \qquad h = 0,1. \tag{9.3.19}$$

The corresponding degrees of freedom for SST(h), SSR(h), and SSE(h) are IJ, I, and $I(J - 1)$, respectively. Table 9.3.2 gives the analysis of variance table for model (9.3.17). Since samples obtained at different temperatures are independent of each other, the sum of squares due to regression under model (9.3.17) can be partitioned into I independent sums of squares, that is, $\text{SSR}_i(h)$, $i = 1, \ldots, I$ which can be obtained separately under model (9.3.3). Under model (9.3.17), statistical inference for the reaction rate can be obtained based on the following estimates for the error variances

$$\hat{\sigma}^2(h) = \text{MSE}(h) = \frac{\text{SSE}(h)}{I(J - 1)}, \tag{9.3.20}$$

which has $I(J - 1)$ degrees of freedom. It should be noted that under model (9.3.17), $\sigma^2(h)$, and the upper quantiles of a central t distribution with $I(J - 1)$ degrees of freedom should be substituted for the estimated standard error, $(1 - \alpha) \times 100\%$ confidence interval, and hypothesis testing about reaction rates $\beta_i(h)$ given in (9.3.10), (9.3.11), (9.3.12), (9.3.14), and (9.3.16), respectively. Although the discussion above assumes the same time points for all temperatures, the methodology described above for estimation and inference about rate constants can easily be applied to the situation where there are different time points at different temperatures without modification.

Once the rate constants are estimated at each temperature, Bohidar and Peace (1988) have suggested obtaining estimates of the unknown parameters in the Arrhenius equation given in (9.2.14) by fitting a linear regression (or weighted) model to the logarithm of the estimated rate constants $\ln(b_i(h)$ with temperature as the independent variable. Since a typical thermal accelerated

TABLE 9.3.2 ANOVA Table for Simple Regression Without Intercept Corresponding to Model (9.3.17)

Source of variation	df	Sum of squares[a]	Mean squares	F value
Regression	I	$SSR(h)$	$MSR(h) = SSR(h)/I$	$F = MSR(h)/MSE(h)$
Temp. 1	1	$SSR_1(h)$	$MSR_1(h) = SSR_1(h)$	$F_1 = MSR_1(h)/MSE(h)$
.	.	.	.	.
.	.	.	.	.
Temp. I	1	$SSR_I(h)$	$MSR_I(h) = SSR_I(h)$	$F_I = MSR_I(h)/MSE(h)$
Residual	$I(J-1)$	$SSE(h)$	$MSE(h) = SSE(h)/I(J-1)$	
Total	IJ	$SST(h)$		

[a]$SST(h) = \sum SST_i(h)$

$SSR(h) = \sum SSR_i(h)$

$SSE(h) = \sum SSE_i(h)$

See Table 9.3.1 and the text for more details about $SST_i(h)$, $SSR_i(h)$, and $SSE_i(h)$.

stability testing is usually conducted at three or four different elevated temperatures, statistical inference about the unknown parameters in the Arrhenius equation is then based on only one or two degrees of freedom. To overcome this drawback, one may consider utilizing the observed negative degradation rate per time unit, or the observed negative reaction rates $K_{ij}(h)$, $h = 0,1$, $i = 1, \ldots, I$ and $j = 1, \ldots, J$. As a result, all observations are used to estimate the two unknown parameters in the Arrhenius equation and consequently, statistical inference regarding the tentative expiration dating period can be obtained based on an estimate of the error variance with $IJ - 2$ degrees of freedom.

Recall that the negative reaction rates observed are defined as

$$K_{ij}(h) = -\frac{D_{ij}(h)}{t_j} = \begin{cases} \dfrac{100 - Y_{ij}}{t_j} & \text{if } h = 0 \\[2mm] \dfrac{\ln(100/Y_{ij})}{t_j} & \text{if } h = 1. \end{cases} \tag{9.3.21}$$

However, the Arrhenius equation states that the relationship between the reaction rate and absolute temperature is

$$K(h) = A \exp\left(-\frac{E}{RT}\right).$$

Let $\alpha(h) = \ln A$, $\beta(h) = -E/R$, and $X = 1/T$. Then the Arrhenius equation can be rewritten as

$$K(h) = \exp[\alpha(h) + \beta(h)X] \tag{9.3.22}$$

$$\ln[K(h)] = \alpha(h) + \beta(h)X. \tag{9.3.23}$$

For the unknown parameters in (9.3.22), we may apply the following two methods to obtain estimates of $\alpha(h)$ and $\beta(h)$. The first method is to apply the method of ordinary least squares in a simple linear regression model, as described in Sec. 2.3, to the logarithm of the rate constants. The other method is simply to fit a nonlinear regression model directly to the original data of the reaction rates.

Let $K_{ij}^*(h)$ be the logarithm of the observed negative reaction rate, that is,

$$K_{ij}^*(h) = \ln[K_{ij}(h)], \qquad i = 1, \ldots, I, \quad j = 1, \ldots, J.$$

Then, according to (9.2.14), the model for the logarithm of $K_{ij}(h)$ is given by

$$K_{ij}^*(h) = \alpha(h) + \beta(h)X_i + e_{ij}, \tag{9.3.24}$$

where $i = 1, \ldots, I$ and $j = 1, \ldots, J$. Let $a(h)$ and $b(h)$ be the MVUE of $\alpha(h)$ and $\beta(h)$. Also, let $\widehat{\text{var}}[a(h)]$ and $\widehat{\text{var}}[b(h)]$ be the estimates of the variances of $a(h)$ and $b(h)$, respectively, which are obtained from (2.3.9) and (2.3.18) in

Section 2.3. The covariance between $a(h)$ and $b(h)$ can be estimated by

$$\widehat{\text{cov}}[a(h),b(h)] = \hat{\sigma}^2(h) \frac{-\overline{X}}{JS_{XX}}, \qquad (9.3.25)$$

where

$$\overline{X} = \frac{1}{I} \sum_{i=1}^{I} X_i,$$

$$S_{XX} = \sum_{i=1}^{I} (X_i - \overline{X})^2,$$

and $\hat{\sigma}^2(h)$ is an estimate of the error variance that is obtained from the ANOVA table in Table 2.3.1.

To obtain an estimate of the tentative expiration dating period, we need, first, to obtain the predicted mean reaction rates at the marketing storage temperature T for reaction order h. This can be done by considering the following linear regression model:

$$\hat{K}^*(h) = a(h) + b(h)X, \qquad (9.3.26)$$

where $X = 1/T$. An estimate of the variance of $\hat{K}^*(h)$ can be obtained as

$$\widehat{\text{var}}[\hat{K}^*(h)] = \hat{\sigma}^2(h) \{\widehat{\text{var}}[a(h)] + X^2 \widehat{\text{var}}[b(h)]$$

$$+ 2X \widehat{\text{cov}}[a(h), b(h)]\}. \qquad (9.3.27)$$

From (9.3.21) it can be verified that the predicted degradation after time t at the marketing storage temperature T is given by

$$\hat{D}(h) = -\exp[\hat{K}^*(h)]t. \qquad (9.3.28)$$

Let $G(h)$ be the minimum strength required for a drug product to maintain under reaction order h, that is,

$$G(h) = \begin{cases} 100 - P(0) & \text{if } h = 0 \\ \ln \dfrac{100}{100 - P(1)} & \text{if } h = 1, \end{cases} \qquad (9.3.29)$$

where $P(h)$ is the amount of maximum degradation allowed for reaction order h, where $h = 0$ and 1. For the zero-order reaction (i.e., $h = 0$),

$$D(0) = G(0) - 100 = -P(0).$$

It follows that

$$P(0) = \exp[\hat{K}^*(0)]t$$

or

$$\ln[P(0)] = \hat{K}^*(0) + \ln(t)$$
$$= a(0) + b(0)X + \ln(t).$$

Consequently,

$$\ln(\hat{t}) = \ln[P(0)] - [a(0) + b(0)X]. \tag{9.3.30}$$

Since $P(0)$ is a predetermined fixed constant, say $P(0) = 10\%$, the estimate of the variance of $\ln(\hat{t})$ is the same as that for $\hat{K}^*(h)$ given in (9.3.27). The $(1 - \alpha) \times 100\%$ lower confidence limit for the time based on the logarithmic scale is then given by

$$L_t(0) = \ln(\hat{t}) - t(\alpha, IJ - 2) \text{ SE}(\hat{K}^*(0)), \tag{9.3.31}$$

where

$$\text{SE}(\hat{K}^*(0)) = \sqrt{\hat{\text{var}}[\hat{K}^*(0)]},$$

and $t(\alpha, IJ - 2)$ is the αth upper quantile of a central t distribution with $IJ - 2$ degrees of freedom. Thus an estimate of the tentative expiration dating period for a maximum allowable degradation of $P(0)$ at the marketing temperature T under the zero-order reaction is defined as

$$t_T(0) = \exp[L_t(0)]. \tag{9.3.32}$$

Note that the estimated tentative expiration dating period defined in (9.3.32) is not derived from the mean degradation but is based on the 95% lower confidence limit for degradation. Thus the tentative expiration dating period obtained in this manner assures that 95% of future samples at marketing storage temperature T are expected to remain above the specified minimum strength $G(0)$. On the other hand, for the first-order reaction, we have

$$G(1) = \ln \frac{100}{100 - P(1)}$$
$$= -\ln \frac{100 - P(1)}{100}$$
$$= -\ln \frac{Y(t)}{100}$$
$$= -D(1).$$

Thus a similar method can be applied to obtain an estimate of the tentative expiration dating period based on the fact that

$$G(1) = \exp[\hat{K}^*(1)]t.$$

Let $a(1)$ and $b(1)$ be the MVUE of $\alpha(1)$ and $\beta(1)$. Then

$$\ln[G(1)] = \hat{K}^*(1) + \ln(t)$$
$$= a(1) + b(1)X + \ln(t).$$

Following the same arguments, an estimate of the tentative expiration dating period for a maximum allowable degradation of $P(1)$ at the marketing temperature T under the first-order reaction is given by

$$t_T(1) = \exp[L_t(1)], \tag{9.3.33}$$

where $L_t(1)$ is the $(1 - \alpha) \times 100\%$ lower confidence limit for the time based on the logarithmic scale at temperature T, that is,

$$L_t(1) = \ln(\hat{t}) - t(\alpha, IJ - 2)\, \text{SE}(\hat{K}^*(1)),$$

$$\ln(\hat{t}) = \ln[G(1)] - [a(1) + b(1)X],$$

and $\text{SE}(\hat{K}^*(1))$ is defined similarly.

The other method is to fit a nonlinear regression model directly to obtain estimates of $\alpha(h)$ and $\beta(h)$ in the Arrhenius equation. Once estimates of $\alpha(h)$, $\beta(h)$, and their variances and covariance are obtained, an estimate of the tentative expiration dating period at marketing storage temperature T can be obtained similarly using (9.3.32) and (9.3.33). To provide a better understanding, in what follows we provide a brief description of the estimation of the unknown parameters in a nonlinear regression model. More details are given in Draper and Smith (1981).

As suggested by the functional relationship stated in (9.3.22), consider the following nonlinear regression model for the observed negative reaction rate:

$$K_{ij} = \exp(\alpha + \beta X_i) + e_{ij}, \qquad i = 1, \ldots, I, \quad j = 1, \ldots, J. \tag{9.3.34}$$

Note that for simplicity, the index for reaction order was dropped in the model above. Similarly, we assume that random errors e_{ij} are independently identically distributed as a normal distribution with mean zero and varaiance σ^2.

To obtain estimates of α and β, we consider a Taylor series expansion of K_{ij} around K_{ij}^0 with respect to α and β up to the first derivative, where K_{ij}^0 is the value of K_{ij} evaluated at a^0 and b^0, and a^0 and b^0 are some selected initial values of α and β. Thus (9.3.34) can be approximated by the following equation:

$$K_{ij} = K_{ij}^0 + Z_{\alpha ij}^0 (\alpha - a^0) + Z_{\beta ij}^0 (\beta - b^0) + e_{ij},$$

$$i = 1, \ldots, I, \quad j = 1, \ldots, J, \tag{9.3.35}$$

where

$$Z_{\alpha ij}^0 = \left.\frac{\partial K_{ij}}{\partial \alpha}\right|_{\alpha = a^0} = \exp(a^0 + b^0 X_i),$$

$$Z_{\beta ij}^0 = \left.\frac{\partial K_{ij}}{\partial \beta}\right|_{\beta = b^0} = X_i \exp(a^0 + b^0 X_i), \quad (9.3.36)$$

Equation (9.3.35) can be rewritten as

$$k_{ij} = K_{ij} - K_{ij}^0 = Z_{\alpha ij}^0 \delta_0^0 + Z_{\beta ij}^0 \delta_1^0 + e_{ij},$$

$$i = 1, \ldots, I, \quad j = 1, \ldots, J, \quad (9.3.37)$$

where

$$\delta_0^0 = \alpha - a^0,$$
$$\delta_1^0 = \beta - b^0.$$

Let

$$k^0 = (K_{11} - K_{11}^0, \ldots, K_{IJ} - K_{IJ}^0),$$

$$Z^0 = (Z_\alpha^0, Z_\beta^0) = \begin{bmatrix} Z_{\alpha 11}^0 & Z_{\beta 11}^0 \\ \vdots & \vdots \\ Z_{\alpha IJ}^0 & Z_{\beta IJ}^0 \end{bmatrix},$$

$$\delta_0 = (\alpha - a^0, \beta - b^0).$$

The ordinary least-squares estimator of δ_0, which minimizes the sum of squares

$$\sum_{i=1}^I \sum_{j=1}^J (K_{ij} - K_{ij}^0 - Z_{\alpha ij}^0 \delta_0^0 - Z_{\beta ij}^0 \delta_1^0)^2,$$

is given by

$$\hat{\delta}_0 = (Z_0' Z_0)^{-1} Z_0' k^0. \quad (9.3.38)$$

After $\hat{\delta}_0$ is obtained, we can repeat the steps from (9.3.36) to (9.3.38) to improve the linear approximation. Denote $\beta = (\alpha, \beta)'$ and let $b = (a, b)'$ be an estimator of β. At the uth iteration, the resulting estimator of β is given by

$$b_u = b_{u-1} + \hat{\delta}_{u-1}$$

$$= b_{u-1} + (Z_{u-1}' Z_{u-1})^{-1} Z_{u-1}' k^{u-1}, \quad (9.3.39)$$

where

$$\mathbf{b}_u = (a_u, b_u)',$$

$$\mathbf{Z}_{u-1} = (\mathbf{Z}_\alpha^{u-1}, \mathbf{Z}_\beta^{u-1})',$$

$$\mathbf{k}^{u-1} = (K_{11} - K_{11}^{u-1}, \ldots, K_{IJ} - K_{IJ}^{u-1})'. \tag{9.3.40}$$

Let λ be some prespecified small number (e.g., 10^{-5}). Then the iterative procedure continues until the following criteria are met:

$$\left| \frac{a_u - a_{u-1}}{a_{u-1}} \right| < \lambda,$$

$$\left| \frac{b_u - b_{u-1}}{b_{u-1}} \right| < \lambda. \tag{9.3.41}$$

Note that currently, many statistical software packages for nonlinear regression are available. For example, the PROC NLIN in SAS (SAS, 1990) provides estimates for the unknown parameters and their variances and covariance and 95% confidence intervals for the unknown parameters. Once estimates of the unknown parameters in the Arrhenius equation are obtained from the nonlinear regression model, as mentioned before, an estimate of the tentative expiration dating period at the marketing storage temperature can be obtained using (9.3.32) and (9.3.33) for the zero- and first-order reactions, respectively.

9.4. EXAMINATIONS OF MODEL ASSUMPTIONS

In Sec. 9.3 we demonstrated how to apply statistical models, including a simple linear regression model and a nonlinear regression model for obtaining an estimate of the tentative expiration dating period under the assumption that the reaction is either zero- or first-order. The order of the reaction has an impact on the estimate of the tentative expiration dating period. One of the primary objectives of accelerated stability testing at the early stage of drug development is to empirically determine the order of reaction. As indicated earlier, the number of elevated temperatures examined at an accelerated stability testing study is usually between three and five. Thus at each elevated temperature, the degradation of the drug product is evaluated at three to five time points, including time zero. Based on these few observations, it is difficult to ensure the accuracy and precision of the empirically determined order of reactions for the drug product. After the reaction order of the degradation of the drug product is determined, the next step is to apply the Arrhenius equation. It is then important to evaluate whether the Arrhenius equation can adequately describe the relationship between degradation and temperature. In practice, it is suggested that the adequacy of the two postulated models be examined. It is necessary to check whether the models of the zero- or first-order reaction can adequately describe the relationship between degradation and time. In addition, it is of interest to determine which model provides a better description of the relationship.

At each temperature, a zero-order reaction is generally used to describe a linear relationship between strength and time based on the original scale, while a first-order reaction dictates a linear relationship between log(strength) and time. To provide a visual inspection of the linear relationship, scatter plots of the strength and log(strength) against time points by temperatures are often employed as a useful graphical presentation of reaction orders. If the scatter plots reveal that linearity exists for the strength on the original (or log) scale, the reaction for the degradation of an ingredient of the drug product may be of order zero (or first). In practice, however, if the degradation is not sufficient, it is very difficult to determine the order of reaction either by graphical or by other sophisticated statistical methods. Carstensen (1990) showed that if degradation is less than 15%, we may not be able to distinguish a first-order reaction from a zero-order reaction. Let $P(t)$ denote the amount of strength that has been decomposed after time t. The remaining strength at time t is then given by $Y(t) = 100 - P(t)$, or, equivalently,

$$\frac{Y(t)}{100} = 1 - \frac{P(t)}{100}.$$

If the reaction is of first order, we have

$$\ln \frac{Y(t)}{100} = -K_1 t$$

or

$$\ln \left[1 - \frac{P(t)}{100} \right] = -K_1 t.$$

If $P(t)/100 < 15\%$, we can approximate

$$\ln \left[1 - \frac{P(t)}{100} \right]$$

by $-P(t)/100$, that is,

$$\ln \left[1 - \frac{P(t)}{100} \right] \cong - \frac{P(t)}{100}. \tag{9.4.1}$$

Consequently,

$$\frac{P(t)}{100} = 1 - \frac{Y(t)}{100} = K_1 t. \tag{9.4.2}$$

On the other hand, for the zero-order reaction, we have

$$Y(t) - 100 = -K_0 t \tag{9.4.3}$$

or

$$1 - \frac{Y(t)}{100} = \frac{K_0}{100} t.$$

By comparing (9.4.2) and (9.4.3), it appears that the first-order reaction is similar to a zero-order reaction with a rate constant equal to that of the first-order reaction normalized by the initial strength at time zero. As a result, when the degradation is small, it is very difficult to differentiate these two orders.

As indicated earlier, model (9.3.17) is employed to describe the relationship between degradation and time. Suppose that there are r_{ij} replicates at time t_j and temperature T_i. Then the test statistic for lack of fit discussed in Sec. 2.6.1 can be directly applied to model (9.3.17). The sum of squares of pure error, denoted by SSPE(h), can be computed by (2.6.2). The sum of squares of lack of fit, denoted by SSLF(h), can then be obtained by subtracting the sum of squares of residuals from SSPE(h). The degrees of freedom for SSPE(h) and SSLF(h) are given by

$$\text{df}(\text{SSPE}(h)) = \sum_{i=1}^{I} \sum_{j=1}^{J} (r_{ij} - 1) = N - IJ,$$

$$\text{df}(\text{SSLF}(h)) = (N - I) - (N - IJ) = I(J - 1),$$

where

$$N = \sum_{i=1}^{I} \sum_{j=1}^{J} r_{ij}.$$

Similarly, the mean squares of pure error and lack of fit can be obtained by dividing the respective sums of squares by their corresponding degrees of freedom as follows:

$$\text{MSPE}(h) = \frac{\text{SSPE}(h)}{N - IJ},$$

$$\text{MSLF}(h) = \frac{\text{SSLF}(h)}{I(J - 1)}.$$

Table 9.4.1 provides the ANOVA table, which partitions the residual sum of squares into SSPE and SSLF. Model (9.3.17) is considered adequate for a description of the relationship between degradation and time if we fail to reject the null hypothesis of no lack of fit. The null hypothesis of no lack of fit is

TABLE 9.4.1 ANOVA Table for Lack of Fit for Model (9.3.17)

Source of variation	df	Sum of squares	MeanYd squares	F value
Regression	I	SSR(h)	MSR(h) = SSR(h)/I	$F = \dfrac{\text{MSR}(h)}{\text{MSE}(h)}$
Residual	$N - I$	SSE(h)	MSE(h) = SSE(h)/($N - I$)	
Lack of fit	$I(J - 1)$	SSLF(h)	MSLF(h) = SSLF(h)/[($J - 1$)]	$F_{LF} = \dfrac{\text{MSLF}(h)}{\text{MSPE}(h)}$
Pure error	$N - IJ$	SSPE(h)	MSPE(h) = SSPE(h)/($N - IJ$)	
Total	N	SST(h)		

rejected at the α level of significance if

$$F_{LF} = \frac{\text{MSLF}(h)}{\text{MSPE}(h)} > F(\alpha, I(J - 1), N - IJ), \tag{9.4.4}$$

where $F(\alpha, I(J - 1), N - IJ)$ is the αth upper quantile of a central F distribution with $I(J - 1)$ and $N - IJ$ degrees of freedom. If we fail to reject the null hypothesis of no lack of fit at the α level of significance, then $\hat{\sigma}^2(h)$ given in (9.3.20) provides an unbiased estimate for the error variance. However, if the null hypothesis of no lack of fit is rejected, model (9.3.17) is considered inadequate. In this case one needs to, at least, examine residual plots as described in Sec. 2.6.1 for possible outliers. Residual plots may also provide useful information for alternative models.

If model (9.3.17) is considered adequate for a linear relationship between degradation and time, the next step is to investigate whether the Arrhenius equation can provide a satisfactory description for the relationship between degradation and temperature. Note that there are I unknown parameters in model (9.3.17), while the Arrhenius equation (9.3.22) or (9.3.23) consists of only two unknown parameters. Therefore, if the Arrhenius equation is adequate, no statistically significant increase in sum of squares of residuals would occur. The sum of squares of residuals under the Arrhenius equation is given by

$$\text{SSE}_A(h) = \sum_{i=1}^{I} \sum_{j=1}^{J} [D_{ij}(h) - \hat{D}_{ij}(h)]^2, \tag{9.4.5}$$

where $\hat{D}_{ij}(h)$ is as given in (9.3.28).

Let $\text{SSE}_L(h)$ be the residual sum of squares obtained from model (9.3.17). The sum of squares due to the lack of fit under the Arrhenius equation is then given by

$$\text{SSLF}_A(h) = \text{SSE}_A(h) - \text{SSE}_L(h). \tag{9.4.6}$$

It follows that the null hypothesis of no lack of fit for the Arrhenius equation is rejected at the α level of significance if

$$F_A = \frac{\text{SSLF}_A(h)/(I - 2)}{\text{MSL}_L(h)} > F(\alpha, I - 2, I(J - 1)), \qquad (9.4.7)$$

where $\text{MSE}_L(h)$ is as defined in (9.3.20) and $F(\alpha, I - 2, I(J - 1))$ is the αth upper quantile of a central F distribution with $I - 2$ and $I(J - 1)$ degrees of freedom.

Finally, it is suggested that the residuals from fitting the Arrhenius equation be examined thoroughly for special patterns. When the null hypothesis of no lack of fit is rejected, it is useful to examine the nature of inadequacy and the departure from the Arrhenius equation by plotting the logarithm of the estimates of the rate constants obtained from model (9.3.17) versus the inverse of the absolute temperature.

9.5. EXAMPLE

In this section we use the data set adopted from Carstensen (1990) to illustrate statistical methods discussed in previous sections for determination of a tentative expiration dating period. This data set was obtained from an accelerated stability testing study which consists of three temperatures: 35, 45, and 55°C. Different time points were used for different temperatures: 0, 1, 2, and 3 months at 35°C; 0, 1, and 3 months at 45°C; and 0, 0.5, and 2 months at 55°C. All data except those at initial time points (which are 100%) are reproduced in Table 9.5.1 along with log(strength), $D_{ij}(0)$, $D_{ij}(1)$, $K_{ij}^*(0)$, and $K_{ij}^*(1)$. The scatter plot of assay results versus time by temperature is provided in Fig. 9.5.1 for the zero-order reaction. The scatter plot of logarithm of assay results versus time given in Fig.

TABLE 9.5.1 Strength of an Accelerated Stability Testing Study

Temperature (°C)	Time (months)	Strength (mg/mL)	ln(strength)	$D_{ij}(0)$	$D_{ij}(1)$	$K_{ij}^*(0)$	$K_{ij}^*(1)$
35	1	99.5	4.600	−0.5	−0.005	−0.693	−5.296
35	2	98.0	4.585	−2.0	−0.020	0.000	−4.595
35	3	97.0	4.575	−3.0	−0.031	0.000	−4.590
45	1	98.0	4.585	−2.0	−0.020	0.693	−3.902
45	3	95.2	4.556	−4.8	−0.049	0.470	−4.111
55	0.5	97.5	4.580	−2.5	−0.025	1.609	−2.983
55	1	95.1	4.555	−4.9	−0.050	1.589	−2.991
55	2	90.4	4.504	−9.6	−0.101	1.569	−2.987

Source: Carstensen (1990).

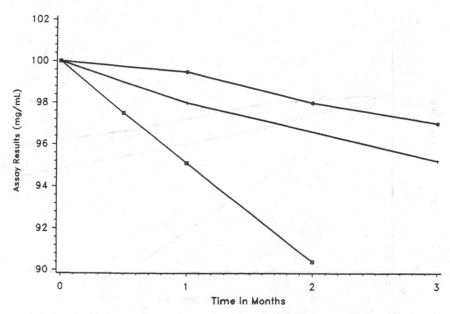

FIGURE 9.5.1 Assay results (mg/mL) versus time in months. Circle, 35°C; plus, 45°C; square, 55°C.

9.5.2 is used to examine a possible first-order reaction. Both plots reveal that a simple linear regression model can provide a better description of the relationship between strengths and time points at higher temperature than at lower temperature. This can be explained in part by the fact that at most 3% was decomposed for the first 3 months at 35°C.

Test results for estimation of the rate constants under model (9.3.17) for both orders are summarized in Table 9.5.2. Also included in the table are their standard errors, t statistics, and p values for the null hypothesis of a negative reaction rate. It can be seen from the table that all rate constants are negative and all p values are less than 0.0001. Hence the null hypothesis of (9.3.13) for each rate constant is rejected at the 5% level of significance. As a result, we conclude that all rate constants are statistically significantly smaller than 0. Table 9.5.3 also gives the ANOVA tables for both orders. Note that although both orders under model (9.3.17) yield a R^2 value greater than 99%, this does not guarantee that it gives a good fit. It can easily be verified that the studentized residual at time point 1 month and temperature 35°C exceeds 1.7 for both orders. Since no replicate tests were conducted at all combinations between time point and temperature, we are unable to perform a lack-of-fit test for this data set. However, to demonstrate the techniques, three strengths after 1 month at each

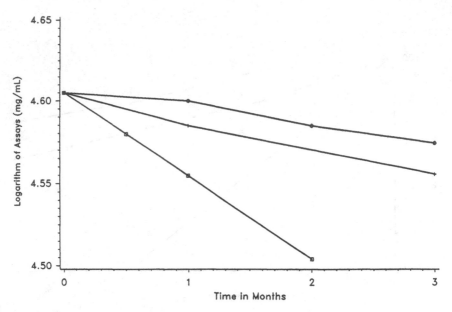

FIGURE 9.5.2 Logarithm of assay results (mg/mL) versus time in months. Circle, 35°C; plus, 45°C; square, 55°C.

TABLE 9.5.2 Results of Estimation of Rate Constants by Model (9.3.18)

Order of reaction	Temperature (°C)	Estimate	SE	T_b	p value
Zero	35	−0.9643	0.0748	−12.888	<0.0001
	45	−1.6400	0.0885	−18.525	<0.0001
	55	−4.8286	0.1222	−39.520	<0.0001
First	35	−0.0098	0.0007	−13.353	<0.0001
	45	−0.0168	0.0009	−19.378	<0.0001
	55	−0.0504	0.0012	−42.203	<0.0001

of three temperatures were added artificially to the data set. The values are 99.2, 97.8, and 96.1 for 35, 45, and 55°C, respectively. The ANOVA table for this modified data set of 1 data points under a zero-order reaction and model (9.3.17) is given in Table 9.5.4. The residual sum of squares is given by 1.426 with 8 degrees of freedom and the sum of squares for pure error is 0.565. Since there are only two replicates available at three combinations of time point and temperature, the degrees of freedom for the sum of squares of pure error is 3.

TABLE 9.5.3 ANOVA Table Under Model (9.3.17)

Order of reaction	Source of variation	df	Sum of squares	Mean squares	F value	p value	R^2
Zero	Regression	3	162.318	54.106	690.380	<0.0001	99.76%
	Residual	5	0.392	0.078			
	Total	8	162.710				
First	Regression	3	0.0175	0.0058	778.296	<0.0001	99.79%
	Residual	5	3.75×10^{-5}	7.496×10^{-6}			
	Total	8	0.0175				

TABLE 9.5.4   ANOVA Table for the Modified Data for Zero-Order Reaction Under Model (9.3.17)

Source of variation	df	Sum of squares	Mean squares	F value	p value
Regression	3	181.974	60.658	340.195[a]	<0.0001
Residual	8	1.426	0.178		
Lack of fit	5	0.861	0.172		
Pure error	3	0.565	0.188	0.914	0.433
Total	11	183.400			

[a]Use the sum of squares of residuals as the error term.

Therefore, the sum of squares for lack of fit is equal to 0.861 with 5 degrees of freedom. As a result, the F value for the lack-of-fit test is 0.914, with a p value of 0.433. Hence we conclude that there is no evidence of inadequacy for model (9.3.17) with respect to the modified data set.

The original data set is used to estimate the unknown parameters in the Arrhenius equation by a nonlinear regression technique. The estimates of $\alpha(h)$ and $\beta(h)$ obtained from simple linear regression model (9.3.24) can be used as initial values for nonlinear regression. These values are 29.57 and -9193.75 for the zero-order reaction and 25.30 and -9294.54 for the first-order reaction. Figures 9.5.3 and 9.5.4 display the fitted simple regression lines for the zero and first-order reactions, respectively. Estimates for $\alpha(h)$, $\beta(h)$, and their standard errors for model (9.3.34) are presented in Table 9.5.5. The resulting estimates, which were obtained by fewer than seven iterations, are quite close to those obtained from a simple linear regression. Readers should note that the correlation between the two estimates is close to 1.

Suppose that one wishes to establish a tentative expiration dating period at a marketing temperature 25°C such that the strength of the drug product is at least 90% of the label claim within the tentative expiration dating period. We may extrapolate temperature in the Arrhenius equation to a marketing temperature of 25°C with the estimates provided in Table 9.5.5. Table 9.5.6 provides 95% lower confidence limits for the time on the logarithmic scale, and hence the tentative expiration dating period at 25°C. Note that both orders produce a very similar tentative expiration dating period. Under the zero-order reaction, the tentative expiration dating period is 26.6 months, while it is 28.6 months for the first-order reaction. The adequacy of the Arrhenius equation can be examined by testing for lack of fit. The residuals from the Arrhenius equation are given in Table 9.5.7 for both orders of reaction. Table 9.5.8 provides the results for the tests of lack of fit. It can be seen from Table 9.5.8 that the p values of the tests for lack of fit are less than 0.05 for both orders. Hence at the 5% level

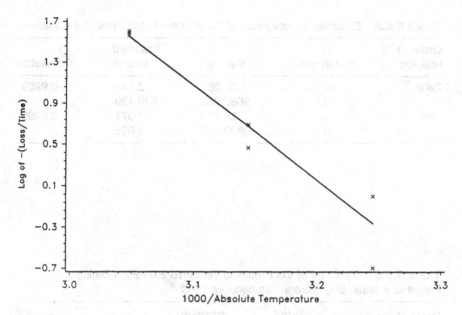

FIGURE 9.5.3 Regression of logarithm of minus loss divided by time versus temperature. Log of $-(loss/time) = log[-(y - 100)/time]$.

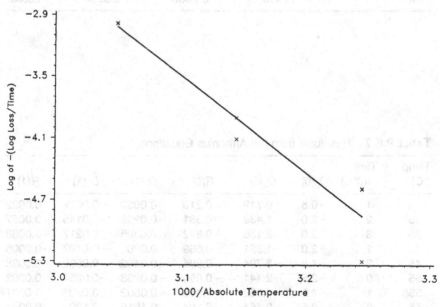

FIGURE 9.5.4 Regression of logarithm of minus log loss divided by time versus temperature. Log of $-(log \ loss/time) = log[-log(y/100)/time]$.

TABLE 9.5.5 Summary of Estimates of Parameters in the Arrhenius Equation

Order of reaction	Parameter	Estimate	Standard error	Correlation
Zero	α	31.091	2.140	−0.9999
	β	−9682.682	699.439	
First	α	26.883	2.071	−0.9999
	β	−9803.517	676.885	

TABLE 9.5.6 Summary of the Predicted Tentative Expiration Dating Period at a Marketing Storage Temperature 25°C

Order of reaction	$\ln(\hat{t})$	$SE((\ln(\hat{t}))$	L_t	$\exp(L_t)$
Zero	3.6856	0.2071	3.2832	26.66
First	3.7458	0.2008	3.3556	28.66

TABLE 9.5.7 Residuals from the Arrhenius Equation[a]

Temp. (°C)	Time (months)	$D_{ij}(0)$	$\hat{D}_{ij}(0)$	$R(0)$	$D_{ij}(1)$	$\hat{D}_{ij}(1)$	$R(1)$
35	1	−0.5	−0.719	0.219	−0.0050	−0.0072	0.0022
35	2	−2.0	−1.439	−0.561	−0.0202	−0.0145	−0.0057
35	3	−3.0	−2.158	−0.842	−0.0305	−0.0217	−0.0088
45	1	−2.0	−1.931	−0.069	−0.0202	−0.0197	−0.0005
45	3	−4.8	−5.794	0.994	−0.0492	−0.0590	0.0098
55	0.5	−2.5	−2.441	−0.059	−0.0253	−0.0251	0.0002
55	1	−4.9	−4.882	−0.018	−0.0502	−0.0503	0.0001
55	2	−9.6	−9.764	0.164	−0.1010	−0.1005	0.0004

[a] $R(0)$ and $R(1)$ are residuals for reaction of order 0 and 1, respectively.

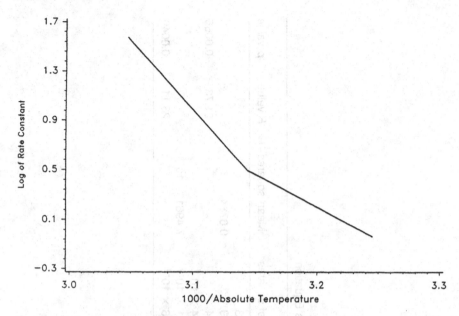

FIGURE 9.5.5 Regression of logarithm of zero-order rate constant by time versus temperature.

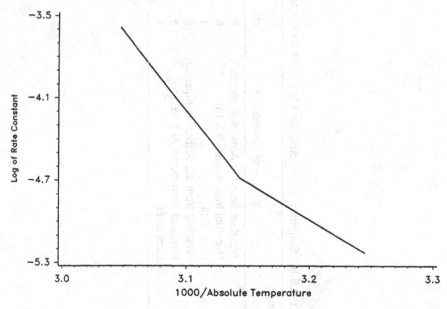

FIGURE 9.5.6 Regression of logarithm of first-order rate constant versus temperature.

TABLE 9.5.8 Summary of Residuals for Lack of Fit for the Arrhenius Equation

Order of reaction	Source of variation	df	Sum of squares	Mean squares	F value	p value
Zero	Residual from the Arrhenius equation	6	2.0953			
	Residual from model (9.3.18)	5	0.3919	0.0784		
	Lack of fit	1	1.7034		21.73	0.0055
First	Residual from the Arrhenius equation	6	2.1074×10^{-4}			
	Residual from model (9.3.18)	5	3.7481×10^{-5}	7.4961×10^{-6}		
	Lack of fit	1	1.7326×10^{-4}		23.11	0.0049

of significance, the null hypothesis of no lack of fit is rejected for both orders. As a result, for this data set, the Arrhenius equation is inadequate for describing the relationship between reaction rates and temperature. Failure of the Arrhenius equation for both orders becomes clear in Figs. 9.5.5 and 9.5.6 when the logarithm of rate constants is plotted against the inverse of the absolute temperature. Figures 9.5.5 and 9.5.6 indicate that the relationship between rate constant and inverse of the absolute temperature is not linear.

9.6. DISCUSSION

For the numerical example presented in Sec. 9.5, the null hypothesis of no lack of fit for the Arrhenius equation is rejected at the 5% level of significance for both reaction orders. One possible explanation for failure of the Arrhenius equation is that the study was not designed properly. This may be because no proper prior information regarding the rate of degradation was available for the selection of time points and temperature. For example, the maximum degradation in this data set is only 9.6% after a storage period of 2 months at 55°C. As indicated earlier, if the proportion of degradation is less than 15% of the initial strength, it is difficult to distinguish a zero-order reaction from a first-order reaction. Davies and Hudson (1981) presented an example which showed that the departure from linearity of strengths versus time for a zero-order reaction does not become apparent until the degradation exceeds at least 40%. Therefore, unless the strength has decreased by more than 40%, one is unable to distinguish the first order from the zero order; and consequently, is unable to describe adequately the relationship among degradation, time, and temperature.

As indicated earlier, the primary objective of an accelerated stability testing study is to provide an accurate and reliable estimate of the tentative expiration dating period. To achieve this objective it is important to select an efficient design that will provide the maximum information to an accelerated stability testing. Since the amount of information provided by a design is a function of the inverse of the variance, in practice it is recommended that the design generate an estimate of time on the logarithmic scale based on (9.3.30) with the smallest possible variance.

Relationships among the amount of degradation, temperature, and time stated in (9.2.15) and (9.2.16) imply that the difference between the degradation and time on the logarithmic scale is a linear function of the absolute temperature. Hence the time on the logarithmic scale can be viewed as the residual, on the logarithmic scale, between the prespecified maximum allowable degradation and that predicted by the Arrhenius equation. Consequently, the information from an accelerated stability testing study may be defined as the inverse of the variance for the estimate of the time on the logarithmic scale, which is a function of the variances of the estimates for the unknown parameters in the Arrhenius equation.

In general, the principles and sample-size determination for designing a calibration experiment presented in Chapter 2 can be applied separately to the selection of time points and temperatures in an accelerated stability testing study. For example, to examine the possible departure from linearity, at least three design points should be used for both time and temperature. The range of time and temperature should be chosen for maximum degradation to determine the correct order of reaction. On the other hand, since the technique for determination of the tentative expiration dating period is the extrapolation of temperature, it is preferable to select the lowest temperature in a stressed test: either lower than or as close to the marketing storage temperature as possible. As a rule of thumb, in the following we provide some recommendations for temperatures and time points in the design selection of an accelerated stability testing program:

1. Use at least three design points separately for time and temperature.
2. Select the highest temperature such that accurate discrimination of the degradation of a first-order reaction at this temperature from a zero-order reaction can be reached in a short period of time, say within 3 months.
3. Select the lowest temperature possible close to the marketing storage temperature, which will be used in long-term stability studies under ambient conditions.
4. The lowest and highest temperatures should be selected as far apart as scientifically and physically possible. This defines the range of temperatures.
5. The lower limit for time points is the initial point, at zero. The upper limit of the range for time points is suggested as the time point at which the amount of degradation for an adequate determination of reaction rates can be reached at the highest temperature selected in item 2.
6. Select at least one more data point within the range of temperatures and time points such that at least three data points are available for an investigation of a departure from linearity with respect to both time and temperature. Techniques such as factorial or fractional designs and designs for a response surface (e.g., central composite design, discussed in Chapter 4) can also be applied here provided that the time and temperature ranges have been determined.
7. Replicates should be obtained at various combinations to test lack of fit. The number of replicates can be determined based on $\beta(h)$ in (9.3.24) using the method described in Sec. 2.6.2.

Equation (9.2.15) and (9.2.16) is a combination of linear and nonlinear functions. For example, degradation relates to time points in a linear fashion

TABLE 9.6.1   Means and Variances of Logarithmic Strengths by Temperature

Temperature (°C)	Mean	Variance
35	4.5866	0.00016
45	4.5705	0.00042
55	4.5463	0.01485

but depends on temperature in a nonlinear fashion. The recommendations discussed above fall under the assumption that the relationship between degradation and temperature is also linear. As a result, the recommendations above will not actually provide optimal designs. However, if one only considers the nonlinear relationship between reaction rate and temperature in (9.3.34), the method for construction of a design for nonlinear regression proposed by Box and Lucas (1959) might be useful. Let I be the number of temperatures employed in an accelerated stability testing study. Define a matrix Z of order $I \times 2$ as

$$Z = (Z_\alpha, Z_\beta),$$

where

$$Z_\alpha = (Z_{\alpha 1}, \ldots, Z_{\alpha I})',$$
$$Z_\beta = (Z_{\beta 1}, \ldots, Z_{\beta I})',$$

and $Z_{\alpha i}$ and $Z_{\beta i}$ are as defined in (9.3.36). Box and Lucas (1959) suggested selecting temperatures that maximize the determinant of matrix $Z'Z$. When $I = 2$ it can be shown that the temperatures that maximize $|Z'Z|$ are lower and upper limits of the temperature range. However, more research is needed for the selection of optimal designs that can accommodate both linear and nonlinear parts of (9.2.15) and (9.2.16).

The means and variances of the logarithm of strengths for the data set given in Table 9.5.1 are presented in Table 9.6.1 by temperature. Table 9.6.1 reveals that the variance of the logarithm of strengths increases as the temperature increases. This indicates that the assumption of a constant error variance might be violated. In addition, it can be seen from Table 9.5.5 that the correlation between the estimates of the two unknown parameters in the Arrhenius equation is close to -1. Therefore, the nonlinear technique may not converge to obtain estimates due to the almost perfect correlation. To alleviate these problems, Davies and Hudson (1981) suggested that the strengths be weighted by the inverse of sample variance at each temperature. In addition, the inverse of the absolute temperature in (9.3.22) and (9.3.23) needs to be centralized to avoid high correlation. For more details, see Davies and Hudson (1981).

10

Design for Long-Term Stability Studies

10.1. INTRODUCTION

In the pharmaceutical industry, stability programs are usually applied at various stages of drug development. For example, at the early stage of drug development, a stability program is necessarily carried out to study the stability of bulk drug substances. The purpose is to evaluate excipient compatibility under various storage factors, such as heat, humidity, light, and container. At a later stage, it is also required to conduct a stability program for the formulations used in preclinical and/or clinical studies to make sure that the drug product is within USP/NF specifications during the entire study. For the proposed market formulation, a stability program is required to establish an expiration dating period applicable to all future batches of the drug product. For the production batches, it is a common practice to have a stability monitoring program in place to assure that all drug characteristics remain within USP/NF specifications prior to the established expiration date. The success of a stability program requires an approved stability study protocol in which reasons for choosing an appropriate stability design should be described in detail.

The FDA guideline indicates that a stability study protocol must describe (1) how the stability study is to be designed and carried out, and (2) statistical methods to be used in analyzing the data. The design of a stability study is intended to establish an expiration dating period, which is based on testing a limited number of batches of a drug product, applicable to all future batches of the drug product manufactured under similar circumstances. Therefore, the study design should be chosen so that it can reduce bias and identify and control any expected and/or unexpected sources of variations. The goal for selection of an appropriate stability design is to improve the accuracy and precision of the established shelf life. On the other hand, statistical methods used for analysis of the data collected should reflect the nature of the design to provide a valid statistical inference for the established shelf life. In this chapter we focus on designs for long-term stability studies. Statistical methods for the analysis of stability data are provided in Chapters 11 and 12.

For estimation of drug shelf life, an ideal design is a design that can provide an unbiased estimate with the minimum variance. In practice, a stability study usually involves three batches, which may be stored under different storage conditions, of different strengths, which may be packed in different packaging types, such as bottle, blister, and tube. The terms *batch, strength, package*, and *storage condition* are usually referred to as *design factors*. In the interest of establishing an expiration dating period for a drug product across all design factors, It is important to select a design that can avoid possible confounding and interaction effects among design factors. The effects due to the confounding and interaction among design factors may have an impact on the variability used for statistical inference of the true shelf life. In addition, to ensure that there is a valid statistical inference for the true shelf life based on testing a small number of batches, tested batches must be representative in all respects, including the manufacturing process and age of bulk material of the population of all production batches. Thest test batches must be representative of the drug product and conform to all USP/NF specifications. Therefore, it is suggested that a stability design, which can account for variabilities from various sources, such as individual dosage units, containers within a batch, and batches, be chosen. Since the degree of variability affects the confidence that one might have in the ability of a future batch to remain within USP/NF specifications until its expiration date, it is important to ensure that the resulting data for each batch be truly representative of the batch as a whole and to quantify the variability from batch to batch.

The remainder of this chapter is organized as follows. In the next section we provide some basic design considerations for planning a stability design. In Sec. 10.3 we introduce various stability designs, including factorial, matrixing, and bracketing designs. Also included in this section are some useful commonly used NDA stability designs proposed by Nordbrock (1992). These designs are classified into three categories, depending on whether stability tests are done at every sampling time point or at partial points. Some criteria for design selection are given in Sec. 10.5.

10.2. BASIC DESIGN CONSIDERATIONS

10.2.1. Background Information

In stability study design, background information is obtained to ensure the success of the study. In practice, it is helpful to have some knowledge regarding marketing requirements, manufacturing practice, previous formulation study results, and the variability of the assay method. For marketing requirements, the following questions may affect the direction of a stability study:

1. What package types will be used for the drug product?
2. What are the USP/NF specifications for the drug product?
3. What is the desired shelf life?
4. When will the stability data be filed with the FDA?
5. Where is the drug product to be marketed?

In practice, it is recognized that degradation of a drug product may differ from one package type to another. The specifications for the characteristics of the drug product can usually be found in the USP/NF. The information regarding which package type is to be used for the drug product is useful in determining whether the desired shelf life can be achieved. Moreover, if a pharmaceutical company wishes to file a submission in a short period of time, a short-term stability study such as accelerated testing may be desirable to establish a tentative shelf life. Therefore, knowledge of the lead time prior to FDA submission is critical in planning an appropriate stability study. Finally, different regulatory agencies in different countries (e.g., EC and Japan) may have different requirements on stability. Information on where the drug product is to be marketed is useful in devising strategy at an early stage of planning a stability study.

In addition, knowledge of manufacturing practices is usually helpful in the design of a stability study. For example, answers to the following questions provide crucial information for the selection of an appropriate stability design.

1. How many strengths of the same formulation will be manufactured?
2. Will multiple strengths be made out of a common granulation batch?
3. Will a common encapsulation batch be made into multiple package types?

An adequate stability study should be designed to evaluate the stability of the drug product across batch, strength, and package type.

Other information, such as previous formulation study results and the variability of the assay method, are also helpful in the design of a stability study. Previous formulation study results may provide important information about factors that might affect the stability of drug products of this kind under certain storage conditions. The variability of an assay method, such as that between and within run CVs are useful for sample-size determination, which assures the establishment of a reliable drug shelf life.

10.2.2. FDA Considerations

When conducting a stability study, the FDA requires that pharmaceutical companies describe how the stability study is to be designed and carried out. An appropriate stability design can help to achieve the objective of a stability study. FDA guideline provides design considerations for long-term stability studies under ambient conditions. These design considerations include:

1. Batch sampling considerations
2. Container-closure and drug product sampling
3. Sampling-time considerations

It can be seen that these design considerations focus primarily on how data are to be collected. The purpose of these considerations is to ensure that the data be representative of the population of all future production batches.

For batch sampling considerations, the FDA guidelines recommend that at least three batches, and preferably more, be tested to allow for batch-to-batch variability and to test the hypothesis that a single expiration dating period for all batches is justifiable. For a consideration of container-closure and drug product sampling, the FDA emphasizes that the selection of containers from the batches chosen for inclusion in the study should be carried out so as to ensure that the samples chosen represent the batch as a whole. For sampling time, the FDA guideline suggests that stability testing be done at 3-month intervals during the first year, 6-month intervals during the second year, and annually thereafter. For drug products predicted to degrade rapidly, more frequent sampling is necessary.

Note that in Chapter 9 we provided some statistical considerations regarding the design and analysis of stability studies which are related to the design considerations above. In addition, specific considerations when planning a design for a stability study are given below.

10.2.3. Design Factors

In practice, several strengths of a drug product may be developed to fulfill different medical needs. The various strengths may be packed in different containers (package types). In such a case, stability designs for long-term stability studies will typically involve the following design factors: batch, strength, package type, and storage condition. Suppose it is recommended that the drug product be stored at room temperature. Pharmaceutical companies usually find it necessary to investigate the effect of strength, package, and batch on the stability of the drug product at room temperature. In other words, it is of interest to examine the following scientific questions (Nordbrock, 1992).

1. Do all package-by-strength combinations have the same stability at room temperature?
2. Do all packages have the same stability at room temperature?
3. Do all batches have the same stability at room temperature?
4. Do all strengths have the same stability at room temperature?

5. Do all storage conditions have the same stability for all packages?
6. Do all storage conditions have the same stability for all batches?
7. Do all storage conditions have the same stability for all strengths?

An appropriate stability design can provide useful information to address these scientific questions. For example, questions 1 to 4 can be examined by testing the following hypotheses at room temperature.

1. Degradation rates among packages are consistent across strengths.
2. Degradation rates are the same for all packages.
3. Degradation rates are the same for all strengths.
4. Degradation rates are the same for all batches.

If we fail to reject the hypotheses above, stability data may be pooled to establish a single shelf life that can reflect the expiration period for all batches manufactured under similar circumstances. The establishment of a single shelf life applicable to all future batches is the primary objective of a stability study. On the other hand, if hypothesis 1 is rejected, the differences in degradation rate between package types are not consistent across strengths. In this case there is a significant interaction between package type and strength. Thus the data cannot be pooled and shelf lives for each combination of package types and strengths should be established. In addition to interaction, as indicated in Chapter 4, an appropriate design should be able to separate any possible confounding effects.

10.2.4. Sample Size

Suppose that the desired shelf life of a drug product is 4 years. Then it is easy to determine the number of stability tests for a given combination of design factors according to the FDA suggestions for sampling intervals. In practice, however, it may be too costly and/or time consuming to perform stability tests at every time point for each combination of design factors. Therefore, pharmaceutical companies often have an interest in reducing the total number of stability tests by either reducing the combinations of design factors or performing stability tests at the selected time points. This is often done provided that the reduction of stability tests can reach an acceptable degree of precision for the established shelf life without losing much information.

Basically, before the sample can be chosen in an appropriate stability design, the following issues should be addressed.

1. How many observations are to be taken?
2. How large a difference in degradation rate is to be detected between design factors?
3. How much variation is present?

For the first issue, if stability tests are to be performed at every sampling interval, the total number of assays can be determined. In some cases, as indicated earlier, the pharmaceutical companies may not be able to perform stability tests at every time point, due to limited resources available. Instead, stability tests may be done at selected time points. Suppose that a pharmaceutical company is able to handle N assays according to its capacity. These N assays may not be large enough to cover every time point but to cover some selected time points or a few time points twice. In other words, we may test the stability at some time points once or have replicates at a few time points. In this case it is important to determine how many observations are to be taken at each time point, which can certainly have an impact on the estimated shelf life.

When there are a number of design factors in a stability study, it is often of interest to investigate the impact of these design factors on stability. For example, it is of interest to determine whether degradation rates are the same for all packages. To address this question, the sample size should be chosen so that there is sufficient statistical power for detection of a meaningful difference in stability loss between packages. Therefore, it is important to determine how large a difference in degradation rate detected between packages is meaningful. The sample size selected should have sufficient power for detection of meaningful difference in degradation rate among design factors under study.

Finally, since sample-size determination and justification are usually based on a prestudy power analysis which is very sensitive to the variability, it is important to have some prior knowledge regarding the variation. The variation may include variabilities from different sources, such as location, analyst, and manufacturing process. For example, with large containers, dosage units near the cap of a bottle may have different stability properties from dosage units in other parts of the container. Thus it may be desirable to sample dosage units from all parts of the container. In this case the location within the container from which they are drawn should be identified and taken into consideration for sample-size justification.

10.2.5. Statistical Analysis

For a given stability design, statistical methods used for data analysis should reflect the design to provide a valid statistical inference for the established shelf life. As an example, if the hypotheses listed in Sec. 10.2.1 are of particular interest, we may test these hypotheses based on a linear model using PROC GLM in SAS. Let Y be the potency (expressed as percent of claim) and A be the time (in months), which is a continuous covariate. Also, let B, S, and P denote the batch, strength, and package, respectively. Note that B, S, and P are class variables. Then the PROC GLM models are as follows:

Model 1: $Y = B\ S\ B*S\ A\ A*B\ A*S\ A*P\ A*P*S$;
Model 2: $Y = B\ S\ B*S\ A\ A*B\ A*S\ A*P$.

Note that the term P is not included in the models above because there is no reason to believe that the initial potency will be different for different package types. Each model has separate intercepts for each batch-by-strength combination. Model 1 has separate slopes for each package-by-strength combination and has separate slopes for each batch. Model 2 has separate slopes for each batch, for each strength, and for each package. Model 1 is used to test the $A*P*S$ term and associated contrasts and thus to address the first hypothesis listed in Sec. 10.2.2. If the $A*P*S$ term and associated contrasts are not significant, model 2 is used for further analysis (i.e., to test hypotheses 2 to 4).

In the models above, we assume that the term B is a fixed class variable. However, Chow and Shao (1991) indicated that the term B should be considered as a random variable in order to establish an expiration dating period that can reflect the shelf life for all future batches. In the next two chapters, statistical methods for estimation of drug shelf life are discussed under the assumptions that (1) the term *batch* is a fixed effect (Chapter 11) and that (2) the term *batch* is a random effect (Chapter 12).

10.2.6. Other Issues

The FDA guideline indicates that an appropriate stability design should take into consideration the variability of individual dosage units, of containers within a batch, and of batches, to ensure that the resulting data for each batch are truly representative of the batch as a whole and to quantify the variability from batch to batch. We should be aware that other sources of variation may also affect the efficiency of the stability design selected. These sources of variation may include variabilities from different assay methods, different analysts, different laboratories, and different locations or sites. In addition, expected and/or unexpected variabilities that may occur during each stage of the manufacturing process can also have an impact on the stability design selected. An appropriate stability design should be able to avoid bias and achieve the minimum variability.

10.3. DESIGNS FOR STABILITY STUDIES

In this section we introduce some stability designs that are commonly used when conducting stability studies. These designs include complete (or full) factorial design, fractional factorial design, matrixing design, and bracketing design. To illustrate these designs, consider the following example.

Suppose that a newly developed pharmaceutical compound is to be manufactured in the dosage form of tablets with three different strengths: 15 mg, 30 mg, and 60 mg. To fulfill the needs from various markets, it is suggested that three different packaging types be taken into consideration: glass bottle, PVC blister, and PE tubes. In addition, to study the impact of heat and moisture on the product over the desired expiration dating period (say, 60 months), we have to store three different batches of the finished product under different conditions simulating the adverse effects of storage under the conditions to which the product might be subjected during distribution, shipping, handling, and dispensing. The storage conditions of interest are listed below.

1. 21°C and 45% relative humidity
2. 25°C and 60% relative humidity
3. 30°C and 35% relative humidity
4. 30°C and 70% relative humidity

In other words, we store three batches of three different strengths kept in three types of packages under four different conditions.

In this section we assume that the degradation curve is linear. If there is an exponential decay, it may be linearized by transformation. The drug characteristic of interest is the potency (percent of label claim). For stability testing, the FDA guideline also recommends that the drug product be tested at 3-month intervals during the first year, 6-month intervals during the second year, and annually thereafter. In other words, it is recommended that stability testing be done at the following times if we only consider stability testing up to 4 years:

$$T_1 = \{0, 3, 6, 9, 12, 18, 24, 36, 48\}.$$

In the interest of balance, we assume that sampling times are fixed across all factors.

10.3.1. Factorial Design

Suppose that we are interested in conducting a stability study under ambient conditions (e.g., 60% relative humidity and 25°C room temperature). A full factorial design consists of $3^3 = 27$ combinations (see Table 10.3.1). If each combination is to be tested at T_1 time points, there are a total of

$$N = 3 \times 3 \times 3 \times 10 = 270$$

assays.

In practice, if every batch by strength-by-package combination is tested (i.e., a complete factorial design is used), a substantial expense is involved. Besides, it is in the best interest of the pharmaceutical companies that a longer shelf life can be claimed by testing fewer batches as to strength-by-package combinations within a short period of time. Therefore, for considerations of time and cost, a fractional factorial design is often used to reduce the total number of tests (or assays).

Although a fractional factorial design is preferred in the interest of reducing the number of tests (i.e., cost), it has the following disadvantages:

TABLE 10.3.1 3^3 Complete Factorial Design

Combination	Batch	Strength	Package
1	1	15	Bottle
2	1	15	Blister
3	1	15	Tube
4	1	30	Bottle
5	1	30	Blister
6	1	30	Tube
7	1	60	Bottle
8	1	60	Blister
9	1	60	Tube
10	2	15	Bottle
11	2	15	Blister
12	2	15	Tube
13	2	30	Bottle
14	2	30	Blister
15	2	30	Tube
16	2	60	Bottle
17	2	60	Blister
18	2	60	Tube
19	3	15	Bottle
20	3	15	Blister
21	3	15	Tube
22	3	30	Bottle
23	3	30	Blister
24	3	30	Tube
25	3	60	Bottle
26	3	60	Blister
27	3	60	Tube

1. If there are interactions such as a strength-by-package interaction, the data cannot be pooled to establish a single shelf life. In this case it is recommended that individual shelf lives be established for each combination of strength and package. However, we may not have three batches for each combination of strength and package for a fractional factorial design.
2. We may not have sufficient precision for the estimated drug shelf life.

10.3.2. Matrixing and Bracketing Designs

Generally, a reduction of stability tests could be achieved if we applied a different method, such as bracketing and matrixing, which are also special cases of fractional factorial designs. There is no universal definition for a matrixing design. For example, the ICH (1993) defines a matrixing design as a statistical design of a stability schedule so that only a fraction of the total number of samples are tested at any specified sampling point. At a subsequent sampling point, different sets of samples of the total number would be tested. The underlying assumption is that the stability of the samples tested represents the stability of all samples. The ICH indicates that matrixing can cover reduced testing when more than one design factor is being evaluated. As a result, the design of the matrix will be dictated by the factors needing to be covered and evaluated. For a matrixing design, the ICH suggests that in every case all batches be tested initially and at the end of long-term testing. The definition of ICH, however, may not best reflect matrixing. As an alternative, Chow (1992) gave a definition of a matrixing design. He suggested that any subset of a complete factorial design be considered as matrixing design. For example, in Table 10.2.1, if we only consider two packages per strength and batch or two strengths per package and batch, these two types of designs are considered matrixing designs.

Helboe (1992) discussed some examples of applications of matrixing designs for long-term stability studies. For example, he considered an example concerning a drug product that was manufactured at three dosage strengths from three different batches of granulation. The same granulations *A*, *B*, and *C*, were used in all three dosage strengths. Three types of containers, one blister pack and two sizes of high-density polyethylene (HDPE) bottle, were considered. As a result, the stability study involves three design factors, with three levels in each. In this case, if a full factorial design is adopted, a total of 27 combinations need to be tested at each sampling time point. Instead, one may consider a matrixing design to reduce the total number of tests. Table 10.3.2 presents a *two-thirds matrixing design*. Helboe (1992) indicated that this design was actually implemented at one major pharmaceutical company in the United States. In Table 10.3.2, at each time point, the combinations in parentheses were not

TABLE 10.3.2 Two-Thirds Matrixing Design

Package type	Dosage strength/lot of granulation[a]								
	50 mg			75 mg			100 mg		
	A	*B*	*C*	*A*	*B*	*C*	*A*	*B*	*C*
Blister	+	+	(+)	(+)	+	+	+	(+)	+
HDPE1	(+)	+	+	+	(+)	+	+	+	(+)
HDPE2	+	(+)	+	+	+	(+)	(+)	+	+

Source: Helboe (1992).
[a](+), not tested at this time point.

tested. It can be seen from Table 10.3.2 that only two-thirds of 27 combinations of the full factorial design were tested. At each sampling time point, each container, dosage strength, and granulation was tested six times. Helboe (1992) referred to a design of this kind as a two-thirds matrixing design.

Another design of particular interest is *bracketing design.* The ICH defines a bracketing design as the design of a stability schedule such that at any time point only the samples on the extremes of container size and/or dosage strengths, for example, are tested. The design assumes that the stability of the intermediate condition samples are represented by those at the extremes. Where there are several strengths to be tested, bracketing designs may be applicable if the strengths are very closely related in composition: for example, for the range of tablets made with different compression weights of a similar basic granulation, or the range of capsules made by filling different plug fill weights of the same basic composition into different-size capsule shells. In this case it is believed that testing the highest and lowest strengths will provide sufficient stability information for the drug product. Therefore, there is no need to test the middle strengths. The samples for the middle strengths, which are bracketed, are kept as backup in case there is a significant difference in stability loss between the highest and lowest strengths. The same idea can be applied to packaging. We may only test for the largest and smallest package sizes and leave the middle-size samples as backup. When we have a stable active ingredient in the form of tablets, if we take the example given at the beginning of Sec. 10.3, we would test samples kept at 25°C/60% relative humidity and 30°C/70% relative humidity over the expiration dating period. The other samples, which are bracketed, are kept as a backup in case one condition is found to be too severe. The details of this bracketing design are given in Table 10.3.3. For strength, we may only test the lowest and highest strengths (i.e., 15 mg and 60 mg) and bracket the 30-mg tablets. As a result, the design achieves a 50% reduction in total tests. It

TABLE 10.3.3   Example of Bracketing Design

Storage condition		Testing interval[a] (months)							
Temp. (°C)	Relative humidity (%)	3	6	9	12	18	24	36	48
21	45	(+)	(+)	(+)	(+)	(+)	(+)	(+)	(+)
25	60	+	+	+	+	+	+	+	+
30	35	(+)	(+)	(+)	(+)	(+)	(+)	(+)	(+)
30	70	+	+	+	+	+	+	+	+

[a]The parentheses indicate that the corresponding stability tests are omitted.

should be noted that this design cannot provide stability information for 75-mg strength and for HDPE/100.

Note that the bracketing design given in Table 10.3.3 does not use the lower extremes of temperature 21°C and relative humidity 35% to bracket temperature and relative humidity factors. Hence, strictly speaking, it is not a bracketing design with respect to temperature and relative humidity. To provide a better understanding of bracketing design, consider the example given in Helboe (1992). This stability study considers three strengths; three batches of granulations, with each granulation used in all three strengths; and one size of blister pack and three sizes of HDPE bottles. If this study is bracketed on strength and bottle size, the resulting bracketing design is as given in Table 10.3.4. Helboe (1992) pointed out that the fundamental assumption for the validity of a bracketing design is that the stability of multiple levels for a design factor can be determined by the stability of the extremes. According to Chow's definition, a bracketing design is in fact a special case of matrixing designs.

10.3.3. Classification of Designs

Earlier, stability tests have been assumed to be done at every time point suggested by the FDA: that is,

$$T_1 = \{0, 3, 6, 9, 12, 18, 24, 36, 48\}.$$

The total number of stability tests can be further reduced if stability tests are done only at certain time points (e.g., a subset of T_1). For the selection of a subset of T_1, Nordbrock (1992) consider the following subsets:

$$
\begin{aligned}
T_2 &= \{0, \quad 3, \qquad\quad 9, \qquad\quad 18, \qquad\quad 36, \quad 48\}, \\
T_3 &= \{0, \qquad 6, \qquad 12, \qquad\quad 24, \qquad\qquad\quad 48\}, \\
T_5 &= \{0, \quad 3, \qquad\quad 12, \qquad\qquad\qquad 36, \quad 48\}, \\
T_6 &= \{0, \qquad 6, \qquad\qquad 18, \qquad\qquad\qquad\quad 48\}, \\
T_7 &= \{0, \qquad\qquad 9, \qquad\qquad\quad 24, \qquad\qquad 48\}, \\
T_8 &= \{0, \quad 3, \qquad\quad 9, \quad 12, \qquad 24, \quad 36, \quad 48\}, \\
T_9 &= \{0, \quad 3, \quad 6, \qquad 12, \quad 18, \qquad\quad 36, \quad 48\}, \\
T_A &= \{0, \qquad 6, \quad 9, \qquad\quad 18, \quad 24, \qquad\qquad 48\}.
\end{aligned}
$$

In practice, the subsets above can be divided into three groups: (1) T_2 and T_3; (2) T_5, T_6, and T_7; and (3) T_8, T_9, and T_A. For a given stability design, if the first group of subsets is applied, half of the stability tests will be done at 3, 9, 18, 36, and 48 months, and the other half will be done at 6, 12, 24, and 48 months. It can be seen that half of the stability tests will be done at each time point except at 48 months. A design of this type is usually referred to as a ⟨one-half design⟩. For example, if the first group of subsets is applied to a complete factorial design, we will refer to the design as a complete-$\frac{1}{2}$ design. Similarly,

TABLE 10.3.4 Example of Bracketing Design

| Package type | Dosage strength/raw material lot[a] | | | | | | | | |
| | 50 mg | | | 75 mg | | | 100 mg | | |
	A	B	C	A	B	C	A	B	C
Blister	+	+	+	(+)	(+)	(+)	+	+	+
HDPE/15	+	+	+	(+)	(+)	(+)	+	+	+
HDPE/100	(+)	(+)	(+)	(+)	(+)	(+)	(+)	(+)	(+)
HDPE/500	+	+	+	(+)	(+)	(+)	+	+	+

Source: Helboe (1992).
[a] (+), not tested at this time point.

for a given design, if the second group of subsets (i.e., $\{T_5, T_6, T_7\}$), is applied, one-third of stability tests will be done at 3, 12, 36, and 48 months; one-third will be tested at 6, 18, and 48 months; and one-third will be tested at 9, 24, and 48 months. The design then becomes a ⟨*one-third design*⟩. For the third group of subsets (i.e., $\{T_8, T_9, T_A\}$) the resulting design is a ⟨*two-thirds design*⟩ because each group consists of two-thirds of the total time points.

Note that the idea for applying the three groups of subsets above to a design is to reduce the total number of stability tests by $\frac{1}{2}, \frac{1}{3}, \frac{2}{3}$, respectively, at each time point except the last. In such a case, the test results obtained at each time point are balanced.

In practice, it may be too closely and/or time consuming to conduct a complete factorial design by testing every time point. Consequently, it may not be practical for pharmaceutical companies to conduct such a study. As an alternative, the companies are interested in a reduced stability design. A reduced stability design is a stability design that tests only a reduced number of combinations of factors of interest, such as strength, package type, and batch, at either all or a reduced number of sampling time points. Basically, reduced stability designs can be classified into the following categories:

Design	Factors	Sampling times
Type I	Complete	Partial
Type II	Matrixing	All
Type III	Matrixing	Partial

Note that a reduced stability design should be used only when it can achieve a similar degree of precision for the estimation of drug shelf life. If a reduced stability design were to lose a lot of information and/or the degree of accuracy and precision of the estimated shelf life, the relative benefit and risk should be evaluated carefully.

10.3.4. Examples

Based on appropriate choice of a subset of T_1, Nordbrock (1992) provided some useful reduced stability designs for long-term stability studies at room temperature. These designs are summarized below.

Design 1: Complete. Every batch-by-strength-by-package combination is chosen. All combinations chosen are tested at every time point.

Design 2: Complete-$\frac{2}{3}$ (type I design). Every batch-by-strength-by-package combination is chosen. Two-thirds of the combinations chosen are tested at each time point. One-third of the combinations chosen are tested at 3, 9, 12, 24, 36, and 48 months; one-third are tested at 3, 6, 12, 18, 36, 48 months; and one-third are tested at 6, 9, 18, 24, and 48 months.

Design 3: Complete-$\frac{1}{2}$ (type I design). Every batch-by-strength-by-package combination is chosen. Half the combinations chosen are tested at 3, 9, 18, 36 and 48 months, and the other half are tested at 6, 12, 24, and 48 months.

Design 4: Complete-$\frac{1}{3}$ (type I design). Every batch-by-strength-by-package combination is chosen. One-third of the combinations chosen are tested at 3, 12, 24, and 48 months; one-third are tested at 6, 18, 36, and 48 months; and one-third are tested at 9, 24, and 48 months.

Design 5: Fractional (type II design). Two-thirds of the batch-by-strength-by-package combinations are chosen. All combinations chosen are tested at every time point.

Design 6: Two strengths per batch (type II design). Two strengths per batch are selected, and then all packages for this selection are chosen. All combinations chosen are tested at every time point.

Design 7: Two packages per strength (type II design). Two packages per strength are selected, and then all batches for this selection are chosen. All combinations chosen are tested at every time point.

Design 8: Fractional-$\frac{1}{2}$ (type III design). Two-thirds of the batch-by-strength-by-package combinations are chosen. Half the chosen combinations are tested at 3, 9, 18, 36, and 48 months, and the other half are tested at 6, 12, 24, and 48 months.

Design 9: Two strengths per batch-$\frac{1}{2}$ (type III design). Two strength per lot are selected, and then all packages for this selection are chosen. Half the combinations chosen are tested at 3, 9, 18, 36, and 48 months, and the other half are tested at 6, 12, 24, and 48 months.

Design 10: Two packages per strength-$\frac{1}{2}$ (type III design). Two packages per strength are selected, and then all batches for this selection are chosen. Half the combinations chosen are tested at 3, 9, 18, 36, and 48 months, and the other half are tested at 6, 12, 24, and 48 months.

Details of the designs above are given in Table 10.3.5. For each reduced stability design, the total number of stability tests required and the relative percentage of reducing stability tests as compared to the full design (i.e., the complete factorial design, including every time point) are summarized in Table 10.3.6. It can be seen from the table that type III designs may reduce the total number of stability tests as much as 59.3%.

Note that sample sizes in terms of the number of assays for designs 2, 5, 6, and 7 are all the same except at 48 months, and sample sizes for designs 4, 8, 9, and 10 are all the same except at 48 months. The reduced stability designs described above can easily be modified if the four storage conditions stated at the beginning of Sec. 10.3 are to be incorporated.

10.4. DESIGN SELECTION

Nordbrock (1992) proposed a criterion for design selection based on the power of detection of a significant difference between slopes (stability losses). For a fixed sample size, the design with the highest power of detection of a significant difference between slopes is the best design. On the other hand, for a fixed desired power, the design with the smallest sample size is the best design. Consider the following model for a single batch:

$$Y_i = \alpha + \beta X_i + e_i \qquad i = 1, \ldots, n, \tag{10.4.1}$$

where Y_i is the assay result at time X_i. Then the power for detection of a significant degradation (say, $\beta = \Delta$) for the null hypothesis of $\beta = 0$ is given by

$$\text{power} = P\left\{ |\hat{\beta}| > z(1 - \alpha/2) \frac{\sigma}{\sqrt{S_{XX}}} \mid \beta = \Delta \right\}, \tag{10.4.2}$$

where $\hat{\beta}$ is the least-squares estimator of β, which follows a normal distribution with mean β and variance:

$$\frac{\sigma^2}{S_{XX}},$$

where

$$S_{XX} = \sum_{i=1}^{n} (X_i - \overline{X})^2.$$

TABLE 10.3.5   NDA Stability Designs

Batch	Strength	Bottle	Blister	Tube	Bottle	Blister	Tube
		Design 1: Complete factorial design			Design 2: Complete-$\frac{2}{3}$ design		
1	15	T_1	T_1	T_1	T_8	T_9	T_A
	30	T_1	T_1	T_1	T_9	T_A	T_8
	60	T_1	T_1	T_1	T_A	T_8	T_9
2	15	T_1	T_1	T_1	T_A	T_8	T_9
	30	T_1	T_1	T_1	T_8	T_9	T_A
	60	T_1	T_1	T_1	T_9	T_A	T_8
3	15	T_1	T_1	T_1	T_9	T_A	T_8
	30	T_1	T_1	T_1	T_A	T_8	T_9
	60	T_1	T_1	T_1	T_8	T_9	T_A
		Design 3: Complete-$\frac{1}{2}$ design			Design 4: Complete-$\frac{1}{3}$ design		
1	15	T_2	T_3	T_2	T_5	T_6	T_7
	30	T_3	T_3	T_2	T_6	T_7	T_5
	60	T_3	T_2	T_3	T_7	T_5	T_6
2	15	T_2	T_2	T_3	T_7	T_5	T_6
	30	T_2	T_3	T_3	T_5	T_6	T_7
	60	T_3	T_3	T_2	T_6	T_7	T_5
3	15	T_3	T_2	T_3	T_6	T_7	T_5
	30	T_3	T_2	T_2	T_7	T_5	T_6
	60	T_2	T_3	T_2	T_5	T_6	T_7
		Design 5: Fractional factorial design			Design 6: Two strength per batch design		
1	15	T_1	T_1	—	T_1	T_1	T_1
	30	T_1	—	T_1	T_1	T_1	T_1
	60	—	T_1	T_1	—	—	—
2	15	—	T_1	T_1	—	—	—
	30	T_1	T_1	—	T_1	T_1	T_1
	60	T_1	—	T_1	T_1	T_1	T_1
3	15	T_1	—	T_1	T_1	T_1	T_1
	30	—	T_1	T_1	—	—	—
	60	T_1	T_1	—	T_1	T_1	T_1

TABLE 10.3.5 Continued

Batch	Strength	Bottle	Blister	Tube	Bottle	Blister	Tube
		Design 7: Two packages per strength design			Design 8: Fractional-$\frac{1}{2}$ design		
1	15	T_1	—	T_1	T_2	T_3	—
	30	T_1	T_1	—	T_3	—	T_2
	60	—	T_1	T_1	—	T_2	T_3
2	15	T_1	—	T_1	—	T_2	T_3
	30	T_1	T_1	—	T_2	T_3	—
	60	—	T_1	T_1	T_3	—	T_2
3	15	T_1	—	T_1	T_3	—	T_3
	30	T_1	T_1	—	—	T_2	T_2
	60	—	T_1	T_1	T_2	T_3	—
		Design 9: Two strength per batch-$\frac{1}{2}$ design			Design 10: Two packages per strength-$\frac{1}{2}$ design		
1	15	T_2	T_3	T_2	T_2	—	T_3
	30	T_3	T_3	T_2	T_3	T_2	—
	60	—	—	—	—	T_3	T_2
2	15	—	—	—	T_2	—	T_3
	30	T_2	T_2	T_3	T_2	T_3	—
	60	T_3	T_3	T_2	—	T_2	T_0
3	15	T_3	T_2	T_3	T_3	—	T_2
	30	—	—	—	T_3	T_2	—
	60	T_2	T_3	T_2	—	T_3	T_0

Thus

$$\text{power} = P\left\{ \frac{\hat{\beta} - \Delta}{\sigma/\sqrt{S_{XX}}} < -z(1 - \tfrac{1}{2}\alpha) - \frac{\Delta}{\sigma}\sqrt{S_{XX}} \right\}$$

$$+ P\left\{ \frac{\hat{\beta} - \Delta}{\sigma/\sqrt{S_{XX}}} > z(1 - \tfrac{1}{2}\alpha - \frac{\Delta}{\sigma}\sqrt{S_{XX}} \right\}$$

$$= 1 - \Phi\left[z(1 - \tfrac{1}{2}\alpha) - \frac{\Delta}{\sigma}\sqrt{S_{XX}} \right]$$

$$+ \Phi\left[-z(1 - \tfrac{1}{2}\alpha) - \frac{\Delta}{\sigma}\sqrt{S_{XX}} \right]. \qquad (10.4.3)$$

TABLE 10.3.6 Number of Stability Tests Required for
Various Designs

Type	Design description	Number of assays	Percent reduced[a]
—	Complete	243	—
I	Complete$-\frac{2}{3}$	180	25.9
I	Complete$-\frac{1}{2}$	142	41.6
I	Complete$-\frac{1}{3}$	117	51.9
II	Fractional	162	33.3
II	Two strengths per batch	162	33.3
II	Two packages per strength	162	33.3
III	Fractional$-\frac{1}{2}$	99	59.3
III	Two strengths per batch$-\frac{1}{2}$	99	59.3
III	Two packages per strength$-\frac{1}{2}$	99	59.3

[a] Compared to the complete factorial design.

It can be seen from the above that the power increases as S_{xx} increases. When there are two batches, statistical power for detection of a significant difference in degradation rate per time unit can be obtained similarly. Let Y_{ij} be the assay result of the jth batch at time X_i. Then Y_{ij} can be described by the following linear model:

$$Y_{ij} = \alpha_j + \beta_j X_{ij} + e_{ij}, \quad i = 1, \ldots, n, \quad j = 1, 2, \qquad (10.4.4)$$

where it is assumed that e_{ij} are i.i.d. normal with mean zero and variance σ^2. Power for detection of a significant difference between β_1 and β_2 (i.e., $\beta_1 - \beta_2 = \Delta$) can be obtained similarly, as follows:

$$\text{power} = 1 - \Phi\left[z(1 - \tfrac{1}{2}\alpha) - \frac{\Delta}{\sigma}\left(\frac{1}{S_1^2} + \frac{1}{S_2^2}\right)^{-1/2} \right]$$

$$+ \Phi\left[-z(1 - \tfrac{1}{2}\alpha) - \frac{\Delta}{\sigma}\left(\frac{1}{S_1^2} + \frac{1}{S_2^2}\right)^{-1/2} \right], \qquad (10.4.5)$$

where

$$S_j^2 = \sum_{i=1}^{n} (X_{ij} - \overline{X}_j)^2,$$

$$\overline{X}_j = \frac{1}{n}\sum_{i=1}^{n} X_{ij}.$$

Note that when $S_1^2 = S_2^2 = S_{xx}$, (10.4.3) reduces to

$$\text{power} = 1 - \Phi\left[z(1 - \tfrac{1}{2}\alpha) - \frac{\Delta}{\sqrt{2}\sigma} \sqrt{S_{xx}} \right]$$
$$+ \Phi\left[-z(1 - \tfrac{1}{2}\alpha) - \frac{\Delta}{\sqrt{2}\sigma} \sqrt{S_{xx}} \right].$$

The criterion proposed by Nordbrock (1992), however, may not be appropriate because the primary objective of a stability study is to establish drug shelf life rather than to examine the effect of strength, package, batch, and storage time. Information regarding the differences in stability losses among packages, across strengths, between packages, between strengths, and between batches is useful for decision making as to whether or not the data should be pooled to establish a single shelf life. As an alternative, Chow (1992) and Ju and Chow (1994b) propose the following criterion: For a fixed sample size, the design with the best precision for shelf-life estimation is the best design. For a fixed desired precision of shelf-life estimation, the design with the smallest sample size is the best design.

Let Y denote the assay result of a drug characteristic: say, potency. For a given batch, the degradation of the drug characteristic can be described by model (10.4.1), which can be rewritten as the following general linear model:

$$Y_j = x(t_j)' \beta + e_j, \qquad j = 1, \ldots, n, \tag{10.4.6}$$

where $x(t_j)$ is a p vector of the jth value of the regressor, t_j is the sampling time at $X_j = t_j$, β is a $p \times 1$ vector of the parameter, and e_j is the random error in observing Y_j. Note that $x(t_j)$ may be of the form $(1, t_j, t_j w_j)'$ or $(1, t_j, w_j, t_j w_j)$, where w_j is a class variable for package type (e.g., w_j = bottle or blister), $t_j = X_j$, $j = 1, \ldots, n$ (number of sampling time points). When there are K batches, model (10.4.6) can be extended as follows

$$Y_{ij} = x(t_{ij})' \beta_i + e_{ij}, \qquad j = 1, \ldots, n_i, \quad i = 1, \ldots, k. \tag{10.4.7}$$

Note that $x(t_{ij})' \beta_i$ is the mean drug characteristics for the ith batch at $x(t_{ij})$. The primary assumptions of the model above are:

1. β_i are independent and identically distributed (i.i.d.) as N_p (β, Σ_β), where b is an unknown p vector and Σ is an unknown $p \times p$ nonnegative definite matrix.
2. e_{ij} are i.i.d. as $N(0, \sigma_e^2)$ and $\{e_{ij}\}$ and $\{\beta_i\}$ are independent.
3. $n_i > p$.

Model (10.4.6) can be expressed in the form of a matrix as follows:

$$Y_i = X_i \beta_i + \epsilon_i, \qquad i = 1, \ldots, K, \tag{10.4.8}$$

where

$$
\mathbf{Y}_i = \begin{bmatrix} Y_{i1} \\ \vdots \\ Y_{in_i} \end{bmatrix}, \quad \mathbf{X}_i = \begin{bmatrix} \mathbf{x}(t_{i1})' \\ \vdots \\ \mathbf{x}(t_{in_i})' \end{bmatrix}_{n_i \times p}, \quad \text{and} \quad \boldsymbol{\epsilon}_i = \begin{bmatrix} e_{i1} \\ \vdots \\ e_{in_i} \end{bmatrix}.
$$

Let η be the approved lower specification limit. Then if the definition of the true shelf-life for batch i is given by

$$
t_{\text{true}} = \inf\{t: \mathbf{x}(t)'\,\boldsymbol{\beta}_i \le \eta\},
$$

where $\mathbf{x}(t)'\,\boldsymbol{\beta}_i$ is the average drug characteristic at time t and $\boldsymbol{\beta}_i$ is a random vector distributed as $N_p\,(\boldsymbol{\beta},\boldsymbol{\Sigma}_\beta)$. When there is a batch-to-batch variation (i.e., $\boldsymbol{\Sigma}_\beta \ne 0$), t_{true} is random since $\boldsymbol{\beta}_i$ is random. In this case, Shao and Chow (1994) suggested taking an $1 - \alpha$ lower confidence bound of the ϵth quantile of t_{true} as the labeled shelf life. This leads to

$$
t_\epsilon = \inf\{t: \mathbf{x}(t)'\boldsymbol{\beta} - \eta = z_\epsilon \sigma(t)\},
$$

where t_ϵ satisfies

$$
P_\beta\,\{t_{\text{true}} \le t_\epsilon\} = \epsilon
$$

and $z_\epsilon = \Phi^{-1}(1 - \epsilon)$. Note that $t_{\text{label}} \le t_\epsilon$ if and only if

$$
P_\beta\{t_{\text{true}} \le t_{\text{label}}\} \le \epsilon.
$$

For the balanced case (i.e., $n_i = n$ and $\mathbf{X}_i = \mathbf{X}$), Shao and Chow (1994) proposed using $\tilde{t}$ as the labeled shelf life, where

$$
\tilde{t} = \inf\{t: \mathbf{x}(t)'\,\hat{\mathbf{b}} \le \bar{\eta}(t)\},
$$

$\hat{\mathbf{b}}$ is the least-squares estimator of $\boldsymbol{\beta}$, and

$$
\bar{\eta}(t) = \eta + c_k(\epsilon,\alpha)z_\epsilon \sqrt{v(t)},
$$
$$
c_k(\epsilon,\alpha) = t(\alpha, k - 1, \sqrt{K}z_\epsilon)/\sqrt{K}z_\epsilon,
$$
$$
v(t) = \frac{\mathbf{x}(t)'\,(\mathbf{X}'\mathbf{X})^{-1}\,\mathbf{X}'\mathbf{S}\mathbf{X}(\mathbf{X}'\mathbf{X})^{-1}\mathbf{x}(t)}{K - 1},
$$

where $t(\alpha, k - 1, \sqrt{K}z_\epsilon)$ is the αth upper quantile of the noncentral t distribution with degrees of freedom $k - 1$ and noncentral parameter $\sqrt{K}z_\epsilon$. Thus to assess the precision of the estimation of drug shelf life, we may consider the following quantity:

$$
\nabla = E\,|\tilde{t} - t_\epsilon| = \int_{t_\epsilon}^{\infty} P\{\tilde{t} > t\}\,dt + \int_{0}^{t_\epsilon} P\{\tilde{t} < t\}\,dt.
$$

A smaller ∇ indicates that the estimate is closer to the true shelf life. Therefore, a design with a smaller ∇ is considered a better design. An optimal design can then be obtained by minimizing $E \mid \hat{t} - t_\epsilon \mid$. However, it seems difficult to minimize $E \mid \hat{t} - t_\epsilon \mid$. Since

$$\int_0^{t_\epsilon} P\{\hat{t} < t\} \, dt \leq t_\epsilon P\{\hat{t} < t_\epsilon\} \leq t_\epsilon \alpha$$

is usually small, Ju and Chow (1994b) propose to minimize

$$\int_{t_\epsilon}^{\infty} P\{\hat{t} > t\} \, dt = \int_{t_\epsilon}^{\infty} P\{I_\epsilon > \sqrt{K}z_\epsilon c_k(\epsilon, \alpha)\} \, dt,$$

where

$$I_\epsilon \sim t\left(K - 1, \frac{\sqrt{K}(x(t)' \, \beta - \eta)}{\sqrt{a(t)}}\right),$$

$$a(t) = x(t)' \, [\Sigma + \sigma_e^2 \, (X'X)^{-1}]x(t).$$

Minimizing $\displaystyle\int_{t_\epsilon}^{\infty} P\{\hat{t} > t\} \, dt$ is equivalent to minimizing $a(t)$ or

$$x(t)' \, (X'X)^{-1}x(t)$$

by choosing a suitable design matrix X. As a result, design X_A may be considered to be better than design X_B if

$$x(t) \, (X'_A \, X_A)^{-1}x(t) < x(t)' \, (X'_B \, X_B)x(t) \qquad \text{for } t \geq t_\epsilon.$$

Therefore, for an arbitrary $p \times 1$ vector x, the efficiency of a design D can be defined as

$$E[D] = \frac{1}{x' \, (X'X)^{-1}x}.$$

Thus the relative efficiency of design A to design B is given by

$$\lambda = \frac{E[A]}{E[B]} = \frac{x(t)'(X'_B \, X_B)^{-1}x(t)}{x(t)' \, (X'_A \, X_A)^{-1}x(t)}. \tag{10.4.9}$$

As a result, λ can be viewed as a relative efficiency index of design B as compared to design A. For example, if $\lambda < 1$, we conclude that design B is at least as efficient as design A. On the other hand, if $\lambda > 1$, design A is superior to design B in terms of its relative efficiency.

Example 10.4.1

To illustrate the foregoing proposed criteria for the evaluation of stability designs, consider the following two designs for a stability study with three strengths and three package types:

Design A: complete factorial design
Design B: two packages per strength design

For design A, all chosen combinations are tested at $T_2 = (0,3,9,18,36,48)'$. For design B, all chosen combinations are tested at every time point [i.e., at $T_1 = 0,3,6,9,12,18,24,36,48)'$]. Note that design A is in fact a type I design and design B is a type II design. To evaluate $x(t)' (X'X)^{-1}x(t)$ at various $x(t)$, it is important to lay out the design matrix. Design matrices X_A and X_B are given in Table 10.4.1. The first row in the design matrix is the overall mean, the second and third rows refer to the comparisons between strengths, and the fourth and fifth rows refer to the comparisons between package types, and the last row consists of time points. Based on these design matrices $(X_A'X_A)^{-1}$ and $(X_B'X_B)^{-1}$ can be obtained easily (see Table 10.4.2). Consequently, $x(t)' (X_A'X_A)^{-1}x(t)$ and $x(t)' (X_B'X_B)^{-1}x(t)$ can be evaluated at various $x(t)$. For example, in the interest of a single shelf life, $x(t) = (1,0,0,0,0,t)$ was used. The following $x(t)$ were evaluated for different shelf lives for packages or strengths:

1. $(1,1,0,0,0,t)$
2. $(1,0,1,0,0,t)$
3. $(1,-1,-1,0,0,t)$
4. $(1,0,0,1,0,t)$
5. $(1,0,0,0,1,t)$
6. $(1,0,0,-1,-1,t)$

Note that 1 to 3 can be used for estimation of shelf lives for different strengths, while 4 to 6 can be used for estimation of shelf lives for different package types. Other combinations of strength and package can be evaluated similarly. For example, $x(t) = (1, 1, 0, 1, 0, t)$ is used to estimate the shelf life for the combination of the first level between strength and package type.

Table 10.4.3 gives $x(t)' (X'X)^{-1}x(t)$ values of the two designs and their relative efficiency λ evaluated at $t = 12, 18, 24, 36, 48$, and 60 for single shelf life. The results indicate that design B is more efficient than design A at times 12 and 18. However, design A becomes more efficient than design B after time $t = 24$. These results suggest that design A is an appropriate stability design for a long-term marketing stability monitoring program. Fewer time points are tested at all combinations. In case of package-to-package and/or strength-to-strength variations, Tables 10.4.4 and 10.4.5 summarize the values of $x(t)' (X'X)^{-1}x(t)$ and the relative efficiencies of the two designs, which allow different shelf lives

TABLE 10.4.1 Design Matrices[a]

	Design A						Design B				

$$X_A = \begin{bmatrix}
1 & 1 & 0 & 1 & 0 & 0 \\
1 & 1 & 0 & 0 & 1 & 0 \\
1 & 1 & 0 & -1 & -1 & 0 \\
1 & 0 & 1 & 1 & 0 & 0 \\
1 & 0 & 1 & 0 & 1 & 0 \\
1 & 0 & 1 & -1 & -1 & 0 \\
1 & -1 & -1 & 1 & 0 & 0 \\
1 & -1 & -1 & 0 & 1 & 0 \\
1 & -1 & -1 & -1 & -1 & 0 \\
1 & 1 & 0 & 1 & 0 & 3 \\
1 & 1 & 0 & 0 & 1 & 3 \\
1 & 1 & 0 & -1 & -1 & 3 \\
1 & 0 & 1 & 1 & 0 & 3 \\
1 & 0 & 1 & 0 & 1 & 3 \\
1 & 0 & 1 & -1 & -1 & 3 \\
1 & -1 & -1 & 1 & 0 & 3 \\
1 & -1 & -1 & 0 & 1 & 3 \\
1 & -1 & -1 & -1 & -1 & 3 \\
1 & 1 & 0 & 1 & 0 & 9 \\
1 & 1 & 0 & 0 & 1 & 9 \\
1 & 1 & 0 & -1 & -1 & 9 \\
1 & 0 & 1 & 1 & 0 & 9 \\
1 & 0 & 1 & 0 & 1 & 9 \\
1 & 0 & 1 & -1 & -1 & 9 \\
1 & -1 & -1 & 1 & 0 & 9 \\
1 & -1 & -1 & 0 & 1 & 9 \\
1 & -1 & -1 & -1 & -1 & 9 \\
1 & 1 & 0 & 1 & 0 & 18 \\
1 & 1 & 0 & 0 & 1 & 18 \\
1 & 1 & 0 & -1 & -1 & 18 \\
1 & 0 & 1 & 1 & 0 & 18 \\
1 & 0 & 1 & 0 & 1 & 18 \\
1 & 0 & 1 & -1 & -1 & 18 \\
1 & -1 & -1 & 1 & 0 & 18 \\
1 & -1 & -1 & 0 & 1 & 18 \\
1 & -1 & -1 & -1 & -1 & 18 \\
1 & 1 & 0 & 1 & 0 & 36 \\
1 & 1 & 0 & 0 & 1 & 36 \\
1 & 1 & 0 & -1 & -1 & 36 \\
1 & 0 & 1 & 1 & 0 & 36 \\
1 & 0 & 1 & 0 & 1 & 36 \\
1 & 0 & 1 & -1 & -1 & 36 \\
1 & -1 & -1 & 1 & 0 & 36 \\
1 & -1 & -1 & 0 & 1 & 36 \\
1 & -1 & -1 & -1 & -1 & 36 \\
1 & 1 & 0 & 1 & 0 & 48 \\
1 & 1 & 0 & 0 & 1 & 48 \\
1 & 1 & 0 & -1 & -1 & 48 \\
1 & 0 & 1 & 1 & 0 & 48 \\
1 & 0 & 1 & 0 & 1 & 48 \\
1 & 0 & 1 & -1 & -1 & 48 \\
1 & -1 & -1 & 1 & 0 & 48 \\
1 & -1 & -1 & 0 & 1 & 48 \\
1 & -1 & -1 & -1 & -1 & 48
\end{bmatrix}
\qquad
X_B = \begin{bmatrix}
1 & 1 & 0 & 1 & 0 & 0 \\
1 & 1 & 0 & -1 & -1 & 0 \\
1 & 0 & 1 & 1 & 0 & 0 \\
1 & 0 & 1 & 0 & 1 & 0 \\
1 & -1 & -1 & 0 & 1 & 0 \\
1 & -1 & -1 & -1 & -1 & 0 \\
1 & 1 & 0 & 1 & 0 & 3 \\
1 & 1 & 0 & -1 & -1 & 3 \\
1 & 0 & 1 & 1 & 0 & 3 \\
1 & 0 & 1 & 0 & 1 & 3 \\
1 & -1 & -1 & 0 & 1 & 3 \\
1 & -1 & -1 & -1 & -1 & 3 \\
1 & 1 & 0 & 1 & 0 & 6 \\
1 & 1 & 0 & -1 & -1 & 6 \\
1 & 0 & 1 & 1 & 0 & 6 \\
1 & 0 & 1 & 0 & 1 & 6 \\
1 & -1 & -1 & 0 & 1 & 6 \\
1 & -1 & -1 & -1 & -1 & 6 \\
1 & 1 & 0 & 1 & 0 & 9 \\
1 & 1 & 0 & -1 & -1 & 9 \\
1 & 0 & 1 & 1 & 0 & 9 \\
1 & 0 & 1 & 0 & 1 & 9 \\
1 & -1 & -1 & 0 & 1 & 9 \\
1 & -1 & -1 & -1 & -1 & 9 \\
1 & 1 & 0 & 1 & 0 & 12 \\
1 & 1 & 0 & -1 & -1 & 12 \\
1 & 0 & 1 & 1 & 0 & 12 \\
1 & 0 & 1 & 0 & 1 & 12 \\
1 & -1 & -1 & 0 & 1 & 12 \\
1 & -1 & -1 & -1 & -1 & 12 \\
1 & 1 & 0 & 1 & 0 & 18 \\
1 & 1 & 0 & -1 & -1 & 18 \\
1 & 0 & 1 & 1 & 0 & 18 \\
1 & 0 & 1 & 0 & 1 & 18 \\
1 & -1 & -1 & 0 & 1 & 18 \\
1 & -1 & -1 & -1 & -1 & 18 \\
1 & 1 & 0 & 1 & 0 & 24 \\
1 & 1 & 0 & -1 & -1 & 24 \\
1 & 0 & 1 & 1 & 0 & 24 \\
1 & 0 & 1 & 0 & 1 & 24 \\
1 & -1 & -1 & 0 & 1 & 24 \\
1 & -1 & -1 & -1 & -1 & 24 \\
1 & 1 & 0 & 1 & 0 & 36 \\
1 & 1 & 0 & -1 & -1 & 36 \\
1 & 0 & 1 & 1 & 0 & 36 \\
1 & 0 & 1 & 0 & 1 & 36 \\
1 & -1 & -1 & 0 & 1 & 36 \\
1 & -1 & -1 & -1 & -1 & 36 \\
1 & 1 & 0 & 1 & 0 & 48 \\
1 & 1 & 0 & -1 & -1 & 48 \\
1 & 0 & 1 & 1 & 0 & 48 \\
1 & 0 & 1 & 0 & 1 & 48 \\
1 & -1 & -1 & 0 & 1 & 48 \\
1 & -1 & -1 & -1 & -1 & 48
\end{bmatrix}$$

[a]Design A, complete factorial design with $T_2 = (0,3,9,18,36,48)'$; design B, two packages per strength design with $T_1 = (0,3,6,9,12,18,24,36,48)'$.

TABLE 10.4.2 $(X'X)^{-1}$ for Designs A and B

$$(X'_A X_A)^{-1}$$

$$
\begin{bmatrix}
0.0402 & 0.0000 & 0.0000 & 0.0000 & 0.0000 & -0.0011 \\
0.0000 & 0.0370 & -0.0185 & 0.0000 & 0.0000 & 0.0000 \\
0.0000 & -0.0185 & 0.0370 & 0.0000 & 0.0000 & 0.0000 \\
0.0000 & 0.0000 & 0.0000 & 0.0370 & -0.0185 & 0.0000 \\
0.0000 & 0.0000 & 0.0000 & -0.0185 & 0.0370 & 0.0000 \\
-0.0011 & 0.0000 & 0.0000 & 0.0000 & 0.0000 & 0.0001
\end{bmatrix}
$$

$$(X'_B X_B)^{-1}$$

$$
\begin{bmatrix}
0.0428 & 0.0000 & 0.0000 & 0.0000 & 0.0000 & -0.0014 \\
0.0000 & 0.0494 & -0.0247 & -0.0123 & 0.0247 & 0.0000 \\
0.0000 & -0.0247 & 0.0494 & -0.0123 & -0.0123 & 0.0000 \\
0.0000 & -0.0123 & -0.0123 & 0.0494 & -0.0247 & 0.0000 \\
0.0000 & 0.0247 & -0.0123 & -0.0247 & 0.0494 & 0.0000 \\
-0.0014 & 0.0000 & 0.0000 & 0.0000 & 0.0000 & 0.0001
\end{bmatrix}
$$

TABLE 10.4.3   Relative Efficiencies for Comparing Designs A and B[a] (Single Shelf Life)

Time (months)	$x(t)'\,(X'X)^{-1}x(t)$ Design A	$x(t)'\,(X'X)^{-1}x(t)$ Design B	λ
12	0.0215	0.0208	0.9696
18	0.0186	0.0186	0.9987
24	0.0200	0.0221	1.1040
36	0.0359	0.0466	1.2990
48	0.0691	0.0944	1.3662
60	0.1196	0.1654	1.3829

[a] Design A, complete factorial design with T_2; design B, two packages per strength design with T_1.

for different package types or strengths, and different combinations of package and strength, respectively. The results reveal that design A is almost uniformly superior to design B. This can be explained by the fact that a fraction of a complete factorial design may lose the degrees of freedom for testing two-factor and/or high-factor interactions and consequently, lose its efficiency in estimating drug shelf life.

TABLE 10.4.4 Relative Efficiencies for Comparing Designs A and B^a (Different Shelf Lives for Different Packages or Strengths)

Time (months)	$x(t)'$ $(X'X)^{-1}x(t)$		λ
	Design A	Design B	
12	0.0585	0.0702	1.1999
18	0.0556	0.0679	1.2215
24	0.0571	0.0715	1.2529
36	0.0729	0.0960	1.3164
48	0.1061	0.1438	1.3548
60	0.1566	0.2148	1.3712

[a] Design A, complete factorial design with T_2; design B, two packages per strength design with T_1.

To provide a better understanding, the results with single shelf life given in Table 10.4.3 are summarized in Fig. 10.4.1. As can be seen from the figure, the difference in efficiency for estimation of drug shelf life between the two designs becomes significant as t increases. In practice, it is often of interest to reduce the number of tests by either cutting down the number of combinations or testing the product at fewer time points. In either case it is suggested that the relative efficiency of the reduced stability design as compared to the complete design be carefully evaluated to assure the reliability of the estimated shelf life.

10.5. DISCUSSION

For a long-term stability study it is of interest to adopt a complete factorial design by testing stability at every time point. A complete factorial design cannot only provide valid statistical tests for main effects of design factors under study but can provide estimates for interactions with the maximum precision. As a result, it improves the precision of the estimated drug shelf life. A complete factorial design is considered an ideal design if applied to more homogeneous drug products. However, a complete factorial design is usually too costly and time consuming to perform. In practice, it is of interest to consider a matrixing or bracketing design. It should be noted that a matrixing or bracketing design may not be able to evaluate interaction effects. For example, for a 2^{4-1} fractional factorial design, two-factor effects are confounded with each other. In this case we may not be able to determine whether the data should be pooled.

In practice it is preferred to have a single shelf life applicable to all future batches. For this purpose it is desirable to pool the data across all design factors to achieve a better statistical inference on the estimated shelf life. It is suggested, however, that some preliminary tests for interactions be tested to determine

TABLE 10.4.5 Relative Efficiencies for Comparing Designs A and B^a (Different Shelf Lives for Different Combinations of Package and Strength)

| Time (months) | $\mathbf{x}(t)'\ (\mathbf{X'X})^{-1}\mathbf{x}(t)$ | | λ |
	Design A	Design B	
12	0.0955	0.0949	0.9932
18	0.0927	0.0926	0.9997
24	0.0941	0.0962	1.0221
36	0.1100	0.1207	1.0976
48	0.1432	0.1685	1.1767
60	0.1937	0.2395	1.2364

[a] Design A, complete factorial design with T_2; design B, two packages per strength design with T_1.

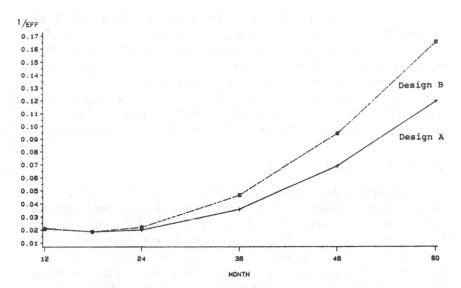

FIGURE 10.4.1 Efficiencies for designs A and B with single shelf life. $1/EFF = \mathbf{x}(t)'\ (\mathbf{X'X})^{-1}\mathbf{x}(t)$.

whether the data should be pooled. If a significant interaction is observed, the data should not be pooled. On the contrary, individual shelf lives for each combination of the factors with significant interaction should be carefully evaluated. Thus to achieve a better statistical inference on the estimated shelf life, a design should be chosen to avoid possible confounding and/or interaction effects. Once the design is chosen, statistical analysis should reflect the nature of the design selected.

Since the primary objective of a stability is to establish an expiration dating period, the selection of an appropriate design should be based on the precision of shelf life estimation rather than statistical power for detection of a meaningful difference. The relative efficiency index λ proposed by Ju and Chow (1994b) can be applied to evaluate the efficiency of a stability design. If two designs have the same efficiencies, the relative merits and disadvantages should be taken into account for design selection. In practice, since all the reduced stability designs can be classified into one of the three type of designs (i.e., types I, II, and III) for a given sample size N (e.g., the total number of assays), it is of interest to determine an optimal design within each type of designs. This needs further investigation.

As mentioned earlier, a complete factorial design for any stability study is fully efficient in the sense that it provides 100% information regarding the design factors considered in a stability program. On the other hand, matrixing and bracketing designs are different versions of fractional factorial designs which will not provide full efficiency for all design factors. If previous experience showed that the variability in degradation is small across different strengths that might be manufactured by increasing the size of the tablets but they were made from the same granulation by the same manufacturing process, the strength category might be a candidate for matrixing or bracketing. However, the relative efficiency of such fractional factorial design should be evaluated carefully based on the criterion given in (10.4.9).

Lin (1994) studied the applicability of matrixing and bracketing to stability study designs. She indicated that a matrixing design may be applicable to strength if there is no change in proportion of active ingredients, container size, and intermediate sampling time points. The application of a matrixing design to situations such as (1) closure systems; (2) orientation of container during storage; (3) packaging form, such as glass, plastic, and foil; (4) manufacturing process (e.g., mixing times); and (5) batch size (e.g., proportion of container filled, such as liquid) should be evaluated carefully. Lin (1994) also discussed some situations where a matrixing design is not applicable. For example, if there is a significant change in proportions of active ingredients, the matrixing design is not suitable for strength. Lin (1994) indicated that a matrixing design should not be applied to sampling times at two endpoints (i.e., the initial and the last) and at any time points beyond the desired expiration date. If the drug product is sensitive to temperature, humidity, and light, the matrixing design should be avoided.

Although the relative efficiency discussed in Sec. 10.4 was derived based on the assumption that β_i are random, it does not contain any random components. As an alternative, we may derive the efficiency as follows. As discussed in detail in Chapters 11 and 12 under the assumption that the drug characteristic decreases linearly with time, the FDA guideline suggests estimating the expiration dating period as the time point at which a 95% lower confidence limit for the mean degradation line intersects the acceptable lower specification limit, η. As a result, the precision (or efficiency) of the estimated shelf life is actually a function of the precision (or efficiency) for the mean degradation line. Under the sample linear regression with fixed batch effects, the variance of the least-squares estimate of the regression line at a particular time point x, $\hat{Y} = a + bx$, is given as (Draper and Smith, 1981)

$$V(\hat{Y}) = \sigma_e^2 \left[\frac{1}{n} + \frac{(x - \bar{X})^2}{\Sigma (X_i - \bar{X})^2} \right]. \tag{10.5.1}$$

Note that for a simple linear regression

$$X = \begin{bmatrix} 1 & \cdots & 1 \\ X_1 & \cdots & X_n \end{bmatrix},$$

$$X'X = \begin{bmatrix} n & n\bar{X} \\ n\bar{X} & \Sigma X_i^2 \end{bmatrix}.$$

Hence

$$(X'X)^{-1} = \frac{1}{n\Sigma(X_i - \bar{X})^2} \begin{bmatrix} \Sigma X_i^2 & -n\bar{X} \\ -n\bar{X} & n \end{bmatrix}.$$

Let $x = (1,x)'$; then it is easy to show that

$$V(\hat{Y}) = \sigma_e^2 \left[\frac{1}{n} + \frac{(x - \bar{X}^2}{\Sigma (X_i - \bar{X})^2} \right] \tag{10.5.2}$$

$$= \sigma_e^2 \, x' \, (X'X)^{-1}x.$$

Thus the variance of the least-squares estimate of the mean degradation line is the inverse of the efficiency. Examination of $V(\hat{Y})$ in (10.5.1) reveals that it is a decreasing function of $\Sigma (X_i - \bar{X})^2$ and an increasing function of $(x - \bar{X})^2$. This information is helpful in planning a stability study for estimating a shelf life with high efficiency. From the accelerated stability testing program, a tentative shelf life is obtained from the methods described in Chapter 9. Then the sampling-time points should be selected such that the average time point is close (or equal) either to the targeted tentative shelf life or to the estimate of $(\eta - \alpha)/\beta$. However, as indicated by the FDA guideline, the initial and final time points should always be included in the design. Furthermore, the last time point should be chosen as far away as physically possible. Some estimates of degradation rate per time unit are usually available at the planning stage of a long-term stability program. If the degradation rate is quite small and it is not expected that significant stability loss will occur at an early stage of a stability study, fewer sampling-time points should be allocated at the early period of the study. On the other hand, more sampling-time points should be selected near the time point at which the estimated shelf life is likely to occur. In summary, one should allocate the sampling time points at initial time point zero; at the last time point, which is as far as physically possible; and at the average time point, which should be chosen to be as close as possible to the targeted shelf life. Stability studies with this type of allocation of sampling time points not only maximize the efficiency of design but also allow for examination of lack of fit of the postulated linear regression model in (10.4.1). Hence selection of such sampling time points will provide an estimated expiration dating period with a higher precision than the one suggested in the FDA guideline. It should be noted, however, that when different time points are used for different batches or other combinations, the definition of the efficiency of a design D at time x should be modified. For example, we might modify the definition as follows:

$$E[D] = \left\{ \frac{1}{K} \mathbf{x}' \left[\sum_{i=1}^{K} (\mathbf{X}_i'\mathbf{X}_i)^{-1} \right] \mathbf{x} \right\}^{-1}. \tag{10.5.3}$$

Then the relative efficiency for comparing two designs can be defined similarly as

$$\lambda = \frac{E[A]}{E[B]} = \frac{K_A \mathbf{x}' \left[\sum_{i=1}^{K_A} (\mathbf{X}_{Ai}'\mathbf{X}_{Ai})^{-1} \right] \mathbf{x}}{K_B \mathbf{x}' \left[\sum_{i=1}^{K_B} (\mathbf{X}_{Bi}'\mathbf{X}_{Bi})^{-1} \right] \mathbf{x}}. \tag{10.5.4}$$

It should be noted that in this chapter, our discussions are restricted only to the assumption that the storage conditions are fixed. In practice, the study of stability of a drug product under various storage conditions may be necessary due to different market needs from different countries (e.g., EC and Japan). The inclusion of storage condition as a design factor may complicate the planning of a stability program.

11

Stability Analysis with Fixed Batches

11.1. INTRODUCTION

As mentioned in Chapter 8, the labeled expiration dating period or shelf life of
a drug product is usually established based on the primary stability data obtained
from long-term stability studies that are conducted under ambient conditions.
For the determination of a labeled shelf life, the FDA guideline requires that at
least three batches, and preferably more, be tested to allow for a reliable estimate
of batch-to-batch variability and to test the hypothesis that a single expiration
dating period for all batches is justifiable. In addition to individual shelf lives
estimated from each batch, it is desirable to establish a single shelf life for a
drug product based on combined stability data from all batches. As indicated
by the FDA guideline, this single labeled expiration dating period should be
applicable to all future batches. Before one can combine stability data from all
batches, it is required by the FDA guideline to perform preliminary tests for
batch similarity. Batch similarity is usually evaluated by testing the equality of
intercepts and the equality of slopes of degradation lines among different
batches. For testing the hypotheses of the equality of intercepts and the equality
of slopes among batches, the FDA guideline suggests the 0.25 level of significance be used. If the hypotheses of equal intercepts and equal slopes are not
rejected at the 0.25 level of significance, a single expiration dating period can
be estimated by fitting a single degradation curve based on pooled stability data
of all batches under the assumption that batch effects are fixed. On the other
hand, if the hypotheses of equal intercepts and equal slopes are rejected at the

0.25 level of significance, the FDA suggests that a single expiration dating period of the drug product be determined based on the minimum of individual shelf lives obtained from each batches. This method, however, lacks of statistical justification (Chow and Shao, 1991). Under the assumption of fixed batch effects, as an alternative, Ruberg and Hsu (1992) proposed a method for estimation of an expiration dating period using multiple comparison technique for pooling stability data with the worst batch.

In Chapters 11 and 12 we consider only the estimation of drug shelf life for a single active ingredient of a drug product. In addition, we assume that the strength of the drug product decreases linearly with time. Furthermore, as indicated in the FDA guideline, the percent of label claim on the original scale, not percent of initial value, is used as the primary variable for determination of shelf life of the drug product. In this chapter we focus on statistical analysis for estimation of drug shelf life with fixed batch effects. The case where batch effects are assumed random is discussed in Chapter 12.

In the next section the method for determination of an expiration dating period for a single batch suggested in the FDA guideline is described. An alternative method for estimation of drug shelf life based on the lower 95% confidence interval of the slope of the degradation line rather than mean degradation is also presented (Rahman, 1992). Statistical properties and relative merits and disadvantages of the two methods are compared in Sec. 11.2. In Sec. 11.3 the ANCOVA technique is applied to derive tests for the hypotheses of equal intercepts and equal slopes for batch similarity. The minimum approach for estimation of a single expiration dating period for multiple batches described in the FDA guideline is given in Sec. 11.4. In Sec. 11.5 we describe the multiple comparison procedures proposed by Ruberg and Hsu (1992) for pooling stability data with the worst batch. A numerical example is provided in Sec. 11.6 to illustrate various methods for determination of drug shelf life with fixed batch effects. A brief discussion is given in Sec. 11.7, including a discussion on the choice between the original and logarithmic scale of percent of label claim for determination of drug shelf life.

11.2. DRUG SHELF LIFE FOR A SINGLE BATCH

For a single batch, the FDA guideline suggests that an acceptable approach for drug characteristics that are expected to decrease with time is to determine the time at which the 95% one-sided lower confidence limit for the mean degradation curve intersects the lower acceptable specification limit (see Fig. 8.3.1). The lower acceptable specification limit, η, is usually adopted from the USP/NF. For many drug products, η is 90%.

Under the assumption that the strength of a drug product decreases linearly with time, the degradation of the strength over time for a batch can be described by the following simple linear regression model:

$$Y_j = \alpha + \beta X_j + e_j, \qquad j = 1, \ldots, n, \tag{11.2.1}$$

where Y_j is the assay result (percent of label claim) at sampling time X_j; α is the intercept, which is the value of the percent of label claim at the initial time point (i.e., $X_j = 0$); β is the slope, which is the degradation rate per time unit; and e_j are i.i.d. normal random variables with mean zero and variance σ^2. Since β is the degradation rate per time unit, the stability loss over a time interval t is βt. The expected value of Y_j under model (11.2.1) is given by

$$E(Y_j) = \alpha + \beta X_j.$$

Note that α is sometimes referred to as the batch effect at the initial time point. It can be seen that model (11.2.1) is the same as model (2.3.10). Therefore, statistical inference such as estimation and hypothesis testing derived in Sec. 2.3 can be applied directly. Recall that under model (2.3.1) [or equivalently, model (11.2.1)], the least-squares estimates for slope, intercept, and error variance are given, respectively, by

$$b = \frac{S_{XY}}{S_{XX}},$$

$$a = \bar{Y} - b\bar{X},$$

$$s^2 = \frac{S_{YY} - bS_{XY}}{n - 2}, \tag{11.2.2}$$

where $\bar{X}$ and $\bar{Y}$, S_{XX}, S_{YY}, and S_{XY} are as defined in (2.3.7) and (2.3.8), respectively.

At a particular time point $t = x$, the least-squares estimate of mean degradation $E(Y(x)) = \alpha + \beta x$ is then given by

$$y(x) = a + bx, \tag{11.2.3}$$

with the variance

$$V[y(x)] = \sigma^2 \left[\frac{1}{n} + \frac{(x - \bar{X})^2}{S_{XX}} \right]. \tag{11.2.4}$$

From (11.2.2), the least-squares estimate of $V[y(x)]$ can be obtained as

$$\hat{V}[y(x)] = s^2 \left[\frac{1}{n} + \frac{(x - \bar{X})^2}{S_{XX}} \right]. \tag{11.2.5}$$

Consequently, the standard error of the estimated mean degradation line and the 95% lower confidence limit of the mean degradation line are given, respectively, by

$$SE(x) = \left\{ s^2 \left[\frac{1}{n} + \frac{(x - \overline{X})^2}{S_{xx}} \right] \right\}^{1/2}, \tag{11.2.6}$$

$$L(x) = a + bx - t(0.05, n - 2)SE(x), \tag{11.2.7}$$

and $t(0.05, n - 2)$ is the 5% upper quantile of a central t distribution with $n - 2$ degrees of freedom. Thus the points where (11.2.7) intersects the acceptable lower specification limit η (if exist) are the two roots of the following quadratic equation:

$$[\eta - (a + bx)]^2 = t^2(0.05, n - 2)s^2 \left[\frac{1}{n} + \frac{(x - \overline{X})^2}{S_{xx}} \right]. \tag{11.2.8}$$

The two roots, denoted by x_L and x_U, of (11.2.8) constitute the lower and upper limits of the 90% confidence interval for $(\eta - \alpha)/\beta$.
    Let

$$T_a = \frac{a - \eta}{SE(a)} \quad \text{and} \quad T_b = \frac{b}{SE(b)}, \tag{11.2.9}$$

where $SE(a)$ and $SE(b)$ are as defined in Sec. 2.3. If the slope is statistically significantly smaller than zero and the intercept is statistically significantly larger than η, which is the acceptable lower specification limit at the 0.05 level of significance, that is,

$$(i) \quad \frac{b}{SE(b)} < -t(0.05, n - 2), \tag{11.2.10}$$

$$(ii) \quad \frac{a - \eta}{SE(a)} > t(0.05, n - 2), \tag{11.2.11}$$

then the 90% confidence interval for $(\eta - \alpha)/\beta$ is an inclusive and close interval (x_L, x_U). In this case, the expiration dating period of a single batch is defined as $t = x_L$ (Kohberger, 1988). However, in other cases, the 90% confidence intervals for $(\eta - \alpha)/\beta$ is either the entire real line or two disjoint open intervals; consequently, the expiration dating period is not defined.
    Note that the foregoing approach is based on the 95% lower confidence limit for mean degradation line. Its interpretation in terms of hypothesis testing is given below (Easterling, 1969). Under model (11.2.1), the pth upper quantile of the distribution for the percent of label claim at a given time point $t = x$ is $\alpha + \beta x + z_p \sigma$, where x_p is the pth upper quantile of a standard normal distribution. The null hypothesis that the pth upper quantile of the distribution for the percent of label claim at time point $t = x_0$ is larger than the acceptable lower

specification limit η can be stated as

$$H_0: \alpha + \beta x_0 + \sigma z_p \geq \eta \quad \text{vs.} \quad H_a: \alpha + \beta x_0 + \sigma z_p < \eta,$$

$$(11.2.12)$$

which can be rewritten as

$$H_0: \eta - (\alpha + \beta x_0 + \sigma z_p) \leq 0$$

$$\text{vs.} \quad H_a: \eta - (\alpha + \beta x_0 + \sigma z_p) > 0. \quad (11.2.13)$$

Furthermore, the hypotheses can be expressed in terms of time point $t = x_0$ as follows (with $\beta < 0$):

$$H_0: \frac{\eta - \alpha - \sigma z_p}{\beta} \leq x_0 \quad \text{vs.} \quad H_a: \frac{\eta - \alpha - \sigma z_p}{\beta} > x_0. \quad (11.2.14)$$

For estimation of the shelf life of a drug product, as specified in the FDA guideline, the mean degradation line is to be used. Hence $p = 0.5$ is chosen. When $p = 0.5$ and $z_p = 0$, the hypotheses (11.2.14) reduce to

$$H_0: \frac{\eta - \alpha}{\beta} \leq x_0 \quad \text{vs.} \quad H_a: \frac{\eta - \alpha}{\beta} > x_0. \quad (11.2.15)$$

Note that $(\eta - \alpha)/\beta$ is in fact the time point at which the mean degradation line intersects the acceptable lower specification limit η. The null hypothesis of (11.2.14) is to test whether this time point is less than $t = x_0$. Therefore, if the null hypothesis is tested at the 5% level of significance, the corresponding set of x for which the null hypothesis (11.2.14) is not rejected at the 5% significance level constitutes the 95% one-sided confidence interval [i.e., (x_L, ∞)] for $(\eta - \mu)/\beta$. The lower limit of the 95% one-sided confidence interval for $(\eta - \alpha)/\beta$ is x_L, which can be obtained as the smaller root of the quadratic equation (11.2.8).

For the method suggested by the FDA, the probability of a mean degradation line greater than $L(x)$, where x denotes a given time point t, is 0.95, that is,

$$P\{\alpha + \beta x \geq L(x)\} = 0.95.$$

In addition, for any time point $x \leq x_L$, it follows that

$$P\{\alpha + \beta x \geq \eta\} \geq P\{\alpha + \beta x \geq L(x)\} \geq 0.95. \quad (11.2.16)$$

The probability statement above can easily be verified from Fig. 8.3.1. As a result, the expiration dating period for a single batch provides a 95% confidence that the average drug characteristic of the dosage units in the batch is within specifications up to the end of the expiration dating period.

Rahman (1992) indicated that some drug companies used the following alternative method for estimation of drug shelf life based on the 95% confidence interval of the slope of the true mean degradation line, that is,

$$b_L = b - t(0.05, n - 2)SE(b).$$ (11.2.17)

Thus a new estimated degradation line may be constructed from the same estimated intercept and b_L, that is,

$$y'(x) = a + b_L x.$$ (11.2.18)

The expiration dating period can then be estimated as the time interval at which the new estimated degradation line intersects the acceptable lower specification limit η. In other words, $t = x'_L$ is the time point such that

$$y'(x'_L) = \eta$$

$$a + b_L x'_L = \eta$$

$$a + [b - t(0.05, n - 2)SE(b)]x'_L = \eta.$$ (11.2.19)

Equation (11.2.19) is a linear function of x'_L. Hence the solution for x'_L always exists and is given by

$$x'_L = \frac{\eta - a}{b - t(0.05, n - 2)SE(b)}.$$ (11.2.20)

Rahman (1992) showed that there exists one and only point of intersection between $L(x)$ and $y'(x)$, which is given as

$$x^* = \frac{\sum X_i^2}{2\sum X_i}.$$ (11.2.21)

If the sampling time points in a stability study are those recommended in the FDA guideline up to 5 years (i.e., 0, 3, 6, 9, 12, 18, 24, 36, 48, and 60 months), x^* is about 19.4 months, which is about one-third of the entire length of the study period. Rahman (1992) also pointed out that when $x \leq x^*$,

$$P\{y(x) > y'(x)\} < 0.95,$$ (11.2.22)

and when $x > x^*$,

$$P\{y(x) > y'(x)\} > 0.95.$$ (11.2.23)

Furthermore, under usual practical situations, x_L is always longer than x'_L. Hence, x'_L is much more conservative than x_L.

Note that the estimated expiration dating period derived from the 95% lower confidence interval for the degradation rate is not based on the mean degradation line as suggested in the FDA guideline. Furthermore, the probability statement about the relationship among time points, observed percent of label claim, and the acceptable lower specification limit cannot be made by this method. Therefore, this approach may not be appropriate for estimation of the expiration dating period.

11.3. PRELIMINARY TEST FOR BATCH SIMILARITY

The FDA guideline requires that at least three batches and preferably more be tested to allow some estimate of batch-to-batch variability and at the same time to allow us to test the hypothesis that a single expiration dating period for all batches is justifiable. Justification for a single expiration dating period estimated from the pooled stability data of all batches can be verified, as suggested in the FDA guideline, by testing batch similarity. The FDA guideline also points out that batch similarity of the degradation lines can be evaluated in terms of the equality of slopes and the equality of intercepts obtained from the stability data of individual batches.

Let Y_{ij} be the assay result (percent of label claim) of the ith batch for a drug product at sampling time X_{ij}. If the degradation is to decrease linearly over time for all batches, model (11.2.1) for a single batch can be extended to describe the degradation for multiple batches as follows:

$$Y_{ij} = \alpha_i + \beta_i X_{ij} + e_{ij}, \quad i = 1, \ldots, K; \quad j = 1, \ldots, n_i, \tag{11.3.1}$$

where α_i and β_i are the intercept and slope of the degradation line for batch i, and e_{ij} are assumed to be i.i.d. as a normal distribution with mean zero and variance σ^2. Note that α_i can be viewed as the ith batch effect at time zero, and β_i is the degradation rate per time unit.

Tests for the hypotheses of equality of slopes and the equality of intercepts are in essence the tests for homogeneity of the degradation lines among batches, which can be examined by testing the following hypotheses for slopes and intercepts, respectively,

$$H_{0\beta}: \beta_i = \beta_{i'} \text{ for all } i \neq i', \tag{11.3.2}$$

$$H_{0\alpha}: \alpha_i = \alpha_{i'} \text{ for all } i \neq i'. \tag{11.3.3}$$

The typical analysis of covariance (ANCOVA) for a completely randomized design can be applied to obtain test statistics for both hypotheses (11.3.2) and (11.3.3) [see, e.g., Snedecor and Cochran (1980) and Wang and Chow (1994)].

Let $S_{XX}(i)$, $S_{YY}(i)$, and $X_{XY}(i)$ be the sum of squares of time points, percent of label claim, and the sum of cross products between time points and percent of label claims for batch i individually and

$$S_{XX}(W) = \sum_{i=1}^{K} S_{XX}(i),$$

$$S_{YY}(W) = \sum_{i=1}^{K} S_{YY}(i),$$

$$S_{XY}(W) = \sum_{i=1}^{K} S_{XY}(i). \tag{11.3.4}$$

The degrees of freedom for $S_{XX}(i)$, $S_{YY}(i)$, and $S_{XY}(i)$ and $S_{XX}(W)$, $S_{YY}(W)$, and $S_{XY}(W)$ are $n_i - 1$ and $N - K$, where $N = \Sigma n_i$. The least-squares estimate of the slope and the intercept for batch i are given, respectively, by

$$b_i = \frac{S_{XY}(i)}{S_{XX}(i)},$$

$$a_i = \overline{Y}_{i\cdot} - b_i \overline{X}_{i\cdot}, \tag{11.3.5}$$

where

$$\overline{X}_{i\cdot} = \frac{1}{n_i} \sum_{j=1}^{n_i} X_{ij} \quad \text{and} \quad \overline{Y}_{i\cdot} = \frac{1}{n_i} \sum_{j=1}^{n_i} Y_{ij}.$$

The residual sum of squares for batch i is given as

$$\text{SSE}(i) = S_{YY}(i) - \frac{[S_{XY}(i)]^2}{S_{XX}(i)}. \tag{11.3.6}$$

The combined residual sum of squares is the sum of individual residual sum of squares over all batches, that is,

$$\text{SSE} = \sum_{i=1}^{K} \text{SSE}(i), \tag{11.3.7}$$

which has $N - 2K$ degrees of freedom. On the other hand, the residual sum of squares computed from $S_{XX}(W)$, $S_{XY}(W)$, and $S_{YY}(W)$ is given by

$$\text{SSE}(W) = S_{YY}(W) - \frac{[S_{XY}(W)]^2}{S_{XX}(W)}, \tag{11.3.8}$$

which has $N - K - 1$ degrees of freedom. It follows that the sum of squares for the difference in slopes is given by

$$SS(\beta) = SSE(W) - SSE. \qquad (11.3.9)$$

Therefore, the null hypothesis of equality of slopes is rejected at the α level of significance if

$$F_\beta = \frac{MS(\beta)}{MSE} > F(\alpha, K - 1, N - 2K), \qquad (11.3.10)$$

where

$$MS(\beta) = \frac{SS(\beta)}{K - 1} \quad \text{and} \quad MSE = \frac{SSE}{N - 2K}$$

and $F(\alpha, K - 1, N - 2K)$ is the αth upper quantile of a central F distribution with $K - 1$ and $N - 2K$ degrees of freedom.

Let $w_i = 1/S_{xx}(i)$ and $\bar{b}$ be the weighted mean of the least squares estimates of slopes, that is,

$$\bar{b} = \frac{\sum_{i=1}^{K} w_i b_i}{\sum_{i=1}^{K} w_i}. \qquad (11.3.11)$$

The sum of squares for the differences of slopes can be obtained as

$$SS(\beta) = \sum_{i=1}^{K} w_i(b_i - \bar{b})^2. \qquad (11.3.12)$$

If the null hypothesis of equal slopes is not rejected at the α level of significance, β_i in model (11.3.1) can be replaced by a common slope β and model (11.3.1) reduces to

$$Y_{ij} = \alpha_i + \beta X_{ij} + e_{ij}, \quad i = 1, \ldots, K, \quad j = 1, \ldots, n_i. \qquad (11.3.13)$$

The null hypothesis of equal intercepts can be treated as the null hypothesis of equal batch effects after adjustment for the linear regression between time and percent of label claim. This can be obtained by a direct application of the analysis of covariance. Define

$$S_{XX}(T) = \sum_{i=1}^{K} \sum_{j=1}^{n_i} (X_{ij} - \bar{X}_{..})^2,$$

$$S_{YY}(T) = \sum_{i=1}^{K} \sum_{j=1}^{n_i} (Y_{ij} - \bar{Y}_{..})^2,$$

$$S_{XY}(T) = \sum_{i=1}^{K} \sum_{j=1}^{n_i} (X_{ij} - \bar{X}_{..}) (Y_{ij} - \bar{Y}_{..}),$$

$$S_{XX}(B) = \sum_{i=1}^{K} n_i (\bar{X}_{i\cdot} - \bar{X}_{..})^2,$$

$$S_{YY}(B) = \sum_{i=1}^{K} n_i (\bar{Y}_{i\cdot} - \bar{Y}_{..})^2,$$

$$S_{XY}(B) = \sum_{i=1}^{K} n_i (\bar{X}_{i\cdot} - \bar{X}_{..}) (\bar{Y}_{i\cdot} - \bar{Y}_{..}), \tag{11.3.14}$$

where

$$\bar{X}_{..} = \frac{1}{N} \sum_{i=1}^{K} \sum_{j=1}^{n_i} X_{ij},$$

$$\bar{Y}_{..} = \frac{1}{N} \sum_{i=1}^{K} \sum_{j=1}^{n_i} Y_{ij}.$$

The total sum of deviations from regression is given as

$$\text{SST} = S_{YY}(T) - \frac{[S_{XY}(T)]^2}{S_{XX}(T)}. \tag{11.3.15}$$

Similarly, the within-batch sum of deviations from regression is SSE(*W*) given in (11.3.8). The between-batch sum of deviations from regression can be obtained by subtraction as

$$\text{SSB} = \text{SST} - \text{SSE}(W). \tag{11.3.16}$$

The degrees of freedom associated with SST, SSW, and SSB are $N - 2$, $N - K - 1$, and $K - 1$, respectively. Hence the corresponding between- and within-batch mean squares after adjustment for regression are given by

$$\text{MSB} = \frac{\text{SSB}}{K - 1} \quad \text{and} \quad \text{MSW} = \frac{\text{SSE}(W)}{N - K - 1}, \tag{11.3.17}$$

respectively. The null hypothesis of equality of intercepts is rejected if

$$F'_\alpha = \frac{\text{MSB}}{\text{MSW}} > F(\alpha, K - 1, N - K - 1), \tag{11.3.18}$$

where $F(\alpha, K - 1, N - K - 1)$ is the αth upper quantile of a central F distribution with $K - 1$ and $N - K - 1$ degrees of freedom.

Note that the least-squares estimate of the common slope in model (11.3.13) is given by

$$b = \frac{S_{XY}(W)}{S_{XX}(W)}. \qquad (11.3.19)$$

The inference about β in model (11.3.13) can be obtained based on b and

$$SE(b) = \frac{MSW}{S_{XX}(W)}. \qquad (11.3.20)$$

Note that test statistic F'_α is derived under the assumption that there is a common slope as described in model (11.3.13). Therefore, F'_α is the test statistic for the following hypotheses:

$$H_0: \alpha_i = \alpha_{i'}; \beta_i = \beta_{i'} \text{ for all } i \ne i'$$
$$\text{vs. } H_a: \alpha_i \ne \alpha_{i'} \text{ for some } i \ne i' \text{ and } \beta_i = \beta_{i'} \text{ for all } i \ne i' \qquad (11.3.21)$$

On the other hand, test statistic for the unrestricted null hypotheses (11.3.3) can be obtained as

$$F_\alpha = \frac{MSB}{MSE}. \qquad (11.3.22)$$

We then reject the unrestricted null hypothesis of equal intercepts if

$$F_\alpha > F(\alpha, K - 1, N - 2K). \qquad (11.3.23)$$

These results are summarized in the ANCOVA table (see Table 11.3.1). Note that the sum of squares due to the common slope is given by

$$SSS = \frac{[S_{XY}(W)]^2}{S_{XX}(W)}. \qquad (11.3.24)$$

It can easily be verified that the sum of squares for the sum of the differences of slopes in (11.3.12) is also the sum of squares due to the interaction between time and batch.

Note that the FDA guideline indicates that the preliminary tests for the equality of slopes and the equality of intercepts be performed at the 0.25 level of significance as suggested by Bancroft (1964). Bancroft (1964) suggested that one preliminary test be performed for the two commonly used models: the two-stage nested model and the two-way cross-classification mixed model. However, as discussed above, testing for batch similarity on degradation lines basically involves two preliminary tests: one for the equality of slopes and the other for the equality of intercepts. In the FDA guideline it is not stated clearly whether

TABLE 11.3.1   ANCOVA Table for Model (11.3.1)

Source variation	df	Sum of squares	Mean square	F statistic
Intercept (batch)	$k - 1$	SSB	MSB	F_α = MSB/MSE
Time (common slope)	1	SSS[a]	MSS	F_s = MSS/MSE
Different in slope (batch-by-time)	$k - 1$	SS(β)	MS(β)	F_β = MS(β)/MSE
Error	$N - 2k$	SSE	MSE	
Total	$N - 1$	SST		

[a]SSS = $[S_{xy}(W)]^2/S_{xx}(W)$.

the 0.25 level of significance should be applied to each of the two preliminary tests separately or should be used as the overall significance level for the following joint hypotheses:

$$H_0: \alpha_i = \alpha_{i'} \text{ and } \beta_i = \beta_{i'} \text{ for all } i \neq i'$$

vs. $$H_a: \alpha_i \neq \alpha_{i'} \text{ or } \beta_i \neq \beta_{i'} \text{ for some } i \neq i'. \qquad (11.3.25)$$

11.4. MINIMUM APPROACH FOR MULTIPLE BATCHES

If the preliminary tests for the equality of slopes and the equality of intercepts are not rejected at the 0.25 level of significance for the null hypothesis of batch similarity of the degradation lines among batches, all batches are considered from the same population of production batches with a common degradation pattern. As a result, model (11.3.1) reduces to

$$Y_{ij} = \alpha + \beta X_{ij} + e_{ij}, \qquad i = 1, \ldots, K, \quad j = 1, \ldots, n_i, \qquad (11.4.1)$$

where α and β are the common intercept and slope for model (11.4.1) and the same normality assumption is posed for e_{ij}.

The procedure for estimating an expiration dating period of single batch described in Sec. 11.2 can be applied directly to the pooled stability data from all batches. The least-squares estimates of β, α, and σ^2 are then given by

$$b_c = \frac{S_{XY}(T)}{S_{XX}(T)},$$

$$a_c = \overline{Y}_{..} - b\overline{X}_{..},$$

$$s_c^2 = \frac{S_{YY}(T) - bS_{XY}(T)}{N - 2}, \qquad (11.4.2)$$

where $S_{XX}(T)$, $S_{YY}(T)$, $S_{XY}(T)$, $\bar{X}_{..}$, $\bar{Y}_{..}$, and N are as defined in (11.3.14). The least-squares estimate of the mean degradation line at time point $t = x$ is given as

$$y(x) = a_c + b_c x \tag{11.4.3}$$

with its least-squares estimate of the variance

$$\hat{V}[y(x)] = s_c^2 \left[\frac{1}{N} + \frac{(x - \bar{X})^2}{S_{XX}(T)} \right]. \tag{11.4.4}$$

Therefore, the 95% lower confidence limit for the mean degradation line is given as

$$L_c(x) = a_c + b_c x - t(0.05, N - 2)\text{SE}(x), \tag{11.4.5}$$

where

$$\text{SE}(x) = \sqrt{\hat{V}[y(x)]},$$

and $t(0.05, N - 2)$ is the 5% upper quantile of a central t distribution with $N - 2$ degrees of freedom. Hence the overall expiration dating period can be estimated as the small root $x_L(c)$ of the following quadratic equation:

$$[\eta - (a_c + b_c x)]^2 = t^2(0.05, N - 2)s_c^2 \left[\frac{1}{N} + \frac{(x - \bar{X})^2}{S_{XX}(T)} \right]. \tag{11.4.6}$$

The conditions for the existence of the root $x_L(c)$ for the quadratic equation above are the same as those given in (11.2.10) and (11.2.11) for a single batch. However, the standard error of slope and intercept estimated from the pooled stability data should be used to evaluate the two conditions.

Since under the assumption that all batches come from a population for which the degradation pattern can be described accurately by model (11.4.1) with the common slope and intercept, the pooled stability data from all batches provide more precise least-squares estimates of slope, intercept, and variability. Hence the 95% confidence limit for the mean degradation line becomes much narrower because they are based on the pooled stability data with $N - 2$ degrees of freedom. Therefore, if model (11.4.1) is adequate, the expiration dating period estimated from the pooled stability data is longer than those estimated from individual batches.

On the other hand, if preliminary tests based on (11.3.10) and (11.3.22) are rejected at the 0.25 level of significance, the degradation lines of individual batches can not be considered the same because of different slopes and/or different intercepts. In this case, according to the FDA guideline, the overall expiration dating period may depend on the minimum time that a batch is expected to remain within acceptable limits. Therefore, let $x_L(i)$ be the estimated shelf life for batch i, $i = 1, \ldots, K$. Then an intuitive estimate of the overall expiration dating period which meets the FDA requirements may be obtained as follows:

$$x_L(\min) = \min\{x_L(1), \ldots, x_L(K)\}. \tag{11.4.7}$$

Since $x_L(\min)$ is the shortest shelf life among all batches, this estimate will provide a 95% confidence that the strength of the drug product will remain above the acceptable lower specification limit η until $x_L(\min)$ for all batches. However, $x_L(\min)$ is a conservative estimate of the overall expiration dating period because it provides more than 95% confidence for all batches except the batch from which it is estimated. The approach above is usually referred to as the minimum approach.

The minimum approach for estimation of the overall shelf life of a drug product is elected when the preliminary tests for batch similarity are rejected (i.e., there are different intercepts and different slopes) at the 0.25 level of significance. However, the procedure for testing the batch similarity of degradation lines and the minimum approach for determination of shelf life as the estimated overall expiration dating period have received considerable criticisms because of their shortcomings. For example, Chow and Shao (1991) indicated that the minimum approach lacks statistical justification. Ruberg and Stegeman (1991) and Ruberg and Hsu (1992) illustrated the disadvantages for using the minimum approach through two numerical data sets of six batches. The ANCOVA tables for the two stability data sets in Ruberg and Stegeman (1991) are reported in Tables 11.4.1 and 11.4.2, respectively. The results of fitting the least squares to individual batches and to the pooled stability data with the estimated shelf lives for both data sets are summarized in Tables 11.4.3 and 11.4.4. Figures 11.4.1 and 11.4.2. give the stability data and individual regression lines. Note that the overall shelf life presented in Tables 11.4.3. and 11.4.4 were obtained under model (11.3.13) with a common slope and different intercepts in Ruberg and Stegeman (1991).

From Table 11.4.1, the F statistic for overall difference in slopes obtained from stability data set 1 is 1.64 with a p value of 0.186. Hence the null hypothesis of equal slopes is rejected at the 0.25 level of significance. According

TABLE 11.4.1 ANCOVA Table for Data Set 1

Source variation	df	Sum of squares	F statistic	p value
Intercepts	5	0.60	2.85	0.038
Time	1	21.52	503.24	<0.001
Different in slopes	5	0.35	1.64	0.186
Error	25	1.07		

Source: Ruberg and Stegeman (1991).

TABLE 11.4.2 ANCOVA Table for Data Set 2

Source variation	df	Sum of squares	F statistic	p value
Intercepts	5	15.93	4.01	0.009
Time	1	4.14	5.21	0.032
Different in slopes	5	4.60	1.16	0.359
Error	25	18.28		

Source: Ruberg and Stegeman (1991).

TABLE 11.4.3 Results of Least-Squares Regression for Stability Data Set 1

Batch	n	Intercept	Slope	s^2	S_{xx}	Shelf life
1	9	100.49	−1.515	0.019	14.63	6.7
2	7	100.66	−1.449	0.043	7.83	6.8
3	7	100.25	−1.682	0.062	5.14	5.5
4	6	100.45	−1.393	0.035	1.38	6.2
5	4	100.45	−1.999	0.011	0.61	4.4
6	4	99.98	−1.701	0.124	0.61	3.5
Pooled		99.90	−1.534	0.047		6.2

Source: Ruberg and Stegeman (1991).

TABLE 11.4.4 Results of Least-Squares Regression for Stability Data Set 2

Batch	n	Intercept	Slope	s^2	S_{xx}	Shelf life
1	9	100.48	−0.109	0.343	14.63	32.3
2	6	103.63	−0.449	0.703	2.96	9.6
3	7	101.24	−0.778	1.189	5.14	7.0
4	5	102.21	0.194	0.221	1.26	16.2
5	4	102.21	−2.218	0.256	0.61	3.2
6	4	100.07	−1.045	2.973	0.61	1.7
Pooled		100.41	−0.330	0.628		18.2

Source: Ruberg and Stegeman (1991).

to the FDA guideline, the stability data of six batches in data set 1 cannot be pooled. Hence the overall expiration dating period was determined using the minimum approach. Since batch 6 gives the minimum shelf life among the six batches, the estimated shelf life of 3.5 years from batch 6 is then used as the overall expiration dating period. On the other hand, for data set 2, the null

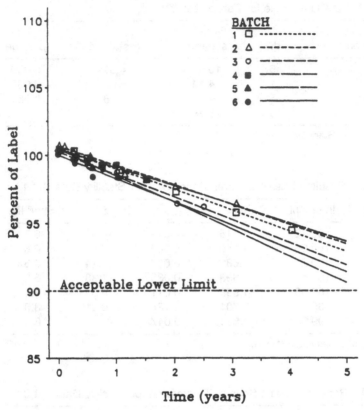

FIGURE 11.4.1   Stability data and individual regression lines for data set 1. [From Ruberg and Stegeman (1991).]

hypothesis of equal slopes is not rejected at the 0.25 level of significance because the p value for the difference in slopes is 0.359 as shown in Table 11.4.2. Ruberg and Stegeman (1991) then pooled the stability data over six batches to estimate the overall expiration dating period, which gives a shelf life of 18.2 years under model (11.3.13).

It is quite evident from Figs. 11.4.1. and 11.4.2 that the variability of stability data set 1 is much smaller than that of data set 2. However, following the FDA guideline for the use of the significance level of 0.25 for the null hypothesis of the equality of slopes, stability data set 2, with a much larger variability, can be pooled, but stability data set 1, with a smaller variability, cannot be pooled over batches. Therefore, a paradox occurs. As indicated by Ruberg and Stegeman (1991), well-designed and carefully executed stability

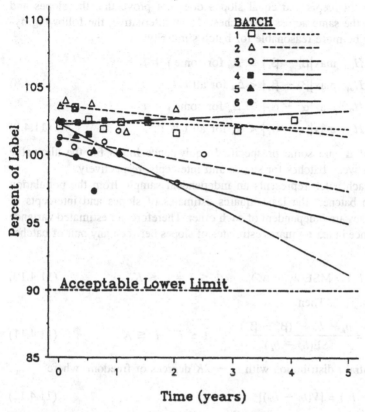

FIGURE 11.4.2 Stability data and individual regression lines for data set 2. [From Ruberg and Stegeman (1991).]

studies generate reliable and less variable data to provide least-squares estimates of the mean degradation lines and their variances with high precision and efficiency, yet the accuracy, precision, and efficiency of these estimates cannot be utilized for estimation of the overall expiration dating period simply because the less variable data are able to detect smaller differences of no practical importance in slopes as being of statistical significance due to a quite arbitrary choice of a significance level of 0.25. Therefore, good stability studies are in fact penalized for their small variability by the recommendation as to the choice of the significance level in the FDA guideline.

Another reason which might explain the paradox is that the null hypotheses of equal slopes and equal intercepts are in fact wrong hypotheses for batch similarity of degradation lines among batches. Failure to reject the null hypotheses of equal intercepts and equal slopes does not prove that the slopes and intercepts are the same across all batches. As an alternative, the following hypotheses may be more reasonable for batch similarity:

$$H_{0\beta}: \max|\beta_i - \beta_{i'}| \geq \Delta_\beta \text{ for some } i \neq i'$$

vs. $$H_{a\beta}: \max|\beta_i - \beta_{i'}| < \Delta_\beta \text{ for all } i \neq i, \qquad (11.4.8)$$

$$H_{0\alpha}: \max|\alpha_i - \alpha_{i'}| \geq \Delta_\alpha \text{ for some } i \neq i'$$

vs. $$H_{a\alpha}: \max|\alpha_i - \alpha_{i'}| < \Delta_\alpha \text{ for all } i \neq i', \qquad (11.4.9)$$

where Δ_β and Δ_α are some prespecified equivalence limits for the allowable differences between batches for slopes and intercepts, respectively.

Since each batch represents an independent sample from the population of production batches, the least-squares estimates of slopes and intercepts of different batches are independent of each other. Therefore, an estimated variance of the difference in least-squares estimates of slopes between any pair of batches is given by

$$\hat{V}(b_i - b_{i'}) = \text{MSE}(w_i + w_{i'}), \qquad 1 \leq i \neq i' \leq K, \qquad (11.4.10)$$

where $w_i = 1/S_{xx}(i)$. Then

$$T_b(i,i') = \frac{b_i - b_{i'} - (\beta_i - \beta_{i'})}{\text{SE}(b_i - b_{i'})}, \qquad 1 \leq i \neq i' \leq K, \qquad (11.4.11)$$

follows a central t distribution with $N - 2K$ degrees of freedom, where

$$\text{SE}(b_i - b_{i'}) = [\hat{V}(b_i - b_{i'})]^{\frac{1}{2}}. \qquad (11.4.12)$$

Let

$$T_{\max}(\beta) = \max_{1 \leq i < i' \leq K} |T_b(i,i')|. \qquad (11.4.13)$$

Then $\sqrt{2}T_{\max}(\beta)$ is distributed as the range of K independent standard normal random variables divided by the square root of a central chi-square random variable with $N - 2K$ degress of freedom divided by $N - 2K$. Since

$$\max| \beta_i - \beta_{i'}| = \beta_{\max} - \beta_{\min}, \qquad i \leq i \neq i' \leq K,$$

the hypotheses of the similarity for slopes in (11.4.8) can be reformulated as

$$H_{0\beta}: \beta_{\max} - \beta_{\min} > \Delta_\beta \quad \text{vs.} \quad H_{a\beta}: \beta_{\max} < \Delta_\beta, \qquad (11.4.14)$$

where

$$\beta_{\max} = \max\{\beta_1, \ldots, \beta_K\},$$
$$\beta_{\min} = \min\{\beta_1, \ldots, b_K\}. \qquad (11.4.15)$$

Then the $(1 - \alpha) \times 100\%$ upper confidence interval for the maximum of all pairwise differences between β_i and $\beta_{i'}$ for $i \neq i'$ or $\beta_{max} - \beta_{min}$ is given as $U_{max}(\beta)$, where

$$U_{max}(\beta) = b_{max} - b_{min} + (0.5)^{1/2} Q(\alpha, k, N$$
$$- 2K)\text{SE}(b_{max} - b_{min}), \quad (11.4.16)$$

where b_{max}, b_{min}, and $\text{SE}(b_{max} - b_{min})$ are defined similarly to (11.4.15) and (11.4.12), respectively, and $Q(\alpha, K, N - 2K)$ is the αth upper quantile of studentized range distribution with parameter K and $N - 2K$ degrees of freedom (provided in Appendix A.8). A procedure for the interval hypothesis (11.4.8) for testing the similarity of slopes among batches is to reject $H_{0\beta}$ if the $(1 - \alpha) \times 100\%$ upper confidence interval $U_{max}(\beta)$ is smaller than Δ_β. Let

$$T_U(\beta) = \frac{b_{max} - b_{min} - \Delta_\beta}{(0.5)^{1/2} \, \text{SE}(b_{max} - b_{min})}. \quad (11.4.17)$$

Then $H_{0\beta}$ in (11.4.14) is rejected at the α level of significance if

$$T_U(\beta) < -Q(\alpha, K, N - 2K). \quad (11.4.18)$$

Note that the confidence limit approach given in (11.4.16) is operationally equivalent to the hypothesis-testing procedure described in (11.4.17). Similarly, the $(1 - \alpha) \times 100\%$ upper confidence limit and the testing procedure can be applied to hypotheses (11.4.9) for the similarity of intercepts among batches. Note that the estimated variance of the difference in least-squares estimates of intercepts between two batches is given as follows:

$$\hat{V}(a_i - a_{i'}) = \text{MSE} \left[\frac{US_{xx}(i)}{n_i S_{xx}(i)} + \frac{US_{xx}(i')}{n_{i'} S_{xx}(i')} \right], \quad (11.4.19)$$

where $i \leq i \neq i' \leq K$ and $US_{xx}(i)$ is the uncorrected sum of squares of x for batch i.

11.5. MULTIPLE COMPARISON PROCEDURE FOR POOLING BATCHES

As mentioned in Sec. 11.4, the current FDA requirement for pooling data has the following disadvantages:

1. The choice of the significance level of 0.25 for testing batch similarity may penalize good stability studies with small variabilities.
2. The minimum approach ignores the information from other batches for estimation of an overall expiration dating period.
3. The use of wrong hypotheses of equality to test batch similarity in terms of intercepts and slopes of degradation lines among batches.

Under the assumption of fixed batch effects for model (11.3.1), Ruberg and Hsu (1992) proposed an approach using the concept of multiple comparison to derive some criteria for pooling batches with the worst batches. Instead of testing the null hypothesis of the equality of slopes, they suggested investigating a simultaneous confidence interval for

$$\theta_i = \beta_i - \min_{i \neq i'} \beta_{i'} \qquad \text{for } i = 1, \ldots, K \tag{11.5.1}$$

From (11.5.1), the worst batch is defined as the batch with the largest degradation rate or minimum slope. If Δ_β is some equivalence limit for the allowable difference between batches as defined in (11.4.8), the idea of Ruberg and Hsu (1992) for combining stability data from a certain number of batches is to pool the batches:

$$\theta_i = \beta_i - \min_{i \neq i'} \beta_{i'} < \Delta_\beta \tag{11.5.2}$$

In other words, Ruberg and Hsu's procedure is to pool the batches that have slopes similar to the worst degradation rate with respect to the equivalence limit Δ_β.

To illustrate Ruberg and Hsu's procedure, let us start with an arbitary batch, say batch i, as the reference batch. We first calculate all possible lower confidence limits:

$$\ell_{ii'} = (b_i - b_{i'}) - d_i(\alpha)\text{SE}(b_i - b_{i'}) \qquad \text{for } i \leq i \neq i' \leq K, \tag{11.5.3}$$

where $\text{SE}(b_i - b_{i'})$ is as defined in (11.4.12) and $d_i(\alpha)$ is the $(1 - \alpha) \times 100\%$ critical values for the confidence interval of

$$\beta_i - \min_{i \neq i} \beta_{i'},$$

which depends on the degrees of freedom for the combined residual sum of squares and the $(K - 1) \times (K - 1)$ correlation matrix of

$$b_i - b_{i'}, \qquad i = 1, \ldots, K.$$
$$\scriptstyle i \neq i'$$

The lower limit of the $(1 - \alpha) \times 100\%$ confidence interval for θ_i is then given by

$$L_i = \min(\ell_i, 0), \qquad i = 1, \ldots, K, \tag{11.5.4}$$

where

$$\ell_i = \max_{i \neq i'} (\ell_{ii'}), \, i = 1, \ldots, K.$$

We then repeat the procedure above with each batch as the reference batch to compute the lower limit L_i, $i = 1, \ldots, K$. Note that if $\ell_{ii'} > 0$, according to (11.5.4), the lower limit for the $(1 - \alpha) \times 100\%$ confidence interval is zero. Therefore, the degradation rate is statistically significantly different from the true minimum slope, and the ith batch is not the worst batch. On the other hand, let G be the set of all batches with the smallest slope:

$$G = \{i, \ell_i < 0\}.$$

Hence G is the set that contains all possible worst batches. The computation of the upper limit of the $(1 - \alpha) \times 100\%$ confidence interval for θ_i depends on the number of batches in G. If G contains only a single batch g, batch g has the largest degradation rate and the upper limit of the $(1 - \alpha) \times 100\%$ confidence interval for θ_i is then given by

$$U_i = \begin{cases} 0 & \text{if } i = g \\ (b_i - b_g) + d_g(\alpha)\text{SE}(b_i - b_g) & \text{if } i \neq g. \end{cases} \qquad (11.5.5)$$

If G contains more than one batch, calculate all possible upper confidence limits using the batches in G as the candidate batches for the worst batches as follows:

$$u_{ig} = (b_i - b_g) + d_g(\alpha)\text{SE}(b_i - b_g) \qquad \text{for all } g \in G \text{ and } i \neq g.$$

The upper limit of the $(1 - \alpha) \times 100\%$ confidence interval for θ_i is then given by

$$U_i = \max(u_i, 0), \qquad (11.5.6)$$

where

$$u_i = \max_{i \neq g} (u_{ig}).$$

As indicated earlier, calculation of critical values $d_i(\alpha)$ depends on the correlation matrix of

$$\underset{i \neq i'}{b_i - b_{i'}}, \qquad i = 1, \ldots, K.$$

Let

$$\lambda_{i'} = \left[1 + \frac{S_{xx}(i)}{S_{xx}(i')}\right]^{-1/2}. \qquad (11.5.7)$$

Then the off-diagonal elements of the correlation matrix of

$$\underset{i \neq i'}{b_i - b_{i'}}, \qquad i = 1, \ldots, K,$$

are given as

$$r_{i'i''} = \lambda_{i'}\lambda_{i'}, \qquad i' \neq i''. \qquad (11.5.8)$$

If $S_{xx}(i) = S_{xx}(i')$ for $1 \leq i \neq i'$, then $d_i(\alpha)$ is Dunnett's one-sided αth upper quantile with $K - 1$ and $N - 2K$ degrees of freedom (given in Appendix A.9). However, if $S_{xx}(i) \neq S_{xx}(i')$ for some $i \neq i'$, $d_i(\alpha)$ is the solution of integration of the multivariant t distribution which as proved in Ruberg and Hsu (1992). In practice, numerical integration is required to obtain $d_i(\alpha)$. Since numerical integration of the multivariate t distribution is sometimes quite tedious and computer routines for numerical integration may not be available, Ruberg and Hsu (1992) suggested the use of the Tukey–Kramer procedure for all pairwise comparisons of degradation rates. The critical values used in the Tukey–Kramer procedure are the upper quantile of the studentized range distribution $Q(\alpha, K, N - 2K)$ given in (11.4.16), which are available in any introductory statistical textbook. The Tukey–Kramer $(1 - \alpha) \times 100\%$ simultaneous confidence intervals for all pairwise comparison between β_i and $\beta_{i'}$ are given by

$$u_{ii'} \; (\ell_{ii'}) = (b_i - b_{i'}) \pm (0.5)^{1/2} \, Q(\alpha, K, N - 2K)\mathrm{SE}(b_i - b_{i'}), \qquad (11.5.9)$$

where $i \leq i \neq i' \leq K$. Consequently, the lower and upper limits for the $(1 - \alpha) \times 100\%$ confidence interval for

$$\theta_i = \beta_i - \min_{i \neq i'} \beta_{i'}$$

are given, respectively, as

$$L_i = \max_{i \neq i'} (\ell_{ii'}),$$

$$U_i = \max_{i \neq i'} (u_{ii'}). \qquad\qquad (11.5.10)$$

Ruberg and Hsu (1992) also suggested two sets of decision rules for pooling stability data over batches. The first uses an FDA-like approach (FDA, 1987), and the second is a bioequivalence-like approach. (Chow and Liu, 1992). In the FDA-like approach, 75% simultaneous confidence intervals are calculated. The decision rules for pooling batches are as follows:

1. If $L_i = 0$, batch i is not a candidate for the worst batch.
2. Since the event $U_i = 0$ can only occur for at most one batch; therefore, if $U_i = 0$, batch i is the only candidate for the worst batch.
3. If $L_i < 0$ and $U_i > 0$, pool all such batches for slope estimation because they are candidates for the worst batch.

Since this approach is the version of confidence intervals for the null hypothesis of the equality of slopes, as recommended in the FDA guideline, it suffers the same drawbacks. Stability studies with a poor design and large variability will produce a wide simultaneous confidence interval for θ_i and allow too many batches to be pooled. On the other hand, fewer batches from good stability studies cannot be pooled for an accurate, precise, and efficient estimation because of tighter confidence intervals for θ_i due to the small variability.

For the bioequivalence-like approach, we first compute the 95% upper confidence limits U_i for all θ_i, $i = 1, \ldots, K$. Then pool batches with $U_i < \Delta_\beta$, where Δ_β is a prespecified upper allowable specification limit. It all $U_i > \Delta_\beta$, no batch can be pooled. In this case, shelf lives are computed separately for each batch and the minimum among all batches is used to estimate the overall expiration dating period. This is a much more reasonable approach because it is also based on the concept of similarity, as discussed in Sec. 11.4. As a result, good studies with tight upper confidence limit will not be penalized any more by using the bioequivalence-like approach.

11.6. EXAMPLE

A stability study was conducted on 300-mg tablets of a drug product to establish an overall expiration dating period. Tablets from five different batches were stored at room temperature (25°C) in two different types of containers (i.e., high-density polyethylene bottle and blister package). The tablets were tested for potency at 0, 3, 6, 9, 12, and 18 months. The assay results (expressed as percent of label claim) were reported in Shao and Chow (1994). These results are given in Table 11.6.1. Note that this data set contains sampling-time intervals only up to 18 months, which does not cover the entire range of sampling-time points up to 60 months or more. In addition, assays of all batches were performed at the same time points. Therefore, this data set represents the simplest structure of a stability study. Because of its simplicity, assay results from bottle container are

TABLE 11.6.1 Assay Results in Percent of Label Claim

Package	Batch	Sampling time (months)					
		0	3	6	9	12	18
Bottle	1	104.8	102.5	101.5	102.4	99.4	96.5
	2	103.9	101.9	103.2	99.6	100.2	98.8
	3	103.5	102.1	101.9	100.3	99.2	101.0
	4	101.5	100.3	101.1	100.6	100.7	98.4
	5	106.1	104.3	101.5	101.1	99.4	98.2
Blister	1	102.0	101.6	100.9	101.1	101.7	97.1
	2	104.7	101.3	103.8	99.8	98.9	97.1
	3	102.5	102.3	100.0	101.7	99.0	100.9
	4	100.1	101.8	101.4	99.9	99.2	97.4
	5	105.2	104.1	102.4	100.2	99.6	97.5

selected to illustrate statistical concepts and computational procedures discussed in this chapter.

Figure 11.6.1 displays the scatter plot of stability data given in Table 11.6.1 with the acceptable lower specification limit equal to 90%. The stability data of batch 1 using the bottle container in Table 11.6.1 are chosen to demonstrate the computation of the shelf life for a single batch. It can easily be verified that

$$\overline{X} = 8, \quad \overline{Y} = 101.183, \quad S_{XX} = 210, \quad S_{XY} = -88.9, \quad \text{and} \quad S_{YY} = 41.508.$$

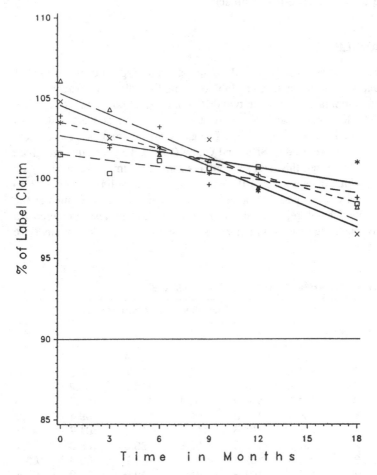

FIGURE 11.6.1   Scatter plot of stability data in Table 11.6.1. x, Batch 1; +, batch 2; *, batch 3; □, batch 4; △, batch 5.

Therefore, the least-squares estimates of slope, intercept, and error variance are given, respectively, as

$$b = -\frac{88.9}{210} = -0.423,$$

$$a = 101.183 - (-0.423)(8) = 104.57,$$

$$s^2 = \frac{41.508 - (-0.423)(-88.9)}{4} = 0.969.$$

Hence the least-squares estimates of the mean degradation line at time $t = x$ is given as

$$y(x) = 104.57 - 0.423x.$$

The corresponding ANOVA table is provided in Table 11.6.2, and the standard error of the least-squares estimates for slope and intercept are given by

$$SE(b) = 0.0679 \quad \text{and} \quad SE(a) = 0.676,$$

respectively. Before we apply (11.2.8) to calculate the shelf life, we need to check conditions (11.2.10) and (11.2.11). Since for $\eta = 90$,

$$T_a = \frac{104.57 - 90}{0.656} = 22.21$$

with a p value less than 0.001 and

$$T_b = \frac{-0.423}{0.0679} = -6.234$$

with a p value of 0.0017, both conditions are met. If $\eta = 90$ is selected to be the acceptable lower specification limit, the shelf life is estimated as the smaller root of the following equation:

$$[90 - [104.57 + (-0.423)x]]^2 = (2.132)^2(0.969)\left[\frac{1}{6} + \frac{(x - 8)^2}{210}\right].$$

TABLE 11.6.2 ANOVA Table for Batch 1 of Bottle Container Stability Data Set in Table 11.6.1

Source variation	df	Sum of squares	Mean squares	F value	p value
Regression	1	37.634	37.634	38.858	0.0034
Residual	4	3.874	0.969		
Total	5	41.508			

Therefore, the estimated expiration dating period for batch 1 with bottle container is 27.5 months. The stability data with estimated regression line, the 95% lower confidence limit for the mean degradation line, and the acceptable lower specification limit of 90% are plotted in Fig. 11.6.2.

A summary of the results on estimation of slopes and intercepts by least-squares regression is provided in Table 11.6.3. along with the corresponding standard errors. It can be verified that conditions (11.2.10) and (11.2.11) are both satisfied for all batches except for batch 3. The slope of batch 3 is estimated as -0.168 with a standard error of 0.08. Therefore, T_b is -2.1 with a p value of 0.053. Therefore, the slope of batch 3 is not statistically significantly smaller

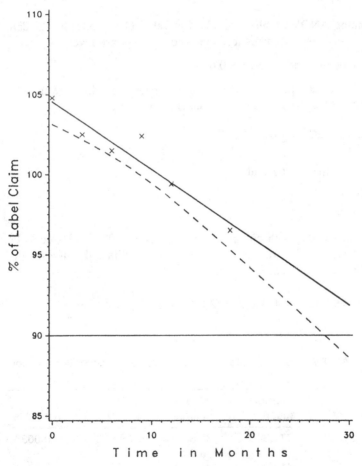

FIGURE 11.6.2. Degradation line and 90% lower confidence limit for batch 1.

than zero at the 0.05 level of significance. Consequently, the shelf life cannot be estimated by the method described in (11.2.8). Table 11.6.4 provides the ANCOVA table for the data set given in Table 11.6.1. The F value for the difference in slopes is 4.36 with a p value of 0.0107. Thus, according to the FDA guideline, the stability data presented in Table 11.6.1 cannot be pooled for estimation of a common slope for all batches.

Suppose from previous experience that the specification for the minimum allowable degradation rate is 0.33% of the label claim per month. From Table 11.6.2, $b_{max} = -0.135$ and $b_{min} = -0.441$. Then

$$T_U(\beta) = \frac{-0.135 - (-0.441) - 0.35}{0.0676} = -0.651,$$

which is larger than $-Q(0.05,5,20) = -4.232$. Hence the null hypothesis of (11.4.8) is not rejected at the 5% level of significance. Hence the stability data given in Table 11.6.1 cannot be pooled with respect to a Δ_β of 0.33% per month. It can be verified that if Δ_β was chosen to be 0.6%, the null hypothesis would have been rejected. Therefore, knowledge and experience with the maximum

TABLE 11.6.3 Summary Results of Least-Squares Estimation of Slopes and Intercepts

Batch	Intercept	SE(a)	Slope	SE(b)	s^2
1	104.57	0.676	−0.423	0.068	0.969
2	103.50	0.742	−0.280	0.075	1.166
3	102.67	0.800	−0.168	0.080	1.358
4	101.51	0.488	−0.135	0.049	0.505
5	105.29	0.614	−0.441	0.062	0.800
Pooled	103.51	0.374	−0.289	0.038	

TABLE 11.6.4 ANCOVA Table for the Stability Data Set in Table 11.6.1

Source variation	df	Sum of squares	Mean squares	F value	p value
Intercept	4	19.09	4.77	4.97	0.0060
Time	1	87.84	87.84	91.53	<0.0001
Difference in slopes	4	16.75	4.19	4.36	0.0107
Error	20	19.19	0.96		
Total	29	129.37			

allowable degradation rate of a drug product is very important and crucial in the decision for pooling stability data.

Since $S_{xx}(i) = S_{xx}(i') = 210$ for all i, the Dunnett's upper 5% one-sided critical value with parameter 5 and degrees of freedom 20 (= 2.39) is used for illustration of Ruberg and Hsu's multiple comparison procedure with the worst batch. The results are summarized in Table 11.6.5 with those computed from the Tukey–Kramer simultaneous confidence intervals. Since $\ell_i > 0$, for batches 3 and 4, the set of all possible worst batches includes batches 1, 2, and 5. Therefore, the upper limits of the 95% confidence interval for θ_i were computed from all possible confidence bounds using batches 1, 2, and 5 as candidates for the worst batches by multiple comparison procedure.

From Table 11.6.5, the 95% confidence intervals of

$$\beta_i - \min_{i \neq i'} \beta_{i'}$$

by a multiple comparison procedure are narrower than those obtained from the Tukey–Kramer method. However, if $\Delta_\beta = 0.33\%$ per month is still selected as the upper allowable degradation rate, by the bioequivalence-like approach, batches 1 and 5 can be pooled for estimation of a common slope and the overall expiration dating period. Table 11.6.6 lists the shelf lives by individual batches. Batch 4 has the longest shelf life; batch 1 produces the shortest shelf life. The shelf life estimation from the data by pooling all five batches is 39.5 months. The pooled data set from batches 1 and 5 generates a shelf life of 30.3 months compared to the minimum approach of 27.5 months from batch 1. On the other

TABLE 11.6.5   95% Confidence Interval of $\theta_i = \beta_i - \min\beta_{i'}$[a]

Method[b]	Batch	95% Confidence interval
MCW	1	(−0.21,0.24)
	2	(−0.07,0.39)
	3	(0.00,0.50)
	4	(0.00,0.53)
	5	(−0.24,0.21)
TK	1	(−0.27,0.30)
	2	(−0.12,0.45)
	3	(−0.01,0.56)
	4	(0.02,0.59)
	5	(−0.30,0.27)

[a]$d_i(\alpha) = 2.39$, the Dunnett's upper one-sided critical value with parameter 5 and 20 degrees of freedom; $Q(0.05,5,20) = 4.232$.
[b]MCW, multiple comparison with the worst; TW, Tukey–Kramer simultaneous confidence intervals.

TABLE 11.6.6 Summary of Estimation of Shelf Lives for Data Set in Table 11.6.1 ($\alpha = 0.05$)

Method	Batch	Shelf life (months)
Individual	1	27.5
	2	33.5
	3	—
	4	51.4
	5	28.6
Pooled	All	39.5
FDA-minimum		27.5
MCW/TK[a]	1,5	30.3
	2,3,4	49.2

[a]MCW-TK, multiple comparison with the worst and Tukey–Kramer simultaneous confidence interval.

hand, the combined data set from the other three batches (2, 3, and 4) gives a shelf life of 49.2 months. Examination of slopes in Table 11.6.3 and Fig. 11.6.1 reveals that those five batches can basically be classified into two groups: one group consists of batches 1 and 5, which have a degradation rate more than 0.4% per month, and the other group contains batches 2, 3, and 4, which have a degradation rate less than 0.3% per month. Therefore, the overall expiration dating period estimated either by batch 1 alone or by batches 1 and 5 combined using the multiple comparison procedure are still quite conservative because the other three batches have much slower degradation rates.

11.7. DISCUSSION

As shown in Table 11.6.6 and Fig. 11.6.1, the estimated shelf lives for all batches for the stability data considered in the example above are beyond the range of observed time intervals. These estimated shelf lives are indeed obtained based on extrapolation from the estimated regression line over the range of the time intervals observed. However, it is not known whether an empirical linear relationship between the strength and time still holds from the last observed time interval to the estimated shelf life. If the true relationship is not linear between these two time points, the shelf life estimated by extrapolation beyond the range of observed time points is seriously biased.

Throughout this chapter, estimation of an expiration dating period for a drug product is based on fitting a linear regression model to the percent of label claim on the original scale. In other words, the assumption of a linear degradation is made for the entire range of time points selected in the stability study.

However, as pointed out in Chapter 9, the true degradation function is generally not linear rather than a simple exponential first-order function. Morris (1992) compares the differences in estimated shelf life between a linear regression and a simple exponential model. The results indicate that if the total amount of degradation over the entire range of time points is less than 15% of the label claim, the difference in estimated shelf life between the two models is quite trivial. On the other hand, if the loss of strength is expected to be greater than 15%, the exponential model should be used for estimation of the expiration dating period. Under the current FDA guideline, the acceptable lower specification limit specified in the USP/NF is usually set to be 90%. This indicates that only a maximum amount of degradation of 10% is allowed. As a result, the current method for fitting a linear regression model to the percent of label claim on the original scale is adequate. However, it is suggested that the use of extrapolation beyond the range of observed time points be carefully evaluated. Thus the FDA guideline requires that an expiration dating period granted on the basis of extrapolation be verified by actual stability data up to the granted expiration time as soon as these data become available.

Comparison of regression lines includes not only examination of the similarity of slopes and intercepts but also the equivalence of the within-batch variability. However, the similarity of within-batch variability is often ignored during the decision making for pooling stability data over batches. Tables 11.4.3 and 11.4.4 indicate that the ratio of the maximum within-batch variability to the minimum is 11.3 and 13.45, respectively, for stability data given in Ruberg and Stegeman (1991), while the same ratio is 2.69 for the data set of the bottle container given in Table 11.6.1. Hence large differences in within-batch variability exist for both data sets of Ruberg and Stegeman (1991). More interestingly, the extremes of within-batch variability occur in the batches with the fewest data points in their data sets. Either Bartlett's chi-square test or Hartley F_{max} test (Gill, 1978) can be applied to examine the null hypothesis of equality of within-batch variability. However, Bartlett's test is quite sensitive to the departure of normality, although it can be generalized to the unequal number of observations with each batch. On the other hand, Hartley's F_{max} test is rather robust against nonnormality. However, it can be applied only to the situation where each batch has the same number of assays. Since the upper 5% quantile of the distribution for F_{max} with five batches and 4 residual degrees of freedom is 25.2 and the observed F_{max} is 2.69 for the stability data of the bottle container for the data set given in Table 11.6.1, the null hypothesis of equal within-batch variability is not rejected at the 5% level of significance. It should be noted that these procedures are for the equality; further research is required for testing the similarity of within-batch variability.

An ideal situation for examination of the similarity of the degradation lines among bottles is that all batches have the same range of time points as shown by the data set given in Table 11.6.1. However, in practice, during the early stage of drug development, the duration of time points may be quite different from batch to batch. For example, in both data sets presented in Ruberg and Stegeman (1991), the duration of time points was more than 4 years for one batch, between 2 to 3 years for two batches, 1.5 years for one batch, and 1 year for two batches. Since the entire degradation pattern is not fully realized for those batches with a short duration, one probably should not test the similarity of degradation lines unless batches also have reached similar ranges of duration.

Under model (11.2.1), the fitted least-squares line is given by

$$y(x) = a + bx.$$

Intuitively, one may consider the time point $t = x$ at which the fitted least-squares line intersects the approved specification limit η as the estimated shelf life; that is, consider

$$x = \frac{\eta - a}{b}$$

as an estimate of the shelf life. However, the FDA guideline clearly indicates that it is not acceptable to determine the allowable expiration dating period by determining where the fitted least-squares line intersects the appropriate specification limit. It should be noted that the lower 95% confidence bound for $E(x)$ is the same as that obtained in (11.2.8).

Similar to the inverse estimator for calibration introduced in Sec. 2.4, an alternative approach for determination of shelf life can be obtained as follows. A fitted least-squares line based on the method of inverse regression is given by

$$x = c + dy,$$

where

$$C = \bar{X} - d\bar{Y},$$
$$d = \frac{S_{XY}}{S_{YY}},$$

and S_{XY} and S_{YY} are as defined before. Therefore, we may construct a 95% confidence interval for the expected value of $x = c + d\eta$. The lower 95% confidence limit can then be used to estimate the shelf life. Note that it may be of interest to study the relative accuracy and precision for determination of drug shelf life based on the classical linear regression model or an inverse linear regression described above.

12

Stability Analysis with Random Batches

12.1. INTRODUCTION

To establish an expiration dating period, as indicated earlier, the FDA guideline requires that at least three batches, and preferably more, be tested in stability analysis to account for batch-to-batch variation so that a single shelf life is applicable to all future batches manufactured under similar circumstances. Under the assumption that the drug characteristic decreases linearly over time, the FDA guideline indicates that if there is no documented evidence for batch-to-batch variation (i.e., all the batches have the same shelf life), the single shelf life can be determined, based on the ordinary least-squares method, as the time point at which the 95% lower confidence bound for the mean degradation curve of the drug characteristic intersects the approved lower specification limit. Along this line, several statistical methods were proposed, as discussed in detail in Chapter 11.

For simplicity, the following notation is used in this chapter. We let t_{label} denote the established expiration dating period that appears on the container label of a drug product. Also, t_{true} is the true shelf life of a particular batch of the drug product. Since t_{true} is unknown, it is reasonable to assume that t_{label} will not be granted by the FDA unless $t_{true} \geq t_{label}$ is statistically justified. According to the FDA guideline, under a fixed effects model, it can be shown that t_{label} is actually a confidence lower bound for t_{true}, and therefore if t_0 is chosen to be less than or equal to t_{label}, $t_{true} \geq t_0$ provides strong statistical evidence. However, as indicated in Chapter 11, the result obtained using this approach should be supported by showing that there is no batch-to-batch variation. If there is batch-to-batch variation, the FDA suggests that the minimum approach be considered. It should be noted, however, that the minimum approach is conservative and does not take into account batch-to-batch variation.

As indicated in the FDA guideline, the batches used in long-term stability studies for establishment of drug shelf life should constitute a random sample from the population of future production batches. In addition, the FDA guideline requires that all estimated expiration dating periods should be applicable to all future batches. In this case, the statistical methods discussed in Chapter 11, which are derived under a fixed effects model, may not be appropriate. This is because statistical inference about the expiration dating period obtained from a fixed effects model can only be made to the batches under study and cannot be applied to future batches. Since the ultimate goal of a stability study is to apply the established expiration dating period to the population of all future production batches, statistical methods based on a random effects model seems more appropriate. In recent years, several statistical methods for the determination of drug shelf life with random batches have been considered [see, e.g., Chow and Shao (1989, 1991), Murphy and Weisman (1990), Chow (1992), Liu (1992), Ho et al. (1992), and Shao and Chow (1994)].

Note that the difference between a random effects model and a fixed effects model is that the batches used in a random effects model for stability analysis are considered a random sample drawn from the population of all future production batches. As a result, the intercepts and slopes, which are often used to characterize the degradation of a drug product as given in (11.3.1), are no longer fixed unknown parameters but random variables. The objectives of this chapter are (1) to derive some statistical tests for batch-to-batch variation and some related fixed effects, such as the effects due to package, strength, and/or nonlinearity over time, and (2) to introduce statistical methods for the determination of drug shelf life under a random effects model.

This chapter is organized as follows. In the next section we introduce linear regression model with random coefficients. Statistical tests for random batch effects and some related fixed effects are derived in Sec. 12.3. In Secs. 12.4 and 12.5, we introduce several methods for estimation of drug shelf life with random batches. These methods include methods proposed by Chow and Shao (1991) and Shao and Chow (1994) (Sec. 12.4) and by Ho et al. (1992) (Sec. 12.5). These methods are compared with the FDA's minimum approach in Sec. 12.6 through a Monte Carlo simulation study. An example concerning a long-term stability study is used to illustrate these methods in Sec. 12.7. A brief discussion is given in the final section.

12.2. LINEAR REGRESSION WITH RANDOM COEFFICIENTS

Under the assumption that batch is a random variable, stability data can be described by a linear regression model with random coefficients. Consider the following model for a stability study with K batches:

$$Y_{ij} = X'_{ij}\beta_i + e_{ij}, \qquad j = 1, \ldots, n_i, \quad i = 1, \ldots, K, \qquad (12.2.1)$$

where Y_{ij} is the jth assay result (percent of label claim) for the ith batch, X_{ij} is a $p \times 1$ vector of the jth value of the regressor for the ith batch and X'_{ij} is its transpose, β_i is a $p \times 1$ vector of random effects for the ith batch, and e_{ij} is the random error in observing Y_{ij}. Note that $X'_{ij}\beta_i$ is the mean drug characteristic for the ith batch at X_{ij} (conditional on β_i). The primary assumptions for model (12.2.1) is the same as those for model (10.4.7), which are summarized below.

Assumption A

1. $\beta_i, i = 1, \ldots, K$, are independent and identically distributed (i.i.d.) as $N_p(\beta, \Sigma_\beta)$, where β is an unknown $p \times 1$ vector and Σ_β is an unknown $p \times p$ nonnegative definite matrix.
2. $e_{ij}, i = 1, \ldots, K, j = 1, \ldots, n_i$, are i.i.d. as $N(0, \sigma_e^2)$ and $\{e_{ij}\}$ and $\{\beta_i\}$ are independent.
3. $n_i > p$ and $X_i = (X_{i1}, \ldots, X_{in_i})'$ is of full rank for all i.

Note that the K batches constitute a random sample from the population of all future batches of the drug product manufactured under similar circumstances. Hence Σ_β reflects batch-to-batch variation. If $\Sigma_\beta = 0$ (i.e., $\beta_i = \beta$ for all i), there is no batch-to-batch variation. In this case, model (12.2.1) reduces to an ordinary regression model. On the other hand, if $\Sigma_\beta \neq 0$, there is batch-to-batch variation and β_i is a $p \times 1$ vector of unobserved random effects.

In long-term stability studies, X_{ij} is usually selected to be equal to x_j for all i (i.e., $X_{ij} = x_j$ for all i, where x_j is a $p \times 1$ vector). In practice, x_j may be of the form $(1, t_j, t_j w_j)'$ or $(1, t_j, w_j, t_j w_j)'$, where w_j could be a class variable denoting package type (e.g., w_j = bottle or blister) and $t_j, j = 1, \ldots, n_i$, are the sampling time points (e.g., $t_j = 0, 3, 6, 9, 12, 18, 24, 36, \ldots$). If different dosage strengths (e.g., 10 mg, 20 mg) are to be considered, x_j can be obtained similarly. Note that if the mean degradation is quadratic over time, we may add a component t_j^2 to x_j.

Model (12.2.1) is known as a linear regression model with random coefficients. If K is large, Hildreth and Houck (1968) recommended that a weighted least-squares (WLS) approach be used to estimate the mean of β_i. In practice, however, K is usually small in long-term stability studies. The current FDA guideline requires that only three batches (i.e., $K = 3$) be tested to establish an expiration dating period of the drug product. Thus the method suggested by Hildreth and Houck (1968) is not applicable. It is interesting to note that model (12.2.1) is in fact a special case of regression model with random coefficients based on the fact that the values of the regressor X_i are the same for each batch i.

12.3. RANDOM BATCH EFFECT AND OTHER FIXED EFFECTS

Under linear regression model (12.2.1) with random coefficients, we are able to test for the random batch effect and other fixed effects, such as the package effect, the stength effect, and the effect due to nonlinearity over time. Let

$$X_i = (X_{i1}, \ldots, X_{in_i})',$$

$$Y_i = (Y_{i1}, \ldots, Y_{in_i})'$$

$$\epsilon_i = (e_{i1}, \ldots, e_{in_i})'.$$

Model (12.2.1) can then be written as follows:

$$Y_i = X_i\beta_i + \epsilon_1, \qquad i = 1, \ldots, K. \tag{12.3.1}$$

Under assumption A, Y_i, $i = 1, \ldots, K$, are independently distributed as

$$N_{n_i}(X_i\beta, D_i),$$

where

$$D_i = X_i\Sigma_\beta X_i' + \sigma_e^2 I_{n_i}$$

and I_{n_i} is the identity matrix of order n.

If $\Sigma_\beta = 0$, then $\beta_i \equiv \beta$ is nonrandom and model (12.3.1) reduces to

$$Y_i = X_i\beta + \epsilon_i, \qquad i = 1, \ldots, K, \tag{12.3.2}$$

which is an ordinary regression model.

If $n_i = n$ and $X_i = X$ for all i, model (12.3.1) or (12.3.2) is called a *balanced model*. The maximum likelihood estimator (MLE) of β in the balanced case is the same as the ordinary least-squares estimator, which is given by

$$\bar{b} = (X' X)^{-1}X' \bar{Y}, \tag{12.3.3}$$

where

$$\bar{Y} = \frac{1}{K} \sum_{i=1}^{K} Y_i.$$

Since the Y_i are normal,

$$\bar{b} \sim N_p\left(\beta, \frac{1}{K} [\Sigma_\beta + \sigma_e^2 (X'X)^{-1}]\right). \tag{12.3.4}$$

The $\ell'\overline{\mathbf{b}}$ is the uniformly minimum variance unbiased estimator (UMVUE) of $\ell'\beta$, where ℓ is any fixed $p \times 1$ vector. In the case where $\Sigma_\beta \neq 0$, $\overline{\mathbf{b}}$ in (12.3.3) is the ordinary least-squares estimator of β and $\ell'\overline{\mathbf{b}}$ is still the UMVUE of $\ell'\beta$ for any fixed $p \times 1$ vector ℓ, since $\overline{\mathbf{b}}$ is, in fact, obtained from

$$\overline{\mathbf{b}} = (\mathbf{X}'\,\mathbf{D}^{-1}\mathbf{X})^{-1}\mathbf{X}'\,\mathbf{D}^{-1}\overline{\mathbf{Y}}. \tag{12.3.5}$$

Result (12.3.5) is known in the literature [see, e.g., Theorem 10.2.1 in Anderson (1971) or Sec. 4.1 in Laird et al. (1987)].

12.3.1. Test for Batch-to-Batch Variation

Special Case

If $\mathbf{X}_{ij} = (1, X_j)'$ and $\beta_i = (\alpha_i, \beta_i)'$, model (12.3.1) reduces to the following model considered by Chow and Shao (1989):

$$Y_{ij} = \alpha_i + \beta_i X_j + e_{ij}, \quad i = 1,\ldots,K, \quad j = 0,1,\ldots,n-1, \tag{12.3.6}$$

where α_i and β_i are random variables with distributions $N(\alpha, \sigma_\alpha^2)$ and $N(\beta, \sigma_\beta^2)$, respectively, and α_i, β_i, and e_{ij} are mutually independent. If $\sigma_\alpha^2 = 0$ and $\sigma_\beta^2 = 0$, model (12.3.6) reduces to

$$Y_{ij} = \alpha + \beta X_j + e_{ij}, \quad i = 1,\ldots,K, \quad j = 0,1,\ldots,n-1. \tag{12.3.7}$$

If $\sigma_\alpha^2 > 0$ but $\sigma_\beta^2 = 0$ (i.e., different intercepts but common slope), the ordinary least-squares method for the estimation of drug shelf life described in Chapter 11 is still valid since

$$Y_{ij} = \alpha + \beta X_j + u_{ij} \tag{12.3.8}$$

with

$$u_{ij} = \alpha_i - \alpha + e_{ij}$$

being independent $N(0, \sigma_\alpha^2 + \sigma_e^2)$. If, however, $\sigma_\beta^2 > 0$, the ordinary least-squares method is not appropriate. A commonly accepted test procedure for the hypothesis that $\sigma_\beta^2 = 0$ is the likelihood ratio test (Lehmann, 1959). Let

$$L = L(\alpha, \beta, \sigma^2, \sigma_\beta^2)$$

denote the log-likelihood function (given the data Y_{ij}), where $\sigma^2 = \sigma_\alpha^2 + \sigma_e^2$. The likelihood ratio test rejects the null hypothesis that $\sigma_\beta^2 = 0$ if

$$A > \chi^2(\alpha, 1),$$

where

$$A = \sup_{\alpha,\beta,\sigma^2} L(\alpha,\beta,\sigma^2,0) - \sup_{\alpha,\beta,\sigma^2,\sigma_\beta^2} L(\alpha,\beta,\sigma^2,\sigma^2\beta)$$

and $\chi^2(\alpha,1)$ is the αth upper quantile of the chi-square distribution with 1 degree of freedom. A straightforward calculation shows that

$$A = K \sum_{j=1}^{n-1} \ln(\hat{\sigma}_\beta^2 X_j^2 + \hat{\sigma}^2) - Kn \ln (\tilde{\sigma}^2),$$

where

$$\tilde{\sigma}^2 = \frac{1}{nK - 2} \sum_{i=1}^{K} \sum_{j=0}^{n-1} (Y_{ij} - a - bX_j)^2,$$

a and b are the ordinary least-squares estimates of α and β under model (12.3.6), and $\hat{\sigma}_\beta^2$ and $\hat{\sigma}^2$ are solutions of the system

$$\sum_{i=1}^{K} \sum_{j=0}^{n-1} \frac{Y_{ij} - \alpha - \beta X_j}{\sigma_\beta^2 X_j^2 + \sigma^2} = 0,$$

$$\sum_{i=1}^{K} \sum_{j=0}^{n-1} X_j \frac{Y_{ij} - \alpha - \beta X_j}{\sigma_\beta^2 X_j^2 + \sigma^2} = 0,$$

$$\sum_{i=1}^{K} \sum_{j=0}^{n-1} \frac{(Y_{ij} - \alpha - \beta X_j)^2}{\sigma_\beta^2 X_j^2 + \sigma^2} = Kn,$$

$$\sum_{i=1}^{K} \sum_{j=0}^{n-1} \left(\frac{Y_{ij} - \alpha - \beta X_j}{\sigma_\beta^2 X_j^2 + \sigma^2}\right)^2 = K \sum_{j=0}^{n-1} \frac{1}{\sigma_\beta^2 X_j^2 + \sigma^2}.$$

In addition to the likelihood ratio test, under the assumption that $\sigma_\alpha^2 = 0$, Chow and Shao (1989) proposed the following three statistics for testing the null hypothesis that $H_0: \sigma_\beta^2 = 0$. Note that the case where $\sigma_\alpha^2 \neq 0$ was examined in Chow and Shao (1991) and will be discussed later in this section. The first test procedure, which was referred to as test procedure I in Chow and Shao (1989), is described below.

Since $X_0 = 0$, Y_{i0}, $i = 1, \ldots, K$, are independently distributed as $N(\alpha,\sigma^2)$, where $\sigma^2 = \sigma_\alpha^2 + \sigma_e^2$. Hence

$$s_0^2 = \frac{1}{K - 1} \sum_{i=1}^{K} (Y_{i0} - \bar{Y}_0)^2,$$

where

$$\bar{Y}_0 = \frac{1}{K} \sum_{i=1}^{K} Y_{i0},$$

is an unbiased and consistent (as $K \to \infty$) estimator of σ^2 and

$$\frac{(K - 1) s_0^2}{\sigma^2}$$

is distributed as a chi-square variable with $K-1$ degrees of freedom. Under the hypothesis that $\sigma_\beta^2 = 0$,

$$Y_{ij} = \alpha + \beta X_j + u_{ij}, \qquad i = 1, \ldots, K \quad j = 1, \ldots, n - 1, \qquad (12.3.9)$$

is a simple linear regression model with errors u_{ij} independently distributed as $N(0, \sigma^2)$. Let

$$\overline{X}_{(0)} = \frac{1}{n-1} \sum_{j=1}^{n-1} X_j, \qquad \overline{Y}_{(0)} = \frac{1}{K(n-1)} \sum_{i=1}^{K} \sum_{j=1}^{n-1} Y_{ij},$$

$$S_1 = K \sum_{j=1}^{n-1} (X_j - \overline{X}_{(0)})^2,$$

$$S_2 = \sum_{i=1}^{K} \sum_{j=1}^{n-1} (X_j - \overline{X}_{(0)})(Y_{ij} - \overline{Y}_{(0)}).$$

Then $b = s_2/s_1$ and $a = \overline{Y}_{(0)} - b\overline{X}_{(0)}$ are the ordinary least-squares estimators of β and α under model (12.3.7). Let

$$r_{ij} = Y_{ij} - a - bX_j, \qquad i = 1, \ldots, K, \quad j = 1, \ldots, n - 1.$$

Then under the null hypothesis that $\sigma_\beta^2 = 0$,

$$s_r^2 = \frac{1}{m-2} \sum_{i=1}^{K} \sum_{j=1}^{n-1} r_{ij}^2, \qquad m = K(n - 1),$$

is an unbiased and consistent estimator of σ^2 and

$$\frac{(m-2)\, s_r^2}{\sigma^2}$$

is distributed as a chi-square variable with $m-2$ degrees of freedom. If $\sigma_\beta^2 > 0$,

$$E(s_r^2) = \frac{1}{m-2} \sum_{i=1}^{K} \sum_{j=1}^{n-1} E(r_{ij}^2)$$

$$= \sigma^2 + \left[\frac{K}{m-2} \sum_{j=1}^{n-1} (1 - w_j) X_j^2 \right] \sigma_\beta^2,$$

where

$$w_j = \frac{\sum_{\ell=1}^{n-1} X_\ell^2 - 2X_j \sum_{\ell=1}^{n-1} X_\ell + (n-1)X_j^2}{K\left[(n-1) \sum_{\ell=1}^{n-1} X_\ell^2 - \left(\sum_{\ell=1}^{n-1} X_\ell \right)^2 \right]}.$$

Since $0 < w_j < 1$ and $X_j^2 > 0$ for $j = 1, \ldots, n - 1$, $E(s_r^2)$ is larger than σ^2 if $\sigma_\beta^2 > 0$. Hence

$$\frac{s_r^2}{s_0^2} \gg 1$$

indicates that $\sigma_\beta^2 > 0$. Since s_0^2 and s_r^2 are independent, under the null hypothesis that $\sigma_\beta^2 = 0$, s_r^2/s_0^2 distributes as an F with $m - 1$ and $K - 1$ degrees of freedom. Hence we reject the null hypothesis that $\sigma_\beta^2 = 0$ at the α level of significance if

$$\frac{s_r^2}{s_0^2} > F(\alpha, m - 2, K - 1),$$

where $F(\alpha, m - 2, K - 1)$ is the αth upper quantile of the F distribution with $m - 2$ and $K - 1$ degrees of freedom.

For the second test procedure (test procedure II), Chow and Shao (1989) considered

$$s_j^2 = \frac{1}{K - 1} \sum_{i=1}^{K} (Y_{ij} - \bar{Y}_j)^2,$$

where

$$\bar{Y}_j = \frac{1}{K} \sum_{i=1}^{K} Y_{ij}.$$

It can be verified that

$$E(s_j^2) = \sigma_\beta^2 X_j^2 + \sigma^2, \qquad j = 1, \ldots, n - 1.$$

The s_j^2 are independent and identically distributed if $\sigma_\beta^2 = 0$.
Note that

$$E(s_0^2) < E(s_1^2) < \cdots < E(s_{n-1}^2)$$

provided that $\sigma_\beta^2 > 0$. Chow and Shao (1989) suggest using the following test procedure, which rejects the null hypothesis that $\sigma_\beta^2 = 0$ if

$$s_0^2 < s_1^2 < \cdots < s_{n-1}^2.$$

Under the hypothesis that $\sigma_\beta^2 = 0$,

$$P\{s_0^2 < s_1^2 < \cdots < s_{n-1}^2\} = \frac{1}{n!}.$$

Hence this test has level $1/n!$. Chow and Shao (1989) indicated that test procedure II is a robust test procedure because it does not require the normality assumptions for e_{ij}, α_i, and β_i. However, this procedure has some disadvantages. First, one cannot choose a desired test level and the p value is unknown. Second, if $n \geq 6$, the test level $1/n!$ is either too small or too large. In this case Chow and Shao (1989) suggested that the test procedure be modified. Finally, test procedure II requires that there be exactly the same number of observations at each X_j. Thus, unlike test procedure I, one cannot use test procedure II when there are missing observations.

When K is small (e.g., $K = 3$) and n is larger than 5, test procedures I and II may not be appropriate. Chow and Shao (1989) suggested the following alternative (test procedure III). Let $h = n/2$ if n is even and $h = (n - 1)/2$ if n is odd. Denote the least-squares estimators of α and β under model

$$Y_{ij} = \alpha + \beta X_j + u_{ij}, \quad i = 1, \dots, K, \quad j = 0, \dots, h - 1,$$

by a_1 and b_1 and under model

$$Y_{ij} = \alpha + \beta X_j + u_{ij}, \quad i = 1, \dots, K, \quad j = h, \dots, n - 1,$$

by a_2 and b_2. Let

$$s_{r1}^2 = \frac{1}{Kh - 2} \sum_{i=1}^{K} \sum_{j=0}^{h-1} (Y_{ij} - a_1 - b_1 X_j)^2,$$

$$s_{r2}^2 = \frac{1}{K(n - h) - 2} \sum_{i=1}^{K} \sum_{j=h}^{n-1} (Y_{ij} - a_2 - b_2 X_j)^2.$$

Under the hypothesis that $\sigma_\beta^2 = 0$,

$$\frac{(Kh - 2) s_{r1}^2}{\sigma^2} \quad \text{and} \quad \frac{[K(n - h) - 2] s_{r2}^2}{\sigma^2}$$

are distributed as chi-square variables with $Kh - 2$ and $K(n - h) - 2$ degrees of freedom, respectively. Since s_{r1}^2 and s_{r2}^2 are independent, s_{r2}^2/s_{r1}^2 distributes as F with $K(n - h) - 2$ and $Kh - 2$ degrees of freedom. Thus we reject the null hypothesis that $\sigma_\beta^2 = 0$ if

$$\frac{s_{r2}^2}{s_{r1}^2} > F(\alpha, K(n - h) - 2, Kh - 2).$$

It can be seen that test procedure III is of level α. Its p value can be calculated as follows:

$$P \left\{ F > \frac{s_{r2}^2}{s_{r1}^2} \right\}.$$

For the use of the three test procedures above, Chow and Shao (1989) have recommended the following:

1. When K is large or moderate, the first test procedure is preferred.
2. When K is small but n is larger than 5, the third test procedure is recommended.

3. When both K and n are small (e.g., $n = 4$ or $n = 5$), it is suggested that the second test procedure be used.

As indicated by Chow and Shao (1989), test procedure II provides a quick examination of batch-to-batch variation and is robust against nonnormality. However, the restriction on n limits its utility.

Note that test procedures I through III proposed by Chow and Shao (1989) are valid only under the assumption that $\sigma_\alpha^2 = 0$. In practice, σ_α^2 may not be zero and there exists variability between batches with respect to other class variables, such as package type or strength. In this case the following test procedures are useful.

General Case

Consider the general case and the following hypotheses:

$$H_0: \Sigma_\beta = 0 \quad \text{vs.} \quad K_0: \Sigma_\beta \neq 0 \tag{12.3.10}$$

If K_0 is concluded, there is batch-to-batch variation. The sum of squared ordinary least-squares residuals can be decomposed as follows:

$$\text{SSR} = \text{tr (S)} + \text{SE},$$

where

$$\text{SE} = K\overline{\mathbf{Y}}'[\mathbf{I}_n - \mathbf{X}(\mathbf{X}'\mathbf{X})^{-1}\mathbf{X}']\overline{\mathbf{Y}}, \tag{12.3.11}$$

and tr (S) is the trace of the matrix

$$\mathbf{S} = \sum_{i=1}^{K} (\mathbf{Y}_i - \overline{\mathbf{Y}}) (\mathbf{Y}_i - \overline{\mathbf{Y}})'. \tag{12.3.12}$$

Theorem 12.3.1 Under model (12.3.1) and assumption A, we have the following:

(i) SE/σ_e^2 is distributed as the $\chi^2 (n - p)$, the chi-square random variable with $n - p$ degrees of freedom.

(ii) $\mathbf{S}$ in (12.3.12) has a Wishart distribution

$$W(K - 1, \mathbf{X}\Sigma_\beta \mathbf{X}' + \sigma_e^2\mathbf{I}_n),$$

$$E[\text{tr}(\mathbf{S})] = (K - 1) [\text{tr} (\mathbf{X}\Sigma_\beta\mathbf{X}') + n\sigma_e^2].$$

(iii) If H_0 in (12.3.10) holds, tr $(\mathbf{S})/\sigma_e^2$ is distributed as $\chi^2(n(K - 1))$.

(iv) Statistics $\overline{\mathbf{b}}$, SE, and $\mathbf{S}$ are independent.

Proof (i) follows directly from (12.3.11). Since $\mathbf{Y}_i$ are i.i.d. normal, $\mathbf{S}$ has a Wishart distribution $W(K - 1, \mathbf{D})$, where

$$\mathbf{D} = \mathbf{X}\Sigma_\beta\mathbf{X}' + \sigma_e^2\mathbf{I}_n.$$

Hence

$$E[\text{tr}(S)] = (K - 1)\text{tr}(D) = (K - 1)[\text{tr}(X\Sigma_\beta X') + n\sigma_e^2].$$

This proves (ii). If H_0 in (12.3.10) holds, $D = \sigma_e^2 I_n$ and therefore the diagonal elements of S are independent. Thus (iii) follows since each diagonal element of S is distributed as $\sigma_e^2 \chi^2(K - 1)$. Since Y_i are i.i.d. normal, $\overline{Y}$ and S are independent. Hence S and (b, SE) are independent. Since

$$(I_n - H) X = 0,$$

where

$$H = X(X'X)^{-1}X',$$
$$E[(I_n - H) \overline{Y}] = (I_n - H) X\beta = 0,$$
$$\text{cov}[(I_n - H) \overline{Y}, X'\overline{Y}] = E[(I_n - H) \overline{Y} \overline{Y}' X]$$
$$= (I_n - H)[D/K + E(\overline{Y})E(\overline{Y}')]X$$
$$= (I_n - H)[(X\Sigma_\beta X' + \sigma_e^2 I_n)/K + X\beta\beta' X']X = 0.$$

Hence $(I_n - H) \overline{Y}$ and $X'\overline{Y}$ are independent. Therefore,

$$SE = K\overline{Y}' (I_n - H) \overline{Y} = K[(I_n - H) \overline{Y}]' (I_n - H) \overline{Y},$$
$$\overline{b} = (X'X)^{-1}X'\overline{Y}$$

are independent. This proves (iv).

From Theorem 12.3.1, $SE/ (n - p)$ estimates σ_e^2. Under H_0,

$$\frac{\text{tr}(S)}{n (K - 1)}$$

also estimates σ_e^2. Therefore, the statistic

$$T = \frac{(n - p)\text{tr}(S)}{n (K - 1) SE} \qquad (12.3.13)$$

should be around 1. If $\Sigma_\beta \neq 0$, there is another positive component,

$$\frac{1}{n} \text{tr}(X\Sigma_\beta X'),$$

in the expectation of

$$\frac{\text{tr}(S)}{n(K - 1)}$$

and T in (12.3.13) would be large. Hence we may use T to test H_0 in (12.3.10). Under H_0, T follows an F distribution with $n (K - 1)$ and $n - p$ degrees of freedom. At the α level of significance, we would reject H_0 if

$$T > F(\alpha, n(K - 1), n - p),$$

where $F(\alpha,u,v)$ is the αth upper quantile of the F distribution with u and v degrees of freedom.

If H_0 is rejected, we conclude that there is significant batch-to-batch variation. In this case it is not appropriate to use the method described in Chapter 11 for determination of drug shelf life.

12.3.2. Estimation of Batch Variation

For the estimation of σ_α^2 and σ_β^2 under model (12.3.6) for the special case, Chow and Shao (1991) considered the following consistent estimators. Let $d_{j\ell}$ be the (j,ℓ)th element of $\hat{D}$, where

$$\hat{D} = \frac{1}{K - 1} \sum_{i=1}^{K} (Y_i - \overline{Y})(Y_i - \overline{Y})'.$$

Then $d_{j\ell}$ is a consistent estimator of $\sigma_{j\ell}$, where

$$\sigma_{j\ell} = \begin{cases} \sigma_\alpha^2 + \sigma_\beta^2 X_j^2 + \sigma_e^2 & \text{if } j = \ell \\ \sigma_\alpha^2 + \sigma_\beta^2 X_j X_\ell & \text{if } j \neq \ell. \end{cases}$$

Since $\sigma_{j\ell}$ is a linear function of σ_α^2, σ_β^2, and σ_e^2, consistent estimators of σ_α^2 and σ_β^2 can be obtained by solving some linear equations, which are given by

$$\hat{\sigma}_\alpha^2 = \frac{1}{n - 1} \sum_{\ell=2}^{n} d_{1\ell},$$

$$\hat{\sigma}_\beta^2 = \frac{\sum_{j=2}^{n} \sum_{\ell=j+1}^{n} d_{j\ell} - (n - 2)/2 \sum_{\ell=1}^{n} d_{1\ell}}{\sum_{j=2}^{n} \sum_{\ell=j+1}^{n} X_j X_\ell}.$$

As an alternative, Chow and Wang (1994) proposed two unbiased estimators for batch-to-batch variation based on a transformed model under certain conditions. The idea can be applied to some general estimation procedures such as a restricted maximum likelihood (REML) estimator.

12.3.3. Test for Fixed Effects

In stability analysis we may need to test the effects of some covariates, such as package type and dosage strength. In practice, we may want to determine the following:

1.   Whether the degradation rate is the same from package type to package type and from strength to strength

2. Whether the differences in degradation rate between strengths are the same across package types
3. Whether the degradation rate is linear or quadratic in t

Each of the questions above can be formulated and tested as follows.

Let m be a fixed integer, $1 \le m < p$, and $i_1, i_2, \ldots, i_m$ be given integers between 1 and p. For any $p \times 1$ vector ℓ, let $\ell_{(m)}$ be the subvector of ℓ containing the (i_1)th, (i_2)th, $\ldots, (i_m)$th components of ℓ. Similarly, for any $p \times p$ matrix A, let $A_{(m)}$ be the $m \times m$ submatrix of A containing elements that are in the (i_1)th, $\ldots, (i_m)$th rows and columns of A.

Since β_i is random, the (i_1)th, (i_2)th, $\ldots, (i_m)$th terms in the model (12.2.1) have no effect if and only if both $\beta_{(m)} = 0$ and $\Sigma_{\beta(m)} = 0$. Hence we consider the following hypotheses:

$$H_m: \beta_{(m)} = 0 \text{ and } \Sigma_{\beta(m)} = 0 \quad \text{vs.} \quad K_m: H_m \text{ does not hold.}$$

Under H_m,

$$\bar{b}_{(m)} \sim N_m(0, K^{-1} \sigma_e^2 A_m),$$

where $\bar{b}_{(m)}$ is the corresponding subvector of $\bar{b}$

$$A_m = [(X'X)^{-1}]_{(m)},$$

$$K(\bar{b}_{(m)})' A_m^{-1} \bar{b}_{(m)} \sim \sigma_e^2 \chi^2(m).$$

Let ζ be the $p \times 1$ vector whose (i_1)th, $\ldots, (i_m)$th components are 1 and the other components are 0. Under H_m, $\zeta' \Sigma_\beta \zeta = 0$. Hence, by Theorem 12.3.1(ii),

$$S_m = \frac{\zeta'(X'X)^{-1}X'SX(X'X)^{-1}\zeta}{\zeta'(X'X)^{-1}\zeta} \sim \sigma_e^2 \chi^2(K-1).$$

Furthermore, from Theorem 12.3.1(iv),

$$SE + S_m \sim \sigma_e^2 \chi^2(n + K - p - 1)$$

and is independent of $(\bar{b}_{(m)})' A_m^{-1} \bar{b}_{(m)}$. Therefore,

$$T_m = \frac{n + K - p - 1}{m} \frac{K\bar{b}_{(m)}' A_m^{-1} \bar{b}_{(m)}}{SE + S_m}$$

has an F distribution with m and $n + K - p - 1$ degrees of freedom. At the α level of significance, we would reject H_m if

$$T_m > F(\alpha, m, n + K - p - 1).$$

12.4. SHELF LIFE ESTIMATION WITH RANDOM BATCHES

As indicated earlier, in long-term stability studies, X_{ij} is usually chosen to be x_j for all i, where x_j is a $p \times 1$ vector of nonrandom covariates which could be of the form $(1,t_j,t_jw_j)'$ or $(1,t_j,w_j,t_jw_j)'$, where t_j is the jth time point and w_j is the jth value of a $q \times 1$ vector of nonrandom covariates (e.g., package type and dosage strength). For convenience sake, denote $x_j = x(t_j,w_j)$, where $x(t,w)$ is a known function of t and w. In practice, most of the time we need a labeled shelf life for a fixed value of covariates (e.g., a fixed package type and a fixed dosage strength). Thus, for simplicity, when w is fixed, we denote $x(t,w)$ by $x(t)$.

In the simple case where $\Sigma_\beta = 0$ (i.e., there is no batch-to-batch variation), the average drug characteristic at time t is $x(t)'\beta$ and the true shelf life is equal to

$$\bar{t}_{true} = \inf\{t: x(t)'\ \beta \le \eta\},$$

which is an unknown but nonrandom quantity, where η is the approved lower specification limit for the drug characteristic. In this case, as indicated in Chapter 11, the labeled shelf life can be determined as follows.

Suppose that $x(t)'\beta$ is continuous and decreasing in t. Under model (12.3.2), for any given t, an $(1 - \alpha) \times 100\%$ lower confidence bound for $x(t)'\beta$ is given by

$$L(t) = x(t)'\ \bar{b} - t(\alpha, nK - p) \left[\frac{x(t)'\ (X'X)^{-1}x(t)}{K(nK - p)} SSR \right]^{1/2}, \qquad (12.4.1)$$

where SSR is the usual sum of squared residuals from the ordinary least-squares regression under model (12.3.2), and $t(\alpha, u)$ is the αth upper quantile of the t distribution with u degrees of freedom. Define.

$$\hat{t} = \inf\{t: L(t) \le \eta\}. \qquad (12.4.2)$$

The FDA guideline suggests that $\hat{t}$ be used as the labeled shelf life (i.e., $t_{label} = \hat{t}$). This is based on the fact that $\hat{t}$ is an $1 - \alpha$ lower confidence bound for $\hat{t}_{true}$, that is,

$$P_Y\{\hat{t} < \bar{t}_{true}\} = P_Y\{L(\bar{t}_{true}) \le \eta\}$$
$$= P_Y\{L(\bar{t}_{true}) \le x(\bar{t}_{true})'b\} = 1 - \alpha, \qquad (12.4.3)$$

where P_Y is the probability with respect to $Y_1,\ldots,Y_k$. the last quantity of (12.4.3) follows from the fact that $\bar{t}_{true}$ is nonrandom when $\Sigma_\beta = 0$ and $L(\bar{t}_{true})$ is an $1 - \alpha$ lower confidence bound for $x(\bar{t}_{true})'\beta$.

12.4.1. Chow and Shao's Approach

Under model (12.3.1), for a given batch i, $x(t)'\beta_i$ is the average characteristic of the drug product at time t, where β_i is random and distributed as $N_p(\beta,\Sigma_\beta)$. The true shelf life for this batch is then

$$t_{true} = \inf\{t: x(t)'\beta_i \le \eta\}.$$

When there is batch-to-batch variation (i.e., $\Sigma_\beta \neq 0$), t_{true} is random since β_i is random. In this case $x(t)'\beta_i$ follows a normal distribution with mean $x(t)'\beta$ and variance

$$\frac{1}{K} x(t)'[\Sigma_\beta + \sigma_e^2(X'X)^{-1}]x(t).$$

Consequently, the procedure described above is not appropriate even if (12.4.3) holds. It should be noted that

$$P_Y\{t_{\text{label}} \leq t_{\text{true}}\}$$

might be much smaller than

$$P_Y\{t_{\text{label}} \leq \bar{t}_{\text{true}}\}$$

since $\bar{t}_{\text{true}}$ is the median of t_{true}. Also, if $t_{\text{label}} \leq \bar{t}_{\text{true}}$,

$$P_{\beta_i}\{t_{\text{label}} \leq t_{\text{true}}\}$$

could be quite high, where P_{β_i} is the probability with respect to β_i. Define

$$\psi(t) = P_{\beta_i}\{t_{\text{true}} \leq t\} = P_{\beta_i}\{x(t)'\beta_i \leq \eta\}$$

$$= \Phi\left(\frac{\eta - x(t)'\beta}{\sigma(t)}\right), \tag{12.4.4}$$

where Φ is the standard normal distribution function and

$$\sigma(t) = [x(t)' \Sigma_\beta x(t)]^{1/2}$$

is the standard deviation of $x(t)'\beta_i$.

Chow and Shao (1991) and Shao and Chow (1994) propose considering an $(1-\alpha) \times 100\%$ lower confidence bound of the ϵth quantile of t_{true} as the labeled shelf life, where ϵ is a given small positive constant. We will refer to this method as Chow and Shao's approach. That is,

$$P_Y\{t_{\text{label}} \leq t_\epsilon\} \geq 1 - \alpha, \tag{12.4.5}$$

where t_ϵ satisfies

$$P_{\beta_i}\{t_{\text{true}} \leq t_\epsilon\} = \epsilon.$$

It follows from (12.4.4) that

$$t_\epsilon = \inf\{t: x(t)'\beta - \eta = z_\epsilon\sigma(t)\}, \tag{12.4.6}$$

where $z_\epsilon = \Phi^{-1}(1 - \epsilon)$.

The use of a labeled shelf life satisfying (12.4.5) can be justified from another point of view. Note that $t_{\text{label}} \leq t_\epsilon$ if and only if

$$P_{\beta_i}\{t_{\text{true}} \leq t_{\text{label}}\} \leq \epsilon.$$

Hence (12.4.5) is equivalent to

$$1 - \alpha \leq P_Y\{P_{\beta_i}\{t_{\text{true}} \leq t_{\text{label}}\} \leq \epsilon\}$$

$$= P_Y\{\psi(t_{\text{label}}) \leq \epsilon\}, \tag{12.4.7}$$

where $\psi(t)$ is as defined in (12.4.4), which can be viewed as the future failure rate (i.e., the percentage of future batches that fail to meet the specification) at time t. Thus (12.4.5) ensures, with $1 - \alpha$ assurance, that the future failure rate at time t_{label} is no more than ϵ. For small K, Shao and Chow (1994) suggested the following improved procedure for both balanced and imbalanced cases. We first consider the balanced case.

Balanced Case

Consider the following balanced model (i.e., $n_i = n$ and $\mathbf{X}_i = \mathbf{X}$ for all i). When model (12.3.1) is balanced, it can be written as

$$\mathbf{Y}_i = \mathbf{X}\boldsymbol{\beta} + \boldsymbol{\epsilon}_i^*, \qquad i = 1, \ldots, K, \tag{12.4.8}$$

where

$$\boldsymbol{\epsilon}_i^* = \mathbf{X}(\boldsymbol{\beta}_i - \boldsymbol{\beta}) + \boldsymbol{\epsilon}_i$$

are independently distributed as $N_n(0, \mathbf{D})$ with $\mathbf{D} = \mathbf{X}\boldsymbol{\Sigma}_\beta\mathbf{X}' + \sigma_e^2\mathbf{I}_n$. Under model (12.4.8), the ordinary least-squares estimator $\bar{\mathbf{b}}$ of $\boldsymbol{\beta}$ is the same as that given in (12.3.3). Since the covariance matrix $\mathbf{D}$ has a special structure, $\mathbf{x}(t)'\bar{\mathbf{b}}$ is the best linear estimator of $\mathbf{x}(t)'\boldsymbol{\beta}$ under model (12.4.8) [see, e.g., Rao (1973, p. 312)].

Note that $\hat{t}$ in (12.4.2) is equal to

$$\hat{t} = \inf\{t\colon \mathbf{x}(t)'\bar{\mathbf{b}} \leq \hat{\eta}(t)\},$$

where

$$\hat{\eta}(t) = \eta + t(\alpha, nK - p)\left[\frac{\mathbf{x}(t)' \ (\mathbf{X}'\mathbf{X})^{-1}\mathbf{x}(t)\text{SSR}}{K(nK - p)}\right]^{1/2}$$

can be viewed as an adjusted lower specification limit. In the case of $\boldsymbol{\Sigma}_\beta \neq 0$, we may apply the same idea to obtain a valid t_{label}. Let

$$v(t) = \frac{1}{K - 1} \mathbf{x}(t)' \ (\mathbf{X}'\mathbf{X})^{-1}\mathbf{X}'\mathbf{S}\mathbf{X}(\mathbf{X}'\mathbf{X})^{-1}\mathbf{x}(t), \tag{12.4.9}$$

where $\mathbf{S}$ is as defined in (12.3.12). From Theorem 12.3.1, $(K - 1)v(t)$ is distributed as $a(t)\chi^2(K - 1)$, where

$$a(t) = \mathbf{x}(t)'[\boldsymbol{\Sigma}_\beta + \sigma_e^2(\mathbf{X}'\mathbf{X})^{-1}]\mathbf{x}(t) \tag{12.4.10}$$

$$\geq \mathbf{x}(t)'\boldsymbol{\Sigma}_\beta\mathbf{x}(t) = [\sigma(t)]^2.$$

Define

$$\tilde{\eta}(t) = \eta + c_K(\epsilon,\alpha)z_\epsilon \sqrt{v(t)}, \tag{12.4.11}$$

$$\tilde{t} = \inf\{t: \mathbf{x}(t)'\overline{\mathbf{b}} \le \tilde{\eta}(t)\}, \tag{12.4.12}$$

where for given ϵ, α, and K,

$$c_K(\epsilon,\alpha) = \frac{1}{\sqrt{K}z_\epsilon} t(\alpha, K - 1, \sqrt{K}z_\epsilon) \tag{12.4.13}$$

and $t(\alpha, K - 1, \sqrt{K}z_\epsilon)$ is the αth upper quantile of the noncentral t distribution with $K - 1$ degrees of freedom and noncentrality parameter $\sqrt{K}z_\epsilon$. Similar to $\hat{\eta}(t)$, $\tilde{\eta}(t)$ is an adjusted lower specification limit. The values of $c_K(\epsilon,\alpha)$ for $\alpha = 0.05$ and some likely choices of K and ϵ are listed in Table 12.4.1. Shao and Chow (1994) proposed using $\tilde{t}$ in (12.4.12) as the labeled shelf life. This is justified by the following result.

Theorem 12.4.1 For any ϵ, α, and K, (12.4.3) holds for $t_{\text{label}} = \tilde{t}$. If we let σ_e tend to zero or $\mathbf{X}'\mathbf{X}$ tend to infinity, the quantity in (12.4.3) holds.
Proof Let $T(K,\lambda)$ denote a noncentral t random variable with K degrees of freedom and noncentrality parameter λ. By Theorem 12.3.1,

$$\frac{\sqrt{K}\,[\mathbf{x}(t_\epsilon)'\mathbf{b} - \eta]}{\sqrt{v(t_\epsilon)}} = T(K - 1, \lambda_\epsilon),$$

where

$$\lambda_\epsilon = \frac{\sqrt{K}\,[\mathbf{x}(t_\epsilon)'\,\boldsymbol{\beta} - \eta]}{\sqrt{a(t_\epsilon)}},$$

TABLE 12.4.1 Values of $c_K(\epsilon,0.05)$ defined by (12.4.13)

ϵ	k							
	3	4	5	6	7	8	9	10
0.01	4.536	3.027	2.468	2.176	1.995	1.872	1.781	1.711
0.02	4.570	3.056	2.493	2.199	2.016	1.891	1.799	1.729
0.03	4.599	3.081	2.515	2.218	2.034	1.907	1.815	1.743
0.04	4.627	3.104	2.535	2.236	2.051	1.923	1.829	1.757
0.05	4.654	3.127	2.555	2.254	2.067	1.938	1.843	1.770
0.10	4.803	3.248	2.658	2.346	2.150	2.015	1.915	1.837
0.15	4.993	3.396	2.784	2.457	2.250	2.107	2.001	1.918

t_ϵ and $a(t)$ are given in (12.4.6) and (12.4.10), respectively. Thus

$$P_Y\{t_\epsilon < \tilde{t}\} = P_Y\{\mathbf{x}(t_\epsilon)'\mathbf{b} > \bar{\eta}\ (t_\epsilon)\}$$

$$= P_Y\left[\frac{\mathbf{x}(t_\epsilon)'\mathbf{b} - \eta}{\sqrt{v(t_\epsilon)}} > c_K(\epsilon,\alpha)z_\epsilon\right]$$

$$= P_Y\{T(K - 1, \lambda_\epsilon) > \sqrt{K}\ c_K(\epsilon,\alpha)z_\epsilon\}$$

$$\leq P_Y\{T(K - 1, \sqrt{K}z_\epsilon) > \sqrt{K}c_K(\epsilon,\alpha)z_\epsilon\}$$

$$= \alpha,$$

where the first equality follows from the definition of $\tilde{t}$; the second and third equalities follow from the definitions of $\bar{\eta}(t)$ and $T(K - 1, \lambda_\epsilon)$; the inequality follows from

$$\lambda_\epsilon \leq \sqrt{K}z_\epsilon$$

under (12.4.6) and (12.4.10); and the last equality follows from (12.4.13). The last assertion follows from the fact that

$$a(t) \rightarrow [\sigma(t)]^2 \qquad \text{as } \sigma_e \rightarrow 0 \quad \text{or} \quad \mathbf{X'X} \rightarrow \infty.$$

This completes the proof.

Figure 12.4.1 gives a graphical presentation of the foregoing procedure.

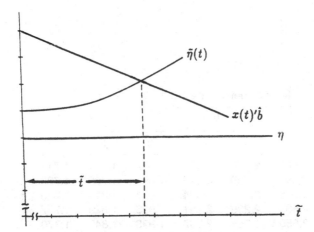

FIGURE 12.4.1 Labeled shelf life. $\tilde{t}$, Labeled shelf life; $x(t)'\hat{b}$, estimated mean degradation curve; η, lower specification limit; $\bar{\eta}(t)$, adjusted lower specification limit.

Unbalanced Case

In the unbalanced case where the n_i are not equal and/or the $\mathbf{X}_i$ are not identical, it is difficult to obtain exact fixed-sample (small K) results without any further assumption. In some cases we may have a large number of observations for each tested batch, and therefore we may assume that

$$n_i \to \infty \quad \text{and} \quad \mathbf{X}'_i \mathbf{X}_i \to \infty, \qquad i = 1, \ldots, K. \tag{12.4.14}$$

Apparently, condition (12.4.14) cannot always be fulfilled. We can, however, adopt an alternative approach, which we will refer to as the small error asymptotic approach, by assuming that

$$\sigma_e^2 \to 0. \tag{12.4.15}$$

Condition (12.4.15) simply means that the assay measurement errors are small, so as to ensure that their variance σ_e^2 is small. This can be done for stability data obtained under well-controlled conditions.

With either condition (12.4.14) or condition (12.4.15), we can extend the result above to the unbalanced case as follows. Let

$$\mathbf{b}_i = (\mathbf{X}'_i \mathbf{X}_i)^{-1} \mathbf{X}'_i \mathbf{Y}_i,$$

where $\mathbf{X}_i$ and $\mathbf{Y}_i$ are as defined in (12.2.1). Under assumption A, the $\mathbf{b}_i$ are independent and

$$\mathbf{b}_i \sim N_p\left(\boldsymbol{\beta}, \ \boldsymbol{\Sigma}_\beta + \sigma_e^2 (\mathbf{X}'\mathbf{X}_i)^{-1}\right). \tag{12.4.16}$$

Under either condition (12.4.14) or (12.4.15), it follows from (12.4.16) that, approximately,

$$\mathbf{b}_i \sim N_p(\boldsymbol{\beta}, \boldsymbol{\Sigma}_\beta).$$

Hence, approximately,

$$\mathbf{b} = \bar{\mathbf{b}} = \frac{1}{K} \sum_{i=1}^{K} \mathbf{b}_i \sim N_p(\boldsymbol{\beta}, \boldsymbol{\Sigma}_b/K), \tag{12.4.17}$$

where

$$\boldsymbol{\Sigma}_b = \boldsymbol{\Sigma}_\beta + \frac{1}{K} \sigma_e^2 \sum_{i=1}^{K} (\mathbf{X}'_i \mathbf{X}_i)^{-1}.$$

Define

$$\tilde{v}(t) = \frac{1}{K-1} \sum_{i=1}^{K} \mathbf{x}(t)' (\mathbf{b}_i - \bar{\mathbf{b}}) (\mathbf{b}_i - \bar{\mathbf{b}})' \mathbf{x}(t). \tag{12.4.18}$$

Let $\tilde{\eta}(t)$ be defined as in (12.4.11) with $v(t)$ replaced by $\tilde{v}(t)$ in (12.4.18) and let $\tilde{t}$ be defined as in (12.4.12) with $\overline{b}$ replaced by $\tilde{b}$ in (12.4.17). Then (12.4.5) still holds approximately for $\tilde{t}$ Therefore, $\tilde{t}$ can be used as the labeled shelf life.

In the balanced case where $n_i = n$ and $X_i = X$ for all i, it follows from (12.4.17) that

$$\tilde{b} = \overline{b} = (X'X)^{-1}X'\overline{Y}, \tag{12.4.19}$$

which is the same as $\overline{b}$ in (12.3.3). Similarly, from (12.4.18) and (12.4.19),

$$\tilde{v}(t) = \frac{1}{K-1} \sum_{i=1}^{K} x(t)' (X'X)^{-1}X' (Y_i - \overline{Y}) (Y_i - \overline{Y})' X(X'X)^{-1}x(t),$$

which is the same as $v(t)$ in (12.4.9). Thus the result in Sec. 12.3 is a special case of that derived in this section, except that the result in Sec. 12.3 is exact.

Note that in the pharmaceutical industry, the imbalance of the model is often caused by missing values. That is, in the original design, $n_i = n$, and $X_i = X$ for all i. But the actual data set, $n_i \leq n$ and X_i is a submatrix of X, $i = 1,\ldots,K$. In such cases, even if neither condition (12.4.14) nor condition (12.4.15) is satisfied, the use of $\tilde{t}$ as the labeled shelf life is still approximately valid as long as

$$(X_i'X_i)^{-1}(X'X) - I_p$$

is nearly equal to the zero matrix for all i.

12.5. HLC METHOD

Chow and Shao's approach described in Sec. 12.4 is based on the concept that the true shelf life is the minimum of the time point at which any observed total stability loss for any future batch randomly chosen from the population of the production batches is equal to or greater than the lower specification limit η with a high degree of confidence. One approach suggested by the FDA guideline for establishment of drug shelf life is to estimate the expiration dating period as the time point at which the 95% one-sided lower confidence limit for mean degradation curve intersects the acceptable lower specification limit. Therefore, statistical concept and procedure for estimating shelf lives described in the FDA guideline is based on the 95% lower confidence limit for the mean degradation curve so that the mean strength of the drug product will remain within specifications until the labeled expiration date for 95% of the future batches.

For an estimation of drug shelf life with multiple batches, there are two major sources of variations: the within-batch variation and between-batch variation. It is suggested that these two sources be taken into account in stability analysis. It should be noted that the statistical methods described in Chapter 11 are derived under a fixed effects model, which considers only the within-batch variability. The consequence of the methods derived from a fixed effects model is that statistical inference can only be made to the batches under study. This is because the satistical inference obtained does not account for the between-batch variability. To account for this problem, Liu (1992) and Ho et al. (1992) suggested an alternative statistical procedure for estimating the expiration dating period. The method suggested not only uses the 95% lower confidence limit approach but also takes into account the between-batch variability. In this chapter we refer to their method as the *HLC method*.

To introduce the HLC method, we first consider a simple linear regression model without covariates for the balanced case where the time points are the same for all batches. Extension to the unbalanced case with different time points will be reviewed later.

For a given batch *i*, consider the following simple linear regression model which was given in (11.3.1):

$$Y_{ij} = \alpha_i + \beta_i X_j + e_{ij}, \qquad i = 1,\ldots,K, \quad j = 1,\ldots,n,$$

where α_i, β_i, and e_{ij} are similarly defined in (11.3.1). Let B_i denote batch *i*, $i = 1, \ldots, K$. Then $\{B_i, i = 1, \ldots, K\}$ represents a random sample from the population of the production batches. Let

$$\beta_i = (\alpha_i, \beta_i), \qquad i = 1,\ldots,K. \tag{12.5.1}$$

Then β_i is a random vector that describes the degradation pattern of drug product characteristic. Under assumption A, β_i, $i = 1, \ldots, K$, are i.i.d. as $N_2(\beta, \Sigma_\beta)$, where

$$\beta = (\alpha, \beta)', \tag{12.5.2}$$

and Σ_β is a 2×2 nonnegative definite covariance matrix. Therefore, model (11.3.1) becomes a regression model with a random coefficient (Gumpertz and Pantula 1989; Carter and Yang, 1986; Vonesh and Carter, 1987). Let

$$b_i = (a_i, b_i)', \qquad i = 1,\ldots,K \tag{12.5.3}$$

be the least-squares estimates of β_i for batch *i*, where a_i and b_i are as defined in (11.3.5). As indicated in (12.3.3) and (12.3.4), under assumption A, the MLE of β is given by

$$\begin{aligned}
\bar{b} &= (X'X)^{-1}X'\bar{Y} \\
&= \frac{1}{K} \sum_{i=1}^{K} (X'X)^{-1}X'Y_i \\
&= \frac{1}{K} \sum_{i=1}^{K} b_i \\
&= (\bar{a}, \bar{b})',
\end{aligned} \tag{12.5.4}$$

where

$$\bar{a} = \frac{1}{K} \sum_{i=1}^{K} a_i \quad \text{and} \quad \bar{b} = \frac{1}{K} \sum_{i=1}^{K} b_i.$$

Hence, under the case above, the MLE for β is simply the average of the ordinary least-squares estimates over the K batches. Since, as indicated in (12.3.4),

$$\bar{b} \sim N_2(\beta, \Sigma_b), \tag{12.5.5}$$

where

$$\Sigma_b = \frac{1}{K} [\Sigma_\beta + \sigma_e^2 (X'X)^{-1}].$$

Note that $\bar{b}$ is also an unbiased estimator of β under the balanced case. In addition, the covariance matrix of $\bar{b}$ consists of the within-batch variability [i.e., $\sigma_e^2 (X'X)^{-1}$] and the between-batch variability (i.e., Σ_β). Therefore, under assumption A, a random effects model can account for both the within-batch and between-batch variabilities for estimation of shelf life.

The unbiased estimators of Σ_b, σ_e^2, and Σ_β are given, respectively, as

$$S_b = \frac{1}{K-1} \sum_{i=1}^{K} (b_i - \bar{b})(b_i - \bar{b})',$$

$$\hat{\sigma}_e^2 = \text{MSE} = \frac{1}{N-2K} \text{SSE} = \frac{1}{N-2K} \sum_{i=1}^{K} \text{SSE }(i),$$

$$\hat{\Sigma}_\beta = S_b - \hat{\sigma}_e^2 (X'X)^{-1}, \tag{12.5.6}$$

where MSE, SSE, and SSE (i) are as defined in (11.3.10), (11.3.7), and (11.3.6), respectively. $\hat{\Sigma}_\beta$ is obtained as the difference between S_b and $\hat{\sigma}_e^2 (X'X)^{-1}$. It, however, should be noted that $\hat{\Sigma}_\beta$ might not be positive definite because the probability that $|\hat{\Sigma}_\beta| < 0$ may be greater than zero. In this case the estimator suggested by Carter and Yang (1986) is recommended to estimate Σ_β. Note that $\hat{\Sigma}_\beta$ is not required for estimation of drug shelf life in balanced case.

For any arbitrary 2 × 1 vector

$$x = (1, x)',$$

the minimum variance unbiased estimator is $x'\bar{b}$, which, under assumption A, follows a univariate normal distribution with mean $x'\beta$ and variance

$$\sigma_x^2 = x' \Sigma_b x.$$

An unbiased estimator for σ_x^2 is given as follows:

$$\hat{\sigma}_x^2 = x' S_b x, \tag{12.5.7}$$

which is distributed as $\sigma_x^2 \chi^2 (K - 1)$. Since $\mathbf{x}'\overline{\mathbf{b}}$ and $\hat{\sigma}_x^2$ are independent of each other,

$$T = \frac{\mathbf{x}'(\overline{\mathbf{b}} - \boldsymbol{\beta})}{\sqrt{\hat{\sigma}_x^2/K}} \tag{12.5.8}$$

follows a central t distribution with $K - 1$ degrees of freedom. Consequently, the 95% lower confidence limit for the mean degradation line $\mathbf{x}'\boldsymbol{\beta}$ at $\mathbf{x}$ is given by

$$L(x) = \mathbf{x}'\overline{\mathbf{b}} - t(0.05, K - 1) \sqrt{\frac{\hat{\sigma}_x^2}{K}}. \tag{12.5.9}$$

Note that

$$\mathbf{x}'\overline{\mathbf{b}} = \overline{a} + \overline{b}x,$$

$$\hat{\sigma}_x^2 = \frac{1}{K-1} \sum_{i=1}^{K} [(a_i - \overline{a})^2 + 2x(a_i - \overline{a})(b_i - \overline{b})$$

$$+ x^2 (b_i - \overline{b})^2]. \tag{12.5.10}$$

The 95% lower confidence limit for the mean degradation curve $\alpha + \beta x$ is constructed from both within- and between-batch variability. Hence statistical inference about the expiration dating period based on $L(x)$ in (12.5.9) can be made to all future production batches.

Similar to the method described in Sec. 11.2, the time points at which (12.5.9) intersects the acceptable lower specification limit η (if exist) are the two roots of the following quadratic equation:

$$[\eta - (\overline{a} + \overline{b}x)]^2 = t^2(0.05, K - 1) \frac{1}{K(K - 1)} \sum_{i=1}^{K} [(a_i - \overline{a})^2$$

$$+ 2x (a_i - \overline{a})(b_i - \overline{b})$$

$$+ x^2 (b_i - \overline{b})^2]. \tag{12.5.11}$$

These two roots, denoted by x_L and x_U, constitute the lower and upper limits of the 90% confidence interval for $(\eta - \alpha)/\beta$. Let

$$SE(\overline{a}) = \left[\frac{1}{K(K-1)} \sum_{i=1}^{K} (a_i - \overline{a})^2 \right]^{1/2},$$

$$SE(\overline{b}) = \left[\frac{1}{K(K - 1)} \sum_{i=1}^{K} (b_i - \overline{b})^2 \right]^{1/2},$$

$$T_{\overline{a}} = \frac{\overline{a} - \eta}{SE(\overline{a})},$$

$$T_{\overline{b}} = \frac{\overline{b}}{SE(\overline{b})}. \tag{12.5.12}$$

If the slope is statistically significantly smaller than zero and the intercept is statistically greater than η at the 5% level of significance, that is,

(i) $T_{\bar{b}} < -t(0.05, K - 1)$,

(ii) $T_{\bar{a}} > t(0.05, K - 1)$,　　　　　　　　　　　　　　　　　　　(12.5.13)

the 90% confidence interval for $(\eta - \alpha)/\beta$ is a close interval (x_L, x_U). Hence x_L is defined as the estimated expiration period for all futue production batches. In other cases, however, the 90% confidence interval for $(\eta - \alpha)/\beta$ is either the entire real line or two disjoint open intervals. Consequently, the estimated expiration dating period is undefined.

The estimated expiration dating period based on the 95% confidence limit for the mean degradation line has the same interpretation in terms of hypothesis testing as discussed in Sec. 11.1. However, in this chapter, the 95% confidence limit is constructed based on both the within- and between-batch variabilities.

When the number of time points is the same for all batches but the time points are different from batch to batch, model (11.3.1) can be expressed in the following matrix form:

$$\mathbf{Y}_i = \mathbf{X}_i\boldsymbol{\beta}_i + \boldsymbol{\epsilon}_i, \qquad i = 1, \ldots, K, \tag{12.5.14}$$

where

$$\mathbf{Y}_i = (Y_{i1}, \ldots, Y_{in}),$$

$$\mathbf{X}_i = \begin{bmatrix} 1 & X_{i1} \\ \vdots & \vdots \\ 1 & X_{in} \end{bmatrix},$$

$\boldsymbol{\beta}_i$ and $\boldsymbol{\epsilon}_i$ are as defined in (12.5.1) and (12.3.1), respectively. Under model (12.5.14) and assumption A, $\bar{\mathbf{b}}$ is also distributed as a bivariate normal vector with mean vector $\boldsymbol{\beta}$ and covariance matrix

$$\boldsymbol{\Sigma}_b = \boldsymbol{\Sigma}_\beta + \frac{1}{K} \sigma^2 \sum_{i=1}^{K} (\mathbf{X}'_i\mathbf{X}_i)^{-1}. \tag{12.5.15}$$

Hence $\bar{\mathbf{b}}$ is still unbiased for $\boldsymbol{\beta}$ and $\mathbf{S}_b$ defined in (12.5.6) is an unbiased estimator of $\boldsymbol{\Sigma}_b$. However, for any arbitrary 2×1 vector $\mathbf{x}$,

$$\hat{\sigma}_x^2 = \mathbf{x}' \, \mathbf{S}_b \mathbf{x}$$

is no longer distributed as a χ^2 random variable. As a result, T statistic defined in (12.5.8) does not have a central t distribution. Gumpertz and Pantula (1989) showed that when the product of the number of batches and number of time points (i.e., nK) becomes large, T follows approximately a central t distribution with v degrees of freedom, where

$$v = \frac{v_N}{v_D},$$

$$v_N = \left\{ \mathbf{x}' \mathbf{\Sigma}_\beta \mathbf{x} + \frac{1}{K} \sigma_e^2 \left[\sum_{i=1}^{K} \mathbf{x}' \, (\mathbf{X}_i' \mathbf{X}_i)^{-1} \mathbf{x} \right] \right\}^2,$$

$$v_D = \left(\frac{1}{K-1} \mathbf{x}' \mathbf{\Sigma}_\beta \mathbf{x} \right)^2 + \left\{ \frac{\sigma_e^2}{K^2(n-2)} \left[\sum_{i=1}^{K} \mathbf{x}' \, (\mathbf{X}_i' \mathbf{X}_i)^{-1} \mathbf{x} \right] \right\}^2. \tag{12.5.16}$$

If the condition in (12.5.13) is satisfied, the expiration dating period can be estimated by the smaller root x_L of the quadratic equation:

$$[\eta - (\bar{a} + \bar{b}x)]^2 = t^2(0.05, v)\hat{\sigma}_x^2, \tag{12.5.17}$$

where $\hat{\sigma}_x^2$ is defined in (12.5.7).

Note that application of (12.5.16) to estimate the degrees of freedom v involves the unknown time point at which the mean degradation line intersects the lower specification limit η, the unknown between batch covariance matrix $\mathbf{\Sigma}_\beta$, and the unknown within-batch variability σ_e^2. However, σ_e^2 and $\mathbf{\Sigma}_\beta$ can be estimated by their unbiased estimators, which are given, respectively, as

$$\hat{\sigma}_e^2 = \text{MSE} = \frac{1}{N - 2K} \sum_{i=1}^{K} \text{SSE}(i),$$

$$\hat{\mathbf{\Sigma}}_\beta = \mathbf{S}_b \sim \hat{\sigma}_e^2 \frac{1}{K} \sum_{i=1}^{K} (\mathbf{X}_i' \mathbf{X}_i)^{-1} \tag{12.5.18}$$

It is suggested that the unknown time point be estimated by its maximum likelihood estimate

$$\hat{x}_0 = \frac{\eta - \bar{a}}{\bar{b}}. \tag{12.5.19}$$

For $\mathbf{\Sigma}_\beta$, as indicated earlier, $\hat{\mathbf{\Sigma}}_\beta$ might not be positive definite. In this case the estimator suggested by Carter and Yang (1986) can be used.

Note that when $n_i = n$ and $\mathbf{X}_i = \mathbf{X}$ for $i = 1, \ldots, K$, the exact inference of the shelf life is based on the number of batches. However, the approximation by a central t distribution with v degrees of freedom can still be applied as long as nK is large. When the number of time points are different from batch to batch, the estimated generalized least-squares (EGLS) estimator for β suggested by Carter and Yang (1986) and Vonesh and Carter (1987) might be useful for construction of the 95% lower confidence limit for mean degradation line $\alpha + \beta x$. However, the statistical inference of their methods is based on the asympotic results as either the number of batches become large or the minimum of the number of time points goes large.

12.6. COMPARISON OF METHODS FOR MULTIPLE BATCHES

Under assumption A for the random effects model, two methods for estimation of expiration dating period were presented in Secs. 12.4 and 12.5. Chow and Shao's method was derived from the probability statement for a given future batch selected randomly from the population of the production batches. On the other hand, the HLC method incorporates the between-batch variability into the construction of the 95% lower confidence limit for the mean degradation curve. Under the simple linear regression model without covariates, for the balanced case where all time points are the same, from (12.4.11), (12.4.12), and (12.4.13), the estimated shelf life by Chow and Shao's method is the solution to the following equation:

$$\bar{a} + \bar{b}x = \eta + c_K(\epsilon,\alpha)z_\epsilon \sqrt{v(t)}. \tag{12.6.1}$$

In other words, the smaller root of the following quadratic equation, if it exists, will be the estimated shelf life provided by Chow and Shao's method:

$$[\eta - (\bar{a} + \bar{b}x)]^2 = [c_K(\epsilon,\alpha)z_\epsilon]^2 v(t). \tag{12.6.2}$$

Note that

$$[c_K(\epsilon,\alpha)z_\epsilon]^2 = \left[\frac{t(\alpha, K - 1, \sqrt{K}\, z_\epsilon)}{\sqrt{K}\, z_\epsilon} z_\epsilon\right]^2$$

$$= \frac{1}{K}[t(\alpha, K - 1, \sqrt{K}\, z_\epsilon]^2. \tag{12.6.3}$$

In addition, from (12.3.10),

$$S = \sum_{i=1}^{K}(\mathbf{Y}_i - \overline{\mathbf{Y}})(\mathbf{Y}_i - \overline{\mathbf{Y}})'.$$

It follows in conjunction with (12.4.9) that

$$(\mathbf{X'X})^{-1}\mathbf{X'SX}(\mathbf{X'X})^{-1}$$

$$= \sum_{i=1}^{K}(\mathbf{X'X})^{-1}\mathbf{X'}(\mathbf{Y}_i - \overline{\mathbf{Y}})(\mathbf{Y} - \overline{\mathbf{Y}})'\mathbf{X}(\mathbf{X'X})^{-1}$$

$$= \sum_{i=1}^{K}(\mathbf{b}_i - \overline{\mathbf{b}})(\mathbf{b}_i - \overline{\mathbf{b}})'$$

$$= (K - 1)\,\mathbf{S}_b, \tag{12.6.4}$$

where S_b is defined in (12.5.6). As a result, for any arbitrary 2×1 fixed vector x, $v(t)$ defined in (12.4.9) gives

$$v(t) = \frac{1}{K-1} x' (X'X)^{-1} X'SX(X'X)^{-1} x$$

$$= \frac{1}{K-1} x'S_b x$$

$$= \hat{\sigma}_x^2.$$

Hence (12.6.2) reduces to

$$[\eta - (\bar{a} + \bar{b}x)]^2 = \frac{1}{K} \hat{\sigma}_x^2 [t(\alpha, K-1, \sqrt{K} z_\epsilon)]^2. \tag{12.6.5}$$

Recall that the estimated shelf life by the HLC method is the smaller root, if it exists, of the following equation:

$$[\eta - (\bar{a} + \bar{b}x)]^2 = \frac{1}{K} \hat{\sigma}_x^2 [t(\alpha, K-1)]^2. \tag{12.6.6}$$

If $\epsilon = 0.5$ and $z(\epsilon) = 0$, (12.6.5) becomes (12.6.6). In addition,

$$\tilde{L}(x) = (\bar{a} + \bar{b}x) - \left(\frac{1}{K} \hat{\sigma}_x^2 \right)^{1/2} t(\alpha, K-1, \sqrt{K} z_\epsilon), \tag{12.6.7}$$

which is the $(1 - \alpha) \times 100\%$ lower ϵ-content tolerance limit. Since for $\epsilon < 0.5$, a $(1 - \alpha) \times 100\%$ lower ϵ-content tolerance limit is the $(1 - \alpha) \times 100\%$ lower confidence limit for the ϵth quantile of the distribution under study (Hahn and Meeker, 1991), the estimated expiration dating period by Chow and Shao's method is the time point at which the $(1 - \alpha) \times 100\%$ lower confidence limit for the ϵth quantile of the distribution of random degradation line $\alpha_i + \beta_i x$ intersects the lower specification limit η. When $\epsilon = 0.5$, the 50% quantile of a normal distribution is the mean. Therefore, the HLC method is in fact a special case of Chow and Shao's method. However, if $\epsilon < 0.5$,

$$t(\alpha, K-1) \leq t(\alpha, K-1, \sqrt{K} z_\epsilon).$$

Hence the estimated expiration dating period by Chow and Shao's method is always shorter than the shelf life given by the HLC method. It should be noted that the interpretation of the estimates are different. The estimate by the HLC method provides a 95% confidence that the average characteristic of the dosage units in future batches will remain within specification up to the end of the estimated shelf life. On the other hand, Chow and Shao's method suggests the use of an estimate which gives a 95% confidence that at least $1 - \epsilon$ proportion of the distribution of the drug characteristic for future batches will be within specifications until the end of the estimated expiration dating period.

Ho et al. (1992) conducted a simulation study to compare four methods for estimation of drug shelf life with multiple batches. These four methods include the FDA's minimum approach, Ruberg and Hsu's method under the fixed effects model discussed in Chapter 11, Chow and Shao's method, and the HLC procedure under the random effects model described in this chapter. Model (11.3.1) was employed to generate random samples. The intercept and slope are chosen to provide true shelf life $t_{true} = (90 - \alpha)/\beta$ to be 4, 6.67, and 20 months. Three sets of sampling time points were selected:

1. 0, 3, 6, 9, 12 months
2. 0, 3, 6, 9, 12, 18, 24 months
3. 0, 3, 6, 9, 12, 18, 24, 36, 48 months

The within-batch variability σ_e^2 were selected to be 0.25, 0.75, and 1.25. The following three between-batch covariance matrices are considered in the simulation:

$$\mathbf{m}_1 = \begin{bmatrix} 0 & 0 \\ 0 & 0 \end{bmatrix}, \quad \mathbf{m}_2 = \begin{bmatrix} 1.00 & 0.03 \\ 0.03 & 0.01 \end{bmatrix}, \quad \text{and} \quad \mathbf{m}_3 = \begin{bmatrix} 1.00 & 0.03 \\ 0.03 & 0.02 \end{bmatrix}.$$

In addition, the impact of sample size was also studied by examining three different numbers of batches: 3, 6, and 9. For each of 81 combinations, 1000 random samples were generated to estimate the shelf life by the four methods. For Ruberg and Hsu's method, the bioequivalence-like approach was used with the upper allowable specification limit Δ_β chosen as recommended by Ruberg and Stegeman (1991). The coverage probability, average bias, and mean-squared error of the corresponding estimates with respect to $(90 - \alpha)/\beta$ were computed. The results are summarized in Tables 12.6.1 through 12.6.3.

In general, if the relationship between drug characteristic and time points is still linear beyond the observed range of time points as assumed in the simulation, the results are consistent even when an extrapolation is required. When both variabilities are large and the number of batches is small, the coverage probabilities of all four methods are relatively lower than those obtained from other combinations which have smaller variability and large number of batches.

Since Chow and Shao's method is not for the mean drug characteristic but rather for the ϵ quantile of the distribution where $\epsilon < 0.5$, not surprisingly, their method has the highest but excessive coverage probability uniformly greater than the nominal level of 0.95. As a consequence, this method has the largest average bias and mean-squared error. This indicates that Chow and Shao's method often underestimates the shelf life and is the most conservative among the four methods under study. On the other hand, the FDA's minimum approach also exhibits a pattern similar to Chow and Shao's method. It provides a coverage probability greater than the 0.95 nominal level for a large number of batches and small within- and between-batches variabilities. However, the

TABLE 12.6.1 Comparison of Methods for Estimating Drug Shelf Life: Study Periods of 0, 3, 6, 9, and 12 Months

(a) True shelf life: 20 months

σ^2	Σ	Batches	Probability coverage				Mean bias				MSE			
			FDA	R&H	C&S	HLC	FDA	R&H	C&S	HLC	FDA	R&H	C&S	HLC
0.25	m_1	3	0.965	0.951	0.997	0.868	−2.001	−1.374	−6.990	−1.459	5.76	2.53	54.12	3.61
		6	0.960	0.951	1.000	0.953	−1.726	−0.942	−6.497	−1.092	5.38	1.20	43.98	1.62
		9	0.977	0.967	1.000	0.964	−1.780	−0.833	−5.549	−0.912	5.99	0.92	31.70	1.08
	m_2	3	0.939	0.867	0.998	0.927	−4.891	−2.872	−14.409	−5.189	31.93	14.65	226.09	38.51
		6	0.981	0.885	1.000	0.937	−6.338	−2.249	−15.467	−3.205	45.54	8.39	246.79	14.28
		9	0.999	0.904	1.000	0.939	−7.152	−1.955	−13.821	−2.590	54.41	5.85	196.09	9.03
	m_3	3	0.952	0.864	0.997	0.939	−5.447	−2.959	−15.235	−5.945	39.95	18.86	246.21	49.87
		6	0.989	0.869	1.000	0.943	−7.187	−2.368	−15.952	−3.812	56.41	9.76	260.68	19.17
		9	1.000	0.883	1.000	0.945	−7.992	−2.111	−14.539	−3.162	66.66	7.50	215.10	13.18
0.75	m_1	3	0.963	0.947	0.998	0.896	−2.962	−2.192	−9.250	−2.340	12.06	6.28	92.53	8.77
		6	0.970	0.953	1.000	0.954	−2.829	−1.540	−8.739	−1.742	12.96	3.16	78.57	4.04
		9	0.970	0.949	1.000	0.952	−2.677	−1.320	−7.616	−1.443	12.75	2.34	59.34	2.79
	m_2	3	0.942	0.900	1.000	0.918	−4.984	−3.224	−14.389	−4.877	33.54	16.48	222.70	35.80
		6	0.968	0.908	1.000	0.938	−6.116	−2.624	−15.525	−3.380	47.21	10.41	248.13	15.78
		9	0.972	0.907	1.000	0.936	−6.895	−2.139	−14.015	−2.668	57.74	6.98	201.60	9.91
	m_3	3	0.942	0.866	0.998	0.825	−5.814	−3.342	−14.805	−5.728	44.78	20.22	233.83	47.12
		6	0.969	0.890	1.000	0.937	−7.295	−2.635	−16.069	−3.850	62.66	11.81	265.06	20.54
		9	0.986	0.884	1.000	0.933	−8.299	−2.288	−14.738	−3.221	76.01	8.87	221.70	14.38
1.25	m_1	3	0.959	0.942	0.998	0.872	−3.625	−2.629	−10.315	−2.699	18.03	9.16	115.20	12.84
		6	0.967	0.959	1.000	0.954	−3.244	−1.929	−9.803	−2.189	16.89	5.06	98.78	6.54
		9	0.948	0.939	1.000	0.951	−3.121	−1.611	−8.688	−1.760	17.33	3.56	76.97	4.14
	m_2	3	0.940	0.905	0.997	0.912	−5.069	−3.531	−14.020	−4.792	36.13	19.70	213.86	37.75
		6	0.964	0.922	1.000	0.941	−6.086	−2.806	−15.545	−3.537	49.27	11.71	249.15	17.18
		9	0.967	0.927	1.000	0.943	−6.658	−2.372	−14.258	−2.861	58.02	8.10	208.65	11.18
	m_3	3	0.930	0.879	1.000	0.895	−5.552	−3.385	−15.076	−5.406	44.53	21.44	242.31	46.72
		6	0.964	0.910	1.000	0.939	−7.121	−2.827	−16.024	−3.891	63.41	12.58	263.04	20.74
		9	0.974	0.902	1.000	0.932	−8.162	−2.441	−14.878	−3.305	77.83	9.46	225.86	14.70

TABLE 12.6.1 (Continued)

(b) True shelf life: 6.67 months

σ^2	Σ	Batches	Probability coverage				Mean bias				MSE			
			FDA	R&H	C&S	HLC	FDA	R&H	C&S	HLC	FDA	R&H	C&S	HLC
0.25	m_1	3	0.961	0.949	1.000	0.882	-0.224	-0.151	-1.782	-0.172	0.07	0.04	3.84	0.05
		6	0.960	0.949	1.000	0.949	-0.213	-0.102	-1.524	-0.119	0.09	0.01	2.51	0.02
		9	0.964	0.951	1.000	0.959	-0.194	-0.085	-1.282	-0.095	0.08	0.02	1.88	0.01
	m_2	3	0.895	0.761	0.997	0.950	-0.867	-0.381	-4.677	-1.214	1.25	0.43	24.22	2.07
		6	0.968	0.791	1.000	0.953	-1.305	-0.289	-4.989	-0.687	2.10	0.22	-26.26	0.64
		9	0.987	0.774	1.000	0.942	-1.524	-0.214	-4.292	-0.512	2.63	0.15	19.25	0.36
	m_3	3	0.914	0.747	1.000	0.946	-1.014	-0.398	-4.705	-1.304	1.56	0.49	24.28	2.37
		6	0.991	0.791	1.000	0.957	-1.420	-0.297	-5.075	-0.720	2.35	0.25	27.04	0.70
		9	0.998	0.767	1.000	0.946	-1.679	-0.256	-4.375	-0.579	3.08	0.18	19.92	0.45
0.75	m_1	3	0.964	0.955	0.100	0.903	-0.397	-0.267	-2.721	-0.310	0.25	0.09	9.16	0.17
		6	0.960	0.950	1.000	0.938	-0.364	-0.175	-2.285	-0.202	0.28	0.05	5.83	0.06
		9	0.962	0.948	1.000	0.953	-0.357	-0.144	-1.784	-0.160	0.29	0.02	3.34	0.04
	m_2	3	0.880	0.797	1.000	0.930	-0.875	-0.455	-4.587	-1.191	1.35	0.52	23.57	2.11
		6	0.936	0.800	1.000	0.945	-1.263	-0.331	-5.088	-0.699	2.32	0.26	27.37	0.67
		9	0.948	0.810	1.000	0.958	-1.511	-0.268	-4.492	-0.548	3.04	0.17	21.12	0.41
	m_3	3	0.901	0.786	0.996	0.938	-1.055	-0.463	-4.515	-1.280	1.80	0.59	22.92	2.39
		6	0.957	0.796	1.000	0.951	-1.537	-0.336	-5.254	-0.746	3.03	0.29	28.87	0.76
		9	0.977	0.768	1.000	0.944	-1.806	-0.248	-4.519	-0.553	3.80	0.18	21.47	0.42
1.25	m_1	3	0.961	0.937	1.000	0.886	-0.514	-0.338	-3.153	-0.390	0.41	0.16	12.19	0.25
		6	0.953	0.940	1.000	0.947	-0.486	-0.230	-2.997	-0.272	0.47	0.07	10.09	0.10
		9	0.966	0.954	1.000	0.959	-0.455	-0.193	-2.229	-0.214	0.46	0.04	5.34	0.05
	m_2	3	0.867	0.788	0.998	0.916	-0.854	-0.432	-4.563	-1.158	1.40	0.51	23.29	2.08
		6	0.908	0.810	1.000	0.920	-1.221	-0.345	-5.159	-0.687	2.41	0.29	28.06	0.69
		9	0.907	0.807	1.000	0.932	-1.346	-0.277	-4.660	-0.534	2.88	0.18	22.94	0.41
	m_3	3	0.913	0.802	0.992	0.945	-1.065	-0.510	-4.623	-1.278	1.91	0.64	23.95	2.43
		6	0.938	0.804	1.000	0.946	-1.534	-0.373	-5.214	-0.756	3.29	0.33	28.51	0.78
		9	0.957	0.822	1.000	0.943	-1.878	-0.303	-4.740	-0.593	4.43	0.21	23.50	0.48

TABLE 12.6.1 (Continued)

(c) True shelf life: 4 months

σ^2	Σ	Batches	Probability coverage				Mean bias				MSE			
			FDA	R&H	C&S	HLC	FDA	R&H	C&S	HLC	FDA	R&H	C&S	HLC
0.25	m_1	3	0.959	0.950	0.998	0.904	−0.150	−0.101	−1.402	−0.119	0.04	0.01	2.31	0.02
		6	0.955	0.937	1.000	0.946	−0.149	−0.068	−1.121	−0.079	0.04	0.01	1.36	0.01
		9	0.966	0.947	1.000	0.955	−0.157	−0.054	−1.002	−0.060	0.05	0.00	1.00	0.00
	m_2	3	0.911	0.797	0.998	0.914	−0.519	−0.252	−2.845	−0.652	0.44	0.16	9.07	0.66
		6	0.979	0.816	1.000	0.960	−0.777	−0.192	−3.155	−0.366	0.74	0.07	10.52	0.18
		9	0.990	0.828	1.000	0.943	−0.904	−0.156	−2.697	−0.283	0.92	0.05	7.66	0.11
	m_3	3	0.924	0.798	0.997	0.927	−0.576	−0.276	−2.906	−0.689	0.50	0.17	9.35	0.70
		6	0.991	0.833	1.000	0.948	−0.852	−0.215	−3.185	−0.388	0.85	0.10	10.70	0.21
		9	0.998	0.836	1.000	0.951	−0.972	−0.170	−2.748	−0.294	1.03	0.06	7.91	0.12
0.75	m_1	3	0.958	0.945	0.996	0.891	−0.276	−0.180	−2.038	−0.209	0.12	0.05	5.08	0.08
		6	0.968	0.960	1.000	0.951	−0.266	−0.123	−1.821	−0.144	0.14	0.02	3.70	0.03
		9	0.966	0.956	1.000	0.953	−0.275	−0.099	−1.373	−0.110	0.17	0.01	2.12	0.01
	m_2	3	0.889	0.816	0.996	0.913	−0.533	−0.284	−2.894	−0.635	0.49	0.18	9.39	0.63
		6	0.953	0.859	1.000	0.945	−0.767	−0.233	−3.188	−0.385	0.85	0.10	10.78	0.21
		9	0.963	0.856	1.000	0.946	−0.923	−0.180	−2.838	−0.293	1.14	0.07	8.46	0.12
	m_3	3	0.909	0.830	1.000	0.907	−0.644	−0.337	−2.935	−0.671	0.64	0.22	9.52	0.70
		6	0.971	0.848	1.000	0.937	−0.961	−0.240	−3.257	−0.391	1.15	0.12	11.14	0.22
		9	0.984	0.861	1.000	0.943	−1.132	−0.191	−2.868	−0.300	1.47	0.07	8.64	0.13
1.25	m_1	3	0.954	0.938	0.999	0.868	−0.345	−0.219	−2.330	−0.258	0.20	0.07	6.50	0.13
		6	0.971	0.960	1.000	0.942	−0.352	−0.156	−2.267	−0.180	0.26	0.03	5.73	0.05
		9	0.967	0.957	1.000	0.964	−0.354	−0.125	−1.807	−0.140	0.30	0.02	3.52	0.03
	m_2	3	0.905	0.843	0.950	0.914	−0.598	−0.325	−2.889	−0.639	0.61	0.21	9.35	0.65
		6	0.927	0.859	1.000	0.928	−0.772	−0.233	−3.273	−0.378	0.96	0.10	11.26	0.21
		9	0.947	0.855	1.000	0.939	−0.936	−0.200	−3.023	−0.308	1.32	0.08	9.62	0.14
	m_3	3	0.920	0.858	0.993	0.933	−0.696	−0.370	−2.892	−0.701	0.77	0.25	9.24	0.77
		6	0.959	0.869	1.000	0.941	−0.990	−0.253	−3.249	−0.391	1.33	0.12	11.11	0.23
		9	0.976	0.873	1.000	0.945	−1.154	−0.208	−3.027	−0.311	1.70	0.08	9.63	0.13

TABLE 12.6.2 Comparison of Methods for Estimating Drug Shelf Life: Study Periods of 0, 3, 6, 9, 12, 18, and 24 Months

(a) True shelf life: 20 months

σ^2	Σ	Batches	Probability coverage				Mean bias				MSE			
			FDA	R&H	C&S	HLC	FDA	R&H	C&S	HLC	FDA	R&H	C&S	HLC
0.25	m_1	3	0.962	0.953	0.999	0.890	-0.814	-0.574	-4.176	-0.633	0.99	0.42	20.14	0.66
		6	0.967	0.953	1.000	0.949	-0.788	-0.409	-3.705	-0.462	1.12	0.24	14.64	0.28
		9	0.962	0.952	1.000	0.951	-0.730	-0.326	-2.991	-0.348	1.12	0.14	9.37	0.14
	m_2	3	0.914	0.722	0.997	0.942	-4.081	-1.395	-14.686	-5.434	24.86	9.74	232.67	39.80
		6	0.993	0.744	1.000	0.932	-5.625	-1.107	-15.459	-3.204	35.97	5.08	246.97	14.17
		9	1.000	0.759	1.000	0.941	-6.342	-0.984	-13.705	-2.570	43.68	3.27	193.44	8.91
	m_3	3	0.922	0.729	0.997	0.949	-4.677	-1.531	-15.187	-6.202	32.41	14.19	244.11	50.75
		6	0.994	0.729	1.000	0.934	-6.350	-1.210	-16.124	-3.774	45.54	7.65	266.73	19.68
		9	0.998	0.758	1.000	0.956	-7.354	-1.247	-14.565	-3.240	57.70	5.30	216.32	13.63
0.75	m_1	3	0.964	0.946	0.997	0.889	-1.339	-0.953	-6.227	-1.069	2.64	1.22	45.73	1.93
		6	0.955	0.941	1.000	0.940	-1.213	-0.672	-5.454	-0.764	2.59	0.61	31.54	0.81
		9	0.972	0.959	1.000	0.953	-1.189	-0.559	-4.462	-0.594	2.78	0.42	20.66	0.46
	m_2	3	0.923	0.733	0.995	0.929	-4.245	-1.448	-14.516	-5.129	26.65	9.37	228.05	37.52
		6	0.986	0.763	1.000	0.954	-6.122	-1.283	-15.692	-3.302	42.47	5.12	254.73	14.56
		9	0.998	0.764	1.000	0.954	-6.898	-1.061	-14.105	-2.625	50.66	3.31	204.12	9.08
	m_3	3	0.922	0.727	0.998	0.941	-5.054	-1.691	-15.099	-6.244	36.40	14.04	243.75	52.27
		6	0.994	0.743	1.000	0.958	-6.882	-1.361	-16.144	-3.886	52.61	7.40	267.34	20.00
		9	1.000	0.764	1.000	0.961	-7.747	-1.269	-14.675	-3.224	63.23	5.31	219.71	13.52
1.25	m_1	3	0.960	0.949	0.998	0.878	-1.655	-1.203	-7.391	-1.302	3.90	1.91	64.41	2.88
		6	0.968	0.958	1.000	0.953	-1.564	-0.866	-6.607	-0.966	4.30	0.99	46.59	1.27
		9	0.969	0.954	1.000	0.961	-1.426	-0.715	-5.325	-0.762	3.92	0.69	29.42	0.77
	m_2	3	0.912	0.796	0.998	0.930	-4.519	-1.942	-14.54	-5.319	30.06	10.49	227.98	39.12
		6	0.969	0.761	1.000	0.937	-6.059	-1.225	-15.626	-3.130	43.63	5.53	253.01	13.95
		9	0.988	0.779	1.000	0.935	-7.180	-1.225	-14.272	-2.707	56.21	4.18	209.71	10.02
	m_3	3	0.915	0.740	0.997	0.940	-5.223	-1.754	-15.056	-6.117	39.26	14.23	241.36	51.84
		6	0.990	0.769	1.000	0.939	-7.235	-1.500	-16.321	-3.933	58.15	7.85	273.18	20.45
		9	1.000	0.770	1.000	0.938	-8.064	-1.356	-14.935	-3.243	68.72	5.78	227.96	14.13

TABLE 12.6.2 (Continued)

(b) True shelf life: 6.67 months

σ^2	Σ	Batches	Probability coverage				Mean bias				MSE			
			FDA	R&H	C&S	HLC	FDA	R&H	C&S	HLC	FDA	R&H	C&S	HLC
0.25	m_1	3	0.967	0.955	1.000	0.887	−0.190	−0.134	−1.663	−0.153	0.05	0.02	3.37	0.03
		6	0.962	0.954	1.000	0.944	−0.193	−0.095	−1.503	−0.106	0.07	0.01	2.45	0.02
		9	0.952	0.939	1.000	0.948	−0.193	−0.076	−1.247	−0.083	0.08	0.01	1.78	0.01
	m_2	3	0.926	0.767	1.000	0.940	−0.978	−0.429	−4.710	−1.232	1.42	0.51	24.53	2.18
		6	0.996	0.783	1.000	0.949	−1.384	−0.308	−5.071	−0.669	2.21	0.25	27.10	0.63
		9	0.999	0.820	1.000	0.957	−1.562	−0.278	−4.315	−0.536	2.69	0.18	19.46	0.39
	m_3	3	0.930	0.792	0.998	0.942	−1.042	−0.495	−4.726	−1.306	1.58	0.64	24.77	2.41
		6	0.999	0.828	1.000	0.948	−1.447	−0.373	−5.142	−0.719	2.38	0.32	27.71	0.70
		9	0.999	0.812	1.000	0.949	−1.660	−0.314	−4.382	−0.565	3.01	0.22	19.98	0.43
0.75	m_1	3	0.965	0.959	1.000	0.896	−0.350	−0.237	−2.706	−0.272	0.18	0.08	9.11	0.12
		6	0.967	0.956	1.000	0.951	−0.347	−0.167	−2.267	−0.189	0.22	0.04	5.62	0.05
		9	0.952	0.939	1.000	0.950	−0.341	−0.133	−1.805	−0.145	0.26	0.03	3.44	0.03
	m_2	3	0.930	0.788	1.000	0.927	−1.082	−0.460	−4.721	−1.211	1.73	0.54	24.73	2.16
		6	0.990	0.807	1.000	0.941	−1.562	−0.349	−5.076	−0.674	2.84	0.28	27.20	0.64
		9	0.995	0.817	1.000	0.946	−1.801	−0.286	−4.446	−0.525	3.54	0.19	20.73	0.39
	m_3	3	0.936	0.787	1.000	0.924	−1.219	−0.540	−4.645	−1.256	2.08	0.71	24.00	2.36
		6	0.996	0.817	1.000	0.941	−1.723	−0.420	−5.156	−0.746	3.37	0.39	27.96	0.78
		9	1.000	0.831	1.000	0.940	−1.906	−0.349	−4.506	−0.582	3.92	0.26	21.20	0.48
1.25	m_1	3	0.963	0.955	1.000	0.924	−0.476	−0.319	−3.299	−0.372	0.35	0.13	13.29	0.22
		6	0.952	0.938	1.000	0.951	−0.434	−0.209	−2.875	−0.239	0.37	0.07	9.27	0.08
		9	0.960	0.946	1.000	0.952	−0.438	−0.177	−2.192	−0.193	0.42	0.04	5.15	0.06
	m_2	3	0.910	0.810	1.000	0.926	−1.144	−0.506	−4.567	−1.180	1.99	0.58	23.30	2.11
		6	0.984	0.815	1.000	0.924	−1.713	−0.375	−5.180	−0.689	3.51	0.32	28.29	0.70
		9	0.996	0.818	1.000	0.942	−1.957	−0.290	−4.595	−0.519	4.20	0.20	22.12	0.39
	m_3	3	0.933	0.830	1.000	0.923	−1.314	−0.580	−4.702	−1.281	2.44	0.74	24.67	2.45
		6	0.989	0.837	1.000	0.945	−1.842	−0.427	−5.205	−0.724	3.88	0.38	28.57	0.75
		9	0.998	0.802	1.000	0.932	−2.072	−0.328	−4.690	−0.555	4.64	0.24	22.99	0.44

TABLE 12.6.2 (Continued)

(c) True shelf life: 4 months

σ^2	Σ	Batches	Probability coverage				Mean bias				MSE			
			FDA	R&H	C&S	HLC	FDA	R&H	C&S	HLC	FDA	R&H	C&S	HLC
0.25	m_1	3	0.964	0.952	1.000	0.885	-0.143	-0.0958	-1.334	-0.111	0.03	0.01	2.05	0.02
		6	0.962	0.952	1.000	0.939	-0.140	-0.0685	-1.096	-0.078	0.04	0.00	1.29	0.01
		9	0.963	0.952	1.000	0.957	-0.134	-0.056	-1.000	-0.061	0.04	0.00	1.00	0.00
	m_2	3	0.940	0.829	0.993	0.938	-0.556	-0.286	-2.877	-0.649	0.45	0.17	9.25	0.63
		6	0.998	0.873	1.000	0.956	-0.800	-0.224	-3.165	-0.361	0.73	0.09	10.58	0.17
		9	1.000	0.876	1.000	0.954	-0.893	-0.194	-2.664	-0.284	0.88	0.06	7.47	0.11
	m_3	3	0.950	0.864	0.988	0.932	-0.607	-0.361	-2.864	-0.675	0.51	0.24	9.22	0.69
		6	0.996	0.870	1.000	0.935	-0.812	-0.261	-3.166	-0.362	0.76	0.11	10.57	0.18
		9	1.000	0.902	1.000	0.948	-0.946	-0.238	-2.748	-0.302	0.98	0.09	7.92	0.12
0.75	m_1	3	0.963	0.954	1.000	0.912	-0.254	-0.172	-1.994	-0.202	0.11	0.04	4.67	0.07
		6	0.968	0.953	1.000	0.949	-0.239	-0.116	-1.682	-0.131	0.11	0.02	3.12	0.02
		9	0.966	0.955	1.000	0.957	-0.235	-0.093	-1.305	-0.101	0.12	0.01	1.91	0.01
	m_2	3	0.934	0.833	1.998	0.913	-0.647	-0.313	-2.911	-0.609	0.60	0.20	9.44	0.59
		6	0.989	0.875	1.000	0.944	-0.935	-0.256	-3.230	-0.370	0.99	0.11	10.94	0.19
		9	0.998	0.887	1.000	0.950	-1.083	-0.207	-2.803	-0.288	1.27	0.07	8.26	0.11
	m_3	3	0.957	0.878	0.998	0.929	-0.737	-0.389	-2.930	-0.671	0.73	0.27	9.54	0.69
		6	0.997	0.901	1.000	0.937	-1.025	-0.298	-3.256	-0.387	1.17	0.14	11.13	0.21
		9	1.000	0.907	1.000	0.942	-1.125	-0.243	-2.845	-0.299	1.36	0.09	8.51	0.13
1.25	m_1	3	0.962	0.956	0.998	0.876	-0.321	-0.216	-2.286	-0.250	0.16	0.06	6.19	0.11
		6	0.948	0.938	1.000	0.944	-0.312	-0.150	-2.080	-0.174	0.19	0.03	4.76	0.04
		9	0.956	0.943	1.000	0.943	-0.299	-0.119	-1.666	-0.130	0.20	0.02	3.02	0.02
	m_2	3	0.950	0.880	0.994	0.928	-0.724	-0.368	-2.893	-0.659	0.73	0.23	9.35	0.68
		6	0.984	0.884	1.000	0.943	-1.0456	-0.272	-3.305	-0.383	1.29	0.12	11.46	0.20
		9	0.994	0.875	1.000	0.937	-1.209	-0.223	-2.929	-0.298	1.61	0.08	9.02	0.13
	m_3	3	0.957	0.857	0.995	0.909	-0.786	-0.392	-2.936	-0.638	0.83	0.28	9.59	0.67
		6	0.997	0.905	1.000	0.942	-1.127	-0.312	-3.310	-0.391	1.42	0.15	11.50	0.22
		9	1.000	0.931	1.000	0.947	-1.286	-0.271	-2.995	-0.325	1.77	0.10	9.43	0.14

TABLE 12.6.3 Comparison of Methods for Estimating Drug Shelf Life: Study Periods of 0, 3, 6, 9, 12, 18, 24, 36, and 48 Months

(a) True shelf life: 20 months

σ^2	Σ	Batches	Probability coverage				Mean bias				MSE			
			FDA	R&H	C&S	HLC	FDA	R&H	C&S	HLC	FDA	R&H	C&S	HLC
0.25	m_1	3	0.955	0.944	0.996	0.891	−0.466	−0.321	−3.267	−0.372	0.33	0.13	12.85	0.24
		6	0.961	0.951	1.000	0.955	−0.438	−0.225	−2.655	−0.252	0.37	0.07	7.62	0.09
		9	0.961	0.944	1.000	0.945	−0.419	−0.181	−2.120	−0.196	0.36	0.03	4.76	0.08
	m_2	3	0.911	0.688	0.997	0.949	−3.975	−1.237	−14.557	−5.463	23.45	8.95	230.66	39.66
		6	0.994	0.704	1.000	0.961	−5.527	−1.026	−15.533	−3.293	35.02	4.98	249.38	14.41
		9	0.998	0.712	1.000	0.954	−6.287	−0.850	−13.864	−2.601	43.10	3.47	197.02	9.20
	m_3	3	0.888	0.692	0.999	0.944	−4.495	−1.271	−15.160	−6.151	31.80	15.75	245.28	50.87
		6	0.983	0.706	1.000	0.947	−6.438	−1.174	−16.194	−3.929	47.31	8.46	268.46	20.63
		9	1.000	0.729	1.000	0.953	−7.205	−1.127	−14.610	−3.233	55.79	5.28	217.31	13.44
0.75	m_1	3	0.965	0.949	0.999	0.890	−0.789	−0.565	−5.356	−0.653	0.91	0.42	36.22	0.71
		6	0.965	0.950	1.000	0.950	−0.766	−0.396	−4.245	−0.445	1.07	0.20	19.89	0.28
		9	0.956	0.943	1.000	0.943	−0.755	−0.323	−3.335	−0.345	1.17	0.15	11.78	0.17
	m_2	3	0.918	0.692	0.997	0.937	−4.259	−1.238	−14.419	−5.376	26.91	10.31	226.23	39.73
		6	0.996	0.666	1.000	0.950	−5.884	−0.937	−15.708	−3.173	39.21	4.90	255.43	13.63
		9	1.000	0.716	1.000	0.951	−6.656	−0.844	−14.012	−2.570	47.80	3.41	201.79	8.90
	m_3	3	0.916	0.695	0.995	0.939	−4.992	−1.542	−15.013	−6.351	36.55	16.87	241.96	53.54
		6	0.992	0.704	1.000	0.950	−6.790	−1.171	−16.136	−3.885	51.99	8.60	266.92	20.19
		9	0.998	0.723	1.000	0.944	−7.649	−1.156	−14.767	−3.203	62.98	5.75	222.91	13.59
1.25	m_1	3	0.969	0.946	0.998	0.895	−1.041	−0.706	−6.863	−0.830	1.61	0.71	60.03	1.12
		6	0.966	0.955	1.000	0.946	−0.964	−0.511	−5.395	−0.570	1.70	0.37	32.29	0.47
		9	0.969	0.959	1.000	0.953	−0.927	−0.422	−4.274	−0.456	1.82	0.26	19.41	0.30
	m_2	3	0.915	0.700	0.995	0.938	−4.599	−1.392	−14.370	−5.553	30.75	10.64	225.73	42.09
		6	0.996	0.736	1.000	0.948	−6.405	−1.136	−16.011	−3.370	45.84	5.49	264.37	15.13
		9	1.000	0.716	1.000	0.947	−7.031	−0.934	−14.241	−2.634	52.93	3.78	208.44	9.38
	m_3	3	0.922	0.697	0.997	0.935	−5.087	−1.332	−15.033	−6.155	38.87	17.41	240.63	52.37
		6	0.992	0.705	1.000	0.934	−6.926	−1.143	−16.104	−3.770	54.06	8.44	267.06	19.75
		9	1.000	0.742	1.000	0.949	−7.926	−1.207	−14.850	−3.238	67.08	5.75	225.35	13.76

TABLE 12.6.3 (Continued)

(b) True shelf life: 6.67 months

σ^2	Σ	Batches	Probability coverage				Mean bias				MSE			
			FDA	R&H	C&S	HLC	FDA	R&H	C&S	HLC	FDA	R&H	C&S	HLC
0.25	m_1	3	0.966	0.956	1.000	0.881	−0.193	−0.132	−1.635	−0.151	0.06	0.02	3.20	0.03
		6	0.964	0.956	1.000	0.932	−0.181	−0.091	−1.442	−0.102	0.07	0.02	2.30	0.01
		9	0.971	0.955	1.000	0.949	−0.183	−0.078	−1.169	−0.083	0.06	0.01	1.62	0.01
	m_2	3	0.940	0.830	1.000	0.930	−0.977	−0.560	−4.703	−1.208	1.38	0.66	24.71	2.14
		6	0.995	0.874	1.000	0.956	−1.377	−0.459	−5.045	−0.682	2.18	0.37	26.81	0.64
		9	1.000	0.896	1.000	0.958	−1.523	−0.387	−4.230	−0.522	2.54	0.25	18.68	0.38
	m_3	3	0.944	0.865	1.000	0.947	−1.070	−0.756	−4.780	−1.310	1.61	1.03	24.99	2.42
		6	0.998	0.924	1.000	0.957	−1.471	−0.605	−5.152	−0.750	2.44	0.55	27.82	0.74
		9	1.000	0.914	1.000	0.944	−1.625	−0.499	−4.371	−0.576	2.90	0.38	19.92	0.46
0.75	m_1	3	0.958	0.945	1.000	0.899	−0.350	−0.238	−2.568	−0.266	0.19	0.08	8.02	0.12
		6	0.972	0.952	1.000	0.943	−0.325	−0.158	−2.145	−0.180	0.21	0.03	5.04	0.04
		9	0.962	0.948	1.000	0.950	−0.319	−0.131	−1.727	−0.140	0.22	0.03	3.14	0.02
	m_2	3	0.953	0.851	0.998	0.919	−1.165	−0.594	−4.727	−1.171	1.83	0.71	25.03	2.08
		6	0.998	0.883	1.000	0.943	−1.576	−0.491	−5.116	−0.687	2.79	0.41	27.56	0.66
		9	1.000	0.884	1.000	0.948	−1.778	−0.394	−4.401	−0.522	3.43	0.26	20.30	0.38
	m_3	3	0.966	0.881	0.997	0.932	−1.299	−0.787	−4.573	−1.286	2.20	1.08	23.53	2.49
		6	0.998	0.894	1.000	0.940	−1.658	−0.573	−5.193	−0.703	3.08	0.53	28.32	0.70
		9	1.000	0.929	1.000	0.953	−1.880	−0.512	−4.489	−0.578	3.82	0.39	21.04	0.46
1.25	m_1	3	0.977	0.964	1.000	0.912	−0.457	−0.314	−3.058	−0.357	0.32	0.13	11.36	0.20
		6	0.967	0.947	1.000	0.936	−0.403	−0.196	−2.646	−0.227	0.32	0.06	7.69	0.09
		9	0.969	0.960	1.000	0.966	−0.411	−0.178	−2.087	−0.190	0.35	0.05	4.65	0.05
	m_2	3	0.961	0.872	0.998	0.935	−1.287	−0.649	−4.644	−1.191	2.17	0.77	24.16	2.15
		6	0.998	0.875	1.000	0.919	−1.741	−0.491	−5.191	−0.677	3.40	0.42	28.42	0.67
		9	1.000	0.907	1.000	0.947	−1.957	−0.421	−4.572	−0.545	4.10	0.29	21.87	0.41
	m_3	3	0.968	0.879	0.997	0.921	−1.396	−0.765	−4.763	−1.233	2.52	1.07	25.13	2.27
		6	0.999	0.918	0.999	0.941	−1.875	−0.634	−5.261	−0.747	3.88	0.61	29.04	0.79
		9	1.000	0.928	1.000	0.947	−2.069	−0.532	−4.652	−0.593	4.58	0.41	22.64	0.48

TABLE 12.6.3 (Continued)

(c) True shelf life: 4 months

σ^2	Σ	Batches	Probability coverage				Mean bias				MSE			
			FDA	R&H	C&S	HLC	FDA	R&H	C&S	HLC	FDA	R&H	C&S	HLC
0.25	m_1	3	0.959	0.948	0.998	0.902	−0.129	−0.088	−1.231	−0.100	0.03	0.01	1.70	0.02
		6	0.953	0.938	1.000	0.933	−0.116	−0.058	−1.032	−0.064	0.03	0.01	1.10	0.01
		9	0.968	0.952	1.000	0.947	−0.117	−0.048	−1.000	−0.052	0.03	0.01	1.00	0.01
	m_2	3	0.940	0.860	0.995	0.917	−0.558	−0.365	−2.887	−0.648	0.43	0.25	9.27	0.62
		6	1.000	0.927	1.000	0.949	−0.766	−0.306	−3.137	−0.365	0.66	0.13	10.40	0.18
		9	1.000	0.923	1.000	0.951	−0.882	−0.252	−2.681	−0.282	0.86	0.09	7.56	0.11
	m_3	3	0.954	0.889	0.998	0.930	−0.588	−0.477	−2.880	−0.670	0.48	0.37	9.19	0.68
		6	0.999	0.938	1.000	0.935	−0.807	−0.396	−3.190	−0.381	0.75	0.22	10.73	0.21
		9	1.000	0.955	1.000	0.944	−0.899	−0.332	−2.662	−0.294	0.89	9.85	7.47	0.12
0.75	m_1	3	0.966	0.951	0.999	0.889	−0.243	−0.150	−1.851	−0.176	0.09	0.03	4.02	0.05
		6	0.966	0.951	1.000	0.945	−0.205	−0.105	−1.525	−0.117	0.09	0.01	2.60	0.02
		9	0.956	0.945	1.000	0.943	−0.202	−0.082	−1.144	−0.088	0.09	0.01	1.44	0.02
	m_2	3	0.964	0.883	0.998	0.908	−0.699	−0.397	−2.947	−0.628	0.64	0.27	9.59	0.63
		6	0.999	0.908	1.000	0.938	−0.931	−0.311	−3.258	−0.367	0.97	0.14	11.17	0.19
		9	1.000	0.920	1.000	0.933	−1.032	−0.255	−2.775	−0.281	1.15	0.10	8.13	0.11
	m_3	3	0.981	0.906	1.997	0.928	−0.737	−0.505	−2.955	−0.652	0.70	0.40	9.63	0.68
		6	1.000	0.963	1.000	0.953	−0.986	−0.417	−3.255	−0.398	1.08	0.23	11.13	0.22
		9	1.000	0.953	1.000	0.928	−1.070	−0.330	−2.812	−0.294	1.24	0.15	8.29	0.12
1.25	m_1	3	0.965	0.953	0.998	0.882	−0.299	−0.197	−2.158	−0.230	0.14	0.05	5.44	0.10
		6	0.963	0.953	1.000	0.950	−0.267	−0.132	−1.852	−0.149	0.13	0.02	3.72	0.03
		9	0.955	0.935	1.000	0.937	−0.275	−0.109	−1.520	−0.116	0.17	0.02	2.57	0.01
	m_2	3	0.972	0.892	0.998	0.921	−0.785	−0.420	−2.956	−0.635	0.78	0.30	9.68	0.64
		6	0.988	0.912	1.000	0.927	−1.033	−0.325	−3.269	−0.370	1.19	0.17	11.27	0.20
		9	0.999	0.922	1.000	0.931	−1.162	−0.271	−2.884	−0.294	1.45	0.10	8.75	0.12
	m_3	3	0.980	0.921	0.996	0.931	−0.825	−0.525	−2.964	−0.658	0.85	0.43	9.64	0.67
		6	1.000	0.947	1.003	0.930	−1.079	−0.418	−3.290	−0.388	1.27	0.24	11.35	0.21
		9	1.000	0.996	1.000	0.930	−1.200	−0.350	−2.912	−0.311	1.54	0.16	8.90	0.13

coverage probability can drop below 0.95 in the presence of a large variability with a small number of batches. If the observed range is 12 months, the coverage probability can be below 0.90. It can be seen from Table 12.6.3a that with an observed range of 48 months and a true shelf life of 20 months, the coverage probability for three batches decreases to about 0.90. Although the FDA's minimum approach is conservative, it may not provide enough coverage probability for some cases with three batches. In summary, the FDA's minimum approach results in large average bias and mean-squared errors. Ruberg and Hsu's method yields an adequate coverage probability near the nominal level of 0.95 in the absence of between-batch variability. However, the coverage probability provided by Ruberg and Hsu's method is the lowest among the four methods if there is batch-to-batch variation. Although both the FDA's minimum approach and Ruberg and Hsu's method were both derived from the fixed effects model, the FDA's minimum approach is more robust with respect to the between-batch variability than Ruberg and Hsu's procedure. It should be noted that the performance of Ruberg and Hsu's method depends on the choice of Δ_β.

Since the sampling distribution (exact or asymptotic) of the HLC method is based on the number of batches rather than the number of total assays, the coverage probability decreases to 0.87 in some cases when the number of batches is small (say, $K = 3$). However, when the number of batches becomes large (say, $K = 6$ or 9), the HLC method provides adequate coverage probability around 0.95, which is within the 95% confidence interval $(0.9365, 0.9635)$ obtained from the 1000 random samples with respect to a nominal level of 0.95. The average bias and mean-squared error is relatively smaller than Chow and Shao's method and the FDA's minimum procedure.

12.7. EXAMPLE

To illustrate Chow and Shao's approach and the HLC method for the determination of drug shelf life, consider the stability data given in Table 11.6.1. The lower specification limit for the drug product is $\eta = 90\%$. For simplicity, consider the following random effects model:

$$Y_{ij} = X_j' \beta_i + e_{ij},$$

where $i = 1, \ldots, 5$, $j = 1, \ldots, 12$, and $x_j = (1, t_j, w_j, t_j w_j)'$, in which $w_j = 0$ for bottle container and $w_j = 1$ for blister package, and t_j are sampling times, which are as follows:

j	1	2	3	4	5	6	7	8	9	10	11	12
t_j	0	3	6	9	12	18	0	3	6	9	12	18
w_j	0	0	0	0	0	0	1	1	1	1	1	1

We first use T statistic given in (12.3.13) to examine the random effect. The data set given in Table 11.6.1 gives tr(S) = 88.396 and SE = 4.376. Since $n = 12$, $p = 4$, and $K = 5$, we have

$$T = \frac{(n - p)\text{tr}(S)}{n(K - 1)\text{SE}} = \frac{(12 - 4)(88.396)}{(12)(5 - 1)(4.376)} = 3.367,$$

which is greater than $F(0.05,48,9) = 2.8$. Hence we conclude that there is a batch-to-batch variation at the 5% level of significance.

It should be noted that although all of the assay results at 18 months are clearly higher than the lower specification limit $\eta = 90\%$, it does not imply that $t_{label} \geq 18$ months can be used as the labeled shelf life, since the assay results are from five batches, which should be considered as a random sample from the population of all future batches. A labeled shelf life should be determined through statistically analyzing the assay results by using the procedures described in Sec. 12.4.

For Chow and Shao's method, since the unit of the shelf life is a month, we need to evaluate $x(t)'\mathbf{b}$ and $\bar{\eta}(t)$ for integer values of t in a reasonable range in order to calculate $\bar{t}$ in (12.4.12). The results of the calculation for both package types are shown in Table 12.7.1. It shows that if ϵ is selected to be 0.05, we may use 22 months (with $\alpha = 5\%$) as the labeled shelf life for the bottle container and 21 months as the labeled shelf life for the blister package. If ϵ is chosen to be 0.01, then 19 months can be used as the labeled shelf life for both bottle container and blister package. Note that in this example the trade-off for reducing ϵ from 0.05 to 0.01 is 2 to 3 months of shelf life.

We now compare the minimum approach with Chow and Shao's method using the assay results for bottle container in this example. The difference between the two methods is significant, since

$$\hat{t}_{min} = 27.5 \text{ months.}$$

For $\epsilon = 0.05$, $\hat{t}_{min} - \bar{t}$ is 5.5 months, and for $\epsilon = 0.01$, $\hat{t}_{min} - \bar{t}$ is 8.5 months. However, the minimum approach is not justifiable since it only ensures that the shelf lives of five batches, rather than the shelf lives of future batches, are longer than the lower specification limit with certain assurance. As a matter of fact, $\bar{t} = 27.5$ if ϵ is selected to be greater than 0.2. This indicates that $t = 27.5$ months is a valid labeled shelf life if we allow the future failure rate at the indicated date of expiration to be as large as 20%. A risk of 20% future failure rate is usually too high for the drug product company.

TABLE 12.7.1 Results from Stability Analysis

Values of statistics[a]

	Bottle container		Blister package	
t (months)	$x(t)'\mathbf{b}$	$\sqrt{v(t)}$	$x(t)'\mathbf{b}$	$\sqrt{v(t)}$
18	98.304	1.140	98.057	1.220
19	98.015	1.275	97.779	1.350
20	97.725	1.411	97.501	1.482
21	97.437	1.548	97.222	1.615
22	97.147	1.686	96.944	1.749
23	96.858	1.825	96.666	1.885
24	96.569	1.963	96.387	2.020
25	96.280	2.102	96.109	2.157
26	95.990	2.242	95.381	2.294

Labeled shelf life $\tilde{t}$ (months; $\alpha = 0.05$)

ϵ	Bottle container	Blister package
0.01	19	19
0.02	20	19
0.03	21	20
0.04	21	21
0.05	22	21
0.10	23	23
0.15	25	24

[a]$x(t)'\mathbf{b}$, estimated mean degradation curve; $\sqrt{v(t)}$, estimated standard deviation of $\sqrt{k}x(t)'\mathbf{b}$.

From Table 11.6.3 it can be verified that

$$\bar{\mathbf{b}} = (\bar{a}, \bar{b})' = (103.51, -0.289),$$

$$\mathbf{S}_b = \begin{bmatrix} 2.250 & -0.2058 \\ -0.2058 & 0.01994 \end{bmatrix}$$

$$\hat{\sigma}_e^2 = 0.9597,$$

$$\hat{\sigma}_e^2(\mathbf{X}'\mathbf{X})^{-1} = \begin{bmatrix} 0.452 & -0.0366 \\ -0.0366 & 0.00457 \end{bmatrix},$$

$$\hat{\mathbf{\Sigma}}_\beta = \mathbf{S}_b - \hat{\sigma}_e^2 (\mathbf{X}'\mathbf{X})^{-1}$$

$$= \begin{bmatrix} 1.798 & -0.1692 \\ -0.1692 & 0.0154 \end{bmatrix}.$$

Hence

$$SE(\bar{a}) = 0.671 \quad \text{and} \quad SE(\bar{b}) = 0.0632.$$

Since

$$T_{\bar{a}} = \frac{103.51 - 90}{0.671} = 20.141 > t(0.05,4) = 2.132,$$

$$T_{\bar{b}} = \frac{-0.289}{0.0632} = -4.58 < -t(0.05,4) = -2.132,$$

both conditions in (12.5.13) are satisified and the estimate of the shelf life by the HLC method is the smaller root of the following equation:

$$[90 - (103.51 - 0.289x)]^2 = (2.132)(\tfrac{1}{5})[2.250 - 0.4116x + (0.01994)^2x^2],$$

which is 35.1 months.

If the asymptotic procedure of the HLC method is applied, then

$$\hat{x}_0 = \frac{90 - 103.51}{-0.289} = 46.71,$$

$$\hat{v}_N = 703.42 \quad \text{and} \quad \hat{v}_D = 97.657.$$

Hence the estimated degrees of freedom is given as

$$\hat{v} = \frac{\hat{v}_N}{\hat{v}_D} = \frac{703.42}{97.657} = 7.2$$

and the estimated expiration dating period is 36.1 months.

12.8. DISCUSSION

For the estimation of drug shelf life with random batches, in addition to Chow and Shao's method and the HLC method, Murphy and Weisman (1990) proposed the use of random slopes to determine drug shelf life. Their idea is outlined briefly below. For the simple linear regression model considered in (11.3.1), the slope β_i, $i = 1, \ldots, K$, is assumed to be i.i.d. as a normal random variable with mean zero and variance σ_β^2. Hence the expected value of $MS(\beta)$ in the ANCOVA table presented in Table 11.3.1 is then given by

$$E(MS(\beta)) = \sigma_e^2 + R\sigma_\beta^2, \tag{12.8.1}$$

where

$$R = \frac{1}{K-1}\left[S_{xx}(W) - \frac{\sum\limits_{i=1}^{K} S_{xx}^2(i)}{S_{xx}(W)}\right],$$

and $S_{xx}(i)$ and $S_{xx}(W)$ are as defined in (11.3.4). The same F statistic $F_\beta = MS(\beta)/MSE$ can be applied to test the following hypotheses:

$$H_0: \sigma_\beta^2 = 0 \quad \text{vs.} \quad H_a: \sigma_\beta^2 > 0. \tag{12.8.2}$$

Depending on whether the null hypothesis of (12.8.2) is rejected at the 0.25 level of significance or $MS(\beta)$ is larger than MSE, Murphy and Weisman (1990) proposed three methods to estimate shelf life. Basically, their methods assume the initial value of the strength at time zero is a fixed nonrandom quantity (i.e., 100% of label claim) for all three batches. Then use slope to determine drug shelf life. In other words, Murphy and Weisman's method totally ignore the information observed at the initial (i.e., time 0). As a result, their method suffers from the same drawbacks as those of the method suggested in Rahman (1992), which were discussed in Sec. 11.2. Note that even in the situation where the batch effect is assumed random, the same disadvantages remain in Murphy and Weisman's methods. It should be noted that Murphy and Weisman's methods are not based on the mean degradation line. Therefore, no probability statements can be made regarding the estimated shelf life, observed strength, and the lower specification limit. Moreover, in their simulation study, the FDA's minimum approach was not considered as the referenced method for comparison. In addition, no coverage probabilities of their methods were reported.

Lin (1990) investigated statistical analysis of stability data in terms of the intercept and slope of the degradation curve. Under the assumption of a fixed effects model, he described the possible situations about the slopes and intercepts encountered in the analysis of stability data: that is common slope and common intercept, different slopes and common intercept, common slope and different intercepts, and different slopes and different intercepts. As an alternative approach, Lin (1990) also described the possible use of a confidence limit (interval) approach for determination of an expiration dating period when the drug characteristic increases or decreases with time. In addition, Lin (1990) also pointed out some common deficiencies/concerns of statistical analyses that the FDA reviewers often have in their reviews of the submission of stability data.

For Chow and Shao's method, in practice, it may be difficult to choose an appropriate ϵ. Too large an ϵ can certainly increase the chance of being recalled prior to the expiration date, whereas too small an ϵ may increase the cost. By calculating $\tilde{t}$ for various values of ϵ's, we may determine a labeled shelf life by balancing the relative merits and disadvantages of having a longer labeled shelf life against the risk of being recalled. In the situation where the final decision is made by the FDA, the research scientist/statistician may report $\tilde{t}$ for several values of ϵ in a reasonable range. When $\Sigma_\beta = 0$ is true, both $\tilde{t}$ and $\hat{t}$ are valid labeled shelf lives, but $\hat{t}$ is usually longer than $\tilde{t}$. When $\Sigma_\beta \neq 0$, however, $\hat{t}$ could be much too large. In practice it is usually difficult to justify $\Sigma_\beta = 0$, since controlling the type II error for any procedure testing the null hypothesis H_0 is difficult due to the complexity of the alternative hypothesis K_0. Thus even if we cannot reject the hypothesis H_0, the use of $\hat{t}$ is still questionable. In this situation, however, the estimated shelf lives by $\hat{t}$ and $\tilde{t}$ are close to each other because of the small contribution of Σ_β due to no evidence for the presence of batch-to-batch variability.

Appendix A: Statistical Tables

Appendix A.1 Areas of Upper Tail of the Standard Normal Distribution

z	0.00	0.01	0.02	0.03	0.04	0.05	0.06	0.07	0.08	0.09
0.0	0.5000	0.4960	0.4920	0.4880	0.4840	0.4801	0.4761	0.4721	0.4681	0.4641
0.1	0.4602	0.4562	0.4522	0.4483	0.4443	0.4404	0.4364	0.4325	0.4286	0.4247
0.2	0.4207	0.4168	0.4129	0.4090	0.4052	0.4013	0.3974	0.3936	0.3897	0.3859
0.3	0.3821	0.3783	0.3745	0.3707	0.3669	0.3632	0.3594	0.3557	0.3520	0.3483
0.4	0.3446	0.3409	0.3372	0.3336	0.3300	0.3264	0.3228	0.3192	0.3156	0.3121
0.5	0.3085	0.3050	0.3015	0.2981	0.2946	0.2912	0.2877	0.2843	0.2810	0.2776
0.6	0.2743	0.2709	0.2676	0.2643	0.2611	0.2578	0.2546	0.2514	0.2483	0.2451
0.7	0.2420	0.2389	0.2358	0.2327	0.2296	0.2266	0.2236	0.2206	0.2177	0.2148
0.8	0.2119	0.2090	0.2061	0.2033	0.2005	0.1977	0.1949	0.1922	0.1894	0.1867
0.9	0.1841	0.1814	0.1788	0.1762	0.1736	0.1711	0.1685	0.1660	0.1635	0.1611
1.0	0.1587	0.1562	0.1539	0.1515	0.1492	0.1469	0.1446	0.1423	0.1401	0.1379
1.1	0.1357	0.1335	0.1314	0.1292	0.1271	0.1251	0.1230	0.1210	0.1190	0.1170
1.2	0.1151	0.1131	0.1112	0.1093	0.1075	0.1056	0.1038	0.1020	0.1003	0.0985
1.3	0.0968	0.0951	0.0934	0.0918	0.0901	0.0885	0.0869	0.0853	0.0838	0.0823
1.4	0.0808	0.0793	0.0778	0.0764	0.0749	0.0735	0.0721	0.0708	0.0694	0.0681
1.5	0.0668	0.0655	0.0643	0.0630	0.0618	0.0606	0.0594	0.0582	0.0571	0.0559
1.6	0.0548	0.0537	0.0526	0.0516	0.0505	0.0495	0.0485	0.0475	0.0465	0.0455
1.7	0.0446	0.0436	0.0427	0.0418	0.0409	0.0401	0.0392	0.0384	0.0375	0.0367
1.8	0.0359	0.0351	0.0344	0.0336	0.0329	0.0322	0.0314	0.0307	0.0301	0.0294
1.9	0.0287	0.0281	0.0274	0.0268	0.0262	0.0256	0.0250	0.0244	0.0239	0.0233
2.0	0.02275	0.02222	0.02169	0.02118	0.02068	0.02018	0.01970	0.01923	0.01876	0.01831
2.1	0.01786	0.01743	0.01700	0.01659	0.01618	0.01578	0.01539	0.01500	0.01463	0.01426
2.2	0.01390	0.01355	0.01321	0.01287	0.01255	0.01222	0.01191	0.01160	0.01130	0.01101
2.3	0.01072	0.01044	0.01017	0.00990	0.00964	0.00939	0.00914	0.00889	0.00866	0.00842
2.4	0.00820	0.00798	0.00776	0.00755	0.00734	0.00714	0.00695	0.00676	0.00657	0.00639
2.5	0.00621	0.00604	0.00587	0.00570	0.00554	0.00539	0.00523	0.00508	0.00494	0.00480
2.6	0.00466	0.00453	0.00440	0.00427	0.00415	0.00402	0.00391	0.00379	0.00368	0.00357
2.7	0.00347	0.00336	0.00326	0.00317	0.00307	0.00298	0.00289	0.00280	0.00272	0.00264
2.8	0.00256	0.00248	0.00240	0.00233	0.00226	0.00219	0.00212	0.00205	0.00199	0.00193
2.9	0.00187	0.00181	0.00175	0.00169	0.00164	0.00159	0.00154	0.00149	0.00144	0.00139

Source: Table 2 of *Statistical Tables for Science, Engineering and Management* by J. Murdoch and J. A. Barnes (Macmillan, London, 1968).

Appendix A.2 Upper Quantiles of a χ^2 Distribution

v/α	0.995	0.990	0.975	0.950	0.900	0.100	0.050	0.025	0.010	0.005
1	392704.10^{-10}	157088.10^{-9}	982069.10^{-9}	393214.10^{-8}	0.0157908	2.70554	3.84146	5.02389	6.63490	7.87944
2	0.0100251	0.0201007	0.0506356	0.102587	0.210720	4.60517	5.99147	7.37776	9.21034	10.5966
3	0.0717212	0.114832	0.215795	0.351846	0.584375	6.25139	7.81473	9.34840	11.3449	12.8381
4	0.206990	0.297110	0.484419	0.710721	1.063623	7.77944	9.48773	11.1433	13.2767	14.8602
5	0.411740	0.554300	0.831211	1.145476	1.61031	9.23635	11.0705	12.8325	15.0863	16.7496
6	0.675727	0.872085	1.237347	1.63539	2.20413	10.6446	12.5916	14.4494	16.8119	18.5476
7	0.989265	1.239043	1.68987	2.16735	2.83311	12.0170	14.0671	16.0128	18.4753	20.2777
8	1.344419	1.646482	2.17973	2.73264	3.48954	13.3616	15.5073	17.5346	20.0902	21.9550
9	1.734926	2.087912	2.70039	3.32511	4.16816	14.6837	16.9190	19.0228	21.6660	23.5893
10	2.15585	2.55821	3.24697	3.94030	4.86518	15.9871	18.3070	20.4831	23.2093	25.1882
11	2.60321	3.05347	3.81575	4.57481	5.57779	17.2750	19.6751	21.9200	24.7250	26.7569
12	3.07382	3.57056	4.40379	5.22603	6.30380	18.5494	21.0261	23.3367	26.2170	28.2995
13	3.56503	4.10691	5.00874	5.89186	7.04150	19.8119	22.3621	24.7356	27.6883	29.8194
14	4.07468	4.66043	5.62872	6.57063	7.78953	21.0642	23.6848	26.1190	29.1413	31.3193
15	4.60094	5.22935	6.26214	7.26094	8.54675	22.3072	24.9958	27.4884	30.5779	32.8013
16	5.14224	5.81221	6.90766	7.96164	9.31223	23.5418	26.2962	28.8454	31.9999	34.2672
17	5.69724	6.40776	7.56418	8.67176	10.0852	24.7690	27.5871	30.1910	33.4087	35.7185
18	6.26481	7.01491	8.23075	9.39046	10.8649	25.9894	28.8693	31.5264	34.8053	37.1564
19	6.84398	7.63273	8.90655	10.1170	11.6509	27.2036	30.1435	32.8523	36.1908	38.5822

Appendix A.2   Upper Quantiles of a χ^2 Distribution (Continued)

v/α	0.995	0.990	0.975	0.950	0.900	0.100	0.050	0.025	0.010	0.005
20	7.43386	8.26040	9.59083	10.8508	12.4426	28.4120	31.4104	34.1696	37.5662	39.9968
21	8.03366	8.89720	10.28293	11.5913	13.2396	29.6151	32.6705	35.4789	38.9321	41.4010
22	8.64272	9.54249	10.9823	12.3380	14.0415	30.8133	33.9244	36.7807	40.2894	42.7956
23	9.26042	10.19567	11.6885	13.0905	14.8479	32.0069	35.1725	38.0757	41.6384	44.1813
24	9.88623	10.8564	12.4011	13.8484	15.6587	33.1963	36.4151	39.3641	42.9798	45.5585
25	10.5197	11.5240	13.1197	14.6114	16.4734	34.3816	37.6525	40.6465	44.3141	46.9278
26	11.1603	12.1981	13.8439	15.3791	17.2919	35.5631	38.8852	41.9232	45.6417	48.2899
27	11.8076	12.8786	14.5733	16.1513	18.1138	36.7412	40.1133	43.1944	46.9630	49.6449
28	12.4613	13.5648	15.3079	16.9279	18.9392	37.9159	41.3372	44.4607	48.2782	50.9933
29	13.1211	14.2565	16.0471	17.7083	19.7677	39.0875	42.5569	45.7222	49.5879	52.3356
30	13.7867	14.9535	16.7908	18.4926	20.5992	40.2560	43.7729	46.9792	50.8922	53.6720
40	20.7065	22.1643	24.4331	26.5093	29.0505	51.8050	55.7585	59.3417	63.6907	66.7659
50	27.9907	29.7067	32.3574	34.7642	37.6886	63.1671	67.5048	71.4202	76.1539	79.4900
60	35.5346	37.4848	40.4817	43.1879	46.4589	74.3970	79.0819	83.2976	88.3794	91.9517
70	43.2752	45.4418	48.7576	51.7393	55.3290	85.5271	90.5312	95.0231	100.425	104.215
80	51.1720	53.5400	57.1532	60.3915	64.2778	96.5782	101.879	106.629	112.329	116.321
90	59.1963	61.7541	65.6466	69.1260	73.2912	107.565	113.145	118.136	124.116	128.299
100	67.3276	70.0648	74.2219	77.9295	82.3581	118.498	124.342	129.561	135.807	140.169

Source: Tables of Percentage Points of the χ^2-Distribution by C. M. Thompson, *Biometrika* (1941), Vol. 32, pp. 188–189.

438

Appendix A.3   Upper Quantiles of a Central t Distribution

ν/α	0.050	0.025	0.010	0.005
1	6.3138	12.706	25.452	63.657
2	2.9200	4.3027	6.2053	9.9248
3	2.3534	3.1825	4.1765	5.8409
4	2.1318	2.7764	3.4954	4.6041
5	2.0150	2.5706	3.1634	4.0321
6	1.9432	2.4469	2.9687	3.7074
7	1.8946	2.3646	2.8412	3.4995
8	1.8595	2.3060	2.7515	3.3554
9	1.8331	2.2622	2.6850	3.2498
10	1.8125	2.2281	2.6338	3.1693
11	1.7959	2.2010	2.5931	3.1058
12	1.7823	2.1788	2.5600	3.0545
13	1.7709	2.1604	2.5326	3.0123
14	1.7613	2.1448	2.5096	2.9768
15	1.7530	2.1315	2.4899	2.9467
16	1.7459	2.1199	2.4729	2.9208
17	1.7396	2.1098	2.4581	2.8982
18	1.7341	2.1009	2.4450	2.8784
19	1.7291	2.0930	2.4334	2.8609
20	1.7247	2.0860	2.4231	2.8453
21	1.7207	2.0796	2.4138	2.8314
22	1.7171	2.0739	2.4055	2.8188
23	1.7139	2.0687	2.3979	2.8073
24	1.7109	2.0639	2.3910	2.7969
25	1.7081	2.0595	2.3846	2.7874
26	1.7056	2.0555	2.3788	2.7787
27	1.7033	2.0518	2.3734	2.7707
28	1.7011	2.0484	2.3685	2.7633
29	1.6991	2.0452	2.3638	2.7564
30	1.6973	2.0423	2.3596	2.7500
40	1.6839	2.0211	2.3289	2.7045
60	1.6707	2.0003	2.2991	2.6603
120	1.6577	1.9799	2.2699	2.6174
∞	1.6449	1.9600	2.2414	2.5758

Source: Tables of Percentage Points of the t-Distribution by M. Merrington, *Biometrika* (1941), Vol. 32, p. 300.

Appendix A.4   Upper Quantiles of an F Distribution $\alpha = 0.05$

ν_2 \ ν_1	1	2	3	4	5	6	7	8	9
1	161.45	199.50	215.71	224.58	230.16	233.99	236.77	238.88	240.54
2	18.513	19.000	19.164	19.247	19.296	19.330	19.353	19.371	19.385
3	10.128	9.5521	9.2766	9.1172	9.0135	8.9406	8.8868	8.8452	8.8123
4	7.7086	6.9443	6.5914	6.3883	6.2560	6.1631	6.0942	6.0410	5.9988
5	6.6079	5.7861	5.4095	5.1922	5.0503	4.9503	4.8759	4.8183	4.7725
6	5.9874	5.1433	4.7571	4.5337	4.3874	4.2839	4.2066	4.1468	4.0990
7	5.5914	4.7374	4.3468	4.1203	3.9715	3.8660	3.7870	3.7257	3.6767
8	5.3177	4.4590	4.0662	3.8378	3.6875	3.5806	3.5005	3.4381	3.3881
9	5.1174	4.2565	3.8626	3.6331	3.4817	3.3738	3.2927	3.2296	3.1789
10	4.9646	4.1028	3.7083	3.4780	3.3258	3.2172	3.1355	3.0717	3.0204
11	4.8443	3.9823	3.5874	3.3567	3.2039	3.0946	3.0123	2.9480	2.8962
12	4.7472	3.8853	3.4903	3.2592	3.1059	2.9961	2.9134	2.8486	2.7964
13	4.6672	3.8056	3.4105	3.1791	3.0254	2.9153	2.8321	2.7669	2.7144
14	4.6001	3.7389	3.3439	3.1122	2.9582	2.8477	2.7642	2.6987	2.6458
15	4.5431	3.6823	3.2874	3.0556	2.9013	2.7905	2.7066	2.6408	2.5876
16	4.4940	3.6337	3.2389	3.0069	2.8524	2.7413	2.6572	2.5911	2.5377
17	4.4513	3.5915	3.1968	2.9647	2.8100	2.6987	2.6143	2.5480	2.4943
18	4.4139	3.5546	3.1599	2.9277	2.7729	2.6613	2.5767	2.5102	2.4563
19	4.3808	3.5219	3.1274	2.8951	2.7401	2.6283	2.5435	2.4768	2.4227
20	4.3513	3.4928	3.0984	2.8661	2.7109	2.5990	2.5140	2.4471	2.3928
21	4.3248	3.4668	3.0725	2.8401	2.6848	2.5727	2.4876	2.4205	2.3661
22	4.3009	3.4434	3.0491	2.8167	2.6613	2.5491	2.4638	2.3965	2.3419
23	4.2793	3.4221	3.0280	2.7955	2.6400	2.5277	2.4422	2.3748	2.3201
24	4.2597	3.4028	3.0088	2.7763	2.6207	2.5082	2.4226	2.3551	2.3002
25	4.2417	3.3852	2.9912	2.7587	2.6030	2.4904	2.4047	2.3371	3.2821
26	4.2252	2.3690	2.9751	2.7426	2.5868	2.4741	2.3883	2.3205	2.2655
27	4.2100	3.3541	2.9604	2.7278	2.5719	2.4591	2.3732	2.3053	2.2501
28	4.1960	3.3404	2.9467	2.7141	2.5581	2.4453	2.3593	2.2913	2.2360
29	4.1830	3.3277	2.9340	2.7014	2.5454	2.4324	2.3463	2.2782	2.2229
30	4.1709	3.3158	2.9223	2.6896	2.5336	2.4205	2.3343	2.2662	2.2107
40	4.0848	3.2317	2.8387	2.6060	2.4495	2.3359	2.2490	2.1802	2.1240
60	4.0012	3.1504	2.7581	2.5252	2.3683	2.2540	2.1665	2.0970	2.0401
120	3.9201	3.0718	2.6802	2.4472	2.2900	2.1750	2.0867	2.0164	1.9588
∞	3.8415	2.9957	2.6049	2.3719	2.2141	2.0986	2.0096	1.9384	1.8799

Source: Tables of Percentage Points of the Inverted beta (F)-Distribution by M. Merrington and C. M. Thompson. *Biometrika* (1942), Vol. 33, pp. 73–88.

Appendix A.4 (Continued) $\alpha = 0.05$

v_2 \ v_1	10	12	15	20	24	30	40	60	12	∞
1	241.88	243.91	245.95	248.01	249.05	250.09	251.14	252.20	253.25	254.32
2	19.396	19.413	19.429	19.446	19.454	19.462	19.471	19.479	19.487	19.496
3	8.7855	8.7446	8.7029	8.6602	8.6385	8.6166	8.5944	8.5720	8.5494	8.5265
4	5.9644	5.9117	5.8578	5.8025	5.7744	5.7459	5.7170	5.6878	5.6581	5.6281
5	4.7351	4.6777	4.6188	4.5581	4.5272	4.4957	4.4638	4.4314	4.3984	4.3650
6	4.0600	3.9999	3.9381	3.8742	3.8415	3.8082	3.7743	3.7398	3.7047	3.6688
7	3.6365	3.5747	3.5108	3.4445	3.4105	3.3758	3.3404	3.3043	3.2674	3.2298
8	3.3472	3.2840	3.2184	3.1503	3.1152	3.0794	3.0428	3.0053	2.9669	2.9276
9	3.1373	3.0729	3.0061	2.9365	2.9005	2.8637	2.8259	2.7872	2.7475	2.7067
10	2.9782	2.9130	2.8450	2.7740	2.7372	2.6996	2.6609	2.6211	2.5801	2.5379
11	2.8536	2.7876	2.7186	2.6464	2.6090	2.5705	2.5309	2.4901	2.4480	2.4045
12	2.7534	2.6866	2.6169	2.5436	2.5055	2.4663	2.4259	2.3842	2.3410	2.2962
13	2.6710	2.6037	2.5331	2.4589	2.4202	2.3803	2.3392	2.2966	2.2524	2.2064
14	2.6021	2.5342	2.4630	2.3879	2.3487	2.3082	2.2664	2.2230	2.1778	2.1307
15	2.5437	2.4753	2.4035	2.3275	2.2878	2.2468	2.2043	2.1601	2.1141	2.0658
16	2.4935	2.4247	2.3522	2.2756	2.2354	2.1938	2.1507	2.1058	2.0589	2.0096
17	2.4499	2.3807	2.3077	2.2304	2.1898	2.1477	2.1040	2.0584	2.0107	1.9604
18	2.4117	2.3421	2.2686	2.1906	2.1497	2.1071	2.0629	2.0166	1.9681	1.9168
19	2.3779	2.3080	2.2341	2.1555	2.1141	2.0712	2.0264	1.9796	1.9302	1.8780
20	2.3479	2.2776	2.2033	2.1242	2.0825	2.0391	1.9938	1.9464	1.8963	1.8432
21	2.3210	2.2504	2.1757	2.0960	2.0540	2.0102	1.9645	1.9165	1.8657	1.8117
22	2.2967	2.2258	2.1508	2.0707	2.0283	1.9842	1.9380	1.8895	1.8380	1.7831
23	2.2747	2.2036	2.1282	2.0476	2.0050	1.9605	1.9139	1.8649	1.8128	1.7570
24	2.2547	2.1834	2.1077	2.0267	1.9838	1.9390	1.8920	1.8424	1.7897	1.7331
25	2.2365	2.1649	2.0889	2.0075	1.9643	1.9192	1.8718	1.8217	1.7684	1.7110
26	2.2197	2.1479	2.0716	1.9898	1.9464	1.9010	1.8533	1.8027	1.7488	1.6906
27	2.2043	2.1323	2.0558	1.9736	1.9299	1.8842	1.8361	1.7851	1.7307	1.6717
28	2.1900	2.1179	2.0411	1.9586	1.9147	1.8687	1.8203	1.7689	1.7138	1.6541
29	2.1768	2.1045	2.0275	1.9446	1.9005	1.8543	1.8055	1.7537	1.6981	1.6377
30	2.1646	2.0921	2.1048	1.9317	1.8874	1.8409	1.7918	1.7396	1.6835	1.6223
40	2.0772	2.0035	1.9245	1.8389	1.7929	1.7444	1.6928	1.6373	1.5766	1.5089
60	1.9926	1.9174	1.8364	1.7480	1.7001	1.6491	1.5943	1.5343	1.4673	1.3893
120	1.9105	1.8337	1.7505	1.6587	1.6084	1.5543	1.4952	1.4290	1.3519	1.2539
∞	1.8307	1.7522	1.6664	1.5705	1.5173	1.4591	1.3940	1.3180	1.2214	1.0000

Appendix A.4 Upper Quantiles of an F Distribution (Continued) $\alpha = 0.025$

ν_2 \ ν_1	1	2	3	4	5	6	7	8	9
1	647.79	799.50	864.16	899.58	921.85	937.11	948.22	956.66	963.28
2	38.506	39.000	39.165	39.248	39.298	39.331	39.355	39.373	39.387
3	17.443	16.044	15.439	15.101	14.885	14.735	14.624	14.540	14.473
4	12.218	10.649	9.9792	9.6045	9.3645	9.1973	9.0741	8.9796	8.9047
5	10.007	8.4336	7.7636	7.3879	7.1464	6.9777	6.8531	6.7572	6.6810
6	8.8131	7.2598	6.5988	6.2272	5.9876	5.8197	5.6955	5.5996	5.5234
7	8.0727	6.5415	5.8898	5.5226	5.2852	5.1186	4.9949	4.8994	4.8232
8	7.5709	6.0595	5.4160	5.0526	4.8173	4.6517	4.5286	4.4332	4.3572
9	7.2093	5.7147	5.0781	4.7181	4.4844	4.3197	4.1971	4.1020	4.0260
10	6.9367	5.4564	4.8256	4.4683	4.2361	4.0721	3.9498	3.8549	3.7790
11	6.7241	5.2559	4.6300	4.2751	4.0440	3.8807	3.7586	3.6638	3.5879
12	6.5538	5.0959	4.4742	4.1212	3.8911	3.7283	3.6065	3.5118	3.4358
13	6.4143	4.9653	4.3472	3.9959	3.7667	3.6043	3.4827	3.3880	3.3120
14	6.2979	4.8567	4.2417	3.8919	3.6634	3.5014	3.3799	3.2853	3.2093
15	6.1995	4.7650	4.1528	3.8043	3.5764	3.4147	3.2934	3.1987	3.1227
16	6.1151	4.6867	4.0768	3.7294	3.5021	3.3406	3.2194	3.1248	3.0488
17	6.0420	4.6189	4.0112	3.6648	3.4379	3.2767	3.1556	3.0610	2.9849
18	5.9781	4.5597	3.9539	3.6083	3.3820	3.2209	3.0999	3.0053	2.9291
19	5.9216	4.5075	3.9034	3.5587	3.3327	3.1718	3.0509	2.9563	2.8800
20	5.8715	4.4613	3.8587	3.5147	3.2891	3.1283	3.0074	2.9128	2.8365
21	5.8266	4.4199	3.8188	3.4754	3.2501	3.0895	2.9686	2.8740	2.7977
22	5.7863	4.3828	3.7829	3.4401	3.2151	3.0546	2.9338	2.8392	2.7628
23	5.7498	4.3492	3.7505	3.4083	3.1835	3.0232	2.9024	2.8077	2.7313
24	5.7167	4.3187	3.7211	3.3794	3.1548	2.9946	2.8738	2.7791	2.7027
25	5.6864	4.2909	3.6943	3.3530	3.1287	2.9685	2.8478	2.7531	2.6766
26	5.6586	4.2655	3.6697	3.3289	3.1048	2.9447	2.8240	2.7293	2.6528
27	5.6331	4.2421	3.6472	3.3067	3.0828	2.9228	2.8021	2.7074	2.6309
28	5.6096	4.2205	3.6264	3.2863	3.0625	2.9027	2.7820	2.6872	2.6106
29	5.5878	4.2006	3.6072	3.2674	3.0438	2.8840	2.7633	2.6686	2.5919
30	5.5675	4.1821	3.5894	3.2499	3.0265	2.8667	2.7460	2.6513	2.5746
40	5.4239	4.0510	3.4633	3.1261	2.9037	2.7444	2.6238	2.5289	2.4519
60	5.2857	3.9253	3.3425	3.0077	2.7863	2.6274	2.5068	2.4117	2.3344
120	5.1524	3.8046	3.2270	2.8943	2.6740	2.5154	2.3948	2.2994	2.2217
∞	5.0239	3.6889	3.1161	2.7858	2.5665	2.4082	2.2875	2.1918	2.1136

Appendix A.4 (Continued) $\alpha = 0.025$

v_2 \ v_1	10	12	15	20	24	30	40	60	120	∞
1	968.63	976.71	984.87	993.10	997.25	1001.4	1005.6	1009.8	1014.0	1018.3
2	39.398	39.415	39.431	39.448	39.456	39.465	39.473	39.481	39.490	39.498
3	14.419	14.337	14.253	14.167	14.124	14.081	14.037	13.992	13.947	13.902
4	8.8439	8.7512	8.6565	8.5599	8.5109	8.4613	8.4111	8.3604	8.3092	8.2573
5	6.6192	6.5246	6.4277	6.3285	6.2780	6.2269	6.1751	6.1225	6.0693	6.0153
6	5.4613	5.3662	5.2687	5.1684	5.1172	5.0652	5.0125	4.9589	4.9045	4.8491
7	4.7611	4.6658	4.5678	4.4667	4.4150	4.3624	4.3089	4.2544	4.1989	4.1423
8	4.2951	4.1997	4.1012	3.9995	3.9472	3.8940	3.8398	3.7844	3.7279	3.6702
9	3.9639	3.8682	3.7694	3.6669	3.6142	3.5604	3.5055	3.4493	3.3918	3.3329
10	3.7168	3.6209	3.5217	3.4186	3.3654	3.3110	3.2554	3.1984	3.1399	3.0798
11	3.5257	3.4296	3.3299	3.2261	3.1725	3.1176	3.0613	3.0035	2.9441	2.8828
12	3.3736	3.2773	3.1772	3.0728	3.0187	2.9633	2.9063	2.8478	2.7874	2.7249
13	3.2497	3.1532	3.0527	2.9477	2.8932	2.8373	2.7797	2.7204	2.6590	2.5955
14	3.1469	3.0501	2.9493	2.8437	2.7888	2.7324	2.6742	2.6142	2.5519	2.4872
15	3.0602	2.9633	2.8621	2.7559	2.7006	2.6437	2.5850	2.5242	2.4611	2.3953
16	2.9862	2.8890	2.7875	2.6808	2.6252	2.5678	2.5085	2.4471	2.3831	2.3163
17	2.9222	2.8249	2.7230	2.6158	2.5598	2.5021	2.4422	2.3801	2.3153	2.2474
18	2.8664	2.7689	2.6667	2.5590	2.5027	2.4445	2.3842	2.3214	2.2558	2.1869
19	2.8173	2.7196	2.6171	2.5089	2.4523	2.3937	2.3329	2.2695	2.2032	2.1333
20	2.7737	2.6758	2.5731	2.4645	2.4076	2.3486	2.2873	2.2234	2.1562	2.0853
21	2.7348	2.6368	2.5338	2.4247	2.3675	2.3082	2.2465	2.1819	2.1141	2.0422
22	2.6998	2.6017	2.4984	2.3890	2.3315	2.2718	2.2097	2.1446	2.0760	2.0032
23	2.6682	2.5699	2.4665	2.3567	2.2989	2.2389	2.1763	2.1107	2.0415	1.9677
24	2.6396	2.5412	2.4374	2.3273	2.2693	2.2090	2.1460	2.0799	2.0099	1.9353
25	2.6135	2.5149	2.4110	2.3005	2.2422	2.1816	2.1183	2.0517	1.9811	1.9055
26	2.5895	2.4909	2.3867	2.2759	2.2174	2.1565	2.0928	2.0257	1.9545	1.8781
27	2.5676	2.4688	2.3644	2.2533	2.1946	2.1334	2.0693	2.0018	1.9299	1.8527
28	2.5473	2.4484	2.3438	2.2324	2.1735	2.1121	2.0477	1.9796	1.9072	1.8291
29	2.5286	2.4295	2.3248	2.2131	2.1540	2.0923	2.0276	1.9591	1.8861	1.8072
30	2.5112	2.4210	2.3072	2.1952	2.1359	2.0739	2.0089	1.9400	1.8664	1.7867
40	2.3882	2.2882	2.1819	2.0677	2.0069	1.9429	1.8752	1.8028	1.7242	1.6371
60	2.2702	2.1692	2.0613	1.9445	1.8817	1.8152	1.7440	1.6668	1.5810	1.4822
120	2.1570	2.0548	1.9450	1.8249	1.7597	1.6899	1.6141	1.5299	1.4327	1.3104
∞	2.0483	1.9447	1.8326	1.7085	1.6402	1.5660	1.4835	1.3883	1.2684	1.0000

Appendix A.4   Upper Quantiles of an F Distribution (Continued) $\alpha = 0.010$

ν_2 \ ν_1	1	2	3	4	5	6	7	8	9
1	4052.2	4999.5	5403.3	5624.6	5763.7	5859.0	5928.3	5981.6	6022.5
2	98.503	99.000	99.166	99.249	99.299	99.332	99.356	99.374	99.388
3	34.116	30.817	29.457	28.710	28.237	27.911	27.672	27.489	27.345
4	21.198	18.000	16.694	15.977	15.522	15.207	14.976	14.799	14.659
5	16.258	13.274	12.060	11.392	10.967	10.672	10.456	10.289	10.158
6	13.745	10.925	9.7795	9.1483	8.7459	8.4661	8.2600	8.1016	7.9761
7	12.246	9.5466	8.4513	7.8467	7.4604	7.1914	6.9928	6.8401	6.7188
8	11.259	8.6491	7.5910	7.0060	6.6318	6.3707	6.1776	6.0289	5.9106
9	10.561	8.0215	6.9919	6.4221	6.0569	5.8018	5.6129	5.4671	5.3511
10	10.044	7.5594	6.5523	5.9943	5.6363	5.3858	5.2001	5.0567	4.9424
11	9.6460	7.2057	6.2167	5.6683	5.3160	5.0692	4.8861	4.7445	4.6315
12	9.3302	6.9266	5.9526	5.4119	5.0643	4.8206	4.6395	4.4994	4.3875
13	9.0738	6.7010	5.7394	5.2053	4.8616	4.6204	4.4410	4.3021	4.1911
14	8.8616	6.5149	5.5639	5.0354	4.6950	4.4558	4.2779	4.1399	4.0297
15	8.6831	6.3589	5.4170	4.8932	4.5556	4.3183	4.1415	4.0045	3.8948
16	8.5310	6.2262	5.2922	4.7726	4.4374	4.2016	4.0259	3.8896	3.7804
17	8.3997	6.1121	5.1850	4.6690	4.3359	4.1015	3.9267	3.7910	3.6822
18	8.2854	6.0129	5.0919	4.5790	4.2479	4.0146	3.8406	3.7054	3.5971
19	8.1850	5.9259	5.0103	4.5003	4.1708	3.9386	3.7653	3.6305	3.5225
20	8.0960	5.8489	4.9382	4.4307	4.1027	3.8714	3.6987	3.5644	3.4567
21	8.0166	5.7804	4.8740	4.3688	4.0421	3.8117	3.6396	3.5056	3.3981
22	7.9454	5.7190	4.8166	4.3134	3.9880	3.7583	3.5867	3.4530	3.3458
23	7.8811	5.6637	4.7649	4.2635	3.9392	3.7102	3.5390	3.4057	3.2986
24	7.8229	5.6136	4.7181	4.2184	3.8951	3.6667	3.4959	3.3629	3.2560
25	7.7698	5.5680	4.6755	4.1774	3.8550	3.6272	3.4568	3.3239	3.2172
26	7.7213	5.5263	4.6366	4.1400	3.8183	3.5911	3.4210	3.2884	3.1818
27	7.6767	5.4881	4.6009	4.1056	3.7848	3.5580	3.3882	3.2558	3.1494
28	7.6356	5.4529	4.5681	4.0740	3.7539	3.5276	3.3581	3.2259	3.1195
29	7.5976	5.4205	4.5378	4.0449	3.7254	3.4995	3.3302	3.1982	3.0920
30	7.5625	5.3904	4.5097	4.0179	3.6990	3.4735	3.3045	3.1726	3.0665
40	7.3141	5.1785	4.3126	3.8283	3.5138	3.2910	3.1238	2.9930	2.8876
60	7.0771	4.9774	4.1259	3.6491	3.3389	3.1187	2.9530	2.8233	2.7185
120	6.8510	4.7865	3.9493	3.4796	3.1735	2.9559	2.7918	2.6629	2.5586
∞	6.6349	4.6052	3.7816	3.3192	3.0173	2.8020	2.6393	2.5113	2.4073

Appendix A.4 (Continued) $\alpha = 0.010$

ν_2 \ ν_1	10	12	15	20	24	30	40	60	120	∞
1	6055.8	6106.3	6157.3	6208.7	6234.6	6260.7	6286.8	6313.0	6339.4	6366.0
2	99.399	99.416	99.432	99.449	99.458	99.466	99.474	99.483	99.491	99.501
3	27.229	27.052	26.872	26.690	26.598	26.505	26.411	26.316	26.221	26.125
4	14.546	14.374	14.198	14.020	13.929	13.838	13.745	13.652	13.558	13.463
5	10.051	9.8883	9.7222	9.5527	9.4665	9.3793	9.2912	9.2020	9.1118	9.0204
6	7.8741	7.7183	7.5590	7.3958	7.3127	7.2285	7.1432	7.0568	6.9690	6.8801
7	6.6201	6.6491	6.3143	6.1554	6.0743	5.9921	5.9084	5.8236	5.7372	5.6495
8	5.8143	5.6668	5.5151	5.3591	5.2793	5.1981	5.1156	5.0316	4.9460	4.8588
9	5.2565	5.1114	4.9621	4.8080	4.7290	4.6486	4.5667	4.4831	4.3978	4.3105
10	4.8492	4.7059	4.5582	4.4054	4.3269	4.2469	4.1653	4.0819	3.9965	3.9090
11	4.5393	4.3974	4.2509	4.0990	4.0209	3.9411	3.8596	3.7761	3.6904	3.6025
12	4.2961	4.1553	4.0096	3.8584	3.7805	3.7008	3.6192	3.5355	3.4494	3.3608
13	4.1003	3.9603	3.8154	3.6646	3.5868	3.5070	3.4253	3.3413	3.2548	3.1654
14	3.9394	3.8001	3.6557	3.5052	3.4274	3.3476	3.2556	3.1813	3.0942	3.0040
15	3.8049	3.6662	3.5222	3.3719	3.2940	3.2141	3.1319	3.0471	2.9595	2.8684
16	3.6909	3.5527	3.4089	3.2588	3.1808	3.1007	3.0182	2.9330	2.8447	2.7528
17	3.5931	3.4552	3.3117	3.1615	3.0835	3.0032	2.9205	2.8348	2.7459	2.6530
18	3.5082	3.3706	3.2273	3.0771	2.9990	2.9185	2.8354	2.7493	2.6597	2.5660
19	3.4338	3.2965	3.1533	3.0031	2.9249	2.8442	2.7608	2.6742	2.5839	2.4893
20	3.3682	3.2311	3.0880	2.9377	2.8594	2.7785	2.6947	2.6077	2.5168	2.4212
21	3.3098	3.1729	3.0299	2.8796	2.8011	2.7200	2.6359	2.5484	2.4568	2.3603
22	3.2576	3.1209	2.9780	2.8274	2.7488	2.6675	2.5831	2.4951	2.4029	2.3055
23	3.2106	3.0740	2.9311	2.7805	2.7017	2.6202	2.5355	2.4471	2.3542	2.2559
24	3.1681	3.0316	2.8887	2.7380	2.6591	2.5773	2.4923	2.4035	2.3099	2.2107
25	3.1294	2.9931	2.8502	2.6993	2.6203	2.5383	2.4530	2.3637	2.2695	2.1694
26	3.0941	2.9579	2.8150	2.6640	2.5848	2.5026	2.4170	2.3273	2.2325	2.1315
27	3.0618	2.9256	2.7827	2.6316	2.5522	2.4699	2.3840	2.2938	2.1984	2.0965
28	3.0320	2.8959	2.7530	2.6017	2.5223	2.4397	2.3535	2.2629	2.1670	2.0642
29	3.0045	2.8685	2.7256	2.5742	2.4946	2.4118	2.3253	2.2344	2.1378	2.0342
30	2.9791	2.8431	2.7002	2.5487	2.4689	2.3860	2.2992	2.2079	2.1107	2.0062
40	2.8005	2.6648	2.5216	2.3689	2.2880	2.2034	2.1142	2.0194	1.9172	1.8047
60	2.6318	2.4961	2.3523	2.1978	2.1154	2.0285	1.9360	1.8363	1.7263	1.6006
120	2.4721	2.3363	2.1915	2.0346	1.9500	1.8600	1.7628	1.6557	1.5330	1.3805
∞	2.3209	2.1848	2.0385	1.8783	1.7908	1.6964	1.5923	1.4730	1.3246	1.0000

Appendix A.4   Upper Quantiles of an F Distribution (Continued) $\alpha = 0.005$

v_2 \ v_1	1	2	3	4	5	6	7	8	9
1	16211	20000	21615	22500	23056	23437	23715	23925	24091
2	198.50	199.00	199.17	199.25	199.30	199.33	199.36	199.37	199.39
3	55.552	49.799	47.467	46.195	45.392	44.838	44.434	44.126	43.882
4	31.333	26.284	24.259	23.155	22.456	21.975	21.622	21.352	21.139
5	22.785	18.314	16.530	15.556	14.940	14.513	14.200	13.961	13.722
6	18.635	14.544	12.917	12.028	11.464	11.073	10.786	10.566	10.391
7	16.236	12.404	10.882	10.050	9.5221	9.1554	8.8854	8.6781	8.5138
8	14.688	11.042	9.5965	8.8051	8.3018	7.9520	7.6942	7.4960	7.3386
9	13.614	10.107	8.7171	7.9559	7.4711	7.1338	6.8849	6.6933	6.5411
10	12.826	9.4270	8.0807	7.3428	6.8723	6.5446	6.3025	6.1159	5.9676
11	12.226	8.9122	7.6004	6.8809	6.4217	6.1015	5.8648	5.6821	5.5368
12	11.754	8.5096	7.2258	6.5211	6.0711	5.7570	5.5245	5.3451	5.2021
13	11.374	8.1865	6.9257	6.2335	5.7910	5.4819	5.2529	5.0761	4.9351
14	11.060	7.9217	6.6803	5.9984	5.5623	5.2574	5.0313	4.8566	4.7173
15	10.798	7.7008	6.4760	5.8029	5.3721	5.0708	4.8473	4.6743	4.5464
16	10.575	7.5138	6.3034	5.6378	5.2117	4.9134	4.6920	4.5207	4.3838
17	10.384	7.3536	6.1556	5.4967	5.0746	4.7789	4.5594	4.3893	4.2535
18	10.218	7.2148	6.0277	5.3746	4.9560	4.6627	4.4448	4.2759	4.1410
19	10.073	7.0935	5.9161	5.2681	4.8526	4.5614	4.3448	4.1770	4.0428
20	9.9439	6.9865	5.8177	5.1743	4.7616	4.4721	4.2569	4.0900	3.9564
21	9.8295	6.8914	5.7304	5.0911	4.6808	4.3931	4.1789	4.0128	3.8799
22	9.7271	6.8064	5.6524	5.0168	4.6088	4.3225	4.1094	3.9440	3.8116
23	9.6348	6.7300	5.5823	4.9500	4.5441	4.2591	4.0469	3.8822	3.7502
24	9.5513	6.6610	5.5190	4.8898	4.4857	4.2019	3.9905	3.8264	3.6949
25	9.4753	6.5982	5.4615	4.8351	4.4327	4.1500	3.9394	3.7758	3.6447
26	9.4059	6.5409	5.4091	4.7852	4.3844	4.1027	3.8928	3.7297	3.5989
27	9.3423	6.4885	5.3611	4.7396	4.3402	4.0594	3.8501	3.6875	3.5571
28	9.2838	6.4403	5.3170	4.6977	4.2996	4.0197	3.8110	3.6487	3.5186
29	9.2297	6.3958	5.2764	4.6591	4.2622	3.9830	3.7749	3.6130	3.4832
30	9.1797	6.3547	5.2388	4.6233	4.2276	3.9492	3.7416	3.5801	3.4505
40	8.8278	6.0664	4.9759	4.3738	3.9860	3.7129	3.5088	3.3498	3.2220
60	8.4946	5.7950	4.7290	4.1399	3.7600	3.4918	3.2911	3.1344	3.0083
120	8.1790	5.5393	4.4973	3.9207	3.5482	3.2849	3.0874	2.9330	2.8083
∞	7.8794	5.2983	4.2794	3.7151	3.3499	3.0913	2.8968	2.7444	2.6210

Appendix A.4 (Continued) $\alpha = 0.005$

ν_2 \ ν_1	10	12	15	20	24	30	40	60	12	∞
1	24224	24426	24630	24836	24940	25044	25148	25253	25359	25465
2	199.40	199.42	199.43	199.45	199.46	199.47	199.47	199.48	199.49	199.51
3	43.686	43.387	43.085	42.778	42.622	42.466	42.308	42.149	41.989	41.829
4	20.967	20.705	20.438	20.167	20.030	19.892	19.752	19.611	19.468	19.325
5	13.618	13.384	13.146	12.903	12.780	12.656	12.530	12.402	12.274	12.144
6	10.250	10.034	9.8140	9.5888	9.4741	9.3583	9.2408	9.1219	9.0015	8.8793
7	8.3803	8.1764	7.9678	7.7540	7.6450	7.5345	7.4225	7.3088	7.1933	7.0760
8	7.2107	7.0149	6.8143	6.6082	6.5029	6.3961	6.2875	6.1772	6.0649	5.9505
9	6.4171	6.2274	6.0325	5.8318	5.7292	5.6248	5.5186	5.4104	5.3001	5.1875
10	5.8467	5.6613	5.4707	5.2740	5.1732	5.0705	4.9659	4.8592	4.7501	4.6385
11	5.4182	5.2363	5.0489	4.8552	4.7557	4.6543	4.5508	4.4450	4.3367	4.2256
12	5.0855	4.9063	4.7214	4.5299	4.4315	4.3309	4.2282	4.1229	4.0149	3.9039
13	4.8199	4.6429	4.4600	4.2703	4.1726	4.0727	3.9704	3.8655	3.7577	3.6465
14	4.6034	4.4281	4.2468	4.0585	3.9614	3.8619	3.7600	3.6553	3.5473	3.4359
15	4.4236	4.2498	4.0698	3.8826	3.7859	3.6867	3.5850	3.4803	3.3722	3.2602
16	4.2719	4.0994	3.9205	3.7342	3.6378	3.5388	3.4372	3.3324	3.2240	3.1115
17	4.1423	3.9709	3.7929	3.6073	3.5112	3.4124	3.3107	3.2058	3.0971	2.9839
18	4.0305	3.8599	3.6827	3.4977	3.4017	3.3030	3.2014	3.0962	2.9871	2.8732
19	3.9329	3.7631	3.5866	3.4020	3.3062	3.2075	3.1058	3.0004	2.8908	2.7762
20	3.8470	3.6779	3.5020	3.3178	3.2220	3.1234	3.0215	2.9159	2.8058	2.6904
21	3.7709	3.6024	3.4270	3.2431	3.1474	3.0488	2.9467	2.8408	2.7302	2.6140
22	3.7030	3.5350	3.3600	3.1764	3.0807	2.9821	2.8799	2.7736	2.6625	2.5455
23	3.6420	3.4745	3.2999	3.1165	3.0208	2.9221	2.8198	2.7132	2.6016	2.4837
24	3.5870	3.4199	3.2456	3.0624	2.9667	2.8679	2.7654	2.6585	2.5463	2.4276
25	3.5370	3.3704	3.1963	3.0133	2.9176	2.8187	2.7160	2.6088	2.4960	2.3765
26	3.4916	3.3252	3.1515	2.9685	2.8728	2.7738	2.6709	2.5633	2.4501	2.3297
27	3.4499	3.2839	3.1104	2.9275	2.8318	2.7327	2.6296	2.5217	2.4078	2.2867
28	3.4117	3.2460	3.0727	2.8899	2.7941	2.6949	2.5916	2.4834	2.3689	2.2469
29	3.3765	3.2111	3.0379	2.8551	2.7594	2.6601	2.5565	2.4479	2.3330	2.2102
30	3.3440	3.1787	3.0057	2.8230	2.7272	2.6278	2.5241	2.4151	2.2997	2.1760
40	3.1167	2.9531	2.7811	2.5984	2.5020	2.4015	2.2958	2.1838	2.0635	1.9318
60	2.9042	2.7419	2.5705	2.3872	2.2898	2.1874	2.0789	1.9622	1.8341	1.6885
120	2.7052	2.5439	2.3727	2.1881	2.0890	1.9839	1.8709	1.7469	1.6055	1.4311
∞	2.5188	2.3583	2.1868	1.9998	1.8983	1.7891	1.6691	1.5325	1.3637	1.0000

Appendix A.5 Upper Quantiles of the Distribution of Wilcoxon-Mann-Whitney Statistic

n_1	α	$n_2 = 2$	3	4	5	6	7	8	9	10	11	12	13	14	15	16	17	18	19	20
2	0.001	0	0	0	0	0	0	0	0	0	0	0	0	0	0	0	0	0	0	0
	0.005	0	0	0	0	0	0	0	0	0	0	0	0	0	0	0	0	0	1	1
	0.01	0	0	0	0	0	0	0	0	0	0	0	1	1	1	1	1	1	2	2
	0.025	0	0	0	0	0	0	1	1	1	1	2	2	2	2	2	3	3	3	3
	0.05	0	0	0	1	1	1	2	2	2	2	3	3	4	4	4	4	5	5	5
	0.10	1	1	1	2	2	2	3	3	4	4	5	5	5	6	6	7	7	8	8
3	0.001	0	0	0	0	0	0	0	0	0	0	0	0	0	0	0	1	1	1	1
	0.005	0	0	0	0	0	0	0	1	1	1	2	2	2	3	3	3	3	4	4
	0.01	0	0	0	0	0	1	1	2	2	2	3	3	3	4	4	5	5	5	6
	0.025	0	0	0	1	2	2	3	3	4	4	5	5	6	6	7	7	8	8	9
	0.05	0	1	1	2	3	3	4	5	5	6	6	7	8	8	9	10	10	11	12
	0.10	1	2	2	3	4	5	6	6	7	8	9	10	11	11	12	13	14	15	16
4	0.001	0	0	0	0	0	0	0	0	1	1	1	2	2	2	3	3	4	4	4
	0.005	0	0	0	0	1	1	2	2	3	3	4	4	5	6	6	7	7	8	9
	0.01	0	0	0	1	2	2	3	4	4	5	6	6	7	8	8	9	10	10	11
	0.025	0	0	1	2	3	4	5	5	6	7	8	9	10	11	12	12	13	14	15
	0.05	0	1	2	3	4	5	6	7	8	9	10	11	12	13	15	16	17	18	19
	0.10	1	2	4	5	6	7	8	10	11	12	13	14	16	17	18	19	21	22	23

	α																				
5	0.001	8	8	7	6	6	5	4	4	3	3	2	2	1	0	0	0	0	0	0
	0.005	14	13	12	11	10	9	8	8	7	6	5	4	3	2	2	1	0	0	0
	0.01	17	16	15	14	13	12	11	10	9	8	7	6	5	4	3	2	1	0	0
	0.025	21	20	19	18	16	15	14	13	12	10	9	8	7	6	4	3	2	1	0
	0.05	26	24	23	21	20	19	17	16	14	13	12	10	9	7	6	5	3	2	1
	0.10	31	29	28	26	24	23	21	19	18	16	14	13	11	9	8	6	5	3	2
6	0.001	13	12	11	10	9	8	7	6	5	5	4	3	2	0	0	0	0	0	0
	0.005	19	18	17	16	14	13	12	11	10	8	7	6	5	4	3	2	1	0	0
	0.01	23	21	20	19	17	16	14	13	12	10	9	8	7	5	4	3	2	0	0
	0.025	28	26	25	23	22	20	18	17	15	14	12	11	9	7	6	4	3	2	0
	0.05	33	31	29	27	26	24	22	20	18	17	15	13	11	9	8	6	4	3	1
	0.10	39	37	35	32	30	28	26	24	22	20	18	16	14	12	10	8	6	4	2
7	0.001	17	16	15	14	12	11	10	9	8	7	6	4	3	2	1	0	0	0	0
	0.005	25	23	22	20	19	17	16	14	13	11	10	8	7	5	4	2	1	0	0
	0.01	29	27	25	24	22	20	18	17	15	13	12	10	8	7	5	4	2	1	0
	0.025	35	33	31	29	27	25	23	21	19	17	15	13	11	9	7	6	4	2	0
	0.05	40	38	36	34	31	29	27	25	22	20	18	16	14	12	9	7	5	3	1
	0.10	47	44	42	39	37	34	32	29	27	24	22	19	17	14	12	9	7	5	2
8	0.001	22	21	19	18	16	15	13	12	10	9	7	6	5	3	2	1	0	0	0
	0.005	31	29	27	25	23	21	19	18	16	14	12	10	8	7	5	3	2	0	0
	0.01	35	33	31	29	27	25	23	21	18	16	14	12	10	8	7	5	3	1	0
	0.025	42	39	37	35	32	30	27	25	23	20	18	16	14	11	9	7	5	3	1
	0.05	48	45	42	40	37	34	32	29	27	24	21	19	16	14	11	9	6	4	2
	0.10	55	52	49	46	43	40	37	34	31	28	25	23	20	17	14	11	8	6	3
	0.001	27	26	24	22	20	18	16	15	13	11	9	8	6	4	3	2	0	0	0
	0.005	37	34	32	30	28	25	23	21	19	17	14	12	10	8	6	4	2	1	0

Appendix A.5 (Continued)

n_1	α	$n_2 = 2$	3	4	5	6	7	8	9	10	11	12	13	14	15	16	17	18	19	20
9	0.01	0	2	4	6	8	10	12	15	17	19	22	24	27	29	32	34	37	39	41
	0.025	1	3	5	8	11	13	16	18	21	24	27	29	32	35	38	40	43	46	49
	0.05	2	5	7	10	13	16	19	22	25	28	31	34	37	40	43	46	49	52	55
	0.10	3	6	10	13	16	19	23	26	29	32	36	39	42	46	49	53	56	59	63
10	0.001	0	0	1	2	4	6	7	9	11	13	15	18	20	22	24	26	28	30	33
	0.005	0	1	3	5	7	10	12	14	17	19	22	25	27	30	32	35	38	40	43
	0.01	0	2	4	7	9	12	14	17	20	23	25	28	31	34	37	39	42	45	48
	0.025	1	4	6	9	12	15	18	21	24	27	30	34	37	40	43	46	49	53	56
	0.05	2	5	8	12	15	18	21	25	28	32	35	38	42	45	49	52	56	59	63
	0.10	4	7	11	14	18	22	25	29	33	37	40	44	48	52	55	59	63	67	71
11	0.001	0	1	1	3	5	7	9	11	13	16	18	21	23	25	28	30	33	35	38
	0.005	0	1	3	6	8	11	14	17	19	22	25	28	31	34	37	40	43	46	49
	0.01	0	2	5	8	10	13	16	19	23	26	29	32	35	38	42	45	48	51	54
	0.025	1	4	7	10	14	17	20	24	27	31	34	38	41	45	48	52	56	59	63
	0.05	2	6	9	13	17	20	24	28	32	35	39	43	47	51	55	58	62	66	70
	0.10	4	8	12	16	20	24	28	32	37	41	45	49	53	58	62	66	70	74	79
12	0.001	0	0	1	3	5	8	10	13	15	18	21	24	26	29	32	35	38	41	43
	0.005	0	2	4	7	10	13	16	19	22	25	28	32	35	38	42	45	48	52	55
	0.01	0	3	6	9	12	15	18	22	25	29	32	36	39	43	47	50	54	57	61
	0.025	2	5	8	12	15	19	23	27	30	34	38	42	46	50	54	58	62	66	70
	0.05	3	6	10	14	18	22	27	31	35	39	43	48	52	56	61	65	69	73	78
	0.10	5	9	13	18	22	27	31	36	40	45	50	54	59	64	68	73	78	82	87
	0.001	0	0	2	4	6	9	12	15	18	21	24	27	30	33	36	39	43	46	49
	0.005	0	2	4	8	11	14	18	21	25	28	32	35	39	43	46	50	54	58	61

n	α																			
13	0.01	1	3	6	10	13	17	21	24	28	32	36	40	44	48	52	56	60	64	68
	0.025	2	5	9	13	17	21	25	29	34	38	42	46	51	55	60	64	68	73	77
	0.05	3	7	11	16	20	25	29	34	38	43	48	52	57	62	66	71	76	81	85
	0.010	5	10	14	19	24	29	34	39	44	49	54	59	64	69	75	80	85	90	95
14	0.001	0	0	2	4	7	10	13	16	20	23	26	30	33	37	40	44	47	51	55
	0.005	0	2	5	8	12	16	19	23	27	31	35	39	43	47	51	55	59	64	68
	0.01	1	3	7	11	14	18	23	27	31	35	39	44	48	52	57	61	66	70	74
	0.025	2	6	10	14	18	23	27	32	37	41	46	51	56	60	65	70	75	79	84
	0.05	4	8	12	17	22	27	32	37	42	47	52	57	62	67	72	78	83	88	93
	0.10	5	11	16	21	26	32	37	42	48	53	59	64	70	75	81	86	92	98	103
15	0.001	0	0	2	5	8	11	15	18	22	25	29	33	37	41	44	48	52	56	60
	0.005	0	3	6	9	13	17	21	25	30	34	38	43	47	52	56	61	65	70	74
	0.01	1	4	8	12	16	20	25	29	34	38	43	48	52	57	62	67	71	76	81
	0.025	2	6	11	15	20	25	30	35	40	45	50	55	60	65	71	76	81	86	91
	0.05	4	8	13	19	24	29	34	40	45	51	56	62	67	73	78	84	89	95	101
	0.10	6	11	17	23	28	34	40	46	52	58	64	69	75	81	87	93	99	105	111
16	0.001	0	0	3	6	9	12	16	20	24	28	32	36	40	44	49	53	57	61	66
	0.005	0	3	6	10	14	19	23	28	32	37	42	46	51	56	61	66	71	75	80
	0.01	1	4	8	13	17	22	27	32	37	42	47	52	57	62	67	72	77	83	88
	0.025	2	7	12	16	22	27	32	38	43	48	54	60	65	71	76	82	87	93	99
	0.05	4	9	15	20	26	31	37	43	49	55	61	66	72	78	84	90	96	102	108
	0.10	6	12	18	24	30	37	43	49	55	62	68	75	81	87	94	100	107	113	120

Appendix A.5 (Continued)

n_1	α	$n_2 = 2$	3	4	5	6	7	8	9	10	11	12	13	14	15	16	17	18	19	20
17	0.001	0	1	3	6	10	14	18	22	26	30	35	39	44	48	53	58	62	67	71
	0.005	0	3	7	11	16	20	25	30	35	40	45	50	55	61	66	71	76	82	87
	0.01	1	5	9	14	19	24	29	34	39	45	50	56	61	67	72	78	83	89	94
	0.025	3	7	12	18	23	29	35	40	46	52	58	64	70	76	82	88	94	100	106
	0.05	4	10	16	21	27	34	40	46	52	58	65	71	78	84	90	97	103	110	116
	0.10	7	13	19	26	32	39	46	53	59	66	73	80	86	93	100	107	114	121	128
18	0.001	0	1	4	7	11	15	19	24	28	33	38	43	47	52	57	62	67	72	77
	0.005	0	3	7	12	17	22	27	32	38	43	48	54	59	65	71	76	82	88	93
	0.01	1	5	10	15	20	25	31	37	42	48	54	60	66	71	77	83	89	95	101
	0.025	3	8	13	19	25	31	37	43	49	56	62	68	75	81	87	94	100	107	113
	0.05	5	10	17	23	29	36	42	49	56	62	69	76	83	89	96	103	110	117	124
	0.10	7	14	21	28	35	42	49	56	63	70	78	85	92	99	107	114	121	129	136
19	0.001	0	1	4	8	12	16	21	26	30	35	41	46	51	56	61	67	72	78	83
	0.005	1	4	8	13	18	23	29	34	40	46	52	58	64	70	75	82	88	94	100
	0.01	2	5	10	16	21	27	33	39	45	51	57	64	70	76	83	89	95	102	108
	0.025	3	8	14	20	26	33	39	46	53	59	66	73	79	86	93	100	107	114	120
	0.05	5	11	18	24	31	38	45	52	59	66	73	81	88	95	102	110	117	124	131
	0.10	8	15	22	29	37	44	52	59	67	74	82	90	98	105	113	121	129	136	144
20	0.001	0	1	4	8	13	17	22	27	33	38	43	49	55	60	66	71	77	83	89
	0.005	1	4	9	14	19	25	31	37	43	49	55	61	68	74	80	87	93	100	106
	0.01	2	6	11	17	23	29	35	41	48	54	61	68	74	81	88	94	101	108	115
	0.025	3	9	15	21	28	35	42	49	56	63	70	77	84	91	99	106	113	120	128
	0.05	5	12	19	26	33	40	48	55	63	70	78	85	93	101	108	116	124	131	139
	0.10	8	16	23	31	39	47	55	63	71	79	87	95	103	111	120	128	136	144	152

Source: Table 1 of Extended Tables of Critical Values for Wilcoxon's Test Statistic by L. R. Verdooren, *Biometrika* (1963), Vol. 50, pp. 177–186.

Quantiles of the Wilcoxon Signed-Rank Test Statistic

n^a	$W_{0.005}$	$W_{0.01}$	$W_{0.025}$	$W_{0.05}$	$W_{0.10}$	$W_{0.20}$	$W_{0.30}$	$W_{0.40}$	$W_{0.50}$	$\dfrac{n(n+1)}{2}$
4	0	0	0	0	1	3	3	4	5	10
5	0	0	0	1	3	4	5	6	7.5	15
6	0	0	1	3	4	6	8	9	10.5	21
7	0	1	3	4	6	9	11	12	14	28
8	1	2	4	6	9	12	14	16	18	36
9	2	4	6	9	11	15	18	20	22.5	45
10	4	6	9	11	15	19	22	25	27.5	55
11	6	8	11	14	18	23	27	30	33	66
12	8	10	14	18	22	28	32	36	39	78
13	10	13	18	22	27	33	38	42	45.5	91
14	13	16	22	26	32	39	44	48	52.5	105
15	16	20	26	31	37	45	51	55	60	120
16	20	24	30	36	43	51	58	63	68	136
17	24	28	35	42	49	58	65	71	76.5	153
18	28	33	41	48	56	66	73	80	85.5	171
19	33	38	47	54	63	74	82	89	95	190
20	38	44	53	61	70	83	91	98	105	210
21	44	50	59	68	78	91	100	108	115.5	131
22	49	56	67	76	87	100	110	119	126.5	153
23	55	63	74	84	95	110	120	130	138	176
24	62	70	82	92	105	120	131	141	150	300
25	69	77	90	101	114	131	143	153	162.5	325
26	76	85	99	111	125	142	155	165	175.5	351
27	84	94	108	120	135	154	167	178	189	378
28	92	102	117	131	146	166	180	192	203	406
29	101	111	127	141	158	178	193	206	217.5	435
30	110	121	138	152	170	191	207	220	232.5	465
31	119	131	148	164	182	205	221	235	248	496
32	129	141	160	176	195	219	236	250	204	528
33	139	152	171	188	208	233	251	266	280.5	561
34	149	163	183	201	222	248	266	282	297.5	595
35	160	175	196	214	236	263	283	299	315	630
36	172	187	209	228	251	279	299	317	333	666
37	184	199	222	242	266	295	316	335	351.5	703
38	196	212	236	257	282	312	334	353	370.5	741
39	208	225	250	272	298	329	352	372	390	780
40	221	239	265	287	314	347	371	391	410	820
41	235	253	280	303	331	365	390	411	430.5	861
42	248	267	295	320	349	384	409	431	451.5	903
43	263	282	311	337	366	403	429	452	473	946
44	277	297	328	354	385	422	450	473	495	990
45	292	313	344	372	403	442	471	495	517.5	1035
46	308	329	362	390	423	463	492	517	540.5	1081
47	324	346	379	408	442	484	514	540	564	1128
48	340	363	397	428	463	505	536	563	588	1176
49	357	381	416	447	483	527	559	587	612.5	1225
50	374	398	435	467	504	550	583	611	637.5	1275

Source: Adapted from Harter and Owen (1970), with permission from the Institute of Mathematical Statistics.

[a] For n larger than 50, the pth quantile w_p of the Wilcoxon signed-rank test statistic may be approximated by $w_p = [n(n+1)/4] + x_p \sqrt{n(n+1)(2n+1)/24}$, where x_p is the pth quantile of a standard normal random variable, obtained from Appendix A.1.

	$1 - \alpha = 0.95$			$1 - \alpha = 0.99$		
n	0.90	0.95	0.99	0.90	0.95	0.99
2	32.019	37.674	48.430	160.193	188.491	242.300
3	8.380	9.916	12.861	18.930	22.401	29.055
4	5.369	6.370	8.299	9.398	11.150	14.527
5	4.275	5.079	6.634	6.612	7.855	10.260
6	3.712	4.414	5.775	5.337	6.345	8.301
7	3.369	4.007	5.248	4.613	5.488	7.187
8	3.136	3.732	4.891	4.147	4.936	6.468
9	2.967	3.532	4.631	3.822	4.550	5.966
10	2.839	3.379	4.433	3.582	4.265	5.594
11	2.737	3.259	4.277	3.397	4.045	5.308
12	2.655	3.162	4.150	3.250	3.870	5.079
13	2.587	3.081	4.044	3.130	3.727	4.893
14	2.529	3.012	3.955	3.029	3.608	4.737
15	2.480	2.954	3.878	2.945	3.507	4.605
16	2.437	2.903	3.812	2.872	3.421	4.492
17	2.400	2.858	3.754	2.808	3.345	4.393
18	2.366	2.819	3.702	2.753	3.279	4.307
19	2.337	2.784	3.656	2.703	3.221	4.230
20	2.310	2.752	3.615	2.659	3.168	4.161
25	2.208	2.631	3.457	2.494	2.972	3.904
30	2.140	2.549	3.350	2.385	2.841	3.733
35	2.090	2.490	3.272	2.306	2.748	3.611
40	2.052	2.445	3.213	2.247	2.677	3.518
45	2.021	2.408	3.165	2.200	2.621	3.444
50	1.996	2.379	3.126	2.162	2.576	3.385
55	1.976	2.354	3.094	2.130	2.538	3.335
60	1.958	2.333	3.066	2.103	2.506	3.293
65	1.943	2.315	3.042	2.080	2.478	3.257
70	1.929	2.299	3.021	2.060	2.454	3.225
75	1.917	2.285	3.002	2.042	2.433	3.197
80	1.907	2.272	2.986	2.026	2.414	3.173
85	1.897	2.261	2.971	2.012	2.397	3.150
90	1.889	2.251	2.958	1.999	2.382	3.130
95	1.881	2.241	2.945	1.987	2.368	3.112
100	1.874	2.233	2.934	1.977	2.355	3.096
150	1.825	2.175	2.859	1.905	2.270	2.983
200	1.798	2.143	2.816	1.865	2.222	2.921
250	1.780	2.121	2.788	1.839	2.191	2.880
300	1.767	2.106	2.767	1.820	2.169	2.850
400	1.749	2.084	2.739	1.794	2.138	2.809
500	1.737	2.070	2.721	1.777	2.117	2.783
600	1.729	2.060	2.707	1.764	2.102	2.763
700	1.722	2.052	2.697	1.755	2.091	2.748
800	1.717	2.046	2.688	1.747	2.082	2.736
900	1.712	2.040	2.682	1.741	2.075	2.726
1000	1.709	2.036	2.676	1.736	2.068	2.718
∞	1.645	1.960	2.576	1.645	1.960	2.576

Source: Adapted by permission from *Techniques of Statistical Analysis* by C. Eisenhart, M. W. Hastay, and W. A. Wallis. Copyright 1947, McGraw-Hill Book Company, Inc.

APPENDIX A.8 Upper Quantiles of the Studentized Range Distribution

(a) t = 2 to 10

						t				
ν	α	2	3	4	5	6	7	8	9	10
1	.20	4.353	6.615	8.075	9.138	9.966	10.64	11.21	11.70	12.12
	.10	8.929	13.44	16.36	18.49	20.15	21.51	22.64	23.62	24.48
	.05	17.97	26.98	32.82	37.08	40.41	43.12	45.40	47.36	49.07
	.01	90.03	135.0	164.3	185.6	202.2	215.8	227.2	237.0	245.6
2	.20	2.667	3.820	4.559	5.098	5.521	5.867	6.158	6.409	6.630
	.10	4.130	5.733	6.773	7.538	8.139	8.633	9.049	9.409	9.725
	.05	6.085	8.331	9.798	10.88	11.74	12.44	13.03	13.54	13.99
	.01	14.04	19.02	22.29	24.72	26.63	28.20	29.53	30.68	31.69
3	.20	2.316	3.245	3.833	4.261	4.597	4.872	5.104	5.305	5.481
	.10	3.328	4.467	5.199	5.738	6.162	6.511	6.806	7.062	7.287
	.05	4.501	5.910	6.825	7.502	8.037	8.478	8.853	9.177	9.462
	.01	8.261	10.62	12.17	13.33	14.24	15.00	15.64	16.20	16.69
4	.20	2.168	3.004	3.527	3.907	4.205	4.449	4.655	4.832	4.989
	.10	3.015	3.976	4.536	5.035	5.388	5.679	5.926	6.139	6.327
	.05	3.927	5.040	5.757	6.287	6.707	7.053	7.347	7.602	7.826
	.01	6.512	8.120	9.173	9.958	10.58	11.10	11.55	11.93	12.27
5	.20	2.087	2.872	3.358	3.712	3.988	4.214	4.405	4.570	4.715
	.10	2.850	3.717	4.264	4.664	4.979	5.238	5.458	5.648	5.816
	.05	3.635	4.602	5.218	5.673	6.033	6.330	6.582	6.802	6.995
	.01	5.702	6.976	7.804	8.421	8.913	9.321	9.669	9.972	10.24

APPENDIX A.8 Upper Quantiles of the Studentized Range Distribution (Continued)

(a) $t = 2$ to 10

ν	α	2	3	4	5	6	7	8	9	10
6	.20	2.036	2.788	3.252	3.588	3.850	4.065	4.246	4.403	4.540
	.10	2.748	3.559	4.065	4.435	4.726	4.966	5.168	5.344	5.499
	.05	3.461	4.339	4.896	5.305	5.628	5.895	6.122	6.319	6.493
	.01	5.243	6.331	7.033	7.556	7.973	8.318	8.613	8.869	9.097
7	.20	2.001	2.731	3.179	3.503	3.756	3.962	4.136	4.287	4.419
	.10	2.680	3.451	3.931	4.280	4.555	4.780	4.972	5.137	5.283
	.05	3.344	4.165	4.681	5.060	5.359	5.606	5.815	5.998	6.158
	.01	4.949	5.919	6.543	7.005	7.373	7.679	7.939	8.166	8.368
8	.20	1.976	2.689	3.126	3.440	3.686	3.886	4.055	4.201	4.330
	.10	2.630	3.374	3.834	4.169	4.431	4.646	4.829	4.987	5.126
	.05	3.261	4.041	4.529	4.886	5.167	5.399	5.597	5.767	5.918
	.01	4.746	5.635	6.204	6.625	6.960	7.237	7.474	7.681	7.863
9	.20	1.956	2.658	3.085	3.393	3.633	3.828	3.994	4.136	4.261
	.10	2.592	3.316	3.761	4.084	4.337	4.545	4.721	4.873	5.007
	.05	3.199	3.949	4.415	4.756	5.024	5.244	5.432	5.595	5.739
	.01	4.596	5.428	5.957	6.348	6.658	6.915	7.134	7.325	7.495
10	.20	1.941	2.632	3.053	3.355	3.590	3.782	3.944	4.084	4.206
	.10	2.563	3.270	3.704	4.018	4.264	4.465	4.636	4.783	4.913
	.05	3.151	3.877	4.327	4.654	4.912	5.124	5.305	5.461	5.599
	.01	4.482	5.270	5.769	6.136	6.428	6.669	6.875	7.055	7.213

11	.20	1.928	2.612	3.027	3.325	3.557	3.745	3.905	4.042	4.162
	.10	2.540	3.234	3.658	3.965	4.205	4.401	4.568	4.711	4.838
	.05	3.113	3.820	4.256	4.574	4.823	5.028	5.202	5.353	5.487
	.01	4.392	5.146	5.621	5.970	6.247	6.476	6.672	6.842	6.992
12	.20	1.918	2.596	3.006	3.300	3.529	3.715	3.872	4.007	4.126
	.10	2.521	3.204	3.621	3.922	4.156	4.349	4.511	4.652	4.776
	.05	3.082	3.773	4.199	4.508	4.751	4.950	5.119	5.265	5.395
	.01	4.320	5.046	5.502	5.836	6.101	6.321	6.507	6.670	6.814
13	.20	1.910	2.582	2.988	3.279	3.505	3.689	3.844	3.978	4.095
	.10	2.505	3.179	3.589	3.885	4.116	4.305	4.464	4.602	4.724
	.05	3.055	3.735	4.151	4.453	4.690	4.885	5.049	5.192	5.318
	.01	4.260	4.964	5.404	5.727	5.981	6.192	6.372	6.528	6.667
14	.20	1.902	2.570	2.973	3.261	3.485	3.667	3.820	3.953	4.069
	.10	2.491	3.158	3.563	3.854	4.081	4.267	4.424	4.560	4.680
	.05	3.033	3.702	4.111	4.407	4.639	4.829	4.990	5.131	5.254
	.01	4.210	4.895	5.322	5.634	5.881	6.085	6.258	6.409	6.543
15	.20	1.896	2.560	2.960	3.246	3.467	3.648	3.800	3.931	4.046
	.10	2.479	3.140	3.540	3.828	4.052	4.235	4.390	4.524	4.641
	.05	3.014	3.674	4.076	4.367	4.595	4.782	4.940	5.077	5.198
	.01	4.168	4.836	5.252	5.556	5.796	5.994	6.162	6.309	6.439
16	.20	1.891	2.551	2.948	3.232	3.452	3.631	3.782	3.912	4.026
	.10	2.469	3.124	3.520	3.804	4.026	4.207	4.360	4.492	4.608
	.05	2.998	3.649	4.046	4.333	4.557	4.741	4.897	5.031	5.150
	.01	4.131	4.786	5.192	5.489	5.722	5.915	6.079	6.222	6.349

APPENDIX A.8 Upper Quantiles of the Studentized Range Distribution (Continued)

(a) $t = 2$ to 10

ν	α	2	3	4	5	6	7	8	9	10
17	.20	1.886	2.543	2.938	3.220	3.439	3.617	3.766	3.895	4.008
	.10	2.460	3.110	3.503	3.784	4.004	4.183	4.334	4.464	4.579
	.05	2.984	3.628	4.020	4.303	4.524	4.705	4.858	4.991	5.108
	.01	4.099	4.742	5.140	5.430	5.659	5.847	6.007	6.147	6.270
18	.20	1.882	2.536	2.930	3.210	3.427	3.604	3.753	3.881	3.993
	.10	2.452	3.098	3.488	3.767	3.984	4.161	4.311	4.440	4.554
	.05	2.971	3.609	3.997	4.277	4.495	4.673	4.824	4.956	5.071
	.01	4.071	4.703	5.094	5.379	5.603	5.788	5.944	6.081	6.201
19	.20	1.878	2.530	2.922	3.200	3.416	3.592	3.740	3.867	3.979
	.10	2.445	3.087	3.474	3.751	3.966	4.142	4.290	4.418	4.531
	.05	2.960	3.593	3.977	4.253	4.469	4.645	4.794	4.924	5.038
	.01	4.046	4.670	5.054	5.334	5.554	5.735	5.889	6.022	6.141
20	.20	1.874	2.524	2.914	3.192	3.407	3.582	3.729	3.855	3.966
	.10	2.439	3.078	3.462	3.736	3.950	4.124	4.271	4.398	4.510
	.05	2.950	3.578	3.958	4.232	4.445	4.620	4.768	4.896	5.008
	.01	4.024	4.639	5.018	5.294	5.510	5.688	5.839	5.970	6.087
24	.20	1.864	2.507	2.892	3.166	3.377	3.549	3.694	3.818	3.927
	.10	2.420	3.047	3.423	3.692	3.900	4.070	4.213	4.336	4.445
	.05	2.919	3.532	3.901	4.166	4.373	4.541	4.684	4.807	4.915
	.01	3.956	4.546	4.907	5.168	5.374	5.542	5.685	5.809	5.919

30	.20	1.853	2.430	2.870	3.140	3.348	3.517	3.659	3.781	3.887
	.10	2.400	3.017	3.386	3.648	3.851	4.016	4.155	4.275	4.381
	.05	2.888	3.486	3.845	4.102	4.302	4.464	4.602	4.720	4.824
	.01	3.889	4.455	4.799	5.048	5.242	5.401	5.536	5.653	5.756
40	.20	1.843	2.473	2.848	3.114	3.318	3.484	3.624	3.743	3.848
	.10	2.381	2.988	3.349	3.605	3.803	3.963	4.099	4.215	4.317
	.05	2.858	3.442	3.791	4.039	4.232	4.389	4.521	4.635	4.735
	.01	3.825	4.367	4.696	4.931	5.114	5.265	5.392	5.502	5.599
60	.20	1.833	2.456	2.826	3.089	3.290	3.452	3.589	3.707	3.809
	.10	2.363	2.959	3.312	3.562	3.755	3.911	4.042	4.155	4.254
	.05	2.829	3.399	3.737	3.977	4.163	4.314	4.441	4.550	4.646
	.01	3.762	4.282	4.595	4.818	4.991	5.133	5.253	5.356	5.447
120	.20	1.822	2.440	2.805	3.063	3.260	3.420	3.554	3.669	3.770
	.10	2.344	2.930	3.276	3.520	3.707	3.859	3.987	4.096	4.191
	.05	2.800	3.356	3.685	3.917	4.096	4.241	4.363	4.468	4.560
	.01	3.702	4.200	4.497	4.709	4.872	5.005	5.118	5.214	5.299
∞	.20	1.812	2.424	2.784	3.037	3.232	3.389	3.520	3.632	3.730
	.10	2.326	2.902	3.240	3.478	3.661	3.808	3.931	4.037	4.129
	.05	2.772	3.314	3.633	3.858	4.030	4.170	4.286	4.387	4.474
	.01	3.643	4.120	4.403	4.603	4.757	4.882	4.987	5.078	5.157

APPENDIX A.8 Upper Quantiles of the Studentized Range Distribution (Continued)

(b) $t = 11$ to 19

v	α	11	12	13	14	15	16	17	18	19
10	.20	4.316	4.414	4.503	4.585	4.660	4.730	4.795	4.856	4.913
	.10	5.029	5.134	5.229	5.317	5.397	5.472	5.542	5.607	5.668
	.05	5.722	5.833	5.935	6.028	6.114	6.194	6.269	6.339	6.405
	.01	7.356	7.485	7.603	7.712	7.812	7.906	7.993	8.076	8.153
11	.20	4.270	4.366	4.454	4.534	4.608	4.677	4.741	4.801	4.857
	.10	4.951	5.053	5.146	5.231	5.309	5.382	5.450	5.514	5.573
	.05	5.605	5.713	5.811	5.901	5.984	6.062	6.134	6.202	6.265
	.01	7.128	7.250	7.362	7.465	7.560	7.649	7.732	7.809	7.883
12	.20	4.231	4.327	4.413	4.492	4.565	4.633	4.696	4.755	4.810
	.10	4.886	4.986	5.077	5.160	5.236	5.308	5.374	5.436	5.495
	.05	5.511	5.615	5.710	5.798	5.878	5.953	6.023	6.089	6.151
	.01	6.943	7.060	7.167	7.265	7.356	7.441	7.520	7.594	7.665
13	.20	4.199	4.293	4.379	4.457	4.529	4.596	4.658	4.716	4.770
	.10	4.832	4.930	5.019	5.100	5.176	5.245	5.311	5.372	5.429
	.05	5.431	5.533	5.625	5.711	5.789	5.862	5.931	5.995	6.055
	.01	6.791	6.903	7.006	7.101	7.188	7.269	7.345	7.417	7.485
14	.20	4.172	4.265	4.349	4.426	4.498	4.564	4.625	4.683	4.737
	.10	4.786	4.882	4.970	5.050	5.124	5.192	5.256	5.316	5.373
	.05	5.364	5.463	5.554	5.637	5.714	5.786	5.852	5.915	5.974
	.01	6.664	6.772	6.871	6.962	7.047	7.126	7.199	7.268	7.333
15	.20	4.148	4.240	4.324	4.400	4.471	4.536	4.597	4.654	4.707
	.10	4.746	4.841	4.927	5.006	5.079	5.147	5.209	5.269	5.324
	.05	5.306	5.404	5.493	5.574	5.649	5.720	5.785	5.846	5.904
	.01	6.555	6.660	6.757	6.845	6.927	7.003	7.074	7.142	7.204

16	.20	4.127	4.218	4.301	4.377	4.447	4.512	4.572	4.628	4.681
	.10	4.712	4.805	4.890	4.968	5.040	5.107	5.169	5.227	5.282
	.05	5.256	5.352	5.439	5.520	5.593	5.662	5.727	5.786	5.843
	.01	6.462	6.564	6.658	6.744	6.823	6.898	6.967	7.032	7.093
17	.20	4.109	4.199	4.282	4.357	4.426	4.490	4.550	4.606	4.659
	.10	4.682	4.774	4.858	4.935	5.005	5.071	5.133	5.190	5.244
	.05	5.212	5.307	5.392	5.471	5.544	5.612	5.675	5.734	5.790
	.01	6.381	6.480	6.572	6.656	6.734	6.806	6.873	6.937	6.997
18	.20	4.093	4.182	4.264	4.339	4.407	4.471	4.531	4.586	4.638
	.10	4.655	4.746	4.829	4.905	4.975	5.040	5.101	5.158	5.211
	.05	5.174	5.267	5.352	5.429	5.501	5.568	5.630	5.688	5.743
	.01	6.310	6.407	6.497	6.579	6.655	6.725	6.792	6.854	6.912
19	.20	4.078	4.167	4.248	4.323	4.391	4.454	4.513	4.569	4.620
	.10	4.631	4.721	4.803	4.879	4.948	5.012	5.073	5.129	5.182
	.05	5.140	5.231	5.315	5.391	5.462	5.528	5.589	5.647	5.701
	.01	6.247	6.342	6.430	6.510	6.585	6.654	6.719	6.780	6.837
20	.20	4.065	4.154	4.234	4.308	4.376	4.439	4.498	4.552	4.604
	.10	4.609	4.699	4.780	4.855	4.924	4.987	5.047	5.103	5.155
	.05	5.108	5.199	5.282	5.357	5.427	5.493	5.553	5.610	5.663
	.01	6.191	6.285	6.371	6.450	6.523	6.591	6.654	6.714	6.771
24	.20	4.024	4.111	4.190	4.262	4.329	4.391	4.448	4.502	4.552
	.10	4.541	4.628	4.708	4.780	4.847	4.909	4.966	5.021	5.071
	.05	5.012	5.099	5.179	5.251	5.319	5.381	5.439	5.494	5.545
	.01	6.017	6.106	6.186	6.261	6.330	6.394	6.453	6.510	6.563
30	.20	3.982	4.068	4.145	4.216	4.281	4.342	4.398	4.451	4.500
	.10	4.474	4.559	4.635	4.706	4.770	4.830	4.886	4.939	4.988
	.05	4.917	5.001	5.077	5.147	5.211	5.271	5.327	5.379	5.429
	.01	5.849	5.932	6.008	6.078	6.143	6.203	6.259	6.311	6.361

APPENDIX A.8   Upper Quantiles of the Studentized Range Distribution (Continued)

(b) $t = 11$ to 19

ν	α	11	12	13	14	15	16	17	18	19
40	.20	3.941	4.025	4.101	4.170	4.234	4.293	4.348	4.399	4.447
	.10	4.408	4.490	4.564	4.632	4.695	4.752	4.807	4.857	4.905
	.05	4.824	4.904	4.977	5.044	5.106	5.163	5.216	5.266	5.313
	.01	5.686	5.764	5.835	5.900	5.961	6.017	6.069	6.119	6.165
60	.20	3.900	3.982	4.056	4.124	4.186	4.244	4.297	4.347	4.395
	.10	4.342	4.421	4.493	4.558	4.619	4.675	4.727	4.775	4.821
	.05	4.732	4.808	4.878	4.942	5.001	5.056	5.107	5.154	5.199
	.01	5.528	5.601	5.667	5.728	5.785	5.837	5.886	5.931	5.974
120	.20	3.859	3.938	4.011	4.077	4.138	4.194	4.246	4.295	4.341
	.10	4.276	4.353	4.422	4.485	4.543	4.597	4.647	4.694	4.738
	.05	4.641	4.714	4.781	4.842	4.898	4.950	4.998	5.044	5.086
	.01	5.375	5.443	5.505	5.562	5.614	5.662	5.708	5.750	5.790
∞	.20	3.817	3.895	3.966	4.030	4.089	4.144	4.195	4.242	4.287
	.10	4.211	4.285	4.351	4.412	4.468	4.519	4.568	4.612	4.654
	.05	4.552	4.622	4.685	4.743	4.796	4.845	4.891	4.934	4.974
	.01	5.227	5.290	5.348	5.400	5.448	5.493	5.535	5.574	5.611

APPENDIX A.8 Upper Quantiles of the Studentized Range Distribution (Continued)

(c) t = 20 to 36

ν	α					t				
		20	22	24	26	28	30	32	34	36
19	.20	4.669	4.759	4.840	4.914	4.981	5.044	5.102	5.156	5.206
	.10	5.232	5.324	5.407	5.483	5.552	5.616	5.676	5.732	5.784
	.05	5.752	5.846	5.932	6.009	6.081	6.147	6.209	6.267	6.321
	.01	6.891	6.992	7.082	7.166	7.242	7.313	7.379	7.440	7.498
20	.20	4.652	4.742	4.822	4.895	4.963	5.025	5.082	5.136	5.186
	.10	5.205	5.296	5.378	5.453	5.522	5.586	5.645	5.700	5.752
	.05	5.714	5.807	5.891	5.968	6.039	6.104	6.165	6.222	6.275
	.01	6.823	6.922	7.011	7.092	7.168	7.237	7.302	7.362	7.419
24	.20	4.599	4.687	4.766	4.838	4.904	4.964	5.021	5.073	5.122
	.10	5.119	5.208	5.287	5.360	5.427	5.489	5.546	5.600	5.650
	.05	5.594	5.683	5.764	5.838	5.906	5.968	6.027	6.081	6.132
	.01	6.612	6.705	6.789	6.865	6.936	7.001	7.062	7.119	7.173
30	.20	4.546	4.632	4.710	4.779	4.844	4.903	4.958	5.010	5.058
	.10	5.034	5.120	5.197	5.267	5.332	5.392	5.447	5.499	5.547
	.05	5.475	5.561	5.638	5.709	5.774	5.833	5.889	5.941	5.990
	.01	6.407	6.494	6.572	6.644	6.710	6.772	6.828	6.881	6.932
40	.20	4.493	4.576	4.652	4.720	4.783	4.841	4.895	4.945	4.993
	.10	4.949	5.032	5.107	5.174	5.236	5.294	5.347	5.397	5.444
	.05	5.358	5.439	5.513	5.581	5.642	5.700	5.753	5.803	5.849
	.01	6.209	6.289	6.362	6.429	6.490	6.547	6.600	6.650	6.697

APPENDIX A.8 Upper Quantiles of the Studentized Range Distribution (Continued)

(c) t = 20 to 36

ν	α	20	22	24	26	28	30	32	34	36
60	.20	4.439	4.520	4.594	4.661	4.722	4.778	4.831	4.880	4.925
	.10	4.864	4.944	5.015	5.081	5.141	5.196	5.247	5.295	5.340
	.05	5.241	5.319	5.389	5.453	5.512	5.566	5.617	5.664	5.708
	.01	6.015	6.090	6.158	6.220	6.277	6.330	6.378	6.424	6.467
120	.20	4.384	4.463	4.535	4.600	4.659	4.714	4.765	4.812	4.857
	.10	4.779	4.856	4.924	4.987	5.044	5.097	5.146	5.192	5.235
	.05	5.126	5.200	5.266	5.327	5.382	5.434	5.481	5.526	5.568
	.01	5.827	5.897	5.959	6.016	6.069	6.117	6.162	6.204	6.244
∞	.20	4.329	4.405	4.475	4.537	4.595	4.648	4.697	4.743	4.786
	.10	4.694	4.767	4.832	4.892	4.947	4.997	5.044	5.087	5.128
	.05	5.012	5.081	5.144	5.201	5.253	5.301	5.346	5.388	5.427
	.01	5.645	5.709	5.766	5.818	5.866	5.911	5.952	5.990	6.026

APPENDIX A.8 Upper Quantiles of the Studentized Range Distribution (Continued)

(d) t = 38 to 100

ν	α	38	40	50	60	70	80	90	100
30	.20	5.103	5.146	5.329	5.475	5.597	5.701	5.791	5.871
	.10	5.593	5.636	5.821	5.969	6.093	6.198	6.291	6.372
	.05	6.037	6.080	6.267	6.417	6.543	6.650	6.744	6.827
	.01	6.978	7.023	7.215	7.370	7.500	7.611	7.709	7.796
40	.20	5.037	5.078	5.257	5.399	5.518	5.619	5.708	5.786
	.10	5.488	5.529	5.708	5.850	5.969	6.071	6.160	6.238
	.05	5.893	5.934	6.112	6.255	6.375	6.477	6.566	6.645
	.01	6.740	6.782	6.960	7.104	7.225	7.328	7.419	7.500
60	.20	4.969	5.009	5.183	5.321	5.437	5.535	5.621	5.697
	.10	5.382	5.422	5.593	5.730	5.844	5.941	6.026	6.102
	.05	5.750	5.789	5.958	6.093	6.206	6.303	6.387	6.462
	.01	6.507	6.546	6.710	6.843	6.954	7.050	7.133	7.207
120	.20	4.899	4.938	5.106	5.240	5.352	5.447	5.530	5.603
	.10	5.275	5.313	5.476	5.606	5.715	5.808	5.888	5.960
	.05	5.607	5.644	5.802	5.929	6.035	6.126	6.205	6.275
	.01	6.281	6.316	6.467	6.588	6.689	6.776	6.852	6.919
∞	.20	4.826	4.864	5.026	5.155	5.262	5.353	5.433	5.503
	.10	5.166	5.202	5.357	5.480	5.582	5.669	5.745	5.812
	.05	5.463	5.498	5.646	5.764	5.863	5.947	6.020	6.085
	.01	6.060	6.092	6.228	6.338	6.429	6.507	6.575	6.636

Source: Values were extracted by permission from H. L. Harter, 1969, *Order Statistics and Their Use in Testing and Estimation*, Vol. 1, Aerospace Research Laboratory, USAF, U.S. Government Printing Office, Washington, D.C., pp. 648–657.

APPENDIX A.9 Upper Quantiles of the Dunnett's *t* Distribution: One-Sided
Comparisons with Control

		\multicolumn{9}{c}{*m*}
ν	α	1	2	3	4	5	6	7	8	9
5	.05	2.02	2.44	2.68	2.85	2.98	3.08	3.16	3.24	3.30
	.01	3.37	3.90	4.21	4.43	4.60	4.73	4.85	4.94	5.03
6	.05	1.94	2.34	2.56	2.71	2.83	2.92	3.00	3.07	3.12
	.01	3.14	3.61	3.88	4.07	4.21	4.33	4.43	4.51	4.59
7	.05	1.89	2.27	2.48	2.62	2.73	2.82	2.89	2.95	3.01
	.01	3.00	3.42	3.66	3.83	3.96	4.07	4.15	4.23	4.30
8	.05	1.86	2.22	2.42	2.55	2.66	2.74	2.81	2.87	2.92
	.01	2.90	3.29	3.51	3.67	3.79	3.88	3.96	4.03	4.09
9	.05	1.83	2.18	2.37	2.50	2.60	2.68	2.75	2.81	2.86
	.01	2.82	3.19	3.40	3.55	3.66	3.75	3.82	3.89	3.94
10	.05	1.81	2.15	2.34	2.47	2.56	2.64	2.70	2.76	2.81
	.01	2.76	3.11	3.31	3.45	3.56	3.64	3.71	3.78	3.83
11	.05	1.80	2.13	2.31	2.44	2.53	2.60	2.67	2.72	2.77
	.01	2.72	3.06	3.25	3.38	3.48	3.56	3.63	3.69	3.74
12	.05	1.78	2.11	2.29	2.41	2.50	2.58	2.64	2.69	2.74
	.01	2.68	3.01	3.19	3.32	3.42	3.50	3.56	3.62	3.67
13	.05	1.77	2.09	2.27	2.39	2.48	2.55	2.61	2.66	2.71
	.01	2.65	2.97	3.15	3.27	3.37	3.44	3.51	3.56	3.61
14	.05	1.76	2.08	2.25	2.37	2.46	2.53	2.59	2.64	2.69
	.01	2.62	2.94	3.11	3.23	3.32	3.40	3.46	3.51	3.56
15	.05	1.75	2.07	2.24	2.36	2.44	2.51	2.57	2.62	2.67
	.01	2.60	2.91	3.08	3.20	3.29	3.36	3.42	3.47	3.52
16	.05	1.75	2.06	2.23	2.34	2.43	2.50	2.56	2.61	2.65
	.01	2.58	2.88	3.05	3.17	3.26	3.33	3.39	3.44	3.48
17	.05	1.74	2.05	2.22	2.33	2.42	2.49	2.54	2.59	2.64
	.01	2.57	2.86	3.03	3.14	3.23	3.30	3.36	3.41	3.45
18	.05	1.73	2.04	2.21	2.32	2.41	2.48	2.53	2.58	2.62
	.01	2.55	2.84	3.01	3.12	3.21	3.27	3.33	3.38	3.42
19	.05	1.73	2.03	2.20	2.31	2.40	2.47	2.52	2.57	2.61
	.01	2.54	2.83	2.99	3.10	3.18	3.25	3.31	3.36	3.40

APPENDIX A.9 Continued

ν	α	m								
		1	2	3	4	5	6	7	8	9
20	.05	1.72	2.03	2.19	2.30	2.39	2.46	2.51	2.56	2.60
	.01	2.53	2.81	2.97	3.08	3.17	3.23	3.29	3.34	3.38
24	.05	1.71	2.01	2.17	2.28	2.36	2.43	2.48	2.53	2.57
	.01	2.49	2.77	2.92	3.03	3.11	3.17	3.22	3.27	3.31
30	.05	1.70	1.99	2.15	2.25	2.33	2.40	2.45	2.50	2.54
	.01	2.46	2.72	2.87	2.97	3.05	3.11	3.16	3.21	3.24
40	.05	1.68	1.97	2.13	2.23	2.31	2.37	2.42	2.47	2.51
	.01	2.42	2.68	2.82	2.92	2.99	3.05	3.10	3.14	3.18
60	.05	1.67	1.95	2.10	2.21	2.28	2.35	2.39	2.44	2.48
	.01	2.39	2.64	2.78	2.87	2.94	3.00	3.04	3.08	3.12
120	.05	1.66	1.93	2.08	2.18	2.26	2.32	2.37	2.41	2.45
	.01	2.36	2.60	2.73	2.82	2.89	2.94	2.99	3.03	3.06
∞	.05	1.64	1.92	2.06	2.16	2.23	2.29	2.34	2.38	2.42
	.01	2.33	2.56	2.68	2.77	2.84	2.89	2.93	2.97	3.00

Source: Values taken by permission from C. W. Dunnett, *J. Am. Stat. Assoc.*, 50(1955): 1115–1116.

Appendix B: SAS Programs

```
*******************************************************************************;
*                         Appendix B.1                                       *;
*          Author: J. Bergum, Ph.D. (modified by J.P. Liu, Ph.D.)            *;
*          Date: May 27, 1994                                                *;
*     Description: To Compute In-house Acceptance Limits for the uniformity  *;
*                  of Dosage Units Based on the Two-stage Sampling Plan       *;
*                  in USP/NF(XXII and XVII 1990) with Normal Approximation    *;
*                  to the Noncentral F Distribution.                          *;
*                  n: Number of assay samples per location.                   *;
*                  L: Number of Location.                                     *;
* Low Probability Bound for passing is 50%.                                   *;
*******************************************************************************;
libname out "XXXXX:[XXXXXX.XXXXX]";
data one1;
n=4;L=10;a=(0.95)**(1/3);
z=abs(probit((1-a)/2));a1=1-a;
xe=cinv(1-a, L*(n-1));
xloc=cinv(1-a, L-1);
slbd=7.8*sqrt(xloc/(L-1));
smbd=slbd;sebd=sqrt(n/(n-1))*7.8*sqrt(xe/(L*(n-1)));
c0=0.06;c=0.078;meanL=85.6;
countm=0;do sm=0.1 to 2.5 by 0.1;
countm=countm+1;
if countm gt 1 then mean=meanL-(7 - (countm/4));
else mean=meanL;
do se=0.1 to 3.5 by 0.1;
se2=se**2;
se2u=L*(n-1)*se2/xe;
sloc2=n*sm**2;
sloc2u=(L-1)*sloc2/xloc;
mvar=sloc2u;
yvar=((n-1)/n)*se2+(sloc2/n);
demy=((((n-1)/n)*se2)**2/(L*(n-1)))+((sloc2/n)**2/(L-1));
dfy=yvar**2/demy;
var=(dfy*yvar)/cinv(1-a,dfy);
y1=sqrt(var);
varsq=sqrt(var);
zt=z*sqrt(mvar/(n*L));
count=0;
start:count=count+1;
if count gt 100 then go to stop;
x1=mean-zt;
p1=probnorm((115-x1)/y1)-probnorm((85-x1)/y1);
p2=probnorm((125-x1)/y1)-probnorm((115-x1)/y1)+probnorm((85-x1)/y1)-probnorm((
75-x1)/y1);
pnorm=p1**30+(30*(P1**29)*p2);
pnorm0=p1**10;
k00=1+10*(x1**2/y1**2);
k01=1+(2*10*(x1**2/y1**2));
num01=sqrt((17*10/(c0*c0))/18);
num02=sqrt(2*k00 - (k01/k00));
dem0=sqrt((10/(c0*c0*9))+(k01/k00));
z0=(num01-num02)/dem0;
k10=1+30*(x1**2/y1**2);
k11=1+(2*30*(x1**2/y1**2));
num11=sqrt((57*30/(c*c))/58);
num12=sqrt(2*k10 - (k11/k10));
dem1=sqrt((30/(c*c*29))+(k11/k10));
z1=(num11-num12)/dem1;
pcv=1-probnorm(z1);
pcv0=1-probnorm(z0);
p0=pcv0+pnorm0-1;
p=pcv+pnorm-1;
maxpL=max(p0,p,0);
```

```
pdiff=maxL-0.50;
if abs(pdiff) < 0.005 then goto stop;
else if  pdiff le -0.005 then mean = mean+(zt/(count+3));
else mean=mean-(zt/(count+3));
go to start;
stop: mean1=mean;output;
end;
end;
keep se sm  varsq x1 count mean1 ;
proc sort data=one1;
by sm se;
data outcnt;
set one1;
if count gt 100;
data one2;
n=4;
L=10;
a=(0.95)**(1/3);
z=abs(probit((1-a)/2));
al=1-a;xe=cinv(1-a, L*(n-1));
xloc=cinv(1-a, L-1);
slbd=7.8*sqrt(xloc/(L-1));
smbd=slbd;
sebd=sqrt(n/(n-1))*7.8*sqrt(xe/(L*(n-1)));
c0=0.06;c=0.078;
meanu=114.4;
countm=0;
do sm=0.1 to 2.5 by 0.1;
countm=countm+1;
if countm gt 1 then mean=meanU+(6.8 - (countm/4));
else mean=meanU;
do se=0.1 to 3.5 by 0.1;
se2=se**2;
se2u=L*(n-1)*se2/xe;
sloc2=n*sm**2;
sloc2u=(L-1)*sloc2/xloc;
mvar=sloc2u;
yvar=((n-1)/n)*se2+(sloc2/n);
demy=((((n-1)/n)*se2)**2/(L*(n-1)))+((sloc2/n)**2/(L-1));
dfy=yvar**2/demy;
var=(dfy*yvar)/cinv(1-a,dfy);
y1=sqrt(var);
varsq=sqrt(var);
zt=z*sqrt(mvar/(n*L));
count=0;
start:count=count+1;
if count gt 100 then go to stop;
x1=mean+zt;
p1=probnorm((115-x1)/y1)-probnorm((85-x1)/y1);
p2=probnorm((125-x1)/y1)-probnorm((115-x1)/y1)+probnorm((85-x1)/y1)-probnorm((
75-x1)/y1);
pnorm=p1**30+(30*(P1**29)*p2);
pnorm0=p1**10;k00=1+10*(x1**2/y1**2);
k01=1+(2*10*(x1**2/y1**2));
num01=sqrt((17*10/(c0*c0))/18);
num02=sqrt(2*k00 - (k01/k00));
dem0=sqrt((10/(c0*c0*9))+(k01/k00));
z0=(num01-num02)/dem0;k10=1+30*(x1**2/y1**2);
k11=1+(2*30*(x1**2/y1**2));
num11=sqrt((57*30/(c*c))/58);
num12=sqrt(2*k10 - (k11/k10));
dem1=sqrt((30/(c*c*29))+(k11/k10));
z1=(num11-num12)/dem1;
pcv=1-probnorm(z1);
```

```
pcv0-1-probnorm(z0);p
0-pcv0+pnorm0-1;p-pcv+pnorm-1;
maxpU-max(p,p0,0);
pdiff-maxpU-0.50;
if abs(pdiff) < 0.01 then goto stop;
else if  pdiff le -0.01 then mean - mean-(zt/(count+3));
else mean-mean+(zt/(count+3));
go to start;
stop: meanU-mean;output;
end;
end;
keep se sm a al count meanU x1 maxpU varsq pdiff p0 p pdiff p1 p2;
data one2;  set one2;
x1U-x1;
countu-count;
keep se sm x1U countu meanU ;
proc sort data-one2;  by sm se;
data outcnt;   set one2;
if countu gt 100;
data work;  merge one1 one2;  by sm se;
if meanL < meanU;keep se sm meanL meanU;
print;proc sort data-work;  by se;
proc transpose data-work out-LLimit prefix-L; by se;
var meanL;
proc transpose data-work out-ULimit prefix-U; vy se;
var meanU;
data table;  merge LLimit Ulimit;  by se;
option nodate nonumber linesize-132 pagesize-60 missing-' ';
data page;   set table;  by se;
retain page line;
if _n_-1 then do;
page-1 ;
line-16;
end;
if _n_ > 1 then do;
line+1;
if line gt 52  then do;
page+1;
line-16;
end;
end;
data page;   set page;
if sov-99 then delete;
TDAY-TODAY();
proc sort data-page;  by page line;

data _null_;   set page;  by page line;
file "XXXXX:[XXXXXX.XXXXXX]XXXXXX.XXX" print notitle;
if first.page then link h;
put #line @2 se 3.1 +1  (L1 u1 L2 u2 L3 u3 L4 u4 L5 U5 L6 U6 L7 U7 L8 U8) (6.2
+1 6.2 +2);
return;
h:
put _page_;
put #3 @50 "Table 6.5.4";put #4 @10 "Acceptance Limits for Content Uniformity for
50% Lower Probability Bound for Passing - Dosage Form: Tablet";
put #5 @15 "Table Entries are the 95% Lower(LL) and Upper(UL) Limits Based on the
Mean of 40 Assays";
put #6 @35 "4 Tablets at Each of 10 Different Locations";
put #7 @20 "Model: One-way Nested Random Effect Model with Location as Random
Effect";
put #8 @15 "SE: Pooled Standard Deviation across Locations(Square Root of the
Mean Square Error)";
put #10 @20 "Standard Deviation of Location Means(Square Root of the Mean Square
```

```
for Location Divided by the No. of Assays per Location";
put #12 @10 "0.1" +12 "0.2" +12 "0.3" +12 "0.4" +12 "0.5" +12 "0.6" +12 "0.7" +12
"0.8";put #13 @2 "SE" @8 "LL" @15 "UL" @23 "LL" @30 "UL" @38 "LL" @45 "UL" @53
"LL" @60 "UL"  @68 "LL" @75 "UL" @83 "LL" @90 "UL" @98 "LL" @105 "UL" @113 "LL"
@120 "UL" ;
Put #14 @2 "__" @8 "__" @15 "__" @23 "__" @30 "__" @38 "__" @45 "__" @53 "__" @60
"__" @68 "__" @75 "__" @83 "__" @90 "__" @98 "__" @105 "__" @113 "__" @120 "__";
return;

data _null_;   set page;   by page line;
file "XXXXX:[XXXXXX.XXXXXX]XXXXXX.XXX" print notitle;
if first.page then link h;
put #line @2 se 3.1 +1  (L9 u9 L10 u10 L11 u11 L12 u12 L13 U13 L14 U14 L15 U15
L16 U17); (6.2 +1 6.2 +2);
return;
h:
put _page_;
put #3 @50 "Table 6.5.4";put #4 @10 "Acceptance Limits for Content Uniformity for
50% Lower Probability Bound for Passing - Dosage Form: Tablet";
put #5 @15 "Table Entries are the 95% Lower(LL) and Upper(UL) Limits Based on the
Mean of 40 Assays";
put #6 @35 "4 Tablets at Each of 10 Different Locations";
put #7 @20 "Model: One-way Nested Random Effect Model with Location as Random
Effect";
put #8 @15 "SE: Pooled Standard Deviation across Locations(Square Root of the
Mean Square Error)";
put #10 @20 "Standard Deviation of Location Means(Square Root of the Mean Square
for Location Divided by the No. of Assays per Location";
put #12 @10 "0.9" +12 "1.0" +12 "1.1" +12 "1.2" +12 "1.3" +12 "1.4" +12 "1.5" +12
"1.6";
put #13 @2 "SE" @8 "LL" @15 "UL" @23 "LL" @30 "UL" @38 "LL" @45 "UL" @53 "LL" @60
"UL" @68 "LL" @75 "UL" @83 "LL" @90 "UL" @98 "LL" @105 "UL" @113 "LL" @120 "UL";
Put #14 @2 "__" @8 "__" @15 "__" @23 "__" @30 "__" @38 "__" @45 "__" @53 "__" @60
"__" @68 "__" @75 "__" @83 "__" @90 "__" @98 "__" @105 "__" @113 "__" @120 "__";
return;

data _null_;   set page;   by page line;
file "XXXXXX:[XXXXXX.XXXXXX]XXXXXX.XXX" print notitle;
if first.page then link h;
put #line @2 se 3.1 +1  (L17 u17 L18 u18 L19 u19 L20 u20 L21 U21 L22 U22 L23 U23
L24 U24); (6.2 +1 6.2 +2);
return;
h:
put _page_;
put #3 @50 "Table 6.5.4";put #4 @10 "Acceptance Limits for Content Uniformity for
50% Lower Probability Bound for Passing - Dosage Form: Tablet";
put #5 @15 "Table Entries are the 95% Lower(LL) and Upper(UL) Limits Based on the
Mean of 40 Assays";
put #6 @35 "4 Tablets at Each of 10 Different Locations";
put #7 @20 "Model: One-way Nested Random Effect Model with Location as Random
Effect";
put #8 @15 "SE: Pooled Standard Deviation across Locations(Square Root of the
Mean Square Error)";
put #10 @20 "Standard Deviation of Location Means(Square Root of the Mean Square
for Location Divided by the No. of Assays per Location";
put #12 @10 "1.7" +12 "1.8" +12 "1.9" +12 "2.0" +12 "2.1" +12 "2.2" +12 "2.3" +12
"2.4";put #13 @2 "SE" @8 "LL" @15 "UL" @23 "LL" @30 "UL" @38 "LL" @45 "UL" @53
"LL" @60 "UL" @68 "LL" @75 "UL" @83 "LL" @90 "UL" @98 "LL" @105 "UL" @113 "LL"
@120 "UL" ;
Put #14 @2 "__" @8 "__" @15 "__" @23 "__" @30 "__" @38 "__" @45 "__" @53 "__" @60
"__" @68 "__" @75 "__" @83 "__" @90 "__" @98 "__" @105 "__" @113 "__" @120 "__";
return;
```

Appendix C: Regulations

211.132 Tamper-resistant packaging requirements for over-the-counter human drug products.
211.134 Drug product inspection.
211.137 Expiration dating.

Subpart H—Holding and Distribution

211.142 Warehousing procedures.
211.150 Distribution procedures.

Subpart I—Laboratory Controls

211.160 General requirements.
211.165 Testing and release for distribution.
211.166 Stability testing.
211.167 Special testing requirements.
211.170 Reserve samples.
211.173 Laboratory animals.
211.176 Penicillin contamination.

Subpart J—Records and Reports

211.180 General requirements.
211.182 Equipment cleaning and use log.
211.184 Component, drug product container, closure, and labeling records.
211.186 Master production and control records.
211.188 Batch production and control records.
211.192 Production record review.
211.194 Laboratory records.
211.196 Distribution records.
211.198 Complaint files.

Subpart K—Returned and Salvaged Drug Products

211.204 Returned drug products.
211.208 Drug product salvaging.

AUTHORITY: Secs. 501, 701, 52 Stat. 1049–1050 as amended, 1055–1056 as amended (21 U.S.C. 351, 371).

SOURCE: 43 FR 45077, Sept. 29, 1978, unless otherwise noted.

Subpart A   General Provisions

§211.1 Scope.

(a) The regulations in this part contain the minimum current good manufacturing practice for preparation of drug products for administration to humans or animals.

(b) The current good manufacturing practice regulations in this chapter, as they pertain to drug products, and in Parts 600 through 680 of this chapter, as they pertain to biological products for human use, shall be considered to supplement, not supersede, the regulations in this part unless the regulations explicitly provide otherwise. In the event it is impossible to comply with applicable regulations both in this part and in other parts of this chapter or in Parts 600 through 680 of this chapter, the regulation specifically applicable to the drug product in question shall supersede the regulation in this part.

(c) Pending consideration of a proposed exemption, published in the FEDERAL REGISTER of September 29, 1978, the requirements in this part shall not be enforced for OTC drug products if the products and all their ingredients are ordinarily marketed and consumed as human foods, and which products may also fall within the legal definition of drugs by virtue of their intended use. Therefore, until further notice, regulations under Part 110 of this chapter, and where applicable, Parts 113 to 129 of this chapter, shall be applied in determining whether these OTC drug products that are also foods are manufactured, processed, packed, or held under current good manufacturing practice.

§211.3 Definitions.

The definitions set forth in §210.3 of this chapter apply in this part.

Subpart B   Organization and Personnel

§211.22 Responsibilities of quality control unit.

(a) There shall be a quality control unit that shall have the responsibility and authority to approve or reject all components, drug product containers, closures, in-process materials, packaging material, labeling, and drug products, and the authority to review production records to assure that no errors have occurred or, if errors have occurred, that they have been fully investigated. The quality control unit shall be responsible for approving or rejecting drug products manufactured, processed, packed, or held under contract by another company.

(b) Adequate laboratory facilities for the testing and approval (or rejection) of components, drug product containers, closures, packaging materials, in-process materials, and drug products shall be available to the quality control unit.

(c) The quality control unit shall have the responsibility for approving or rejecting all procedures or specifications impacting on the identity, strength, quality, and purity of the drug product.

(d) The responsibilities and procedures applicable to the quality control unit shall be in writing; such written procedures shall be followed.

§211.25 Personnel qualifications.

(a) Each person engaged in the manufacture, processing, packing, or holding of a drug product shall have education, training, and experience, or any combination thereof, to enable that person to perform the assigned functions. Training shall be in the particular operations that the employee performs and in current good manufacturing practice (including the current good manufacturing practice regulations in this chapter and written procedures required by these regulations) as they relate to the employee's functions. Training in current good manufacturing practice shall be conducted by qualified individuals on a continuing basis and with sufficient frequency to assure that employees remain familiar with CGMP requirements applicable to them.

(b) Each person responsible for supervising the manufacture, processing, packing, or holding of a drug product shall have the education, training, and experience, or any combination thereof, to perform assigned functions in such a manner as to provide assurance that the drug product has the safety, identity, strength, quality, and purity that it purports or is represented to possess.

(c) There shall be an adequate number of qualified personnel to perform and supervise the manufacture, processing, packing, or holding of each drug product.

§211.28 Personnel responsibilities.

(a) Personnel engaged in the manufacture, processing, packing, or holding of a drug product shall wear clean clothing appropriate for the duties they perform. Protective apparel, such as head, face, hand, and arm coverings, shall be worn as necessary to protect drug products from contamination.

(b) Personnel shall practice good sanitation and health habits.

(c) Only personnel authorized by supervisory personnel shall enter those areas of the buildings and facilities designated as limited-access areas.

(d) Any person shown at any time (either by medical examination or supervisory observation) to have an apparent illness or open lesions that may adversely affect the safety or quality of drug products shall be excluded from direct contact with components, drug product containers, closures, in-process materials, and drug products until the condition is corrected or determined by competent medical personnel not to jeopardize the safety or quality of drug products. All personnel shall be instructed to report to supervisory personnel any health conditions that may have an adverse effect on drug products.

§211.34 Consultants.

Consultants advising on the manufacture, processing, packing, or holding of drug products shall have sufficient education, training, and experience, or any combination thereof, to advise on the subject for which they are retained. Records shall be maintained stating the name, address, and qualifications of any consultants and the type of service they provide.

Subpart C Buildings and Facilities

§211.42 Design and construction features.

(a) Any building or buildings used in the manufacture, processing, packing, or holding of a drug product shall be of suitable size, construction and location to facilitate cleaning, maintenance, and proper operations.

(b) Any such building shall have adequate space for the orderly placement of equipment and materials to prevent mixups between different components, drug product containers, closures, labeling, in-process materials, or drug products, and to prevent contamination. The flow of components, drug product containers, closures, labeling, in-process materials, and drug products through the building or buildings shall be designed to prevent contamination.

(c) Operations shall be performed within specifically defined areas of adequate size. There shall be separate or defined areas for the firm's operations to prevent contamination or mixups as follows:

(1) Receipt, identification, storage, and withholding from use of components, drug product containers, closures, and labeling, pending the appropriate sampling, testing, or examination by the quality control unit before release for manufacturing or packaging;

(2) Holding rejected components, drug product containers, closures, and labeling before disposition;

(3) Storage of released components, drug product containers, closures, and labeling;

(4) Storage of in-process materials;

(5) Manufacturing and processing operations;

(6) Packaging and labeling operations;

(7) Quarantine storage before release of drug products;

(8) Storage of drug products after release;

(9) Control and laboratory operations;

(10) Aseptic processing, which includes as appropriate;

(i) Floors, walls, and ceilings of smooth, hard surfaces that are easily cleanable;

(ii) Temperature and humidity controls;

(iii) An air supply filtered through high-efficiency particulate air filters under positive pressure, regardless of whether flow is laminar or nonlaminar;

(iv) A system for monitoring environmental conditions;

(v) A system for cleaning and disinfecting the room and equipment to produce aseptic conditions;

(vi) A system for maintaining any equipment used to control the aseptic conditions.

(d) Operations relating to the manufacture, processing, and packing of penicillin shall be performed in facilities separate from those used for other drug products for human use.

§211.44 Lighting.

Adequate lighting shall be provided in all areas.

§211.46 Ventilation, air filtration, air heating and cooling.

(a) Adequate ventilation shall be provided.

(b) Equipment for adequate control over air pressure, micro-organisms, dust, humidity, and temperature shall be provided when appropriate for the manufacture, processing, packing, or holding of a drug product.

(c) Air filtration systems, including prefilters and particulate matter air filters, shall be used when appropriate on air supplies to production areas. If air is recirculated to production areas, measures shall be taken to control recirculation of dust from production. In areas where air contamination occurs during production, there shall be adequate exhaust systems or other systems adequate to control contaminants.

(d) Air-handling systems for the manufacture, processing, and packing of penicillin shall be completely separate from those for other drug products for human use.

§211.48 Plumbing.

(a) Potable water shall be supplied under continuous positive pressure in a plumbing system free of defects that could contribute contamination to any drug product. Potable water shall meet the standards prescribed in the Environmental Protection Agency's Primary Drinking Water Regulations set forth in 40 CFR Part 141. Water not meeting such standards shall not be permitted in the potable water system.

(b) Drains shall be of adequate size and, where connected directly to a sewer, shall be provided with an air break or other mechanical device to prevent back-siphonage.

[43 FR 45077, Sept. 29, 1978, as amended at 48 FR 11426, Mar. 18, 1983]

§211.50 Sewage and refuse.

Sewage, trash, and other refuse in and from the building and immediate premises shall be disposed of in a safe and sanitary manner.

§211.52 Washing and toilet facilities.

Adequate washing facilities shall be provided, including hot and cold water, soap or detergent, air driers or single-service towels, and clean toilet facilities easily accessible to working areas.

§211.56 Sanitation.

(a) Any building used in the manufacture, processing, packing, or holding of a drug product shall be maintained in a clean and sanitary condition. Any such building shall be free of infestation by rodents, birds, insects, and other vermin (other than laboratory animals). Trash and organic waste matter shall be held and disposed of in a timely and sanitary manner.

(b) There shall be written procedures assigning responsibility for sanitation and describing in sufficient detail the cleaning schedules, methods, equipment, and materials to be used in cleaning the buildings and facilities; such written procedures shall be followed.

(c) There shall be written procedures for use of suitable rodenticides, insecticides, fungicides, fumigating agents, and cleaning and sanitizing agents. Such written procedures shall be designed to prevent the contamination of equipment, components, drug product containers, closures, packaging, labeling materials, or drug products and shall be followed. Rodenticides, insecticides, and fungicides shall not be used unless registered and used in accordance with the Federal Insecticide, Fungicide, and Rodenticide Act (7 U.S.C. 135).

(d) Sanitation procedures shall apply to work performed by contractors or temporary employees as well as work performed by full-time employees during the ordinary course of operations.

§211.58 Maintenance.

Any building used in the manufacture, processing, packing, or holding of a drug product shall be maintained in a good state of repair.

Subpart D   Equipment

§211.63 Equipment design, size, and location.

Equipment used in the manufacture, processing, packing, or holding of a drug product shall be of appropriate design, adequate size, and suitably located to facilitate operations for its intended use and for its cleaning and maintenance.

§211.65 Equipment construction.

(a) Equipment shall be constructed so that surfaces that contact components, in-process materials, or drug products shall not be reactive, additive, or absorptive so as to alter the safety, identity, strength, quality, or purity of the drug product beyond the official or other established requirements.

(b) Any substances required for operation, such as lubricants or coolants, shall not come into contact with components, drug product containers, closures, in-process materials, or drug products so as to alter the safety, identity, strength, quality, or purity of the drug product beyond the official or other established requirements.

§211.67 Equipment cleaning and maintenance.

(a) Equipment and utensils shall be cleaned, maintained, and sanitized at appropriate intervals to prevent malfunctions or contamination that would alter the safety, identity, strength, quality, or purity of the drug product beyond the official or other established requirements.

(b) Written procedures shall be established and followed for cleaning and maintenance of equipment, including utensils, used in the manufacture, processing, packing, or holding of a drug product. These procedures shall include, but are not necessarily limited to, the following:

(1) Assignment of responsibility for cleaning and maintaining equipment;

(2) Maintenance and cleaning schedules, including, where appropriate, sanitizing schedules;

(3) A description in sufficient detail of the methods, equipment, and materials used in cleaning and maintenance operations, and the methods of disassembling and reassembling equipment as necessary to assure proper cleaning and maintenance;

(4) Removal or obliteration of previous batch identification;

(5) Protection of clean equipment from contamination prior to use;

(6) Inspection of equipment for cleanliness immediately before use.

(c) Records shall be kept of maintenance, cleaning, sanitizing, and inspection as specified in §§211.180 and 211.182.

§211.68 Automatic, mechanical, and electronic equipment.

(a) Automatic, mechanical, or electronic equipment or other types of equipment, including computers, or related systems that will perform a function satisfactorily, may be used in the manufacture, processing, packing, and holding of a drug product. If such equipment is so used, it shall be routinely calibrated, inspected, or checked according to a written program designed to assure proper performance. Written records of those calibration checks and inspections shall be maintained.

(b) Appropriate controls shall be exercised over computer or related systems to assure that changes in master production and control records or other records are instituted only by authorized personnel. Input to and output from the computer or related system of formulas or other records or data shall be checked for accuracy. A backup file of data entered into the computer or related system shall be maintained except where certain data, such as calculations performed in connection with laboratory analysis, are eliminated by computerization or other automated processes. In such instances a written record of the program shall be maintained along with appropriate validation data. Hard copy or alternative systems, such as duplicates, tapes, or microfilm, designed to assure that backup data are exact and complete and that it is secure from alteration, inadvertent erasures, or loss shall be maintained.

§211.72 Filters.

Filters for liquid filtration used in the manufacture, processing, or packing of injectable drug products intended for human use shall not release fibers into such products. Fiber-releasing filters may not be used in the manufacture, processing, or packing of these injectable drug products unles it is not possible to manufacture such drug products without the use of such filters. If use of a fiber-releasing filter is necessary, an additional non-fiber-releasing filter of 0.22 micron maximum mean porosity (0.45 micron if the manufacturing conditions so dictate) shall subsequently be used to reduce the content of particles in the injectable drug product. Use of an asbestos-containing filter, with or without subsequent use of a specific non-fiber-releasing filter, is permissible only upon submission of proof to the appropriate bureau of the Food and Drug Administration that use of a non-fiber-releasing filter will, or is likely to, compromise the safety or effectiveness of the injectable drug product.

Subpart E   Control of Components and Drug Product Containers and Closures

§211.80 General requirements.

(a) There shall be written procedures describing in sufficient detail the receipt, identification, storage, handling, sampling, testing, and approval or rejection of components and drug product containers and closures; such written procedures shall be followed.

(b) Components and drug product containers and closures shall at all times be handled and stored in a manner to prevent contamination.

(c) Bagged or boxed components of drug product containers, or closures shall be stored off the floor and suitably spaced to permit cleaning and inspection.

(d) Each container or grouping of containers for components or drug product containers, or closures shall be identified with a distinctive code for each lot in each shipment received. This code shall be used in recording the disposition of each lot. Each lot shall be appropriately identified as to its status (i.e., quarantined, approved, or rejected).

§211.82 Receipt and storage of untested components, drug product containers, and closures.

(a) Upon receipt and before acceptance, each container or grouping of containers of components, drug product containers, and closures shall be examined visually for appropriate labeling as to contents, container damage or broken seals, and contamination.

(b) Components, drug product containers, and closures shall be stored under quarantine until they have been tested or examined, as appropriate, and released. Storage within the area shall conform to the requirements of §211.80.

§211.84 Testing and approval or rejection of components, drug product containers, and closures.

(a) Each lot of components, drug product containers, and closures shall be withheld from use until the lot has been sampled, tested, or examined, as appropriate, and released for use by the quality control unit.

(b) Representative samples of each shipment of each lot shall be collected for testing or examination. The number of containers to be sampled, and the amount of material to be taken from each container, shall be based upon appropriate criteria such as statistical criteria for component variability, confidence levels, and degree of precision desired, the past quality history of the supplier, and the quantity needed for analysis and reserve where required by §211.170.

(c) Samples shall be collected in accordance with the following procedures:

(1) The containers of components selected shall be cleaned where necessary, by appropriate means.

(2) The containers shall be opened, sampled, and resealed in a manner designed to prevent contamination of their contents and contamination of other components, drug product containers, or closures.

(3) Sterile equipment and aseptic sampling techniques shall be used when necessary.

(4) If it is necessary to sample a component from the top, middle, and bottom of its container, such sample subdivisions shall not be composited for testing.

(5) Sample containers shall be identified so that the following information can be determined: name of the material sampled, the lot number, the container from which the sample was taken, the data on which the sample was taken, and the name of the person who collected the sample.

(6) Containers from which samples have been taken shall be marked to show that samples have been removed from them.

(d) Samples shall be examined and tested as follows:

(1) At least one test shall be conducted to verify the identity of each component of a drug product. Specific identity tests, if they exist, shall be used.

(2) Each component shall be tested for conformity with all appropriate written specifications for purity, strength, and quality. In lieu of such testing by the manufacturer, a report of analysis may be accepted from the supplier of a component, provided that at least one specific identity test is conducted on such

component by the manufacturer, and provided that the manufacturer establishes the reliability of the supplier's analyses through appropriate validation of the supplier's test results at appropriate intervals.

(3) Containers and closures shall be tested for conformance with all appropriate written procedures. In lieu of such testing by the manufacturer, a certificate of testing may be accepted from the supplier, provided that at least a visual identification is conducted on such containers/closures by the manufacturer and provided that the manufacturer establishes the reliability of the supplier's test results through appropriate validation of the supplier's test results at appropriate intervals.

(4) When appropriate, components shall be microscopically examined.

(5) Each lot of a component, drug product container, or closure that is liable to contamination with filth, insect infestation, or other extraneous adulterant shall be examined against established specifications for such contamination.

(6) Each lot of a component, drug product container, or closure that is liable to microbiological contamination that is objectionable in view of its intended use shall be subjected to microbiological tests before use.

(e) Any lot of components, drug product containers, or closures that meets the appropriate written specifications of identity, strength, quality, and purity and related tests under paragraph (d) of this section may be approved and released for use. Any lot of such material that does not meet such specifications shall be rejected.

§211.86 Use of approved components, drug product containers, and closures.

Components, drug product containers, and closures approved for use shall be rotated so that the oldest approved stock is used first. Deviation from this requirement is permitted if such deviation is temporary and appropriate.

§211.87 Retesting of approved components, drug product containers, and closures.

Components, drug product containers, and closures shall be retested or reexamined, as appropriate, for identity, strength, quality, and purity and approved or rejected by the quality control unit in accordance with §211.84 as necessary, e.g., after storage for long periods or after exposure to air, heat or other conditions that might adversely affect the component, drug product container, or closure.

§211.89 Rejected components, drug product containers, and closures.

Rejected components, drug product containers, and closures shall be identified and controlled under a quarantine system designed to prevent their use in manufacturing or processing operations for which they are unsuitable.

§211.94 Drug product containers and closures.

(a) Drug product containers and closures shall not be reactive, additive, or absorptive so as to alter the safety, identity, strength, quality, or purity of the drug beyond the official or established requirements.

(b) Container closure systems shall provide adequate protection against foreseeable external factors in storage and use that can cause deterioration or contamination of the drug product.

(c) Drug product containers and closures shall be clean and, where indicated by the nature of the drug, sterilized and processed to remove pyrogenic properties to assure that they are suitable for their intended use.

(d) Standards or specifications, methods of testing, and, where indicated, methods of cleaning, sterilizing, and processing to remove pyrogenic properties shall be written and followed for drug product containers and closures.

Subpart F Production and Process Controls

§211.100 Written procedures; deviations.

(a) There shall be written procedures for production and process control designed to assure that the drug products have the identity, strength, quality, and purity they purport or are represented to possess. Such procedures shall include all requirements in this subpart. These written procedures, including any changes, shall be drafted, reviewed, and approved by the appropriate organizational units and reviewed and approved by the quality control unit.

(b) Written production and process control procedures shall be followed in the execution of the various production and process control functions and shall be documented at the time of performance. Any deviation from the written procedures shall be recorded and justified.

§211.101 Charge-in of components.

Written production and control procedures shall include the following, which are designed to assure that the drug products produced have the identity, strength, quality, and purity they purport or represented to possess:

(a) The batch shall be formulated with the intent to provide not less than 100 percent of the labeled or established amount of active ingredient.

(b) Components for drug product manufacturing shall be weighed, measured, or subdivided as appropriate. If a component is removed from the original container to another, the new container shall be identified with the following information:

(1) Component name or item code;

(2) Receiving or control number;

(3) Weight or measure in new container;

(4) Batch for which component was dispensed, including its product name, strength, and lot number.

(c) Weighing, measuring, or subdividing operations for components shall be adequately supervised. Each container of component dispensed to manufacturing shall be examined by a second person to assure that:

(1) The component was released by the quality control unit.

(2) The weight or measure is correct as stated in the batch production records.

(3) The containers are properly identified.

(d) Each component shall be added to the batch by one person and verified by a second person.

§211.103 Calculation of yield.

Actual yields and percentages of theoretical yield shall be determined at the conclusion of each appropriate phase of manufacturing, processing, packaging, or holding of the drug product. Such calculations shall be performed by one person and independently verified by a second person.

§211.105 Equipment identification.

(a) All compounding and storage containers, processing lines, and major equipment used during the production of a batch of a drug product shall be properly identified at all times to indicate their contents and, when necessary, the phase of processing of the batch.

(b) Major equipment shall be identified by a distinctive identification number or code that shall be recorded in the batch production record to show the specific equipment used in the manufacture of each batch of a drug product. In cases where only one of a particular type of equipment exists in a manufacturing facility, the name of the equipment may be used in lieu of a distinctive identification number or code.

§211.110 Sampling and testing of in-process materials and drug products.

(a) To assure batch uniformity and integrity of drug products, written procedures shall be established and followed that describe the in-process controls, and tests, or examinations to be conducted on appropriate samples of in-process materials of each batch. Such control procedures shall be established to monitor the output and to validate the performance of those manufacturing processes that may be responsible for causing variability in the characteristics of in-process material and the drug product. Such control procedures shall include, but are not limited to, the following, where appropriate:

(1) Tablet or capsule weight variation;

(2) Disintegration time;

(3) Adequacy of mixing to assure uniformity and homogeneity;

(4) Dissolution time and rate;

(5) Clarity, completeness, or pH of solutions.

(b) Valid in-process specifications for such characteristics shall be consistent with drug product final specifications and shall be derived from previous acceptable process average and process variability estimates where possible and determined by the application of suitable statistical procedures where appropriate. Examination and testing of samples shall assure that the drug product and in-process material conform to specifications.

(c) In-process materials shall be tested for identity, strength, quality, and purity as appropriate, and approved or rejected by the quality control unit, during the production process, e.g., at commencement or completion of significant phases or after storage for long periods.

(d) Rejected in-process materials shall be identified and controlled under a quarantine system designed to prevent their use in manufacturing or processing operations for which they are unsuitable.

§211.111 Time limitations on production.

When appropriate, time limits for the completion of each phase of production shall be established to assure the quality of the drug product. Deviation from established time limits may be acceptable if such deviation does not compromise the quality of the drug product. Such deviation shall be justified and documented.

§211.113 Control of microbiological contamination.

(a) Appropriate written procedures, designed to prevent objectionable microorganisms in drug products not required to be sterile, shall be established and followed.

(b) Appropriate written procedures, designed to prevent microbiological contamination of drug products purporting to be sterile, shall be established and followed. Such procedures shall include validation of any sterilization process.

§211.115 Reprocessing.

(a) Written procedures shall be established and followed prescribing a system for reprocessing batches that do not conform to standards or specifications and the steps to be taken to insure that the reprocessed batches will conform with all established standards, specifications, and characteristics.

(b) Reprocessing shall not be performed without the review and approval of the quality control unit.

Subpart G   Packaging and Labeling Control

§211.122 Materials examination and usage criteria.

(a) There shall be written procedures describing in sufficient detail the receipt, identification, storage, handling, sampling, examination, and/or testing of labeling and packaging materials; such written procedures shall be followed. Labeling and packaging materials shall be representatively sampled, and examined or tested upon receipt and before use in packaging or labeling of a drug product.

(b) Any labeling or packaging materials meeting appropriate written specifications may be approved and released for use. Any labeling or packaging materials that do not meet such specifications shall be rejected to prevent their use in operations for which they are unsuitable.

(c) Records shall be maintained for each shipment received of each different labeling and packaging material indicating receipt, examination or testing, and whether accepted or rejected.

(d) Labels and other labeling materials for each different drug product, strength, dosage form, or quantity of contents shall be stored separately with suitable identification. Access to the storage area shall be limited to authorized personnel.

(e) Obsolete and outdated labels, labeling, and other packaging materials shall be destroyed.

(f) Gang printing of labeling to be used for different drug products or different strengths of the same drug product (or labeling of the same size and identical or simliar format and/or color schemes) shall be minimized. If gang printing is employed, packaging and labeling operations shall provide for special control procedures, taking into consideration sheet layout, stacking, cutting, and handling during and after printing.

(g) Printing devices on, or associated with, manufacturing lines used to imprint labeling upon the drug product unit label or case shall be monitored to assure that all imprinting conforms to the print specified in the batch production record.

§211.125 Labeling issuance.

(a) Strict control shall be exercised over labeling issued for use in drug product labeling operations.

(b) Labeling materials issued for a batch shall be carefully examined for identity and conformity to the labeling specified in the master or batch production records.

(c) Procedures shall be utilized to reconcile the quantities of labeling issued, used, and returned, and shall require evaluation of discrepancies found between the quantity of drug product finished and the quantity of labeling issued when such discrepancies are outside narrow preset limits based on historical operating data. Such discrepancies shall be investigated in accordance with §211.192.

(d) All excess labeling bearing lot or control numbers shall be destoryed.

(e) Returned labeling shall be maintained and stored in a manner to prevent mixups and provide proper identification.

(f) Procedures shall be written describing in sufficient detail the control procedures employed for the issuance of labeling; such written procedures shall be followed.

§211.130 Packaging and labeling operations.

There shall be written procedures designed to assure that correct labels, labeling, and packaging materials are used for drug products; such written procedures shall be followed. These procedures shall incorporate the following features:

(a) Prevention of mixups and cross-contamination by physical or spatial separation from operations on other drug products.

(b) Identification of the drug product with a lot or control number that permits determination of the history of the manufacture and control of the batch.

(c) Examination of packaging and labeling materials for suitability and correctness before packaging operations, and documentation of such examination in the batch production record.

(d) Inspection of the packaging and labeling facilities immediately before use to assure that all drug products have been removed from previous operations. Inspection shall also be made to assure that packaging and labeling materials not suitable for subsequent operations have been removed. Results of inspection shall be documented in the batch production records.

§211.132 Tamper-resistant packaging requirements for over-the-counter human drug products.

(a) *General.* Because most over-the-counter (OTC) human drug products are not now packaged in tamper-resistant retail packages, there is the opportunity for the malicious adulteration of OTC drug products with health risks to individuals who unknowingly purchase adulterated products and with loss of consumer confidence in the security of OTC drug product packages. The Food and Drug Administration has the authority and responsibility under the Federal Food, Drug and Cosmetic Act (the act) to establish a uniform national requirement for tamper-resistant packaging of OTC drug products that will improve the security of OTC drug packaging and help assure the safety and effectiveness of OTC drug products. An OTC drug product (except a dermatological, dentifrice, insulin, or lozenge product) for retail sale that is not packaged in a tamper-resistant package or that is not properly labeled under this section is adulterated under section 501 of the act or misbranded under section 502 of the act, or both.

(b) *Requirement for tamper-resistant package.* Each manufacturer and packer who packages an OTC drug product (except a dermatological, dentifrice, insulin or lozenge product) for retail sale, shall package the product in a tamper-resistant package, if this product is accessible to the public while held for sale. A tamper-resistant package is one having an indicator or barrier to entry which, if breached or missing, can reasonably be expected to provide visible evidence to consumers that tampering has occurred. To reduce the likelihood of substitution of a tamper-resistant feature after tampering, the indicator or barrier to entry is required to be distinctive by design (e.g., an aerosol product container) or by the use of an identifying characteristic (e.g., a pattern, name, registered trademark, logo, or picture). For purposes of this section, the term "distinctive by design" means the packaging cannot be duplicated with commonly available materials or through commonly available processes. For purposes of this section, the term "aerosol product" means a product which depends upon the power of a liquified or compressed gas to expel the contents from the container. A tamper-resistant package may involve an immediate-container and closure system or secondary-container or carton system or any combination of systems intended to provide a visual indication of package integrity. The tamper-resistant feature shall be designed to and shall remain intact when handled in a reasonable manner during manufacture, distribution, and retail display.

(c) *Labeling.* Each retail package of an OTC drug product covered by this section, except ammonia inhalant in crushable glass ampules, aerosol products as defined in paragraph (b) of this section, or containers of compressed medical oxygen, is required to bear a statement that is prominently placed so that consumers are alerted to the specific tamper-resistant feature of the package. The labeling statement is also required to be so placed that it will be unaffected if the tamper-resistant feature of the package is breached or missing. If the tamper-resistant feature chosen to meet the requirement in paragraph (b) of this section is one that uses an identifying characteristic, that characteristic is required to be referred to in the labeling statement. For example, the labeling statement on a bottle with a shrink band could say "For your protection, this bottle has an imprinted seal around the neck."

(d) *Requests for exemptions from packaging and labeling requirements.* A manufacturer or packer may request an exemption from the packaging and labeling requirements of this section. A request for an exemption is required to be submitted in the form of a citizen petition under §10.30 of this chapter and should be clearly identified on the envelope as a "Request for Exemption from Tamper-resistant Rule." The petition is required to contain the following:

(1) The name of the drug product or, if the petition seeks an exemption for a drug class, the name of the drug class, and a list of products within that class.

(2) The reasons that the drug product's compliance with the tamper-resistant packaging or labeling requirements of this section is unnecessary or cannot be achieved.

(3) A description of alternative steps that are available, or that the petitioner has already taken, to reduce the likelihood that the product or drug class will be the subject of malicious adulteration.

(4) Other information justifying an exemption.

This information collection requirement has been approved by the Office of Management and Budget under number 0910-0149.

(e) *OTC drug products subject to approved new drug applications.* Holders of approved new drug applications for OTC drug products are required under §314.8 (a) (4)(vi), (5)(xi), or (d)(5) of this chapter to provide for changes in packaging, and under §314.8(a)(5)(xii) to provide for changes in labeling to comply with the requirements of this section.

(f) *Poison Prevention Packaging Act of 1970.* This section does not affect any requirements for "special packaging" as defined under §310.3(1) of this chapter and required under the Poison Prevention Packaging Act of 1970.

(g) *Effective date.* OTC drug products, except dermatological, dentifrice, insulin, and lozenge products, are required to comply with the requirements of this section on the dates listed below except to the extent that a product's manufacturer or packer has obtained an exemption from a packaging or labeling requirement.

(1) *Initial effective date for packaging requirements.* (i) The packaging requirement in paragraph (b) of this section is effective on February 7, 1983 for each affected OTC drug product (except oral and vaginal tablets, vaginal and rectal suppositories, and one-piece soft gelatin capsules) packaged for retail sale on or after that date, except for the requirement in paragraph (b) of this section for a distinctive indicator or barrier to entry.

(ii) The packaging requirement in paragraph (b) of this section is effective on May 5, 1983 for each OTC drug product that is an oral or vaginal tablet, a vaginal or rectal suppository, or one-piece soft gelatin capsules packaged for retail sale on or after that date.

(2) *Initial effective date for labeling requirements.* The requirement in paragraph (b) of this section that the indicator or barrier to entry be distinctive by design and the requirement in paragraph (c) of this section for a labeling statement are effective on May 5, 1983 for each affected OTC drug product packaged for retail sale on or after that date, except that the requirement for a specific label reference to any identifying characteristic is effective on February 6, 1984 for each affected OTC drug product packaged for retail sale on or after that date.

(3) *Retail level effective date.* The tamper-resistant packaging requirement of paragraph (b) of this section is effective on February 6, 1984 for each affected

OTC drug product held for sale on or after that date that was packaged for retail sale before May 5, 1983. This does not include the requirement in paragraph (b) of this section that the indicator or barrier to entry be distinctive by design. Products packaged for retail sale after May 5, 1983, are required to be in compliance with all aspects of the regulations without regard to the retail level effective date.

(Secs. 201(n), 501, 502, 505, 506, 507, 601, 602, 701, 52 Stat. 1049–1056 as amended, 55 Stat. 851, 59 Stat. 463 as amended (21 U.S.C. 321(n), 351, 352, 355, 356, 357, 361, 362, 371))

[47 FR 50499, Nov. 5, 1982; 48 FR 1707, Jan. 14, 1983, as amended at 48 FR 16664, Apr. 19, 1983; 48 FR 37624, Aug. 19, 1983; 48 FR 41579, Sept. 16, 1983]

EFFECTIVE DATE NOTE: Paragraph (g)(3) of §211.132 was added at 47 FR 50449, Nov. 5, 1982, effective February 6, 1984. At 48 FR 41579, Sept. 16, 1983, FDA published an interim stay of the effective date of paragraph (g)(3).

§211.134 Drug product inspection.

(a) Packaged and labeled products shall be examined during finishing operations to provide assurance that containers and packages in the lot have the correct label.

(b) A representative sample of units shall be collected at the completion of finishing operations and shall be visually examined for correct labeling.

(c) Results of these examinations shall be recorded in the batch production or control records.

§211.137 Expiration dating.

(a) To assure that a drug product meets applicable standards of identity, strength, quality, and purity at the time of use, it shall bear an expiration date determined by appropriate stability testing described in §211.166.

(b) Expiration dates shall be related to any storage conditions stated on the labeling, as determined by stability studies described in §211.166.

(c) If the drug product is to be reconstituted at the time of dispensing, its labeling shall bear expiration information for both the reconstituted and unreconstituted drug products.

(d) Expiration dates shall appear on labeling in accordance with the requirements of §201.17 of this chapter.

(e) Homeopathic drug products shall be exempt from the requirements of this section.

(f) Allergenic extracts that are labeled "No U.S. Standard of Potency" are exempt from the requirements of this section.

(g) Pending consideration of a proposed exemption, published in the FEDERAL REGISTER of September 29, 1978, the requirements in this section shall not be enforced for human OTC drug products if their labeling does not bear dosage limitations and they are stable for at least 3 years as supported by appropriate stability data.

(Secs. 502, 505, 512, 701, 52 Stat. 1050–1053 as amended, 1055–1056 as amended, 82 Stat. 343–349 (21 U.S.C. 352, 355, 360b, 371))

[43 FR 45077, Sept. 29, 1978, as amended at 46 FR 56412, Nov. 17, 1981]

Subpart H   Holding and Distribution

§211.142 Warehousing procedures.

Written procedures describing the warehousing of drug products shall be established and followed. They shall include:

(a) Quarantine of drug products before release by the quality control unit.

(b) Storage of drug products under appropriate conditions of temperature, humidity, and light so that the identity, strength, quality, and purity of the drug products are not affected.

§211.150 Distribution procedures.

Written procedures shall be established, and followed, describing the distribution of drug products. They shall include:

(a) A procedure whereby the oldest approved stock of a drug product is distributed first. Deviation from this requirement is permitted if such deviation is temporary and appropriate.

(b) A system by which the distribution of each lot of drug product can be readily determined to facilitate its recall if necessary.

Subpart I   Laboratory Controls

§211.160 General requirements.

(a) The establishment of any specifications, standards, sampling plans, test procedures, or other laboratory control mechanisms required by this subpart, including any change in such specifications, standards, sampling plans, test procedures, or other laboratory control mechanisms, shall be drafted by the appropriate organizational unit and reviewed and approved by the quality control unit. The requirements in this subpart shall be followed and shall be documented at the time of performance. Any deviation from the written specifications, standards, sampling plans, test procedures, or other laboratory control mechanisms shall be recorded and justified.

(b) Laboratory controls shall include the establishment of scientifically sound and appropriate specifications, standards, sampling plans, and test procedures designed to assure that components, drug product containers, closures, in-process materials, labeling, and drug products conform to appropriate standards of identity, strength, quality, and purity. Laboratory controls shall include:

(1) Determination of conformance to appropriate written specifications for the acceptance of each lot within each shipment of components, drug product containers, closures, and labeling used in the manufacture, processing, packing, or holding of drug products. The specifications shall include a description of the sampling and testing procedures used. Samples shall be representative and adequately identified. Such procedures shall also require appropriate retesting of any component, drug product container, or closure this is subject to deterioration.

(2) Determination of conformance to written specifications and a description of sampling and testing procedures for in-process materials. Such samples shall be representative and properly identified.

(3) Determination of conformance to written descriptions of sampling procedures and appropriate specifications for drug products. Such samples shall be representative and properly identified.

(4) The calibration of instruments, apparatus, gauges, and recording devices at suitable intervals in accordance with an established written program containing specific directions, schedules, limits for accuracy and precision, and provisions for remedial action in the event accuracy and/or precision limits are not met. Instruments, apparatus, gauges, and recording devices not meeting established specifications shall not be used.

§211.165 Testing and release for distribution.

(a) For each batch of drug product, there shall be appropriate laboratory determination of satisfactory conformance to final specifications for the drug product, including the identity and strength of each active ingredient, prior to release. Where sterility and/or pyrogen testing are conducted on specific batches of shortlived radiopharmaceuticals, such batches may be released prior to completion of sterility and/or pyrogen testing, provided such testing is completed as soon as possible.

(b) There shall be appropriate laboratory testing, as necessary, of each batch of drug product required to be free of objectionable microorganisms.

(c) Any sampling and testing plans shall be described in written procedures that shall include the method of sampling and the number of units per batch to be tested; such written procedure shall be followed.

(d) Acceptance criteria for the sampling and testing conducted by the quality control unit shall be adequate to assure that batches of drug products meet each appropriate specification and appropriate statistical quality control criteria as a condition for their approval and release. The statistical quality control criteria shall include appropriate acceptance levels and/or appropriate rejection levels.

(e) The accuracy, sensitivity, specificity, and reproducibility of test methods employed by the firm shall be established and documented. Such validation and documentation may be accomplished in accordance with §211.194(a)(2).

(f) Drug products failing to meet established standards or specifications and any other relevant quality control criteria shall be rejected. Reprocessing may be performed. Prior to acceptance and use, reprocessed material must meet appropriate standards, specifications, and any other relevant criteria.

§211.166 Stability testing.

(a) There shall be a written testing program designed to assess the stability characteristics of drug products. The results of such stability testing shall be used in determining appropriate storage conditions and expiration dates. The written program shall be followed and shall include:

(1) Sample size and test intervals based on statistical criteria for each attribute examined to assure valid estimates of stability;

(2) Storage conditions for samples retained for testing;

(3) Reliable, meaningful, and specific test methods;

(4) Testing of the drug product in the same container-closure system as that in which the drug product is marketed;

(5) Testing of drug products for reconstitution at the time of dispensing (as directed in the labeling) as well as after they are reconstituted.

(b) An adequate number of batches of each drug product shall be tested to determine an appropriate expiration date and a record of such data shall be maintained. Accelerated studies, combined with basic stability information on the components, drug products, and container-closure system, may be used to support tentative expiration dates provided full shelf life studies are not available and are being conducted. Where data from accelerated studies are used to project a tentative expiration date that is beyond a date supported by actual shelf life studies, there must be stability studies conducted, including drug product testing at appropriate intervals, until the tentative expiration date is verified or the appropriate expiration date determined.

(c) For homeopathic drug products, the requirements of this section are as follows:

(1) There shall be a written assessment of stability based at least on testing or examination of the drug product for compatibility of the ingredients, and based on marketing experience with the drug product to indicate that there is no degradation of the product for the normal or expected period of use.

(2) Evaluation of stability shall be based on the same container-closure system in which the drug product is being marketed.

(d) Allergenic extracts that are labeled "No U.S. Standard of Potency" are exempt from the requirements of this section.

(Secs. 502, 505, 512, 701, 52 Stat. 1050–1053 as amended, 1055–1056 as amended, 82 Stat. 343–349 (21 U.S.C. 352, 355, 360b, 371))
[43 FR 45077, Sept. 29, 1978, as amended at 46 FR 56412, Nov. 17, 1981]

§211.167 Special testing requirements.

(a) For each batch of drug product purporting to be sterile and/or pyrogen-free, there shall be appropriate laboratory testing to determine conformance to such requirements. The test procedures shall be in writing and shall be followed.

(b) For each batch of ophthalmic ointment, there shall be appropriate testing to determine conformance to specifications regarding the presence of foreign particles and harsh or abrasive substances. The test procedures shall be in writing and shall be followed.

(c) For each batch of controlled-release dosage form, there shall be appropriate laboratory testing to determine conformance to the specifications for the rate of release of each active ingredient. The test procedures shall be in writing and shall be followed.

§211.170 Reserve samples.

(a) An appropriately identified reserve sample that is representative of each lot in each shipment of each active ingredient shall be retained. The reserve sample consists of at least twice the quantity necessary for all tests required to determine whether the active ingredient meets its established specifications, except for sterility and pyrogen testing. The retention time is as follows:

(1) For an active ingredient in a drug product other than those described in paragraphs (a) (2) and (3) of this section, the reserve sample shall be retained for 1 year after the expiration date of the last lot of the drug product containing the active ingredient.

(2) For an active ingredient in a radioactive drug product, except for nonradioactive reagent kits, the reserve sample shall be retained for:

(i) Three months after the expiration date of the last lot of the drug product containing the active ingredient if the expiration dating period of the drug product is 30 days or less; or

(ii) Six months after the expiration date of the last lot of the drug product containing the active ingredient if the expiration dating period of the drug product is more than 30 days.

(3) For an active ingredient in an OTC drug product that is exempt from bearing an expiration date under §211.137, the reserve sample shall be retained for 3 years after distribution of the last lot of the drug product containing the active ingredient.

(b) An appropriately identified reserve sample that is representative of each lot or batch of drug product shall be retained and stored under conditions consistent with product labeling. The reserve sample shall be stored in the same immediate container-closure system in which the drug product is marketed or in one that has essentially the same characteristics. The reserve sample consists of at least twice the quantity necessary to perform all the required tests, except those for sterility and pyrogens. Reserve samples, except those drug products described in paragraph (b)(2), shall be examined visually at least once a year for evidence of deterioration unless visual examination would affect the integrity of the reserve samples. Any evidence of reserve sample deterioration shall be investigated in accordance with §211.192. The results of the examination shall be recorded and maintained with other stability data on the drug product. Reserve samples of compressed medical gases need not be retained. The retention time is as follows:

(1) For a drug product other than those described in paragraphs (b) (2) and (3) of this section, the reserve sample shall be retained for 1 year after the expiration date of the drug product.

(2) For a radioactive drug product, except for nonradioactive reagent kits, the reserve sample shall be retained for:

(i) Three months after the expiration date of the drug product if the expiration dating period of the drug product is 30 days or less; or

(ii) Six months after the expiration date of the drug product if the expiration dating period of the drug product is more than 30 days.

(3) For an OTC drug product that is exempt for bearing an expiration date under §211.137, the reserve sample must be retained for 3 years after the lot or batch of drug product is distributed.

(Secs. 501, 502, 505, 512, 701, 52 Stat. 1049–1053 as amended, 1055–1056 as amended, 82 Stat. 343–351 (21 U.S.C. 351, 352, 355, 360b, 371))

[48 FR 13025, Mar. 29, 1983]

§211.173 Laboratory animals.

Animals used in testing components, in-process materials, or drug products for compliance with established specifications shall be maintained and controlled in a manner that assures their suitability for their intended use. They shall be identified, and adequate records shall be maintained showing the history of their use.

§211.176 Penicillin contamination.

If a reasonable possibility exists that a non-penicillin drug product has been exposed to cross-contamination with penicillin, the non-penicillin drug product shall be tested for the presence of penicillin. Such drug product shall not be marketed if detectable levels are found when tested according to procedures specified in 'Procedures for Detecting and Measuring Penicillin Contamination in Drugs,' which is incorporated by reference. Copies are available from the Division of Drug Biology (HFN-170), Center for Drugs and Biologics, Food and Drug Administration, 200 C St. SW., Washington, DC 20204, or available for inspection at the Office of the Federal Register, 1100 L St. NW., Washington, DC 20408.

[43 FR 45077, Sept. 29, 1978, as amended at 47 FR 9396, Mar. 5, 1982; 50 FR 8996, Mar. 6, 1985]

Subpart J Records and Reports

§211.180 General requirements.

(a) Any production, control, or distribution record that is required to be maintained in compliance with this part and is specifically associated with a batch of a drug product shall be retained for at least 1 year after the expiration date of the batch or, in the case of certain OTC drug products lacking expiration dating because they meet the criteria for exemption under §211.137, 3 years after distribution of the batch.

(b) Records shall be maintained for all components, drug product containers, closures, and labeling for at least 1 year after the expiration date or, in the case of certain OTC drug products lacking expiration dating because they meet the criteria for exemption under §211.137, 3 years after distribution of the last lot of drug product incorporating the component or using the container, closure, or labeling.

(c) All records required under this part, or copies of such records, shall be readily available for authorized inspection during the retention period at the establishment where the activities described in such records occurred. These records or copies thereof shall be subject to photocopying or other means of reproduction as part of such inspection. Records that can be immediately retrieved from another location by computer or other electronic means shall be considered as meeting the requirements of this paragraph.

(d) Records required under this part may be retained either as original records or as true copies such as photocopies, microfilm, microfiche, or other accurate reproductions of the original records. Where reduction techniques, such as microfilming, are used, suitable reader and photocopying equipment shall be readily available.

(e) Written records required by this part shall be maintained so that data therein can be used for evaluating, at least annually, the quality standards of each drug product to determine the need for changes in drug product specifications or manufacturing or control procedures. Written procedures shall be established and followed for such evaluations and shall include provisions for:

(1) A review of every batch, whether approved or rejected, and, where applicable, records associated with the batch.

(2) A review of complaints, recalls, returned or salvaged drug products, and investigations conducted under §211.192 for each drug product.

(f) Procedures shall be established to assure that the responsible officials of the firm, if they are not personally involved in or immediately aware of such actions, are notified in writing of any investigations conducted under §§211.198, 211.204, or 211.208 of these regulations, any recalls, reports of inspectional observations issued by the Food and Drug Administration, or any regulatory actions relating to good manufacturing practices brought by the Food and Drug Administration.

§211.182 Equipment cleaning and use log.

A written record of major equipment cleaning, maintenance (except routine maintenance such as lubrication and adjustments), and use shall be included in individual equipment logs that show the date, time, product, and lot number of each batch processed. If equipment is dedicated to manufacture of one product, then individual equipment logs are not required, provided that lots or batches of such product follow in numerical order and are manufactured in numerical sequence. In cases where dedicated equipment is employed, the records of cleaning, maintenance, and use shall be part of the batch record. The persons performing and double-checking the cleaning and maintenance shall date and sign or initial the log indicating that the work was performed. Entries in the log shall be in chronological order.

§211.184 Component, drug product, container, closure, and labeling records.

These records shall include the following:

(a) The identity and quantity of each shipment of each lot of components, drug product containers, closures, and labeling; the name of the supplier; the supplier's lot number(s) if known; the receiving code as specified in §211.80; and the date of receipt. The name and location of the prime manufacturer, if different from the supplier, shall be listed if known.

(b) The results of any test or examination performed (including those performed as required by §211.82(a), §211.84(d), or §211.122(a)) and the conclusions derived therefrom.

(c) An individual inventory record of each component, drug product container, and closure and, for each component, a reconciliation of the use of each lot of such component. The inventory record shall contain sufficient information to allow determination of any batch or lot of drug product associated with the use of each component, drug product container, and closure.

(d) Documentation of the examination and review of labels and labeling for conformity with established specifications in accord with §§211.122(c) and 211.130(c).

(e) The disposition of rejected components, drug product containers, closure, and labeling.

§211.186 Master production and control records.

(a) To assure uniformity from batch to batch, master production and control records for each drug product, including each batch size thereof, shall be prepared, dated, and signed (full signature, handwritten) by one person and independently checked, dated, and signed by a second person. The preparation of master production and control records shall be described in a written procedure and such written procedure shall be followed.

(b) Master production and control records shall include:

(1) The name and strength of the product and a description of the dosage form;

(2) The name and weight or measure of each active ingredient per dosage unit or per unit of weight or measure of the drug product, and a statement of the total weight or measure of any dosage unit;

(3) A complete list of components designated by names or codes sufficiently specific to indicate any special quality characteristic;

(4) An accurate statement of the weight or measure of each component, using the same weight system (metric, avoirdupois, or apothecary) for each component. Reasonable variations may be permitted, however, in the amount of components necessary for the preparation in the dosage form, provided they are justified in the master production and control records;

(5) A statement concerning any calculated excess of component;

(6) A statement of theoretical weight or measure at appropriate phases of processing;

(7) A statement of theoretical yield, including the maximum and minimum percentages of theoretical yield beyond which investigation according to §211.192 is required;

(8) A description of the drug product containers, closures, and packaging materials, including a specimen or copy of each label and all other labeling signed and dated by the person or persons responsible for approval of such labeling;

(9) Complete manufacturing and control instructions, sampling and testing procedures, specifications, special notations, and precautions to be followed.

§211.188 Batch production and control records.

Batch production and control records shall be prepared for each batch of drug product produced and shall include complete information relating to the production and control of each batch. These records shall include:

(a) An accurate reproduction of the appropriate master production or control record, checked for accuracy, dated, and signed.

(b) Documentation that each significant step in the manufacture, processing, packing, or holding of the batch was accomplished, including:

(1) Dates;

(2) Identity of individual major equipment and lines used;

(3) Specific identification of each batch of component or in-process material used;

(4) Weights and measures of components used in the course of processing;

(5) In-process and laboratory control results;

(6) Inspection of the packaging and labeling area before and after use;

(7) A statement of the actual yield and a statement of the percentage of theoretical yield at appropriate phases of processing;

(8) Complete labeling control records, including specimens or copies of all labeling used;

(9) Description of drug product containers and closures;

(10) Any sampling performed;

(11) Identification of the persons performing and directly supervising or checking each significant step in the operation;

(12) Any investigation made according to §211.192.

(13) Results of examinations made in accordance with §211.134.

§211.192 Production record review.

All drug product production and control records, including those for packaging and labeling, shall be reviewed and approved by the quality control unit to determine compliance with all established, approved written procedures before a batch is released or distributed. Any unexplained discrepancy (including a percentage of theoretical yield exceeding the maximum or minimum percentages established in master production and control records) or the failure of a batch or any of its components to meet any of its specifications shall be thoroughly investigated, whether or not the batch has already been distributed. The investigation shall extend to other batches of the same drug product and other drug products that may have been associated with the specific failure or discrepancy. A written record of the investigation shall be made and shall include the conclusions and followup.

§211.194 Laboratory records.

(a) Laboratory records shall include complete data derived from all tests necessary to assure compliance with established specifications and standards, including examinations and assays, as follows:

(1) A description of the sample received for testing with identification of source (that is, location from where sample was obtained), quantity, lot number or other distinctive code, date sample was taken, and date sample was received for testing.

(2) A statement of each method used in the testing of the sample. The statement shall indicate the location of data that establish that the methods used

in the testing of the sample meet proper standards of accuracy and reliability as applied to the product tested. (If the method employed is in the current revision of the United States Pharmacopeia, National Formulary, Association of Official Analytical Chemists, Book of Methods,[2] or in other recognized standard references, or is detailed in an approved new drug application and the referenced method is not modified, a statement indicating the method and reference will suffice). The suitability of all testing methods used shall be verified under actual conditions of use.

(3) A statement of the weight or measure of sample used for each test, where appropriate.

(4) A complete record of all data secured in the course of each test, including all graphs, charts, and spectra from laboratory instrumentation, properly identified to show the specific component, drug product container, closure, in-process material, or drug product, and lot tested.

(5) A record of all calculations performed in connection with the test, including units of measure, conversion factors, and equivalency factors.

(6) A statement of the results of tests and how the results compare with established standards of identity, strength, quality, and purity for the component, drug product container, closure, in-process material, or drug product tested.

(7) The initials or signature of the person who performs each test and the date(s) the tests were performed.

(8) The initials or signature of a second person showing that the original records have been reviewed for accuracy, completeness, and compliance with established standards.

(b) Complete records shall be maintained of any modification of an established method employed in testing. Such records shall include the reason for the modification and data to verify that the modification produced results that are at least as accurate and reliable for the material being tested as the established method.

(c) Complete records shall be maintained of any testing and standardization of laboratory reference standards, reagents, and standard solutions.

(d) Complete records shall be maintained of the periodic calibration of laboratory instruments, apparatus, gauges, and recording devices required by §211.160(b)(4).

(e) Complete records shall be maintained of all stability testing performed in accordance with §211.166.

§211.196 Distribution records.

Distribution records shall contain the name and strength of the product and description of the dosage form, name and address of the consignee, date

---

[2]Copies may be obtained from: Association of Official Analytical Chemists, P.O. Box 540, Benjamin Franklin Station, Washington, D.C. 20204.

and quantity shipped, and lot or control number of the drug product. For compressed medical gas products, distribution records are not required to contain lot or control numbers.

(Approved by the Office of Management and Budget under control number 0910-0139)

(Secs. 501, 502, 512, 701, 52 Stat. 1049-1051 as amended, 1055-1056 as amended, 82 Stat. 343-351 (21 U.S.C. 351, 352, 360b, 371))

[49 FR 9865, Mar. 16, 1984]

§211.198 Complaint files.

(a) Written procedures describing the handling of all written and oral complaints regarding a drug product shall be established and followed. Such procedures shall include provisions for review by the quality control unit, of any complaint involving the possible failure of a drug product to meet any of its specifications and, for such drug products, a determination as to the need for an investigation in accordance with §211.192. Such procedures shall include provisions for review to determine whether the complaint represents a serious and unexpected adverse drug experience which is required to be reported to the Food and Drug Administration in accordance with §310.305 of this Chapter.

(b) A written record of each complaint shall be maintained in a file designated for drug product complaints. The file regarding such drug product complaints shall be maintained at the establishment where the drug product involved was manufactured, processed, or packed, or such file may be maintained at another facility if the written records in such files are readily available for inspection at that other facility. Written records involving a drug product shall be maintained until at least 1 year after the expiration date of the drug product, or 1 year after the date that the complaint was received, whichever is longer. In the case of certain OTC drug products lacking expiration dating because they meet the criteria for exemption under §211.137, such written records shall be maintained for 3 years after distribution of the drug product.

(1) The written record shall include the following information, where known: the name and strength of the drug product, lot number, name of complainant, nature of complaint, and reply to complainant.

(2) Where an investigation under §211.192 is conducted, the written record shall include the findings of the investigation and followup. The record or copy of the record of the investigation shall be maintained at the establishment where the investigation occurred in accordance with §211.180(c).

(3) Where an investigation under §211.192 is not conducted, the written record shall include the reason that an investigation was found not to be necessary and the name of the responsible person making such a determination.

Subpart K   Returned and Salvated Drug Products

§211.204 Returned drug products.

Returned drug products shall be identified as such and held. If the conditions under which returned drug products have been held, stored, or shipped before or during their return, or if the condition of the drug product, its container, carton, or labeling, as a result of storage or shipping, casts doubt on the safety, identity, strength, quality or purity of the drug product, the returned drug product shall be destroyed unless examination, testing, or other investigations prove the drug product meets appropriate standards of safety, identity, strength, quality, or purity. A drug product may be reprocessed provided the subsequent drug product meets appropriate standards, specifications, and characteristics. Records of returned drug products shall be maintained and shall include the name and label potency of the drug product dosage form, lot number (or control number or batch number), reason for the return, quantity returned, date of disposition, and ultimate disposition of the returned drug product. If the reason for a drug product being returned implicates associated batches, an appropriate investigation shall be conducted in accordance with the requirements of §211.192. Procedures for the holding, testing, and reprocessing of returned drug products shall be in writing and shall be followed.

§211.208 Drug product salvaging.

Drug products that have been subjected to improper storage conditions including extremes in temperature, humidity, smoke, fumes, pressure, age, or radiation due to natural disasters, fires, accidents, or equipment failures shall not be salvaged and returned to the marketplace. Whenever there is a question whether drug products have been subjected to such conditions, salvaging operations may be conducted only if there is (a) evidence from laboratory tests and assays (including animal feeding studies where applicable) that the drug products meet all applicable standards of identity, strength, quality, and purity and (b) evidence from inspection of the premises that the drug products and their associated packaging were not subjected to improper storage conditions as a result of the disaster or accident. Organoleptic examinations shall be acceptable only as supplemental evidence that the drug products meet appropriate standards of identity, strength, quality, and purity. Records including name, lot number, and disposition shall be maintained for drug products subject to this section.

APPENDIX C.2.   ICH GUIDELINE

Introduction

This guideline has been developed within the Expert Working Group (Quality) of the International Conference on Harmonization. Discussions are still being pursued within the Expert Working Group to define and standardize the conditions for light stability testing of active substances and dosages forms. Once agreed, these conditions will be the subject of a separate document.

The Tripartite Guideline for the Stability Testing of New Drug Substances and Products

Preamble

The following guideline sets out the stability testing requirement for a Registration Application within the three areas of the EC, Japan and the USA. It does not seek necessarily to cover the testing that may be required for registration in or export to other areas of the world.

The guideline seeks to exemplify the core stability data package required for new drug substances and products. It is not always necessary to follow this when there are scientifically justifiable reasons for using alternative approaches.

The guideline provides a general indication on the requirements for stability testing, but leaves sufficient flexibility to encompass the variety of different practical situations required for specific scientific situations and characteristics of the materials being evaluated.

The principle that information on stability generated in any one of the three areas of the EC, Japan and the USA would be mutually acceptable in both of the other two areas has been established, provided it meets the appropriate requirements of this guideline and the labelling is in accord with national/regional requirements.

Details of the specific requirements for sampling, test requirements for particular dosage forms/packaging etc., are not covered in this guideline.

Objective

The purpose of stability testing is to provide evidence on how the quality of a drug substance or drug product varies with time under the influence of a variety of environmental factors such as temperature, humidity and light, and enables recommended storage conditions, re-test periods and shelf lives to be established.

Scope

The guideline primarily addresses the information required in Registration Applications for new molecular entities and associated drug products.

This guideline does not currently seek to cover the information required for abbreviated or abridged applications, variations, clinical trial applications, etc.

The choice of test conditions defined in this guideline is based on an analysis of the effects of climatic conditions in the three areas of the EC, Japan and the USA. The mean kinetic temperature in any region of the world can be derived from climatic data [Grimm, W., *Drugs Made in Germany*, 28, 196–202 1985 and 29, 39–47 1986].

Drug Substance

General

Information on the stability of the drug substance is an integral part of the systematic approach to stability evaluation.

Stress Testing

Stress testing helps to determine the intrinsic stability of the molecule by establishing degradation pathways in order to identify the likely degradation products and to validate the stability indicating power of the analytical procedures used.

Formal Studies

Primary stability studies are intended to show that the drug substance will remain within specification during the re-test period if stored under recommended storage conditions.

Selection of Batches

Stability information from accelerated and long term testing is to be provided on at least three batches. The long term testing should cover a minimum of 12 months duration on at least three batches at the time of submission.

The batches manufactured to a minimum of pilot plant scale should be by the same synthetic route and use a method of manufacture and procedure that simulates the final process to be used on a manufacturing scale.

The overall quality of the batches of drug substance placed on stability should be representative of both the quality of the material used in pre-clinical and clinical studies and the quality of material to be made on a manufacturing scale.

Supporting information may be provided using stability data on batches of drug substance made on a laboratory scale.

The first three production batches of drug substance manufactured post approval, if not submitted in the original Registration Application, should be placed on long term stability studies using the same stability protocol as in the approved drug application.

Test Procedures and Test Criteria

The testing should cover those features susceptible to change during storage and likely to influence quality, safety and/or efficacy. Stability information should cover as necessary the physical, chemical and microbiological test characteristics. Validated stability-indicating testing methods must be applied. The need for the extent of replication will depend on the results of validation studies.

Specification

Limits of acceptability should be derived from the profile of the material as used in the pre-clinical and clinical batches. It will need to include individual and total upper limits for impurities and degradation products, the justification for which should be influenced by the levels observed in material used in pre-clinical studies and clinical trials.

Storage Conditions

The length of the studies and the storage conditions should be sufficient to cover storage, shipment and subsequent use. Application of the same storage conditions as applied to the drug product will facilitate comparative review and assessment. Other storage conditions are allowable if justified. In particular, temperature sensitive drug substances should be stored under an alternative, lower temperature condition which will then become the designated long term testing storage temperature. The six months accelerated testing should then be carried out at a temperature at least 15°C above this designated long term storage temperature (together with the appropriate relative humidity conditions for that temperature). The designated long term testing conditions will be reflected in the labeling and re-test date.

Conditions		Minimum time period at submission (months)
Long-term testing	25°C ± 2°C/60% RH ± 5%	12
Accelerated testing	40°C ± 2°C/75% RH ± 5%	6

Where 'significant change' occurs during six months storage under conditions of accelerated testing at 40°C ± 2°C/75 percent RH ± 5 percent, additional testing at an intermediate condition (such as 30°C ± 2°C/60 percent RH ± 5 percent) should be conducted for drug substances to be used in the manufacture of dosage forms tested long term at 25°C/60 percent RH and this information included in the Registration Application. The initial Registration Application should include a minimum of 6 months data from a 12 months study.

'Significant change' at 40°C/75 percent RH or 30°C/60 percent RH is defined as failure to meet the specification.

The long term testing will be continued for a sufficient period of time beyond 12 months to cover all appropriate re-test periods, and the further accumulated data can be submitted to the Authorities during the assessment period of the Registration Application.

The data (from accelerated testing or from testing at an intermediate condition) may be used to evaluate the impact of short term excursions outside the label storage conditions such as might occur during shipping.

Testing Frequency

Frequency of testing should be sufficient to establish the stability characteristics of the drug substance. Testing under the defined long term conditions will normally be every three months, over the first year, every six months over the second year and then annually.

Packaging/Containers

The containers to be used in the long term, real time stability evaluation should be the same as or simulate the actual packaging used for storage and distribution.

Evaluation

The design of the stability study is to establish, based on testing a minimum of three batches of the drug substance and evaluating the stability information (covering as necessary the physical, chemical and microbiological test characteristics), a retest period applicable to all future batches of the bulk drug substance manufactured under similar circumstances. The degree of variability of individual batches affects the confidence that a future production batch will remain within specification until the retest date.

An acceptable approach for quantitative characteristics that are expected to decrease with time is to determine the time at which the 95% one-sided confidence limit for the mean degradation curve intersects the acceptable lower specification limit. If analysis shows that the batch to batch variability is small, it is advantageous to combine the data into one overall estimate and this can be done by first applying appropriate statistical tests (for example, p values for level of significance of rejection of more than 0.25) to the slopes of the regression lines and zero time intercepts for the individual batches. If it is inappropriate to combine data from several batches, the overall retest period may depend on the minimum time a batch may be expected to remain within acceptable and justified limits.

The nature of any degradation relationship will determine the need for transformation of the data for linear regression analysis. Usually the relationship can be represented by a linear, quadratic or cubic function on an arithmetic or logarithmic scale. Statistical methods should be employed to test the goodness of fit of the data on all batches and combined batches (where appropriate) to the assumed degradation line or curve.

The data may show so little degradation and so little variability that it is apparent from looking at the data that the requested retest period will be granted.

Under the circumstances, it is normally unnecessary to go through the formal statistical analysis but merely to provide a full justification for the omission.

Limited extrapolation of the real time data beyond the observed range to extend expiration dating at approval time, particularly where the accelerated data supports this, may be undertaken. However, this assumes that the same degradation relationship will continue to apply beyond the observed data and hence the use of extrapolation must be justified in each application in terms of what is known about the mechanism of degradation, the goodness of fit of any mathematical model, batch size, existence of supportive data etc.

Any evaluation should cover not only the assay, but the levels of degradation products and other appropriate attributes.

Statements/Labeling

A storage temperature range may be used in accordance with relevant national/ regional requirements. The range should be based on the stability evaluation of the drug substance. Where applicable, specific requirements should be stated, particularly for drug substances that cannot tolerate freezing. The use of terms such as 'ambient conditions' or 'room temperature' is unacceptable. A re-test period shuld be derived from the stability information.

Drug Product

General

The design of the stability programme for the finished product should be based on the knowledge of the behavior and properties of the drug substance and the experience gained from clinical formulation studies and from the stability studies on the drug substance. The likely changes on storage and the rationale for the selection of product variables to include in the testing programme should be stated.

Selection of Batches

Stability information from accelerated and long term testing is to be provided on three batches of the same formulation and dosage form in the containers and closure proposed for marketing. Two of the three batches should be at least pilot scale. The third batch may be smaller (e.g., 25,000 to 50,000 tablets or capsules for solid oral dosage forms). The long term testing should cover at least 12 months duration at the time of submission. The manufacturing process to be used should meaningfully simulate that which would be applied to large scale batches for marketing. The process should provide product of the same quality intended for marketing, and meeting the same quality specification as to be applied for release of material. Where possible, batches of the finished product should be manufactured using identifiably different batches of drug substance.

Data on laboratory scale batches is not acceptable as primary stability information. Data on associated formulations or packaging may be submitted as supportive information. The first three production batches manufactured post approval, if not submitted in the original Registration Application, should be placed on accelerated and long term stability studies using the same stability protocols as in the approved drug application.

Test Procedures and Test Criteria

The testing should cover those features susceptible to change during storage and likely to influence quality, safety and/or efficacy. Analytical test procedures should be fully validated and the assays should be stability-indicating. The need for the extent of replication will depend on the results of validation studies.

The range of testing should cover not only chemical and biological stability but also loss of preservative, physical properties and characteristics, organoleptic properties and where required, microbiological attributes. Preservative efficacy testing and assays on stored samples should be carried out to determine the content and efficacy of antimicrobial preservatives.

Specifications

Limits of acceptance should relate to the release limits (where applicable), to be derived from consideration of all the available stability information. The shelf life specification could allow acceptable and justifiable derivations from the release specification based on the stability evaluation and the changes observed on storage. It will need to include specific upper limits for degradation products, the justification for which should be influenced by the levels observed in material used in pre-clinical studies and clinical trials. The justification for the limits proposed for certain other tests such as particle size and/or dissolution rate will require reference to the results observed for batch(es) used in bioavailability and/or clinical studies. Any differences between the release and shelf life specifications for antimicrobial preservatives should be supported by preservative efficacy testing.

Storage Test Conditions

The length of the studies and the storage conditions should be sufficient to cover storage, shipment and subsequent use (e.g., reconstitution or dilution as recommended in the labeling).

See Table below for accelerated and long term storage conditions and minimum times. An assurance that long term testing will continue to cover the expected shelf life should be provided.

Other storage conditions are allowable if justified. Heat sensitive drug products should be stored under an alternative lower temperature condition which will eventually become the designated long term storage temperature.

Special consideration may need to be given to products which change physically or even chemically at lower storage conditions e.g., suspensions or emulsions which may sediment or cream, oils and semi-solid preparations which may show an increased viscosity. Where a lower temperature condition is used, the six months accelerated testing should be carried out at a temperature at least 15°C above its designated long term storage temperature (together with appropriate relative humditiy conditions for that temperature). For example, for a product to be stored long term under refrigerated conditions, accelerated testing should be conducted at 25°C ± 2°C/60 percent RH ± 5 percent RH. The designated long term testing conditions will be reflected in the labelling and expiration date.

Storage under conditions of high relative humidities applies particularly to solid dosage forms. For products such as solutions, suspensions etc., contained in packs designed to provide a permanent barrier to water loss, specific storage under conditions of high relative humidity is not necessary but the same range of temperatures should be applied. Low relative humidity (e.g. 10–20 percent RH) can adversely affect products packed in semi-permeable containers (e.g. solutions in plastic bags, nose drops in small plastic containers etc.) and consideration should be given to appropriate testing under such conditions.

Conditions		Minimum time period at submission (months)
Long-term testing	25°C ± 2°C/60% RH ± 5%	12
Accelerated testing	40°C ± 2°C/75% RH ± 5%	6

Where 'significant change' occurs due to accelerated testing, additional testing at an intermediate condition e.g., 30°C ± 2°C/60 percent ± 5 percent RH should be conducted. 'Significant change' at the accelerated condition is defined as:

1. A 5 percent potency loss from the initial assay value of a batch
2. Any specified degradant exceeding its specification limit
3. The product exceeding its pH limits
4. Dissolution exceeding the specification limits for 12 capsules or tablets
5. Failure to meet specifications for appearance and physical properties e.g., color, phase separation, resuspendibility, delivery per actuation, caking, hardness, etc.

Should significant change occur at 40°C/75 percent RH then the initial Registration Application should include a minimum of 6 months data from an ongoing one year study at 30°C/60 percent RH; the same significant change criteria shall then apply.

The long term testing will be continued for a sufficient time beyond 12 months to cover shelf life at appropriate test periods. The further accumulated data should be submitted to the authorities during the assessment period of the Registration Application.

The first three production batches manufactured post approval, if not submitted in the original Registration Application, should be placed on accelerated and long term stability studies using the same stability protocol as in the approved drug application.

Testing Frequency

Frequency of testing should be sufficient to establish the stability characteristics of the drug product. Testing will normally be every three months over the first year, every six months over the second year and then annually. The use of matrixing or bracketing can be applied, if justified (See Glossary).

Packaging Materials

The testing should be carried out in the final packaging proposed for marketing. Additional testing of unprotected drug product can form a useful part of the stress testing and pack evaluation, as can studies carried out in other related packaging materials in supporting the definitive pack(s).

Evaluation

A systematic approach should be adopted in the presentation and evaluation of the stability information which should cover as necessary physical, chemical, biological, microbiological quality characteristics, including particular properties of the dosage form (for example dissolution rate for oral solid dose forms).

The design of the stability study is to establish, based on testing a minimum of three batches of the drug product, a shelf-life and label storage instructions applicable to all future batches of the dosage form manufactured and packed under similar circumstances. The degree of variability of individual batches affects the confidence that a future production batch will remain within specification until the expiration date.

An acceptable approach for quantitative characteristics that are expected to decrease with time is to determine the time at which the 95% one-sided confidence limit for the mean degradation curve intersects the acceptable lower specification limit. If analysis shows that the batch to batch variability is small, it is advantageous to combine the data into one overall estimate and this can be done by first applying appropriate statistical tests (for example, p values for level of significance of rejection of more than 0.25) to the slopes of the regression lines and zero time intercepts for the individual batches. If it is inappropriate to combine data from several batches, the overall shelf-life may depend on the minimum time a batch may be expected to remain within acceptable and justified limits.

The nature of the degradation relationship will determine the need for transformation of the data for linear regression analysis. Usually the relationship can be represented by a linear, quadratic or cubic function on an arithmetic or logarithmic scale. Statistical methods should be employed to test the goodness of fit on all batches and combined batches (where appropriate) to the assumed degradation line or curve.

Where the data shows so little degradation and so little variability that it is apparent from looking at the data that the requested shelf-life will be granted, it is normally unnecessary to go through the formal statistical analysis but only to provide a justification for the omission.

Limited extrapolation of the real time data beyond the observed range to extend expiration dating at approval time, particularly where the accelerated data supports this, may be undertaken. However, this assumes that the same degradation relationship will continue to apply beyond the observed data and hence the use of extrapolation must be justified in each application in terms of what is known about the mechanisms of degradation, the goodness of fit of any mathematical model, batch size, existence of supportive data, etc.

Any evaluation should consider not only the assay, but the levels of degradation products and appropriate attributes. Where appropriate, attention should be paid to reviewing the adequacy of the mass balance, different stability and degradation performance.

The stability of the drug products after reconstituting or diluting according to labelling, should be addressed to provide appropriate and supportive information.

Statements/Labeling

A storage temperature range may be used in accordance with relevant national/regional requirements. The range should be based on the stability evaluation of the drug product. Where applicable, specific requirements should be stated particularly for drug products that cannot tolerate freezing.

The use of terms such as 'ambient conditions' or 'room temperature' is unacceptable.

There should be a direct linkage between the label statement and the demonstrated stability characteristics of the drug product.

Annex 1: Glossary and Information

The following terms have been in general use and the following definitions are provided to facilitate interpretation of the guideline.

Accelerated testing: studies designed to increase the rate of chemical degradation or physical change of an active drug substance or drug product by using exaggerated storage conditions as part of the formal, definitive, storage programme. These data, in addition to long term stability studes, may also be used to assess longer term chemical effects at nonaccelerated conditions and to evaluate the impact of short term excursions outside the label storage conditions such as might occur during shipping. Results from accelerated testing studies are not always predictive of physical changes.

Active substance; *active ingredient*; *drug substance*; *medicinal substance*: the unformulated drug substance which may be subsequently formulated with excipients to produce the drug product.

Bracketing: the design of a stability schedule so that at any time point only the samples on the extremes, for example of container size and/or dosage strengths, are tested. The design assumes that the stability of the intermediate condition samples are represented by those at the extremes. Where a range of dosage strengths is to be tested, bracketing designs may be particularly applicable if the strengths are very closely related in composition (e.g., for a tablet range made with different compression weights of a similar basic granulation, or a capsule range made by filling different plug fill weights of the same basic composition into different size capsule shells). Where a range of sizes of immediate containers are to be evaluated, bracketing designs may be applicable if the material of composition of the container and the type of closure are the same throughout the range.

Climatic zones: the concept of dividing the world into four zones based on defining the prevalent annual climatic conditions.

Dosage form; *preparation*: a pharmaceutical product type, for example tablet, capsule, solution, cream etc. that contains a drug ingredient generally, but not necessarily, in association with excipients.

Drug product; *finished product*: the dosage form in the final immediate packaging intended for marketing.

Excipient: anything other than the drug substance in the dosage form.

Expiry/expiration date: the date placed on the container/labels of a drug product designating the time during which a batch of the product is expected to remain within the approved shelf-life specification if stored under defined conditions, and after which it must not be used.

Formal (systematic) studies: formal studies are those undertaken to a pre-approval stability protocol which embraces the principles of these guidelines.

Long term (*real time*) *testing*: stability evaluation of the physical, chemical, biological and microbiological characteristics of a drug product and a drug substance, covering the expected duration of the shelf life and re-test period, which are claimed in the submission and will appear on the labeling.

Mass balance; *material balance*: the process of adding together the assay value and levels of degradation products to see how closely these add up to 100 per cent of the initial value, with due consideration of the margin of analytical precision. This concept is a useful scientific guide for evaluating data but it is not achievable in all circumstances. The focus may instead be on assuring the specificity of the assay, the completeness of the investigation of routes of degradation, and the use, if necessary, of identified degradants as indicators of the extent of degradation via particular mechanisms.

Matrixing: the statistical design of a stability schedule so that only a fraction of the total number of samples are tested at any specified sampling point. At a subsequent sampling point, different sets of samples of the total number would be tested. The design assumes that the stability of the samples tested represents the stability of all samples. The differences in the samples for the same drug product should be identified as, for example, covering different batches, different strengths, different sizes of the same container and closure and possibly in some cases different container/closure systems.

Matrixing can cover reduced testing when more than one variable is being evaluated. Thus the design of the matrix will be dictated by the factors needing to be covered and evaluated. This potential complexity precludes inclusion of specific details and examples, and it may be desirable to discuss design in advance with the Regulatory Authority, where this is possible. In every case it is essential that all batches are tested initially and at the end of the long term testing.

Mean kinetic temperature: when establishing the mean value of the temperature, the formula of J. D. Haynes (*J. Pharm. Sci.* 60, 927–929, 1971) can be used to calculate the mean kinetic temperature. It is higher than the arithmetic mean temperature and takes into account the Arrhenius equation from which Haynes derived his formula.

New molecular entity; *new active substance*: a substance which has not previously been registered as a new drug substance with the national or regional authority concerned.

Pilot plant scale: the manufacture of either drug substance or drug product by a procedure fully representative of and simulating that to be applied on a full manufacturing scale. For oral solid dosage forms this is generally taken to be at a minimum scale of one tenth that of full production or 100,000 tablets or capsules, whichever is the larger.

Primary stability data: data on the drug substance stored in the proposed packaging under storage conditions that support the proposed re-test date. Data on the drug product stored in the proposed container-closure for marketing under storage conditions that support the proposed shelf life.

Re-test date: the date when samples of the drug substance should be re-examined to ensure that material is still suitable for use.

Re-test period: the period of time during which the drug substance can be considered to remain within the specification and therefore acceptable for use in the manufacture of a given drug product, provided that it has been stored under the defined conditions; after this period, the batch should be retested for compliance with specification and then used immediately.

Shelf life; expiration dating period: the time interval that a drug product is expected to remain within the approved shelf-life specification provided that it is stored under the conditions defined on the label in the proposed containers and closure.

Specification—release: the combination of physical, chemical, biological and microbiological test requirements that determine a drug product is suitable for release at the time of its manufacture.

Specification—check/shelf-life: the combination of physical, chemical, biological and microbiological test requirements that a drug substance must meet up to its re-test date or a drug product must meet throughout its shelf life.

Storage conditions tolerances: the acceptable variation in temperature and relative humidity of storage facilities.

The equipment must be capable of controlling temperature to a range of ±2°C and Relative Humidity to ±5% RH. The actual temperatures and humidities should be monitored during stability storage. Short term spikes due to opening of doors of the storage facility are accepted as unavoidable. The effect of excursions due to equipment failure should be addressed by the applicant and reported if judged to impact stability results. Excursions that exceed these ranges (i.e. ±2°C and/or ±5 percent RH) for more than 24 hours should be described in the study report and their impact assessed.

Stress testing (drug product): light testing should be an integral part of stress testing. Special test conditions for specific products (e.g., metered dose inhalations and creams and emulsions) may require additional stress studies.

Stress testing (drug substance): these studies are undertaken to elucidate intrinsic stability characteristics. Such testing is part of the development strategy and is normally carried out under more severe conditions than those used for accelerated tests. Stress testing is conducted to provide data on forced decomposition products and decomposition mechanisms for the drug substance. The severe conditions that may be encountered during distribution can be covered by stress testing of definitive batches of drug substance.

These studies should establish the inherent stability characteristics of the molecule, such as the degradation pathways, and lead to identification of degradation products and hence support the suitability of the proposed analytical procedures. The detailed nature of the studies will depend on the individual drug substance and type of drug product.

This testing is likely to be carried out on a single batch of material and to include the effect of temperatures in 10°C increments above the accelerated temperature test condition (e.g., 50°C, 60°C, etc.) humidity where appropriate (e.g., 75 percent or greater); oxidation and photolysis on the drug substance plus its susceptibility to hydrolysis across a wide range of pH values when in solution or suspension.

Results from these studies will form an integral part of the information provided to regulatory authorities.

Light testing should be an integral part of stress testing. [The standard conditions for light testing are still under discussion and will be considered in a further ICH document].

It is recognized that some degradation pathways can be complex and that under forcing conditions decomposition products may be observed which are unlikely to be formed under accelerated or long term testing. This information may be useful in developing and validating suitable analytical methods, but it may not always be necessary to examine specifically for all degradation products, if it has been demonstrated that in practice these are not formed.

Supporting stability data: Data other than primary stability data, such as stability data on early synthetic route batches of drug substance, small scale batches of materials, investigational formulations not proposed for marketing, related formulations, product presented in containers and/or closures other than those proposed for marketing, information regarding test results on containers, and other scientific rationale that support the analytical procedures, the proposed re-test period or shelf life and storage conditions.

APPENDIX C.3.   1987 FDA STABILITY GUIDELINE

GUIDELINE FOR SUBMITTING DOCUMENTATION
FOR THE STABILITY OF HUMAN DRUGS AND BIOLOGICS.

I.   INTRODUCTION
This guideline provides:
-Recommendations for the design of stability studies to establish
appropriate expiration dating period(s) and product storage
requirements (Section II).

Recommendations for submission of stability information and data
to the Center for Drugs and Biologics (CDB) for investigational
new drugs (IND's) and biologics (Section III), new drug
applications (NDA's) (Section IV) and biological product
licence applications (PLA's) (Section V).

The guideline is issued under 21 CFR 10.90.   An applicant may rely
upon the guideline in submitting documentation for the stability of
human drugs and biologics, or may follow a different approach.   When
a different approach is chosen, a person is encouraged to discuss
the matter in advance with the Food and Drug Administration (FDA) to
prevent the expenditure of money and effort on preparing a
submission that may later be determined to be unacceptable.

The intention is to provide a means of meeting the regulatory
requirements as listed below

IND's	21 CFR 312.23(a)(7)
NDA's	21 CFR 314.50
ANDA's	21 CFR 314.55
PLA's	21 CFR 312.23(a)(7)
Supplements	21 CFR 314.70

This guideline provides a means of developing expiration dating from at least three different batches of the drug product, in order to ensure a statistically acceptable level of confidence for the period proposed. It is important, however, to realize that the manufacturer is responsible for confirming estimated expiration dating periods by continual assessment of stability properties. Such continuing confirmation of the expiration dating period should be an important consideration in the manufacturer's stability program.

II. DEFINITIONS

Accelerated Testing: Studies designed to increase the rate of chemical or physical degradation of a drug substance or drug product by using exaggerated storage conditions. The purpose is to determine kinetic parameters, to predict the tentative expiration dating period. The term "accelerated testing" is often used synonymously with "stress testing."

Approved Stability Study Protocol: The detailed plan described in an approved NDA and applied to generate and analyze acceptable stability data in support of the expiration dating period. May also be used in developing similar data to support an extension of that dating period.

Batch: As defined under 21 CFR 210.3(b)(2), "'Batch' means a specific quantity of a drug or other material that is intended to have uniform character and quality, within specified limits, and is produced according to a single manufacturing order during the same cycle of manufacture."

Bulk Drug Substance: The pharmacologically active component of a drug product before formulation.

Commitment: A signed statement by an applicant of an NDA, an ANDA, or a PLA to conduct (or complete) prescribed studies on commercial production lots after approval of an application. A commitment to obtain data may be accepted in lieu of the data themselves when available data do not cover the full expiration dating period for the specific product/container-closure, but there are sufficient supporting data to predict a favorable outcome with a high degree of confidence (e.g., when an NDA is approved with stability data available only from experimental or pilot lots (not production lots), or when a supplement is approved with data that do not cover the full expiration dating period). A commitment constitutes an agreement to:
-Conduct or complete the desired studies.

-Submit results periodically, as specified by the FDA.

Withdraw from the market any lots found to fall outside the approved specifications for the drug product. If the applicant

has evidence that the deviation is a single occurrence that does
not affect the safety and efficacy of the drug product, the
applicant should immediately discuss it with the reviewing
division and provide justification for the continued
distribution of that batch. The change or deterioration in the
distributed drug product (ED) is required to be reported, as required
under 21 CFR 314.81(b)(1)(ii).

Drug Product: As defined under 21 CFR 210.3(b)(4), "drug product"
means a finished dosage form (e.g., tablet, capsule, solution, etc.)
that contains an active drug ingredient generally, but not
necessarily, in association with inactive ingredients.

Expiration Date: The date placed on the immediate container label
of a drug product that designates the date through which the product
is expected to remain within specifications. If the expiration date
includes only a month and year, it is expected that the product will
meet specifications through the last day of the month.

Expiration Dating Period: The interval that a drug product is
expected to remain within the approved specifications after
manufacture. The expiration dating period is used to establish the
expiration date of individual batches. It may be extended in an
annual report only if the criteria set forth in the approved
stability study protocol are met in obtaining the supporting data.
Otherwise, a supplement requiring FDA approval will be necessary
before the change is made (21 CFR 314.70(b)(2)(ix)).

Lot: As defined under 21 CFR 210.3(b)(10): "'Lot' means a batch,
or a specified identified portion of a batch, having uniform
character and quality within specified limits; or, in the case of a
drug product produced by continuous process, it is a specific
identified amount produced in a unit of time or quantity in a manner
that assures its having uniform character and quality within
specific limits."

Primary Stability Data: Data on the drug product stored in the
proposed container-closure for marketing under storage conditions
that support the proposed expiration date.

Random Sample: A selection of units chosen from a larger population
of such units so that the probability of inclusion of any given unit
in the sample is defined. In a simple random sample each unit has
equal chance of being included. Random samples are usually chosen
with the aid of tables of random numbers found in many statistical
texts.

Stability-Indicating Methodology: Quantitative analytical methods
that are based on the characteristic structural, chemical, or
biological properties of each active ingredient of a drug product,
and that will distinguish each active ingredient from its

degradation products so that the active ingredient content can be accurately measured.

Stability: The capacity of a drug product to remain within specifications established to ensure its identity, strength, quality, and purity.

Strength: A quantitative measure of active ingredient, as well as other ingredients requiring quantitation, such as alcohol and preservatives. (See 21 CFR 210.3(b)(16).)

Stress Testing: See "Accelerated Testing."

Supportive Stability Data: Data other than primary stability data, such as stability data on investigational formulations not proposed for marketing, accelerated studies on the bulk drug substance, published stability data, references to other submissions on file with the agency with appropriate letters of authorization, accelerated studies on the proposed drug product for marketing, information regarding test results on containers, and other scientific rationale that supports the proposed expiration dating period and storage conditions.

Tentative Expiration Dating Period: A provisional expiration dating period determined by projecting results from less than full-term data (such as accelerated studies) using the drug product to be marketed in the proposed container-closure.

III. DESIGN AND INTERPRETATION OF STABILITY STUDIES
The design of the stability protocol should include methodology for determining the stability of the bulk drug substance and drug product and the statistics relating to sampling and data analysis.

The stability-indicating methodology should be validated by the manufacturer (and the accuracy and precision established) and described in sufficient detail to permit validation by FDA laboratories (Ref. 1).

The revision of the NDA regulations in 21CFR Section 314.70(d)(5) should direct more attention to the importance of properly designing a stability study, because only by submitting full shelf-life data from an approved stability protocol can an applicant extend an expiration date without supplemental application.

A. Bulk Drug Substance Profile
Stability information on the drug substance before formulation is valuable in identifying characteristics of the intact molecule that can change under defined storage conditions. When such labile characteristics are found, it is advisable to include those storage conditions in the stability study protocols designed for all drug products of the drug substance.

For the purpose of this guideline, studies to define the Drug Substance Stability Profile need be conducted only once for each new drug substance produced by the same manufacturing process. These studies may also be useful in establishing packaging requirements, storage conditions, and an expiration dating period where required (antibiotics).

Stability studies on the bulk drug substance are needed when adequate stability information is unavailable either from prior studies of from the literature (Ref. 2). A program for the stability assessment might include storage at ambient temperature and under stressed conditions. Stress-testing conditions ordinarily include temperature (e.g., 5°, 50°, and 75°C); humidity, where appropriate (e.g., 75 Percent or greater), and exposure to various wavelengths of electromagnetic radiation (e.g., 190–780 nanometers, i.e., ultraviolet and visible ranges) (Refs 3–6), preferably in open containers where applicable.

It is also suggested that the following conditions be evaluated in stability studies on solutions or suspensions of the bulk drug substances:
-Acidic and alkaline pH.

-High oxygen atmosphere.

-The presence of added substances under consideration for product formulation.

It is important to detect, isolate, and identify degradation products. Degradation products should be quantified and the reaction kinetics established, if practicable.

B. Drug Products.
Stability studies on samples prepared under conditions simulating production of the finished drug product, and contained in the market package stored at the temperature stated on the label, and are required to support assignment of an expiration date. Stress testing of the drug product is frequently used to identify potential problems that may be encountered during storage and transportation and to provide an estimate of the expiration-dating period. Other special studies may be of value for specific drug products (see III.B.6.a-m, below).

When designing stability studies, the following should be considered:

1. Container-Closure
    Stability data should be developed for each type of immediate container-closure proposed for marketing the drug

product that differs in composition from other container-closures or design (e.g., wall thickness for plastic container, torque, etc.), including child-resistant and tamper-resistant closures, regardless of similarities in cap liners. Physicians' samples should also be included in the stability studies if their container-closure is different from the market package. The possibility of interaction between drug and container-closure and the introduction of leachables into drug formulations during storage should be assessed by sensitive procedures, quantitative when practicable. This is necessary even if the container-closure meets suitability tests, such as those outlined in the United States Pharmacopeia (U.S.P.) for plastic containers and rubber or plastic closures.

For most solid-dosage drug products, stability data need only be obtained for the smallest and the largest container-closure to be marketed, provided that any intermediate size container-closure is of identical composition. Stability data should, however, be submitted for all sizes of multiple-unit containers such as parenterals, aerosols, etc. (see separate entries under II.B.6 for details).

Where package container sealant integrity is to be assessed in the study protocol, higher than 75 percent relative humidity at 37°C may be appropriate to stress its adhesive properties (e.g. blister units and strip packages).

2. Extreme Temperature Fluctuations
A study of the effects of temperature fluctuations as appropriate for the shipping and storage conditions of the drug products should be considered (i.e. the packaged drug product should be cycled through temperature conditions that simulate the changes that may be encountered once the drug product is in distribution).

3. Storage Temperatures
The actual storage temperatures (numerical) used during stability studies should be specified.

4. Microbial Quality
Drug products containing preservatives to control microbial contamination should have the preservative content monitored at least at the beginning and end of the projected expiration dating period of the drug product. This may be accomplished by performing microbial challenge tests (e.g., Antimicrobial Preservatives Effectiveness test of the U.S.P., which is applicable to unopened containers) or by performing chemical assays for the preservative. When the lower specification level of preservative needed to achieve

effective microbial control has been determined, chemical assays may be adequate provided that periodic challenge tests are performed (Ref. 7). It is particularly important to consider the adequacy of the preservative system under conditions of use for multiple-use containers (e.g., parenterals, syrups, suspension, etc.) (Ref. 8).

Nonsterile preparations that require control of the microbial quality and that do not contain preservatives should be tested at specific intervals throughout the projected expiration dating period according to the release specification for bioburden (e.g., Microbial Limits Tests of the U.S.P.). In addition, it is recommended that topical preparations also be tested for the presence of topical pathogens that may be identified as potentially harmful (e.g, Pseudomonas cepacia, Aspergillus niger and Candida albicans). Simulated use tests on topical preparations packaged in jars and on opthalmics are desirable.

5. Degradation Products
    When degradation products are detected, the following information about them should be submitted when available:
-   Identity and chemical structure.

-   Cross-reference to any available information about biological effect and significance at the concentrations likely to be encountered.

    Procedure for isolation and purification.

    Mechanism of formation, including order of reaction (see II.C.1.c, below)

-   Physical and chemical properties.

-   Spedifications and directions for testing for their presence at the levels or concentrations expected to be present.

-   Indication of pharmacological action or inaction.

6. Generally Acceptable Design Considerations for Specific Drug Products
a. Tablets: A stability study should include tests for the following characteristics of the tablet: Appearance, friability, hardness, color, odor, moisture, strength and dissolution.

b. Capsules: A stability study should include tests for the following characteristics: Strength, moisture,

color, appearance, shape brittleness, and dissolution.
[For soft gelatin capsules, the fill medium should be
examined for precipitate, cloudiness, and pH.]

c. Emulsions: The following characteristics should be
examined: Appearance (such as phase separation), color,
odor, pH, viscosity, and strength. Storage on the side
or inverted is suggested for assessment of the closure
systems. It is recommended that a heating/cooling cycle
be employed (e.g. between 4° and 45°C) (Refs. 9 and
10).

d. Oral solutions and suspensions: The following
characteristics should be examined: appearance
(precipitate, cloudiness), strength, pH, color, odor,
redispersibility, dissolution (suspensions), and clarity
(solutions). Liquids and suspensions should be stored
on their side or inverted in order to determine whether
contact of the drug product with the closure system
affects product integrity.

After storage, samples of suspensions should be prepared for assay
(ED)according to the recommended labeling.

e. Oral powders: Most oral powders are marketed for
reconstitution prior to administration. The following
characteristics of the powder should be examined:
Appearance, strength, color, odor, and moisture. The
reconstituted product should be prepared according to
the recommended labeling. Specific characteristics to
be examined on the reconstituted material should
include: Appearance, pH, dispersibility, and strength
throughout the recommended storage period.

f. Metered-dose inhalation aerosols: Characteristics that
should be examined in a stability study for all
container-closure sizes include the following:
Strength, delivery dose per actuation, number of
(metered) doses, color, clarity (solutions), particle
size distribution (suspension), loss of propellant,
pressure, valve corrosion, and spray pattern (Ref. 11).

Because the container contents are under pressure,
filled containers must be checked for weight loss over
the expiration dating period. For suspensions,
aggregate (or solvate) formation may lead to clogged
valves or to the delivery of a pharmacologically
inactive dose. Corrosion of the metering valve or
gasket deterioration may adversely affect the delivery
of the correct amount of drug substance.

If the drug product is intended for use in the
respiratory system it is important to confirm that the
initial release specifications are maintained to assure
the absence of pathogenic organisms (e.g.,
Staphylococcus aureus, Pseudomonas aeroginosa,
Escherichia coli, and Salmonella species) and the total
microbial limit per cannister.

g. Topical and ophthalmic preparations: Included in this
broad category are ointments, creams, lotions, pastes,
gels, solutions, and nonmeterd aerosols for application
to the skin.   For stability studies of topical
ointments, creams, lotions, solutions, and gels, the
following characteristics should be examined, as
appropriate to the drug product:

Appearance, clarity, color, homogeneity,
odor, pH, resuspendibility (lotions), consistency,
particle size distribution, strength and weight loss
(plastic containers).

Ointments, pastes and creams, in containers larger than
3.5 grams, should be assayed by sampling at the surface,
middle, and bottom of the container.   In addition, tubes
should be sampled near the crimp.

Evaluation of nonmetered aerosols should include the
following: Appearance, odor, strength, pressure, weight
loss, net weight dispensed, delivery rate, and spray
pattern.

Evaluation of ophthalmic preparations (e.g. creams,
ointments, solutions, and suspensions) should include
the following as appropriate to the drug product:
Appearance, odor, consistency, pH, resuspendibility,
particle size, homogeneity (suspensions), creams and
ointments), strength, and sterility.

h. Small-volume parenterals (SVP's): SVP's include an
extremely wide range of preparations and container-
closures, all of which should be included in the
stability study.   Evaluation of these drug products
should include at least the following: Strength,
appearance, color, particulate matter, pH, sterility,
and pyrogenicity (at reasonable intervals).   Stability
studies on powder products should demonstrate that the
residual moisture content remains within acceptable
limits and that the product is stable throughout the
recommended storage period.

The stability of reconstituted products should also be determined after they are constituted according to the recommended labeling. Specific parameters to be examined at appropriate intervals throughout the maximum intended use period of the constituted drug product, stored under condition(s) recommended in labeling, should include: Appearance, odor, color, pH, strength, dispersibility, and particulate matter.

Continued assurance of sterility for all sterile products may be assessed by a variety of means, including evaluation of the container-closure integrity by appropriate challenge test(s), testing for preservatives (if present), and/or sterility testing.

For terminally sterilized drug products, a specification for maximum process parameters should be provided. Stability studies should evaluate and support the adequacy of the maximum release specification for process lethality (e.g., F_0, Mrads, etc.).

Parenterals (except ampules) should be stored inverted or on their sides in order to determine, by comparison, whether contact of the drug product or solvent with the closure system affects product integrity or results in leaching of chemical substances from the closure material.

i. Large-volume parenterals (LVP's): Stability tests for LMP's are similar to those for SVP's. A minimum evaluation should include the following: Strength, appearance, color, clarity, particulate matter (U.S.P. or equivalent), pH, volume (plastic containers), extractables (plastic containers), sterility, and pyrogenicity (at reasonable intervals).

Continued assurance of sterility for all sterile products may be assessed by a variety of means, including evaluation of the container-closure integrity by appropriate challenge test(s), by testing for preservatives (if present), or by sterility testing.

These products should be stored with some inverted and some on their sides in order to determine whether contact of the drug product or solvent with the container-closure system affects product integrity, or results in leaching of chemical substances from the container-closure material.

j. Suppositories: Suppositories should be evaluated for strength, softening range, appearance, and dissolution.

The effect of aging may also be observed from a
hardening of the suppository and a polymorphic
transformation of the drug substance; therfore, control
and stability testing should include dissolution time at
37°C.

k. Drug additive: For any drug product that is intended
    for use as an additive to another drug product, the
    possibility of incompatibilities exists. In such cases,
    the drug product labeled to be administered by addition
    to another drug product (e.g., parenterals, aerosols)
    should be studied for stability and compatibility in
    admixture with the other drug product.

    A suggested stability protocol should provide for tests
    to be conducted at 0-, 6-to 8-, and 24-hour intervals,
    or as appropriate over the intended use period. These
    should include:
    - Assay of the drug product and additive.
    - pH (especially for unbuffered LVP's), color,
       clarity.
    - Particulate matter.
    - Interaction with the container.

l. Intrauterine devices and vaginal devices regulated as
    drugs
    Stability testing for intrauterine devices (IUD's)
    should include the following tests: Deflection of
    horizontal arms or other parts of the frame if it is not
    a T-shaped device (frame memory), tensile strength of
    the withdrawal string, and integrity of the package
    (i.e., seal strength of the pouch and sterility of the
    device).

    If the device contains a drug substance reservoir from
    which drug substance diffuses through a
    controlled-release membrane, it should be tested for
    total drug substance content, decomposition products,
    and in vitro drug product release rate in addition to
    the above tests.

    Vaginal devices such as doughnut-shaped silastic or
    other polymeric matrix containing a drug product
    uniformly dispensed through the matrix must be
    checked for in vitro drug product release rate and
    extraneous extractable substances to establish stability
    and drug product compatibility with the matrix.

m. Biological products: In addition to other parameters
    described for specific drug products, it is required for
    biological products that potency be a measure of

biological activity. Generally, the official potency
test (21 CFR Parts 600-680), or the potency test
described in the manufacturer's approved licence
application for a given product, will be adequate for
potency determination.

C. Statistical Considerations

Under 21 CFR 314.69(d)(5), a new drug applicant may take certain
actions on the basis of an approved stability study protocol,
such as extending an expiration dating period based on full
shelf-life data without prior approval of a supplemental
application by including the change in the next annual report
under §314.81(b)(2). A stability study protocol must describe
not only how the stability study is to be designed and carried out,
but also the statistical methods to be used in analyzing
the data. An acceptable approach is described in part 2,
below. If the sponsor wishes to use an alternative statistical
procedure, it must be described in the stability study
protocol. Part 1 of this section describes specific design
features of stability studies that are pertinent to the
statistical analysis.

1. ## Design Considerations for Long-Term Studies under Ambient
   Conditions (Nonaccelerated Data)

   The design of a stability study is intended to establish,
   based on testing a limited number of batches of a drug
   product, an expiration dating period applicable to all
   future batches of the drug product manufactured under
   similar circumstances. this approach assumes that
   inferences drawn from this small group of tested batches
   extend to all future batches. Tested batches must,
   therefore, be representative in all respects, (e.g.,
   formulation, container-closure system, manufacturing
   process, age of bulk material, etc.) of the population of
   all production batches of that drug product and conform with
   all quality specifications.

   The design of a stability study should take into
   consideration the variability of individual dosage units, of
   containers within a batch, and of batches, in order to
   ensure that the resulting data for each batch are truly
   representative of the batch as a whole and to quantify the
   variability from batch to batch. The degree of variability
   affects the confidence one might have in the ability of a
   future batch to remain within specifications until its
   expirations date.

   a. Batch sampling considerations: Ideally, the batches
      selected for stability studies should constitute a
      random sample from the population of production
      batches. In practice, the batches tested to establish

the expiration dating period are usually the first batches produced, but sometimes they may be research or pilot scale batches. If research or pilot scale batches are used, they should have the same characteristics as production scale batches, including the relative proportions of active and inactive ingredients. It is possible that future changes in the production process will result in the obsolence of the initial stability study conclusions.

At least three batches and preferably more should be tested to allow for some estimate of batch-to-batch variability and to test the hypothesis that a single expiration dating period for all batches is justifiable.

Testing of a single batch does not permit assessment of batch-to-batch variability, and testing of two batches provides an unreliable estimate. Although it is true that more data (batches) result in a more precise estimate, practical considerations prevent unlimited collection of data. The specification that at least three batches be tested is a minimum requirement representing a compromise between statistical and practical considerations.

b. Container-closure and drug product sampling considerations: Selection of containers (bottles, packages, vials, etc.) from the batches chosen for inclusion in the stability study should be carried out so as to ensure that the samples chosen represent the batch as a whole. This may be accomplished by taking a random sample of containers from the finished batch, by using a plan whereby at a random starting point every nth container is taken from the assembly line (n is chosen so the sample is spread over the whole batch), or by some other plan designed to ensure an unbiased selection.

Samples to be assayed at a given sampling time are to be taken from previously unopened containers. For this reason, at least as many containers must be sampled as the number of sampling times in the stability study. In any case, sampling of at least two containers for each sampling time is encouraged.

As a rule, dosage units from a given container should be sampled randomly, with each dosage unit having an equal chance to be included in the sample. If it is believed that the individual units entered the container randomly, then sampling of the units at the opening of the container is acceptable. With large containers, because dosage units near the cap of a bottle may have different stability properties than dosage units in other parts of the container, it may be desirable to sample dosage units from all parts of the container. (For dosage units sampled in this fashion, the location within the container from which they were taken should be identified and this information included with the results.)

Composites may be assayed instead of individual units. If more than one container is sampled at a given sampling time, an equal number of units from each container may be combined into the composite. It is suggested that the same type of composite be used throughout the stability study, e.g. if 20-tablet composites are tested initially, then 20-tablet composites should be used throughout. If it is desired to have a larger sample at a given sampling time, replicated 20-tablet composites would be assayed, not a single assay of a composite made from more than 20 tablets.

If composites are used, their makeup should be described in the stability report.

c. <u>Sampling-time considerations</u>: The sample times should be chosen so that any degradation can be adequately characterized (i.e., at a sufficient frequency to determine with reasonable assurance the nature of the degradation curve.) Usually, the relationship can be adequately represented by a linear, quadratic, or cubic function on an arithmetic or a logarithmic scale (Section III.B.6).

Stability testing generally may be done at 3-month intervals during the first year, 6-month intervals during the second, and yearly thereafter. For drug products predicted to degrade rapidly (e.g., certain radiopharmaceuticals), more frequent sampling is necessary.

The degradation curve is estimated most precisely (in terms of the width of the confidence intervals about the estimated curve, as illustrates in Fig. 1) around the average of the sampling times included in the study. Therefore, testing an increased number of replicates at the later sampling times, particularly the latest sampling time, is encouraged, because it will increase the average sampling time toward the desired expiration dating period.

2. Data Analysis and Interpretation: Long-Term Studies
    The methods described in this section are used to establish,
    with a high degree of confidence, an expiration dating
    period during which the average drug product characteristic
    (e.g., strength) of the batch will remain within
    specifications. This expiration dating period should be
    applicable to all future batches produced by the
    manufacturing process for the drug product. It is not
    sufficient that a proposed expiration dating period ensure
    that the process average is within specifications, if a
    substantial number of individual batch averages are out of
    specifications at the end of the proposed expiration dating
    period.

    If an applicant chose an expiration dating period to ensure
    that the characteristics of a large proportion of the
    individual dosage units are within specifications, different
    statistical methods than those proposed below would be
    needed. For example, see Easterling (Ref. 12). Also, it
    would be necessary to test individual units rather than
    composites. However, as noted before, the following
    represents an acceptable approach.

a. Determining the allowable expiration dating period for
    an individual batch: The time during which a batch may
    be expected to remain within specifications depends not
    only on the degradation rate, but also on the initial
    average value for the batch. Thus any information on
    the initial value for the batch, such as the results of
    release testing on that batch, is relevant to the
    determination of the allowable expiration dating period
    and should be included in the stability study report.
    Also, percent of label claim, not percent of initial
    average value, is the variable of interest.

    When establishing the expiration-dating period for an
    individual batch, support is obtained from the observed
    pattern of degradation for the quantitative drug product
    characteristic under study (e.g., strength) and to the
    precision by which it is estimated. An acceptable
    approach for drug characteristics that are expected to
    decrease with time is to determine the time at which the
    95% one-sided lower confidence limit (sometimes called
    the 95% lower confidence bound) for the mean degradation
    curve intersects the acceptable lower specification
    limit.

    Carstensen and Nelson (ref. 13) proposed an approach
    equally acceptable to this, and the 95% lower confidence limit
    for the mean is described in their paper and is
    illustrated in their Figure 1, labeled Roman Numeral I.

Note, however, that Carstensen and Nelson proposed that the expiration dating period be determined on the basis of a different curve (the so-called "prediction limit," labeled Roman Numeral II in their Figure 1) than is proposed here. In the example shown in our Figure 1 (where the lower specification limit is assumed to be 90% of label claim) an expiration dating period of four years would be granted. For drug product characteristics expected to increase with time (e.g., there may be an upper limit on the amount of certain degradation products), the 95% one-sided upper confidence limit for the mean would be used.

For drug product characteristics with both an upper and lower specification limit, there may be special cases where it would be appropriate to use the two-sided 95% confidence limits. As an example, suppose the drug characteristic of interest was concentration of unchanged active ingredient for a solution. Chemical degradation of the active ingredient would decrease the concentration. On the other hand, evaporation of the solvent (possibly resulting from the characteristics of the closure) would increase the concentration. Since both possibilities must be allowed for, two-sided confidence limits would be appropriate. (If both mechanisms were acting, however, the concentration might decrease initially and then increase. In this case, the degradation pattern would not be linear and more complicated statistical methods would be needed.)

If the approach of this section is used, we may be 95% confident that the average drug product characteristic (e.g. strength) of the dosage units in the batch is within specifications up to the end of the expiration dating period. It is not acceptable to determine the allowable expiration dating period by determining where the fitted least-squares line intersects the appropriate specification limit. This approach is as likely to overestimate the expiration dating period as to underestimate it (i.e., we may only be 50% confident that the batch average is within specifications at expiration if the fitted least-squares line is used).

The statistical assumptions underlying the procedures described above (e.g., the assumption that the variability of the individual units from the batch average remains constant over the several sampling times) are well known and have been discussed in numerous statistical texts. The above procedures will remain valid even when these assumptions are mildly violated. If there is evidence of severe violation of

the assumptions in the data, an alternate approach may
be necessary to accomplish the objective of determining
an allowable expiration dating period with a high degree
of confidence that the period does not overestimate the
true time during which the drug product remains within
specifications.

There may be cases where the data show so little
degradation and so little variability that it is
apparent from looking at the data that the requested
expiration dating period will be confirmed.   Under these
circumstances it would not be necessary to go through
The formal calculations involved in the above analysis.
However, this case is the exception rather than the
rule, and the final judgment on whether the calculations
are necessary lies with the reviewers in the CDB.
Consequently, failure to include the results of the
analysis described above could result in a delay of the
stability review, if the reviewers feel that the
calculations are needed.   Therefore, it is recommended
that the analyses be carried out routinely.

LONG-TERM STABILITY STUDY

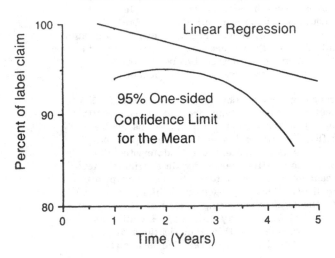

GUIDELINES FIGURE 1

b. Determining the expiration dating period based on the
Information from all of the batches: If bateh-to-batch
variability is small (i.e. the relationship between the
drug product characteristic of interest; e.g., strength
and time is essentially the same from batch to batch),
it would be advantageous to combine the data into one

overall estimate. Combining the data should be
supported by preliminary testing of batch similarity.
The similarity of the degradation curves for each batch
tested should be assessed by applying statistical tests
of equality of slopes and of zero time intercepts.
The level of significance of the tests should be chosen
so that the decision to combine is made only if there is
strong evidence in favor of combining. Bancroft and his
co-workers (Ref. 14) have recommended a level of
significance of 0.25 for preliminary statistical tests
similar to this. If the tests for equality of slopes
and for equality of intercepts do not result in
rejection at a level of significance of 0.25, the data
from the batches would be pooled. If these tests
resulted in p-values less than 0.25, a judgment would be
made by the CDB reviewers as to whether pooling would be
permitted.

If the preliminary statistical test rejects the
hypothesis of batch similarity because of unequal
initial intercept values, it may still be possible to
establish that the lines are parallel (i.e., the slopes
are equal), and in this case the data may be combined
for purpose of estimating the common slope. The
individual allowable expiration dating period for each
batch in the stability study may then be determined by
considering the initial values, using appropriate
statistical methodology. If data from several batches
may be combined, it is advantageous to include as many
batches as feasible, because confidence limits about the
estimated degradation curve will become narrower as the
number of batches increases, usually resulting in
longer allowable expiration dating period.

If it is inappropriate to combine data from several
batches, the overall expiration dating period may depend
on the minimum time a batch may be expected to remain
within acceptable limits.

3. Precautions to Be Observed in Extrapolation Beyond the
   Actual Data Period.
   The statistical methods for determining an expiration dating
   period beyond the range of storage times actually observed
   are the same as for determining an expiration period within
   the observed range. However, the a priori correctness of
   the assumed pattern of degradation as a function of time
   is crucial in the case of extrapolation beyond the observed
   range.

When estimating an assumed degradation line or curve over
the observed range of data, the data themselves provide a

check on the correctness of the assumed relationship, and
statistical methods may be available to test the goodness of
fit of the data to the assumed degradation line or curve.
No such internal check is available beyond the range of
observed data.

As an example, suppose it has been assumed that the
relationship between log strength and time is a straight
line, but in fact the true relationship is a curve. It may
be that over the range of the observed data, the true curve
is close enough to a straight line so that no serious error
is made by approximating the degradation relationship as a
straight line. However, between the last observed data
points and the estimated expiration time, the true curve may
diverge from a straight line enough to have an important
effect on the estimated expiration time.

For extrapolation beyond the observed range to be valid, the
assumed degradation relationship must continue to apply
through the estimated expiration dating period. Thus, an
expiration dating period granted on the basis of
extrapolation should always be verified by actual stability
data up to the granted expiration time as soon as these data become
available.

D. Alternate Stability Study Protocol.
If for any stated reason the approach proposed in these
guidelines is not suitable for the new drug or biological
product under development, a different stability study protocol
should be designed by the sponsor during clinical phases of
phases of investigation (Section III.C.1). The sponsor should ensure
that the stability protocol is acceptable to the CDB reviewers.

IV. INVESTIGATIONAL NEW DRUGS (IND's)
Studies conducted during development of a drug or biological product
do not necessarily follow a rigid separation into Phases 1, 2 and
3, but the following is presented as a general IND development
sequence that is intended to provide guidance for the development of
product stability information during the investigational phases:

A. IND Phase I
The stability characteristics of the bulk drug substances should
be determined at the earliest possible time to support
conditions of use of the bulk drug in toxicity studies (i.e.,
pre-IND studies, mixed with feed, etc.) and the stability of the
drug substance in the initial formulations proposed for use in
clinical pharmacological studies. This information should be
included in the initial IND submission to FDA. Required
stability information would be limited to that needed to

demonstrate that the clinical product would be stable for the
duration of the investigation. If necessary, additional data
may be submitted as they become available during the course of
the clinical study.

B. IND Phase 2.
Stability studies on the investigational formulations should be
well underway by the end of Phase 2.

Drug product or biological formulations developed during Phase 2
(as well as Phase 3) should be based upon the stability
information developed from studies on the bulk drug substance or
on the stability of formulations prepared in experimental
studies. The objectives of stability testing during Phases 1
and 2 are (a) to evaluate the stability of the investigational
formulations used in the clinical trails and (b) to obtain the
additional information needed to develop a final formulation
(e.g. compatibility studies of potential interactive effects
between the drug substance(s) and other components of the
system. This information should be summarized and submitted to
the IND when available.

C. IND Phase 3.
The emphasis in stability testing during Phase 3 is on final
formulations in their probable market packaging, on expiration
dating, and on the study of degradation products when
encountered. Studies to support the proposed expiration dating
period should be completed, where possible, during Phase 3 for
inclusion in the initial NDA, or in the PLA for biological
products.

V. NEW DRUG APPLICATIONS (NDA's)
A. Original Submissions.
Ordinarily, an original NDA submission should contain primary
stability data that, when subjected to appropriate statistical
analysis (Figure 1), support the proposed expiration dating
period. Also, other supportive stability data must clearly
substantiate the time period assigned and the proposed storage
conditions for labeling. This must be accompanied by the
standard commitment to continue the stability study. (See
"Commitment" in Section II.) As a condition for approval, it is
expected that samples of the first three commercial production
lots will be placed in the stability program for the full length
of the expiration dating period for confirmation of the dating
period assigned.

A full report on stability of the bulk drug substance should
provide information outlined in Sections II.A and II.B.5 of the
guidelines on general stability characteristics and degradation
products.

Stability studies conducted for all formulations used during
clinical investigations should be summarized as described in the
introductory paragraph of Section III, in paragraphs B and C of
that section, and in Section VII of these guidelines.

The lots used for stability testing should comply <u>fully</u> with
proposed specifications for the product in its market package.
Studies to support an expiration dating period, under defined
storage conditions using several lots representative of the
product to be marketed, should have been started as
early as possible prior to the NDA.

Because a reviewer cannot make any comparisons with data
contained in another application, stability data submitted must
be complete within themselves.

If an alternate facility is contemplated prior to approval of an
NDA, refer to Section V.D.3.

B. Computation of Expiration Data
The computation of the expiration date of the new drug
production lot in its market package should begin at the time of
quality control release of that lot, and the date of such
release should generally not exceed 30 days from the production
date, regardless of the packaging date.

If the production lot contains reprocessed material, the
expiration dating period should be computed from the date of
manufacture of the oldest reprocessed lot that was made to
conform to the quality standards for identity, strength,
quality, and purity specified in the NDA.
In general proper statistical analysis of long-term stability
data collected as recommended in Section III.C.1.a, and as
exemplified in Figure 1, must support at least a 1-year
expiration period.

C. Abbreviated New Drug Applications (ANDA's)
For drug products that have been approved for marketing under an
ANDA, information such as stress testing, reference to
publications or other sources that describe the stability
profile of the drug substance, and comparative stability data
for the proposed drug product and of the innovator's drug
product, (especially when the comparative data are utilized in
bioavailability/bioequivalence studies) is acceptable.

In the absence of sufficient data at the proposed storage
condition, stress testing will be accepted for the grant of a
tentative expiration dating period, provided adequate
information concerning stability of the drug substance has been
submitted. The recommended stress testing conditions are:

- 40°C, or as appropriate for a particular drug product.
- 75 percent humidity (where appropriate).

Samples should be analyzed initially and at 1, 2, and 3 months. The parameters described under Section III.B. should be considered when collecting stability data for various drug products. Available long-term stability data should be included and reported as outlined in Section VII of the guideline.

If the results are satisfactory, a tentative expiration dating period of up to 24 months may be granted.

When an alternate facility is contemplated prior to approval of an ANDA, refer to Section V.D.3.

The submission should also include the following commitments:
1. The first three commercial production lots of the product will be placed on stability testing as specified in Section II.C.6. Testing at the recommended storage conditions should be done, initially, at 3, 6, 9, 12, 18, and 24 months, and yearly thereafter until the desired expiration date of the product is reached. If more than one package size is marketed, the first three commercial production lots of the smallest and the largest size should be tested. Also, if more than one container-closure is used for a particular size, stability data in each container-closure should be submitted. Yearly, thereafter, at least one production batch should be added to the stability program.

2. Results will be submitted in the next period report or as specified by the FDA.

3. Any lots found to fall outside of the approved specifications for the drug product may be withdrawn from the market. Deviations that do not affect the safety and efficiency of the product will be promptly discussed between the applicant and the reviewing division and must be reported to FDA under 21 CFR 314.81(b)(1)(ii). (Also see "Commitment" Definition.)

D. Supplements to New Drug Applications
A supplement may be classified under several categories as indicated below
1. Changes in Formulation, Supplier, and Container-Closure
   A supplement that proposes a change in the drug product's formulation, in the supplier of a drug substance, or in the container-closure for a marketed drug product will usually require the development of data to show that this change does not adversely affect stability. Usually, accelerated data demonstrating compatability with the previously

approved drug product, plus the standard commitment to
continue the stability study, will suffice. For significant
changes of products known to be relatively unstable,
6 months' data at the normal recommended storage
temperature, as well as the data from accelerated
conditions, may also be required.

If the data give no reason to believe that the proposed
change will alter the stability of the product, the
previously approved expiration dating period may be used.

2. Interchangeability of Polyethylene Containers
    A special case is the interchangeability of polyethylene
    containers for capsules and tablets that meet standards and
    tests described in the U.S.P. In this instance, a
    supplement may be approved with no advance stability data,
    provided there is a commitment to do the stability testing
    in accordance with the previously approved stability study
    protocol or as specified by FDA.

3. New Manufacturing Facilities
    For a change limited to a new manufacturing facility for the
    identical drug product using similar equipment, 3 months'
    accelerated data may be needed, depending on the nature of
    the product, the process involved, and the stability data
    previously generated. A commitment should be made to
    conduct stability studies on at least the first three
    commercial production lots on the approved stability
    study protocol. Ordinarily, the already approved expiration
    dating period may be used under these circumstances.

4. Reprocessed Material
    A supplement providing for the use of reprocessed material
    should include data to demonstrate that the reprocessed
    product has identity, strength, quality, and purity
    comparable to that approved in the NDA for the designated
    expiration dating period. Also, the standard commitment to
    continue the stability study should be submitted.

5. New Container Fabricator
    When a new plastic container fabricator is proposed, with no
    change in materials or specifications, the applicant should
    have full specifications for the approved container to
    supply to the new fabricator. The new fabricator should
    submit manufacturing information to the applicant (or
    directly to FDA), and should agree to inform the drug
    product manufacturer immediately of any change in resin
    designation or supplier. The applicant should provide the
    standard commitment to initiate stability studies on at
    least the first three commercial production lots packaged in

the container from the new fabricator. Under these circumstances, accelerated or preliminary stability data are not required, and the already approved expiration dating period may be used.

VI. PRODUCT LICENCE APPLICATION FOR BIOLOGICAL PRODUCTS (PLA's)

A. General Guidelines for Biological Product Stability Studies

The components of biological products are usually protein derivatives or other organic substances. Such substances are usually heat sensitive and require refrigeration or freezing to protect the potency of the product. Therefore, the methodologies and statistical analyses used for determining the stability characteristics and expiration dating period for drug products are not necessarily applicable to biological drug products.

Because of the complexity and variety of the composition of biological products, requirements for determining their stability may differ markedly among different types of products.

Documentation of biological product stability is required for all new biological products and, when significant changes are made for the composition or to the container-closure, for currently approved biologicals. The descriptions that follow offer guidance regarding when stability data are required for biologicals. All proposals and submissions related to biological product stability should either accompany the product licence application in an original submission for licensure or be submitted as an amendment to an existing product licence application. Each submission will be considered on an individual basis depending on the composition and characteristics of the product.

B. Original Submission

1. Studies Submitted with Application

Studies to support the expiration dating period of a biological product using at least three lots representative of the product to be marketed under defined storage conditions should be submitted at the time of licence application filing. These lots should comply fully with proposed specifications for the product in its market package. Stability data from at least three lots are usually required for licensure approval.

2. Supportive Data

The approved expiration dating period of a biological product is normally based upon the interval of time for which data are available under the storage conditions stated in the labeling. Studies that address the stability of the product when in bulk storage (prior to filling) may be considered to support the expiration dating period of the finished drug product. In addition, the effects of temperature extremes that may be encountered during shipment of the product should be determined.

3. Expiration Dating Period Granted with Commitment
    In some instances, the stability data may not cover the full period desired. It is possible to grant the desired expiration dating period provided that all data and information clearly support this conclusion and there is a sufficient lead time for development of data covering the desired expiration dating period. The standard commitment to continue the stability study at the recommended storage condition, also must be submitted for confirmation.

C. Amendments
1. An amendment to an approved PLA that proposes a change in the product's formulation, including, the culture media for growing live organisms or in the container-closure for the marketed product, will usually require the development of data to show that the proposed change has not adversely affected the product's stability. In certain instances, accelerated storage data demonstrating comparability with the previously approved product plus the standard commitment will suffice. For certain biological products that are known to be relatively unstable, this may require a minimum of 6 months' data at the normal recommended storage temperature together with data from accelerated conditions.

2. New Manufacturing Facility
    For a proposed change to a new manufacturing facility for the same licenced product using similar equipment, accelerated data should be submitted, if feasible. A commitment to conduct stability studies on a minimum of the first three lots produced in the new facility should also be submitted. Ordinarily, the previously approved expiration dating period may be used under these circumstances.

3. Extension of Expiration Dating Period
    An amendment requesting an extension in the expiration dating period should be accompanied by supporting updated stability data.

4. Reprocessed Material
    When appropriate, an amendment providing for the use of reprocessed material should include data to ensure that the reprocessed product will meet final product specifications. The standard commitment to subject any lots of the product made from reprocessed material to stability testing should accompany the amendment.

VII. CONTENT OF STABILITY REPORTS
It is suggested that stability reports include the following
information and data to facilitate decisions concerning the
stability proposals:

A. General Product Information
1. Name of drug substance and drug product or biological
   product.

2. Dosage form and strength, including formulation. (The
   application should provide a table of specific formulations
   under study when more than one formulation has been studied.)

3. Labeling

4. Composition, type, and size of container closure.

B. Specifications and Test Methodology Information
1. Physical, chemical, and microbiological characteristics and
   prior submission specifications (or specific references to
   NDA or USP).

2. Test methodology used (or specific reference to NDA, prior
   submissions, or USP) for each sample tested.

3. Information on accuracy, precision, and suitability of the
   methodology (cited by reference to appropriate sections).

4. For biological products, a description of the potency
   test(s) for measuring biological activity, including
   specifications for potency determination.

C. Study Design and Study Conditions
1. Description of the sampling plan, including:
   a. Batches and numbers selected.
   b. Container-closures and number selected.
   c. Number of dosage units selected and whether tests were
      conducted on individual units or on composites of
      individual units.
   d. Sampling times.
   e. Testing of drug or biological products for
      reconstitution at the time of dispensing (as directed on
      the labeling) as well as after they are reconstituted.

2. Expected duration of the study.

3. Conditions of storage of the product under study
   (temperature, humidity, light).

D. Stability Data/Information
1. Lot number (research, pilot, production) and associated
   manufacturing data.

2. For antibiotic drug products, the age of the bulk active drug substance(s) used in manufacturing the lot.

3. Analytical data and source of each data point (e.g., lot, container, composite, etc.). Pooled estimates may be submitted if individual data points are provided.

4. Summary of information on previous formulations obtained during product development maybe (referenced in previously submitted). Summary should include other container-closures investigated.

E. Data Analysis and Conclusions
1. Documentation of appropriate statitical methods and formulas used in the analysis.

2. Evaluation of data, including calculations, statistical analysis, plots or graphs.

3. Results of statistical test used in arriving at microbiological potency estimates.

4. Proposed expiration dating period and its justification.

5. Release specifications (establishment of acceptable minimum potency at the time of initial release for full expiration dating period to be warranted).

References

1. Debesis, E., J. P. Boehlert, T. E. Givand and J. C. Sheridan, "Submitting HPLC methods to the Compendia and Regulatory Agencies," Pharmaceutical Technology, 6(9), 120–137 (1982)

2. Connors, K. A., G. L. Amidon, and L. Kennon, "Chemical Stability of Pharmaceuticals," John Wiley and Sons, New York, 1979

3. Moore, D. E., Journal of Pharmaceutical Sciences, 66, 1282 (1977); 65, 1447 (1976); 72, 180 (1983)

4. Sanvordeker, D. R., Journal of Pharmaceutical Sciences, 65, 1149 (1976)

5. Lachman, L., C. J. Swartz, and J. Cooper, Journal of the American Pharmaceutical Association, 49, 213 (1960)

6. Kaufman, J. E., "IES Lighting Handbook," (1981)

7. Banker, G. S., and C. T. Rhodes, "Modern Pharmaceutics," Marcel Dekker, Inc., New York and Basel, 7, 454 (1979)

8. Cooper, M. S., "Quality Control in the Pharmaceutical Industry," Academic Press, New York, 1, 118 (1972)

9. Lachman, L., H. A. Lieberman and J. L. Kanig, "The Theory and Practice of Industrial Pharmacy," 2nd Edition, Lea and Febiger, Philadelphia, p. 210 (1976)

10. Zografi, G. "Physical Stability Assessment of Emulsions and Related Disperse Systems: A Critical Review," Journal of Society of Cosmetic Chemists, 33, 345−358 (November 1982)

11. Sharmach, R. E., "Dosage Reproducibility of Inhalation Metering Aerosol Drug Dose Delivery System," presented at the American Pharmaceutical Association Meeting, March 31, 1981, St. Louis

12. Easterling, R. G., "Discrimination Intervals for Percentiles in Regression," Journal of the American Statistical Association, 64, 1031−1041 (1969)

13. Carstensen, J. T., and E. Nelson, "Terminology regarding labeled and contained amounts in dosage forms," Journal of Pharmaceutical Sciences, 65, (2): 311−312 (1976)

14. Bancroft, T. A., "Analysis and Inference for Incompletely Specified Models Involving the Use of Preliminary Test(s) of Significance," Biometrics, 20, (3), 427−442 (1964).

References

Anderson, R. L. (1982). Analysis of variance components. Unpublished lecture notes. University of Kentucky, Lexington, Ky.

Bancroft, T. A. (1964). Analysis and inference for incompletely specified models involving the use of preliminary test(s) of significance. *Biometrics*, 20, 427–442.

Barnard, G. A. (1959). Control charts and stochastic process. *J. Roy. Stat. Soc. B*, 21, 239–271.

Baumert, L. D., Golomb, S. W., and Hall, M. J. (1962). Discovery of an Hadamard matrix of order 92. *Bull. Am. Math. Soc.*, 68, 237–238.

Bergum, J. S. (1990). Constructing acceptance limits for multiple stage tests. *Drug Dev. Ind. Pharm.*, 16, 2153–2166.

Berkson, J. (1969). Estimation of a linear function for a calibration line: consideration of a recent proposal. *Technometrics*, 11, 649–660.

Bissell, A. F. (1969). Cusum techniques for quality control. *Appl. Stat.*, 18, 1–30.

Bohidar, N. R. (1983). Statistical aspects of chemical assay validation. *Proceedings of the Biopharmaceutical Section of the American Statistical Association*, pp. 57–62.

Bohidar, N. R. (1985). Statistical tests of validity for competitive antagonism in drug receptor interaction. *Proceedings of the Biopharmaceutical Section of the American Statistical Association*, pp. 66–71.

Bohidar, N. R., and Peace, K. (1988). Pharmaceutical formulation development. Chapter 4 in *Biopharmaceutical Statistics for Drug Development*, ed. Peace, K. Marcel Dekker, New York, pp. 149–229.

Bohidar, N. R., Restaino, F. A., and Schwartz, J. B. (1975). Selecting key parameters in pharmaceutical factors by principal component analysis. *J. Pharm. Sci.*, 64, 966–969.

Bohidar, N. R., Restaino, F. A., and Schwartz, J. B. (1979). Selecting key parameters in pharmaceutical factors by regression analysis. *Drug Dev. Ind. Pharm.*, 5, 175–216.

Bowker, A. H. (1946). Computation of factors for tolerance limits on a normal distribution when the sample is large. *Ann. Math. Stat.*, 17, 238.

Bowker, A. H. (1947). In *Selected Techniques of Statistical Analysis for Scientific and Industrial Research and Production and Management Engineering*, ed. Eisenhart, C., Hastay, M. W., and Wallis, W. A. McGraw-Hill, New York.

Box, G. E. P., and Behnken, D. W. (1960). Simplex sum designs: a class of second order rotatable design derivable from those of first order. *Ann. Math. Stat.*, 31, 838–864.

Box, G. E. P., and Hunter, J. S. (1961a). The 2^{K-P} fractional factorial designs, Part I. *Technometrics*, 3, 311–351.

Box, G. E. P., and Hunter, J. S. (1961b). The 2^{K-P} fractional factorial designs, Part II. *Technometrics*, 3, 449–458.

Box, G. E. P., and Lucas, H. L. (1959). Design and experiments in non-linear situation. *Biometrics*, 46, 77–90.

Box, G. E. P., Hunter, W. G., and Hunter, J. S. (1978). *Statistics for Experimenters*. Wiley, New York.

Brook, M. A., and Weinfeld, R. E. (1985). A validation process for data from the analysis of drugs in biological fluids. *Drug Dev. Ind. Pharm.*, 11, 1703–1728.

Buonaccorsi, J. P. (1986). Design considerations for calibration. *Technometrics*, 28, 149–155.

Buonaccorsi, J. P., and Iyer, H. K. (1986). Optimal designs for ratios of linear calibrations in the general linear model. *J. Stat. Plann. Inference*, 13, 345–356.

Burr, I. W. (1967). The effect of non-normality on constants for $\overline{X}$ and R charts. *Ind. Quality Control*, 23(2), 563–569.

Carstensen, J. T. (1990). *Drug Stability*. Marcel Dekker, New York.

Carstensen, J. T., and Nelson, E. (1976). Terminology regarding labeled and contained amounts in dosage forms. *J. Pharm. Sci.*, 65, 311–312.

Carter, R. L., and Yang, M. C. K. (1986). Large sample inference in random coefficient regression model. *Commun. Stat. Theory Methods*, 15, 2507–2525.

Cavenaghi, L., Gail, G. G., and Leali, G. M. (1987). Statistical evaluation of the results obtained with the analytical methods used for the quality control of medicines. *Drug Dev. Ind. Pharm.*, 14, 2571–2615.

Chapman, K. G. (1983). A suggested validation lexicon. *Pharm. Technol.*, 7, 51–57.

Chow, S. C. (1989). Procedures for choosing appropriate statistical models for standard curve in assay validation. Unpublished statistical report. Parke-Davis Pharmaceutical Research Division, Warner-Lambert Company, Ann Arbor, Mich.

Chow, S. C. (1992). Statistical design and analysis of stability studies. Presented at the *48th Conference on Applied Statistics*, Atlantic City, N.J., December 1992.

Chow, S. C., and Liu, J. P. (1992). *Design and Analysis of Bioavailability and Bioequivalence Studies*. Marcel Dekker, New York.

Chow, S. C., and Shao, J. (1988). A new procedure for the estimation of variance components. *Stat. Prob. Lett.*, 6, 349–355.

Chow, S. C., and Shao, J. (1989). Test for batch-to-batch variation in stability analysis. *Stat. Med.*, 8, 883–890.

Chow, S. C., and Shao, J. (1990a). Estimating drug shelf-life in NDA stability studies. *Proceedings of the Biopharmaceutical Section of the American Statistical Association*, pp. 190–195.

Chow, S. C., and Shao, J. (1990b). On the difference between the classical and inverse methods of calibration. *J. Roy. Stat. Soc. C*, 39, 219–228.

Chow, S. C., and Shao, J. (1991). Estimating drug shelf-life with random batches. *Biometrics*, 47, 1071–1079.

Chow, S. C., and Tse, S. K. (1991). On variance estimation in assay validation. *Stat. Med.*, 10, 1543–1553.

Chow, S. C., and Wang, S. G. (1994). On the estimation of variance components in stability analysis. *Commun. Stat. Theory Methods*, 23(1), 289–303.

Conover, W. J. (1980). *Practical Nonparametric Statistics*, 2nd edition. Wiley, New York.

Corbeil, R. R., and Searle, S. R. (1976). Restricted maximum likelihood (REML) estimation of variance components in the mixed model. *Technometrics*, 18, 31–38.

Dantzig, G. B. (1963). *Linear Programming and Extensions*. Princeton University Press, Princeton, N.J.

Davies, O. L. (1980). Note on regression with correlated responses. *Biometrics*, 36, 551–552.

Davies, O. L., and Hudson, H. E. (1981). Stability of drugs: accelerated storage tests. Chapter 15 in *Statistics in the Pharmaceutical Industry*, ed. Buncher, C. R., and Tsay, J. Y. Marcel Dekker, New York, pp. 355–395.

Draper, N. R. (1985). Small composite designs. *Technometrics*, 27, 173–180.

Draper, N. R., and Lin, D. K. J. (1990). *Using Plackett and Burman designs with fewer than N − 1 factors*. Working papar 253. University of Tennessee, College of Business Administration, Nashville, Tn.

Draper, N. R., and Smith, H. (1981). *Applied Regression Analysis*, 2nd edition. Wiley, New York.

Duncan, A. J. (1971). The economic design of $\bar{X}$ charts when there is a multiplicity of assignable causes. *J. Am. Stat. Assoc.*, 66, 107–121.

Dunsmore, I. R. (1968). A Bayesian approach to calibration. *J. Roy. Stat. Soc. B*, 31, 160–170.

Easterling, R. G. (1969). Discrimination intervals for percentiles in regression. *J. Am. Stat. Assoc.*, 64, 1031–1041.

EC (1987). Stability tests of active substances and finished products. *Rules Governing Medical Products in the European Community*, Vol. III. Office for Official Publications of the European Community, Brussels, Belgium.

Ewan, W. D. (1963). When and how to use cu-sum charts. *Technometrics*, 5, 1–22.

FDA (1987). *Guideline for Submitting Documentation for the Stability of Human Drugs and Biologics*. Center for Drugs and Biologics, Office of Drug Research and Review, Food and Drug Administration, Rockville, Md.

Fisch, R. D., and Strehlan, G. A. (1993). A simplified approach to calibration confidence set. *Am. Stat.*, 47, 168–171.

Freund, R. A. (1957). Acceptance control charts. *Ind. Quality Control*, 14(4), 13–23.

Fuller, W. A. (1988). *Measurement Error Models*. Wiley, New York.

Gill, J. L. (1978). *Design and Analysis of Experiments in Animal and Medical Sciences*, Vol. 1. Iowa State University Press, Ames, Iowa.

Gitlow, H., Gitlow, S., Oppenheim, A., and Oppenheim, R. (1989). *Tools and Methods for the Improvement of Quality*. Richard D. Irwin, Homewood, Ill.

Goel, A. L., and Wu, S. M. (1973). Economically optimal design of cusum charts. *Management Sci.*, 19, 1271–1282.

Goldsmith, P. L., and Whitfield, H. (1961). Average run lengths in cumulative chart quality control schemes. *Technometrics*, 3, 11–20.

Graybill, F. A. (1976). *Theory and Application of the Linear Model*. Duxbury, Boston.

Gumpertz, M., and Pantula, S. G. (1989). A simple approach to inference in random coefficient models. *Am. Stat.*, 43, 203–210.

Hahn, G. (1970). Statistical intervals for a normal population, Part II: formulas, assumptions, some derivations. *J. Quality Technol.*, 2, 195–206.

Hahn, G. J., and Meeker, W. Q. (1991). *Statistical Intervals: A Guide for the Practitioner*. Wiley, New York.

Halperin, M. (1970). On inverse estimation in linear regression. *Technometrics*, 12, 727–736.

Helboe, P. (1992). New design for stability testing programs: matrix or factorial designs authorities' viewpoint on the predictive value of such studies. *Drug Inf. J.*, 26, 629–634.

Herbach, L. H. (1959). Properties of type II analysis of variance tests. *Ann. Math. Stat.*, 30, 939–959.

Hildreth, G., and Houck, J. R. (1968). Some estimators for a linear model with random coefficients. *J. Am. Stat. Assoc.*, 63, 584–595.

Hinkley, D. V. (1969). Inference about the intersection in two-phase regression. *Biometrika*, 56, 495–504.

Hinkley, D. V. (1971). Inference in two-phase regression. *J. Am. Stat. Assoc.*, 66, 736–743.

Ho, C. H., Liu, J. P., and Chow, S. C. (1992). On analysis of stability data. *Proceedings of the Biopharmaceutical Section of the American Statistical Association*, pp. 198–203.

Hocking, R. R. (1985). *The Analysis of Linear Models*. Brook Lab, Monterey, Calif.

ICH (1993). Stability Testing of New Drug Substances and Products. *Tripartite International Conference on Harmonization Guideline*, September 1, 1993.

John, P. W. M. (1971). *Statistical Design and Analysis of Experiments*. Macmillan, New York.

Johnson, N. L., and Leone, F. C. (1962a). Cumulative sum control charts: mathematical principals applied to construction and use, Part I. *Ind. Quality Control*, 18, 15–21.

Johnson, N. L., and Leone, F. C. (1962b). Cumulative sum control charts: mathematical principals applied to construction and use, Part II. *Ind. Quality Control*, 19, 29–36.

Jones, B., and Kenward, M. G. (1989). *Design and Analysis of Crossover Trials*. Chapman & Hall, London.

Ju, H. L., and Chow, S. C. (1994a). A procedure for weight and model selection in assay development. Submitted for publication.

Ju, H. L., and Chow, S. C. (1994b). On statistical design of stability studies. Currently under revision for *J. Biochem. Stat.*

Kellison, S. G. (1975). *Fundamentals of Numerical Analysis*. Richard D. Irwin, Homewood, Ill.

Kendall, M. G., and Stuart, A. (1961). *The Advanced Theory of Statistics*, Vol. II. Charles Griffin, London.

Kirkwood, T. B. L. (1977). Predicting the stability of biological standards and products. *Biometrics*, 33, 736–742.

Kohberger, R. C. (1988). Manufacturing and quality control. Chapter 14 in *Biopharmaceutical Statistics for Drug Development*, ed. Peace, K. Marcel Dekker, New York, pp. 605–629.

Krutchkoff, R. G. (1967). Classical and inverse methods of calibration. *Technometrics*, 9, 525–539.

Krutchkoff, R. G. (1969). Classical and inverse regression methods of calibration in extrapolation. *Technometrics*, 11, 605–608.

Laird, N., Lange, N., and Stram, D. (1987). Maximum likelihood computations with repeated measures: application of the EM algorithm. *J. Amer. Stat. Assoc.*, 82, 87–105.

Laubscher, N. F. (1960). Normalizing the noncentral t and F distributions. *Ann. Math. Stat.*, 31, 1105–1112.

Lehmann, E. L. (1959). *Testing Statistical Hypotheses*. Wiley, New York.

Lin, K. K. (1990). Statistical analysis of stability study data. *Proceedings of the Biopharmaceutical Section of the American Statistical Association*, pp. 210–215.

Lin, T. Y. D. (1994). Applicability of matrixing and bracketing approach to stability study design. Presented at the *4th ICSA Applied Statistics Symposium*, Food and Drug Administration, Rockville, Md., April 30.

Lin, D. K. J., and Draper, N. R. (1992). Projection properties of Plackett and Burman designs. *Technometrics*, 34, 423–428.

Lindgren, B. W. (1976). *Statistical Theory*. Macmillan, New York.

Liu, J. P. (1992). On analysis of stability data. Presented at the *48th Conference on Applied Statistics*, Atlantic City, N.J.

Lwin, T., and Maritz, J. S. (1982). An analysis of the linear-calibration controversy from the perspective of compound estimation. *Technometrics*, 24, 235–242.

Mandel, J. (1972). Repeatability and reproducibility. *J. Quality Technol.*, 4, 74–85.

Mellon, J. I. (1991). Design and analysis aspects of drug stability studies when the product is stored at several temperatures. Presented at the *12th Annual Midwest Statistical Workshop*, Muncie, Ind.

MHW (1991). *Stability Guidelines*. Ministry of Health and Welfare, Tokyo.

Morris, J. W. (1992). A comparison of linear and exponential models for drug expiry estimation. *J. Biopharm. Stat.*, 2, 83–90.

Murphy, J. R., and Weisman, D. (1990). Using random slopes for estimating shelf-life. *Proceedings of the Biopharmaceutical Section of the American Statistical Association*, pp. 196–203.

Myers, R. H. (1976). *Response Surface Methodology*. Allyn and Bacon, Boston.

Nakagaki, P. (1990). Matrixing and bracketing of solid oral dosage forms for thermal stability studies. *AAPS Annual Meeting*, Las Vegas, Nev.

Nelson, L. S. (1980). The mean square successive difference test. *J. Quality Technol.*, 12, 174–175.

NF XIII (1970). *The National Formulary XIII*, 13th ed. Mack Publishing, Easton, Pa.

Nordbrock E. (1992). Statistical comparison of stability study designs. *J. Biopharm. Stat.*, 2, 91–113.

Oman, S. D. (1985). An exact formula for the mean squared error of the inverse estimator in the linear calibration problem. *J. Stat. Plann. Inference*, 11, 189–196; correction, 12 (1986), 401.

Ott, L. (1984). *An Introduction to Statistical Methods and Data Analysis*, 2nd edition, Duxbury Press, Boston.

Ott, E. R., and Schilling, E. G. (1990). *Process Quality Control*. McGraw-Hill, New York.

Page, E. S. (1954). Continuous inspection schemes. *Biometrika*, 41, 100–115.

Pheatt, C. B. (1980). Evaluation of U.S. Pharmacopeia sampling plans for dissolution. *J. Quality Technol.*, 12, 158–164.

Plackett, R. L., and Burman, J. P. (1946). The design of optimum multifactorial experiments. *Biometrika*, 33, 305–325.

Rahman, R. A. (1992). A comparison of expiration dating period methods. *J. Biopharm. Stat.*, 2, 69–82.

Rao, C. R. (1973). Linear Statistical Inference and Its Applications. 2nd Edition, Wiley, New York.

Reynolds, M. R., Amin, R. W., and Arnold, J. C. (1990). CUSUM charts with variable sampling intervals (with discussion). *Technometrics*, 32, 369–393.

Roberts, C. (1969). Fill weight variation release and control of capsules, tablets, and sterile solids. *Technometrics*, 11, 161–176.

Ruberg, S., and Hsu, J. (1992). Multiple comparison procedures for pooling batches in stability studies. *Technometrics*, 34, 465–472.

Ruberg, S., and Stegeman, J. W. (1991). Pooling data for stability studies: testing the equality of batch degradation slopes. *Biometrics*, 47, 1059–1069.

Sampson, C. B., and Breunig, H. L. (1971). Some statistical aspects of pharmaceutical content uniformity. *J. Quality Technol.*, 3, 170–178.

SAS (1990). *SAS/STAT User's Guide, Version 6*, 4th edition, Vol. 2. SAS Institute, Cary, N.C.

Schilling, E. G. (1982). *Acceptance Sampling in Quality Control*. Marcel Dekker, New York.

Schuirmann, D. J. (1987). A comparison of the two one-sided tests procedure and power approach for assessing the equivalence of average bioavailability. *J. Pharmacokinet. Biopharm.*, 15, 657–680.

Searle, S. R., Casella, G., and McCulloch, C. E. (1992). *Variance Components*. Wiley, New York.

Shaban, S. A. (1980). Change point problem and two-phase regression: an annotated bibliography. *Int. Stat. Rev.*, 48, 83–93.

Shah, V. P., Midha, K. K., Dighe, S., McGilveray, I. J., Skelly, J. P., Yacobi, A., Layloff, T., Viswanathan, C. T., Cook, C. E., McDowall, R. D., Pittman, K. A., and Spector, S. (1992). Analytical methods validation: bioavailability, bioequivalence and pharmaceutical studies. *Pharm. Res.*, 9(4), 588–592.

Shao, J. (1989). Monte Carlo approximations in Bayesian decision theory. *J. Am. Stat. Assoc.*, 84, 727–732.

Shao, J., and Chow, S. C. (1991). Constructing release target for drug products: a decision theory approach. *J. Roy. Stat. Soc. C*, 40, 381–390.

Shao, J., and Chow, S. C. (1993). Two-stage sampling in pharmaceutical applications. *Stat. Med.*, 12, 1999–2008.

Shao, J., and Chow, S. C. (1994). Statistical inference in stability analysis. *Biometrics*, 50, 753–763.

Shewhart, W. A. (1931). *Economic Control of Quality of Manufactured Product*. D. Van Nostrand, New York.

Snedecor, G. W., and Cochran, W. G. (1980). *Statistical Methods*, 7th edition. Iowa State University Press, Ames, Iowa.

Sundberg, R. (1985). When is the inverse regression estimator MSE-superior to the standard regression estimator in multivariate controlled calibration situations? *Stat. Prob. Lett.*, 3, 75–79.

Taylor, H. M. (1968). The economic design of cumulative sum control charts. *Technometrics*, 10, 479–488.

Thompson, W. A. (1962). The problem of negative estimates of variance components. *Ann. Math. Stat.*, 33, 273–289.

Tsong, Y., Hammerstorm, T., Lin, K. K., and Ong, T. E. (1992). Dissolution test acceptance sampling plans. *Proceedings of the Biopharmaceutical Section of the American Statistical Association*, pp. 204–208.

Tukey, J. W. (1951). Components in regression. *Biometrics*, 7, 33–69.

USP XVIII (1970). *The United States Pharmacopeia XVIII*. Mack Printing Company, Easton, Pa.

USP XIX (1974). *The United States Pharmacopeia XIX*. Mack Printing Company, Easton, Pa.

USP/NF (1990). *The United States Pharmacopeia XXII and the National Formulary XVII*. The United States Pharmacopeial Convention, Rockville, Md.

Vasilopoulos, A. V., and Stamboulis, A. P. (1978). Modification of control chart limits in the presence of data correlation. *J. Quality Technol.*, 10, 20–30.

Vonesh, E. F., and Carter, R. L. (1987). Efficient inference for random coefficient growth models with unbalanced data. *Biometrics*, 43, 617–628.

Wallis, W. A. (1951). Tolerance interval for linear regression. *Proceedings of the 2nd Berkeley Symposium on Mathematical Statistics and Probability*. University of California Press.

Wang, S. G., and Chow, S. C. (1994). *Advanced Linear models: Theory and Applications*. Marcel Dekker, New York.

Wheeler, R. E. (1974). Portable power. *Technometrics*, 16, 193–201.

Wheeler, R. E. (1975). The validity of portable power. *Technometrics*, 17, 177–179.

WHO (1993). *World Health Organization Guidelines on Stability Testing of Pharmaceutical Products Containing Well-Established Drug Substances in Conventional Dosage Forms*. Reference WHO/PHARM/92, 158/Rev. 4. WHO, Geneva.

Williams, J. S. (1962). A confidence interval for variance components. *Biometrika*, 49, 278–281.

Index

[Variability]
 interassay, 111
 intraassay, 111
 short-term, 241
 within-batch, 412, 415
 within-run, 10
Variance, 27, 55, 90, 92, 183, 303, 305,
  343, 346, 371, 404
 average asymptotic, 63
 asymptotic, 62
 components, 100, 103, 107
  between-location, 220
  within-location, 220
 maximum asymptotic, 63

Variation
 batch, 402
 batch-to-batch, 391, 393, 395, 400,
  428
 between-batch, 410
 between-location, 174
 weight, 15, 232
 within-batch, 410
 within-location, 174

Weight, 47
Weight selection, 52, 53
Worst case, 206

Printed in the United States
by Baker & Taylor Publisher Services

Printed in the United States
by Baker & Taylor Publisher Services